Practical Guide to the Care of the Geriatric Patient

D1613443

Series Editor

Fred F. Ferri, MD, FACP

Clinical Professor
Warren Alpert Medical School
Brown University
Providence, Rhode Island

OTHER VOLUMES IN THE "PRACTICAL GUIDE SERIES"

Goldberg: *Practical Guide to the Care of the Psychiatric Patient*

Danakas: *Practical Guide to the Care of the Gynecologic/Obstetric Patient*

Alario, et al: *Practical Guide to the Care of the Pediatric Patient*

Ferri: *Practical Guide to the Care of the Medical Patient*

Practical Guide to the Care of the Geriatric Patient

Third Edition

Tom J. Wachtel, MD

Professor of Community Health and Medicine

Brown University School of Medicine

Providence, Rhode Island

President, Rhode Island Medical Directors Association

Marsha D. Fretwell, MD

Clinical Associate Professor of Medicine

University of North Carolina

Chapel Hill, North Carolina

MOSBY

ELSEVIER

MOSBY
ELSEVIER

1600 John F. Kennedy Blvd.
Ste 1800
Philadelphia, PA 19103-2899

PRACTICAL GUIDE TO THE CARE ISBN: 978-0-323-03671-9
OF THE GERIATRIC PATIENT

Notice

Knowledge and best practice in this field are constantly changing. As new research and experience broaden our knowledge, changes in practice, treatment, and drug therapy may become necessary or appropriate. Readers are advised to check the most current information provided (i) on procedures featured or (ii) by the manufacturer of each product to be administered, to verify the recommended dose or formula, the method and duration of administration, and contraindications. It is the responsibility of the practitioners, relying on their own experience and knowledge of the patient, to make diagnoses, to determine dosages and the best treatment for each individual patient, and to take all appropriate safety precautions. To the fullest extent of the law, neither the Publisher nor the Authors assume any liability for any injury and/or damage to persons or property arising out of or related to any use of the material contained in this book.

The Publisher

Library of Congress Cataloging-in-Publication Data
Practical guide to the care of the geriatric patient/[edited by] Tom J. Wachtel, Marsha D. Fretwell. – 3rd ed.
 p. ; cm.
Rev. ed. of: Practical guide to the care of the geriatric patient/Fred F Ferri, Marsha D. Fretwell, Tom J. Wachtel. 2nd ed. ©1997.
 Includes index.
 ISBN 978-0-323-03671-9
 1. Geriatrics–Handbooks, manuals, etc. 2. Older people–Medical care–Handbooks, manuals, etc. I. Wachtel, Tom J. II. Fretwell, Marsha D. III. Ferri, Fred F. Practical guide to the care of the geriatric patient.
 [DNLM: 1. Geriatrics–Handbooks. WT 39 P895 2007]
RC952. 55. F47 2007
618. 97—dc22   2007003815

Acquisitions Editor: Jim Merritt
Developmental Editor: Andrea Deis
Publishing Services Manager: Linda Van Pelt
Project Manager: Joan Nikelsky
Cover and Text Design: Ellen Zanolle

Working together to grow
libraries in developing countries
www.elsevier.com | www.bookaid.org | www.sabre.org

ELSEVIER BOOK AID International Sabre Foundation

Printed in the United States of America

Last digit is the print number: 9 8 7 6 5 4 3 2 1

To our families and friends
Their constant support and encouragement made this book a reality

Contributors

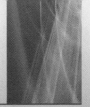

Philip J. Aliotta, MD, MSHA, FACS
Clinical Instructor
Department of Urology
School of Medicine and Biomedical Sciences
State University of New York
Buffalo, New York
Medical Director
Center for Urologic Research of Western New York
Williamsville, New York

George O. Alonso, MD
Instructor in Medicine
Mount Sinai School of Medicine
New York, New York
Director
Department of Infection Control
Elmhurst Hospital Center
Elmhurst, New York

Susan Berner, MD
Geriatrics Fellow
Department of Family Medicine
University of Cincinnati College of Medicine
Cincinnati, Ohio

Lynn Bowlby, MD
Attending Physician
Division of General Internal Medicine
Rhode Island Hospital
Clinical Instructor of Medicine
Warren Alpert Medical School
Brown University
Providence, Rhode Island

John E. Croom, MD, PhD
Clinical Fellow in Neurology
Harvard Medical School
Beth Israel Deaconess Medical Center
Boston, Massachusetts

Claudia L. Dade, MD
Instructor in Medicine
Mount Sinai School of Medicine
New York, New York
Attending Physician
Division of Infectious Diseases
Elmhurst Hospital Center
Elmhurst, New York

George T. Danakas, MD
Clinical Assistant Professor
Department of Gynecology/Obstetrics
School of Medicine and Biomedical Sciences
State University of New York
Buffalo, New York

Mark J. Fagan, MD
Associate Professor of Medicine
Medical School
Brown University
Director
Medical Primary Care Unit
Rhode Island Hospital
Providence, Rhode Island

Mitchell D. Feldman, MD, MPhil
Associate Professor of Clinical Medicine
University of California at San Francisco
Attending Physician
Division of General Internal Medicine
University of California at San Francisco
San Francisco, California

Fred F. Ferri, MD
Clinical Professor
Warren Alpert Medical School
Brown University
Providence, Rhode Island

Marsha D. Fretwell, MD
Associate Professor of Medicine
University of North Carolina
Chapel Hill, North Carolina
Attending Physician
Cape Fear Hospital
New Hanover Medical Center
Medical Director
Elderhaus
Wilmington, North Carolina

Michael P. Gerardo, DO, MPH
Postdoctoral Research Fellow in Community Health
Brown University
Clinical Fellow in Geriatric Medicine
Internal Medicine
Warren Alpert Medical School and Rhode Island Hospital
Brown University
Providence, Rhode Island

Cynthia Holzer, MD, CMD, AGSF
Assistant Professor of Medicine
Boston University School of Medicine
Boston, Massachusetts
Adjunct Assistant Professor of Medicine
Warren Alpert Medical School
Brown University
Providence, Rhode Island
Director, Geriatric Education
Roger Williams Medical Center
Providence, Rhode Island

Richard S. Isaacson, MD
Assistant Professor of Medicine
Leonard M. Miller School of Medicine
Departments of Medical Education, Internal Medicine, and Neurology
Mount Sinai Medical Center
University of Miami
Director, Research Unit in Medical Education
Associate Medical Director
Wien Center for Memory Disorders and Alzheimer's Disease
Miami Beach, Florida

E. Gordon Margolin, MD
Professor of Internal Medicine and Geriatrics
University of Cincinnati College of Medicine
Cincinnati, Ohio

Peter S. Margolis, MD
Clinical Assistant Professor of Medicine
Warren Alpert Medical School
Brown University
Clinical Gastroenterologist
Division of Gastroenterology
Rhode Island Hospital
Providence, Rhode Island

Daniel T. Mattson, MD, MSc (Med)
Clinical Fellow in Neurology
Harvard Medical School
Beth Israel Deaconess Medical Center
Boston, Massachusetts

Lynn McNicoll, MD
Division of Geriatrics
Rhode Island Hospital
Providence, Rhode Island

Lonnie R. Mercier, MD
Clinical Instructor
Department of Orthopedic Surgery
Creighton University School of Medicine
Omaha, Nebraska

Arvind Modawal, MD, MPH, MRCGP
Associate Professor
Department of Family Medicine, Section of Geriatrics
University of Cincinnati College of Medicine
Cincinnati, Ohio

John B. Murphy, MD
Professor of Family Medicine
Brown University
Division of Geriatrics
Rhode Island Hospital
Providence, Rhode Island

Aman Nanda, MD, CMD
Assistant Professor in Medicine
Warren Alpert Medical School
Brown University
Providence, Rhode Island

Pranav M. Patel, MD
Clinical Associate Instructor, Division of Cardiology
Department of Medicine
Warren Alpert Medical School
Brown University
Providence, Rhode Island

Sean I. Savitz, MD
Clinical Fellow in Neurology
Harvard Medical School
Chief Resident in Neurology
Beth Israel Deaconess Medical Center
Boston, Massachusetts

Clifford Milo Singer, MD
Associate Professor of Psychiatry
University of Vermont College of Medicine
Director
Insomnia and Chronobiology Clinic
Vermont Regional Sleep Center
Burlington, Vermont

Michael D. Stein, MD
Associate Professor of Medicine
Warren Alpert Medical School
Brown University
Associate Physician
Division of General Medicine
Rhode Island Hospital
Providence, Rhode Island

Laura Trice, MD
Medical Director
Trihealth SeniorLink
California, Kentucky

Eroboghene E. Ubogu, MD
Assistant Professor of Neurology
Case Western Reserve University School of Medicine
Staff Neurologist
Louis Stokes Cleveland Veterans Affairs Medical Center
Cleveland, Ohio

Tom J. Wachtel, MD
Professor of Community Health and Medicine
Warren Alpert Medical School
Brown University
Division of Geriatrics
Rhode Island Hospital
Providence, Rhode Island

Deborah Adams Wingate, RN, MSN
Nurse Practitioner–Geriatric
New Hanover Medical Center
Davis Healthcare
Wilmington, North Carolina

Wen-Chih Wu, MD
Assistant Professor of Medicine
Warren Alpert Medical School
Brown University
Providence, Rhode Island
Cardiologist
Providence VA Medical Center
Providence, Rhode Island

Beth J. Wutz, MD
Clinical Assistant Professor of Medicine
Division of Internal Medicine/Pediatrics
Kajeida Health – Buffalo General Hospital
State University of New York
Buffalo, New York

Preface

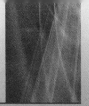

The coexistence of biological and behavioral changes associated with aging and the common presence of multiple acute and chronic diseases make the practice of geriatrics both challenging and time intensive. This manual is intended to be a concise guide for all clinicians involved in the care of elderly patients. In keeping with the style of the *Practical Guides* series, this pocket-size manual provides a compressed yet comprehensive overview of geriatric medicine. Geriatric syndromes such as dementia, delirium, incontinence, pressure ulcers, osteoporosis, and prostatic disease are presented together with internal medicine as applied to the elderly. In particular, the coverage of functional syndromes and system abnormalities has been vastly expanded in this third edition. Specific care issues related to the various settings of geriatrics practice, such as nursing homes and home care, are presented as well. Numerous tables and illustrations are used extensively throughout the text to simplify complex issues and enhance recollection of principal points.

This book's practical approach, with its emphasis on clinical correlations, should make it a useful reference for students and clinicians who are actively involved in the care of the geriatric patient and help those caregivers find answers to most clinical questions at the bedside without having to consult another reference.

Marsha D. Fretwell, MD
Tom J. Wachtel, MD

WHAT DO YOU SEE, NURSE?

What do you see, nurse, what do you see?
What are thinking when you look at me?
A crabbit old woman, not very wise,
Uncertain of habit, with far away eyes,
Who dribbles her food, and makes no reply,
When you say in a loud voice, "I do wish you'd try!"
Who seems not to notice the things that you do,
And forever is losing a stocking or shoe.
Who unresisting or not, lets you do as you will
With bathing and feeding, the long day to fill.
Is that what you're thinking, is that what you see?
Then open your eyes, you're not looking at me.
I'll tell you who I am as I sit here so still,
As I move at your bidding, as I eat at your will.
I am a small child of ten with a father and mother,
Brothers and sisters who love one another.
A young girl of sixteen with wings at her feet
Dreaming that soon now, a lover she'll meet.
A bride soon at twenty, my heart gives a leap,
Remembering the vows that I promised to keep.
At twenty-five now I have young of my own
Who need me to build a secure happy home.
A woman of thirty, my young now grow fast,
Bound to each other with ties that should last.
At forty my young soon will be gone,
But my man stays beside me to see I don't mourn.
At 50 once more babies play 'around my knee,
Again we know children, my loved one and me.
Dark days are upon me, my husband is dead,
I look to the future, I shudder with dread,
For my young are all busy rearing young of their own
And I think of the years and the love I have known.
I'm an old woman now and nature is cruel,
'Tis her jest to make old age look like a fool.
The body it crumbles, grace and vigor depart,
And now there is a stone where I once had a heart.
But inside this old carcass a young girl still dwells.
And now and again my battered heart swells.
I remember the joys, I remember the pain,
And I am loving and living life over again.
I think of the years, all too few, gone too fast,
And accept the stark fact that nothing can last.
So open your eyes, nurse, open and see,
Not a crabbit old woman, look closer, see ME!

Poem found in the belongings of an elderly woman who died in a nursing home in Ireland.
Reproduced from Christiansen JL, Grzybowski JM (eds): *Biology of aging*. St Louis, Mosby, 1993.

Contents

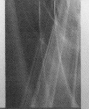

5   Selected Organ System Abnormalities, 137

Biology and Demographics of Aging

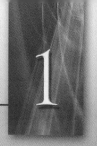

1.1 Physiology of Aging

Fred F. Ferri

1. General comments.
   a. Definitions.
      (1) *Aging* describes the temporal process of growing old.
      (2) The World Health Organization (WHO) characterizes a population between 65 and 75 as *elderly*.
      (3) The term *old* is used for persons between 76 and 90 years of age; *very old* is used for persons older than 90 years.
   b. Aging is associated with a progressive decline in homeostatic control and the ability to respond to stress and/or change.
   c. Elderly persons are heterogeneous with respect to their physiologic function, their burden of illness, and any associated disability.
   d. Normal aging can be subdivided into successful and usual aging (Fig. 1-1).[1]
      (1) *Successful aging* (also known as optimal aging) describes persons who demonstrate minimal physiologic decline from aging alone. Healthful strategies such as exercise, modification of diet, social and intellectual stimulation, and cessation of smoking enhance a person's quality of life and promote successful aging.
      (2) *Usual aging* refers to the more common mode of aging. It is associated, for example, with the observed decline in renal, immune, visual, and hearing function.
2. Rate of age-associated decline in normal function varies with each organ system.
   a. The digestive system is less affected than other organ systems.
   b. The diaphragm and cardiac muscles are not significantly affected by age.
   c. Table 1-1 summarizes physiologic changes associated with aging and their clinical implications.
      (1) Body weight increases in middle age and subsequently decreases in the elderly, especially after 74 years of age.
      (2) Lean body mass decreases (decreased muscle mass).
      (3) The percentage of body fat does not appear to increase significantly after age 40 years. The major reason for the increase in body fat in older persons appears to be weight gain rather than a true age-related increase in percentage of body fat. Previous studies suggesting a marked increase in percentage of body fat

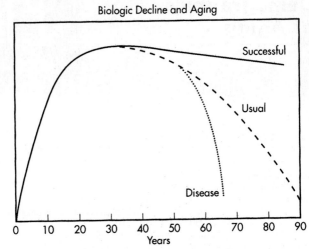

Figure 1-1 Successful and usual patterns of normal aging. Incremental growth (physiologic, functional, or reserve capacities) peaks at age 30 years; thereafter, there is a variable decline, with successful aging showing minimal decrements. (From Yoshikawa TT, Cobbs EL, Brummel-Smith K (eds): *Ambulatory geriatric care*. St Louis, Mosby, 1993, p 171.)

with advancing age did not correct for the increased body mass index that commonly occurs in middle age.[2]
    (4) Plasma volume increases, and interstitial volume decreases.
    (5) Height decreases.
  d. Selected age-related laboratory variations are described in Box 1-1.
3. Theories of aging.
  a. The search for the most likely causes of biological aging has resulted in the following theories:
    (1) Free radicals.
      (a) Free radicals (obtained primarily via metabolism of oxygen) damage cellular protein, DNA, and enzymes, resulting in altered cellular metabolism and accumulation of lipofuscin and other substances. Senescence is caused by the accumulation of irreversible damage.
      (b) Use of antioxidants such as vitamins E and C may be effective in limiting damage from free radicals and extending life.
    (2) Error and somatic mutation: Somatic mutations and errors in DNA and/or RNA synthesis result in abnormal protein synthesis and impaired cellular function. As people age, environmental exposure results in a progressive increase of destructive mutations.
    (3) Wear and tear: Inability to continuously repair damage to crucial cellular components (e.g., DNA) results in declining cellular function and subsequent tissue destruction.

Text continued on page 9

Table 1-1 Comparison of Physiologic Changes in Various Organ Systems and their Clinical Implications

Physiologic Changes with Aging			Clinical Implications		
Increased	Decreased	Other	Increased	Decreased	Other
Cardiovascular System					
Plasma volume	Baroreflex sensitivity	Impaired myocardial diastolic function	Afterload	Cardiac output	High prevalence of sick sinus syndrome and other atrial arrhythmias
Stiffness of aorta and other major arteries	Interstitial volume	Impaired response to sympathetic nervous stimulation	Myocardial hypertrophy	Heart rate	Limited efficacy of direct-acting vasodilators
Total peripheral vascular resistance	Number of pacemaker cells		Risk of orthostatic hypotension	Reflex tachycardia	
	Stroke volume		Susceptibility to hypotensive effect of diuretics		
	Vascular compliance		Systolic blood pressure		
	Ventricular filling time				
Endocrine System					
Atrial natriuretic peptide	Aldosterone concentration	None	None	None	Impaired extracellular volume regulation
Insulin and pancreatic polypeptide	Conversion of thyroxine to triiodothyronine				Impaired glucose tolerance
Norepinephrine levels	Growth hormone response to GHRH				Impaired response to catecholamine stimulation
Parathormone	Metabolism of thyroxine				
Vasopressin secretion					

Continued

Table 1-1 Comparison of Physiologic Changes in Various Organ Systems and their Clinical Implications—cont'd

Physiologic Changes with Aging			Clinical Implications		
Increased	Decreased	Other	Increased	Decreased	Other
Endocrine System—cont'd					
	Plasma renin activity Resistance to insulin-stimulated glucose uptake Secretion of estrogens, androgens, and androgen precursors				Impaired sodium homeostasis
Gastrointestinal System					
None	Amplitude of esophageal contraction during peristalsis Colonic transit time Gastric acid production Hepatic blood flow Hepatic mass Microsomal enzyme activity	Pancreatic acinar atrophy	Constipation Half-life of lipid-soluble drugs	None	None
Hematopoietic System					
Marrow fat RBC mass in women (secondary to end of menstrual loss)	Amount of active bone marrow	None	Functional reserve for hematopoiesis	None	None

Immune System					
Ability of T lymphocytes to proliferate in response to mitogens or antigens Humoral immunity (decreased antibody response to new antigens) Number of newly formed T lymphocytes Secretion of interleukin-2 Suppressor T lymphocytes (OKT5, OKT8)	Helper T lymphocytes (OKT4)	Involution of thymus	Antibody response Killing of intracellular pathogens by macrophages T-cell function	None	Anergy to various skin tests Inadequate response to extrinsic antigens (e.g., pneumococcal vaccine)
Musculoskeletal System					
Bone mass Compliance of chest wall Elasticity of collagen matrix of bone	None	Flattening of arch of feet Osteoblastic activity > osteoclastic activity Trabecular bone > cortical bone	Height Muscle strength	Curvature of spine Gait impairment Muscular work for breathing	Osteoporosis

Continued

Table 1-1   Comparison of Physiologic Changes in Various Organ Systems and their Clinical Implications—cont'd

Physiologic Changes with Aging			Clinical Implications		
Increased	Decreased	Other	Increased	Decreased	Other
Musculoskeletal System—cont'd					
Intervertebral disk space					
Joint space in trunk and extremities					
Lean body mass					
Muscle mass					
Number of muscle fibers					
Repair of microfractures					
Nervous System (Including Ophthalmic and Auditory)					
Binding sites for dopamine	Lipofuscin pigment accumulation (particularly in hippocampus and frontal cortex)	Accumulation of yellow substance in lens	Hearing for pure tones (higher frequencies > lower frequencies)	Risk of glaucoma	Alteration of color perception (e.g., blue appears green-blue)
Blood flow to brain (15%-20%)	Elasticity of lens	Altered baroreflex sensitivity	Olfaction	Risk of syncope	Impaired adaptation to darkness
Brain weight (5%-7%)	Rigidity of iris	Loss of cochlear neurons	Pressure and light touch sensation		Presbyopia
Number of neurons in putamen and locus ceruleus			Size of pupils		Significant impairment of vision in presence of glare
Pacinian and Meissner's corpuscles					
Purkinje cells in cerebellar cortex					
Size of anterior chamber					

Renal and Urologic System					
Bladder capacity	Bladder residual volume	None	Creatinine clearance (8 mL/min/1.73 m²/decade after age 30 y)	None	Facilitation of incontinence
Exchangeable potassium	Nocturnal sodium and fluid excretion		Drug clearance (e.g., digoxin, procainamide, quinidine)		
Glomerular filtration rate	Uninhibited bladder contractions		Maximum urine osmolality		
Renal mass			Renal blood flow		
Renal tubular secretion and concentrating ability					
Reproductive System					
Bactericidal prostatic secretions	Chromosomal abnormalities in germ cells	Prostatic hypertrophy	None	Susceptibility to urinary tract infections	Alteration in vaginal flora
Estrogen levels	Vaginal pH				Impaired micturition
Vaginal secretions					
Respiratory System					
Carbon monoxide diffusion	Alveolar dead space	Alteration of collagen and elastin	Arterial saturation	Risk of infection	None
Expiratory flow rate	Diameter of trachea and central airways	Collapse of small airways	Lung elasticity		
Forced expiratory volume in 1 sec (FEV$_1$)	Residual lung volume (RV)	No change in total lung capacity (TLC)	Maximal oxygen uptake (VO$_{2max}$)		
Forced vital capacity (FVC)					

Continued

Table 1-1 Comparison of Physiologic Changes in Various Organ Systems and their Clinical Implications—cont'd

Physiologic Changes with Aging			Clinical Implications		
Increased	Decreased	Other	Increased	Decreased	Other
Respiratory System—cont'd					
Ratio of FEV₁ to FVC		Ventilation-perfusion imbalance			
Respiratory muscle strength and endurance					
Skin and Connective Tissue					
Collagen	Increased glycosaminoglycans (photoaging secondary to sun exposure)	Cytoarchitectural disarray	Decreased sweating response	Increased blistering	Dry skin
Dermis density		Flattened dermoepidermal junction			Hair graying (graying of axillary hair is one of the most reliable signs of aging)
Epidermal turnover time					Poor insulation
Function of eccrine sweat glands					Prolonged wound healing
Melanocytes					Tendency to neoplasia
Vascularity of dermis					Wrinkled yellowed leathery skin (photoaging)
					Uneven tanning

BOX 1-1 Selected Age-Related Laboratory Variations	
Increased Change	*No Significant Change*
FBS	BUN
T₃	Calcium
TSH	Cortisol
Vasopressin	Free thyroxine index
Decreased Change	GH
Aldosterone	Hemoglobin/hematocrit
Androgens	MCV
Angiotensin II	Platelets
FSH	WBC
LH	
PTH	

BUN, blood urea nitrogen; FBS, fasting blood glucose; FSH, follicle-stimulating hormone; GH, growth hormone; LH, luteinizing hormone; MCV, mean corpuscular volume; PTH, parathyroid hormone; T₃, triiodothyronine; TSH, thyroid-stimulating hormone; WBC, white blood cells.

    (4) Pacemaker: Life span patterns are specific for each animal species. Limitations on cell replication in various organs or organ systems result in cellular damage and death.

    (5) Immunologic: With increasing age, immune system function declines and recognition of one's own cells is reduced. Aging results from active self-destruction mediated by the immune system.

  b. Each theory has its merits; unfortunately, no one theory accounts for all observed phenomena.

  c. Lifestyle factors such as lack of exercise, smoking, alcohol consumption, inadequate diet, and obesity can significantly affect the functional decline of older people (Fig. 1-2).

REFERENCES

1. Walsh J: Successful aging. In Yoshikawa TL Cobbs EL, Brummel-Smith K: *Ambulatory geriatric care.* St Louis, Mosby, 1993.

1.2 Life Expectancy

Tom J. Wachtel

1. Definitions and concepts.
  a. *Life expectancy* is defined as the average length of life expected for a population of persons of a given age. Life expectancy, not otherwise specified, is calculated from birth. Age-specific life expectancy is calculated for a group of persons of a specific age.

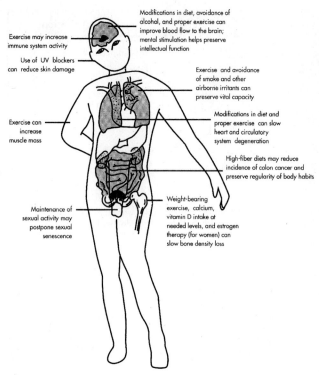

Modifications in diet, avoidance of alcohol, and proper exercise can improve blood flow to the brain; mental stimulation helps preserve intellectual function

Exercise may increase immune system activity

Use of UV blockers can reduce skin damage

Exercise and avoidance of smoke and other airborne irritants can preserve vital capacity

Modifications in diet and proper exercise can slow heart and circulatory system degeneration

Exercise can increase muscle mass

High-fiber diets may reduce incidence of colon cancer and preserve regularity of body habits

Maintenance of sexual activity may postpone sexual senescence

Weight-bearing exercise, calcium, vitamin D intake at needed levels, and estrogen therapy (for women) can slow bone density loss

Figure 1-2   Lifestyle factors can affect the aging process. (From Christiansen JL, Grzybowski JM (eds): *Biology of aging*, St Louis, 1993, Mosby.)

b. U.S. life expectancies based on the 2000 census are presented in Table 1-2.
c. The calculation of life expectancy is based on the age configuration of the population at the time that a census is taken; therefore, life expectancies are calculated as if a person were able to live every year of his or her life in the present state of population mortality. This, of course, is not true; the younger a person is, the more likely he or she will benefit from advances in community health and medical progress or will be penalized by changes in morbidity prevalence (e.g., obesity) or other social calamities such as war.
d. As people age, the differences between men and women or between African Americans and whites attenuate.
e. Maximum life span is defined as the length of the longest-lived members of a species. The longest recorded human life is 122 years

Table 1-2 Life Expectancy by Race, Sex, and Age, United States, 2002*

Age	All Races Total	All Races Male	All Races Female	White Total	White Male	White Female	Black Total	Black Male	Black Female
0	77.3	74.5	79.9	77.7	75.1	80.3	72.3	68.8	75.6
1	76.8	74.1	79.4	77.2	74.6	79.7	72.4	68.8	75.6
5	72.9	70.2	75.4	73.3	70.7	75.8	68.5	65.0	71.7
10	67.9	65.3	70.5	68.3	65.7	70.8	63.6	60.1	66.8
15	63.0	60.3	65.5	63.4	60.8	65.9	58.7	55.2	61.8
20	58.2	55.6	60.7	58.6	56.1	61.0	53.9	50.5	57.0
25	53.5	51.0	55.8	53.8	51.4	56.1	49.3	46.0	52.1
30	48.7	46.3	51.0	49.0	46.7	51.2	44.7	41.6	47.4
35	44.0	41.6	46.1	44.3	42.0	46.4	40.1	37.1	42.7
40	39.3	37.0	41.4	39.6	37.4	41.6	35.6	32.8	38.1
45	34.8	32.6	36.7	35.0	32.9	36.9	31.3	28.5	33.7
50	30.3	29.3	32.2	30.5	28.5	32.4	27.3	24.6	29.5
55	26.1	24.1	27.7	26.2	24.3	27.9	23.4	21.0	25.4
60	22.0	20.2	23.5	22.1	20.3	23.6	19.9	19.6	21.6
65	18.2	16.6	19.5	18.2	16.6	19.5	16.6	14.6	18.0
70	14.7	13.2	15.8	14.7	13.3	15.8	13.5	11.8	14.7
75	11.5	10.3	12.4	11.5	10.3	12.3	10.9	9.5	11.7
80	8.8	7.8	9.4	8.7	7.7	9.3	8.6	7.5	9.2
85	6.5	5.7	6.9	6.4	5.7	6.8	6.6	5.8	7.0
90	4.8	4.2	5.0	4.7	4.1	4.9	5.1	4.5	5.3
95	3.6	3.2	3.7	3.4	3.0	3.5	3.9	3.6	4.0
100	2.7	2.5	2.8	2.4	2.3	2.5	3.0	2.9	3.0

*Race categories are consistent with the 1977 Office of Management and Budget guidelines.
From Arias E: United States life tables, 2002. National vital statistics reports, vol. 53, no. 6. Hyattsville, Maryland, National Center for Health Statistics, 2004.

(a French woman). Current research suggests that average human life span in the absence of premature death from disease or trauma approximates 85 years with a standard deviation of 4 to 5 years. Biotechnology might alter these statistics in the future.

f. Life span is species-specific and is believed to be genetically determined; an almost perfect correlation exists between maximum cell doublings in tissue culture for a given species and the life span for that species. Therefore, it should not be surprising to find longevity running in certain families. However, the mechanism of aging (senescence) has not been identified, and although theories abound (e.g., accumulation of oxygen free radicals, growth hormone deficit), most interventions to correct aging-associated changes (e.g., antioxidants, growth hormone) have not been proved to be effective fountains of youth. The only promising means to increase longevity to date are food restriction (works in rats) and lowering body temperature (works in hamsters).

g. Current thinking attributes the limit on life span to a progressive decline in organ reserve that begins for humans at age 20 to 30 years. Reserve function is needed to respond to lifetime stress. When reserve function has declined to about 20% above basal levels, routine daily perturbations cannot be overcome, homeostasis cannot be maintained, and death will occur with minor illnesses or trauma that would be trivial for vigorous persons.

2. Compression of mortality (and morbidity) and the rectangularization of the population survival curve (Fig. 1-3).

a. Although human life span has not varied during the past millennium, human life expectancy has increased dramatically. For example, life expectancy from birth in the United States in 1900 was 47 years, and in 2002 it was 77.3 years. This gain can be attributed to improvement in infant mortality and primary preventive measures such as sanitation and immunization. Progress in and increased access to medical care can also take some credit for the gains in life expectancy.

b. The combination of a finite limit on life span and an increase in life expectancy results in more persons achieving their maximum life potential of 85 ± 5 years in the population. This trend is demonstrated graphically by a narrowing bell-shaped curve of the number of deaths (see Fig. 1-3B).

3. Future trends.

a. The rectangularization of population survival, the compression of morbidity, and the compression of senescence are predicated on the hypothesis of a finite limit of organ reserve (Fig. 1-4A). As stated by Fries, "As the organ reserve decreases so does the ability to restore homeostasis, and eventually even the smallest perturbation prevents homeostasis to be restored. The inevitable result is natural death, even without disease" or after a short acute illness (e.g., pneumonia).

b. Alternatively, progress in medical technology (e.g., artificial organs) could conceivably halt the trend toward rectangularization and simply move the entire survival curve to the right (Fig. 1-4B).

c. The secular trend toward rectangularization of population survival curves is not inconsistent with a (transient) contemporary widening

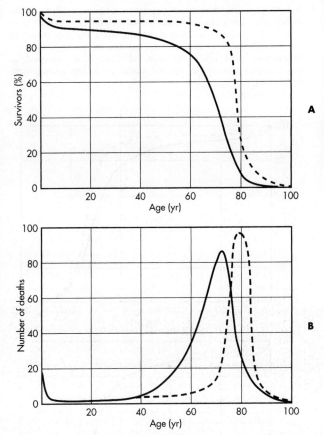

Figure 1-3 **A,** Fraction of survivors in the population (Y axis). **B,** Number of deaths per year in each 1-year age bracket. *Solid line,* present; *dotted line,* future.

of the period of morbidity and mortality associated with recent data that indicate that the elderly citizens of our population are enjoying the greatest decline in mortality (Fig. 1-4C).

d. Possible reasons for the recent downturn in cardiovascular disease and related deaths can be attributed to reduced dietary saturated fat and cholesterol levels, positive developments in medical care for coronary heart disease and stroke, better treatment of hypertension, and improved access to health care for the elderly since 1965 because of the Medicare program.

4. Age-adjusted life expectancy is often underestimated for older individuals because clinicians are familiar with life expectancy figures from birth only. An 80-year-old woman has a life expectancy of 9.5 years. If she is in good general baseline health, an acute life-threatening, but reversible, illness should be treated as aggressively as in a younger person barring specific reasons not to (including patient preference).

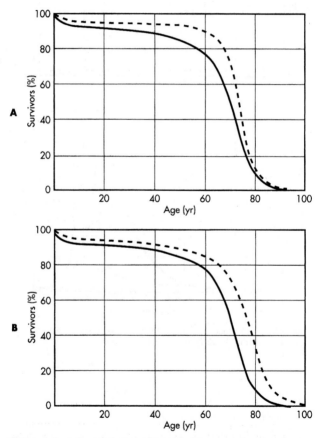

Figure 1-4 A, Rectangularization of the population survival curve as a result of disease prevention and mortality compression. **B,** Prolongation of life expectancy without mortality/morbidity compression in a model where clinical disease is not prevented but only postponed and treated aggressively and successfully in older people.

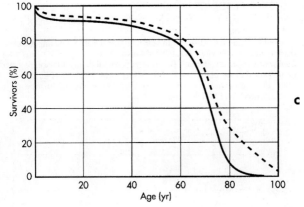

Figure 1-4, cont'd C, Change in a population survival curve where the oldest segment of the population is experiencing the greatest decline in mortality. *Solid lines:* present population survival curve; *broken lines:* conceptual future survival curve.

5. Increasing life expectancy is the reason that the relentless issue of Social Security solvency keeps resurfacing on the political agenda. Indeed, because it is funded by taxing working people, the declining ratio of working-to-retired people in the population can only lead to an increasing tax burden, a decrease in the benefit (payment), raising retirement age, or some combination of those (Fig. 1-5). The same problem applies to the funding of the Medicare system.

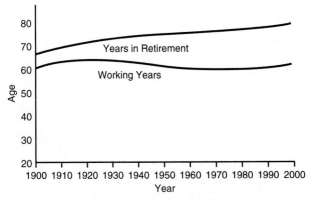

Figure 1-5 Impact of the population's increasing life expectancy on time in retirement and time at work. (From Wachtel TJ: *Geriatric clinical advisor: Instant diagnosis and treatment.* Philadelphia, Mosby, 2006, p 483.)

SUGGESTED READINGS

Fries JF: Aging, natural death, and the compression of morbidity. *N Engl J Med* 303:130-135, 1980.

Olshansky SJ, Carnes BA, Cassel C: In search of Methuselah: Estimating the upper limits to human longevity. *Science* 150:634-640, 1990.

Olshanksy SJ, Passaro DJ, Hershow RC, et al: A potential decline in life expectancy in the United States in the 21st century. *N Engl J Med* 352:1138-1145, 2005.

Wachtel TJ: The connection between health promotion and health care costs. Does it matter? *Am J Med* 94:451-454, 1993.

Comprehensive Geriatric Assessment

Marsha D. Fretwell
Deborah Adams Wingate

2.1 Background

1. Definition: Comprehensive geriatric assessment (CGA) is a systematic approach to collecting patient data that allows the practitioner to evaluate the frail older adult's health status and functional impairments in multiple areas or domains.
2. Purpose: The process of CGA integrates the functional and medical goals of care, allowing physicians to improve clinical outcomes and patient satisfaction.
   a. Older patients often seek or are brought to medical attention because of a nonspecific loss in physical, cognitive, or emotional function.
   b. Frail older persons are subject to multiple physical and mental diseases that interact in complex ways that complicate efforts to achieve satisfactory outcomes.
   c. The goal of the physician is to diagnose and treat the acute medical illness while managing the chronic diseases underlying the loss of function.
   d. The goal of the older patient and family is to regain lost function and maintain independence.
3. Function.
   a. The practitioner collects patient biopsychosocial data.
   b. Findings from the CGA are integrated with the patient's functional capacity.
   c. The CGA allows the practitioner to focus on improving functional impairment and optimize health care outcomes (Box 2-1).

2.2 Steps

Like the traditional SOAP approach (subjective, objective, assessment, plan) to organizing patient information, in CGA we collect the subjective and objective database, integrate that information into an assessment, and create a care plan. The CGA may be done by one person or through an interdisciplinary team approach.

STEP 1. SUBJECTIVE AND OBJECTIVE DATABASE

1. Chief complaint.
   a. The reason for seeking medical attention should be stated in both the patient's and the family or caregiver's words, when possible.

2—Geriatric Assessment

BOX 2-1   **Significant Benefits of Geriatric Assessment Programs**

Process of Care

New diagnoses/problems uncovered
Reduced medications

Patient Outcomes

Improved scores on functional status tests
Improved scores on affective or cognitive function tests
Prolonged survival

Nursing Home Use

Improved placement
Reduction in mean days in nursing homes

Health Care Use and Costs

Increased use of home health care
Reduced use of hospital services (mean days or hospitalized rates)
Reduced medical care costs

Rubenstein LZ, Stuck AE, Siu AL, Wieland D: *J Am Geriatr Soc* 39(9 Pt 2): 8S-16S, 1991.

    b. It should address the specific functional losses that the patient is experiencing.
    c. It should address the more traditional medical complaints.
2. Initial screen of vision, hearing, and cognition.
    a. Before beginning, it is important that the patient be able to see and hear the examiner, pay attention to questions, and give an accurate history.
    b. A brief check of vision (Fig. 2-1), hearing, and cognitive function is suggested.
3. Biomedical data.
    a. Medical diagnosis, present and past, with a statement of duration and impact on patient's physical and mental function.
    b. Nutritional data, including any changes in weight and appetite.
    c. Medications.
        (1) List medications and include duration of use.
        (2) List and describe any adverse drug reactions.
        (3) Estimate creatinine clearance to evaluate appropriate dosing.

$$\text{Creatinine clearance (mL/min)} = \frac{(140 - \text{age in years}) \times \text{weight (kg)}}{\text{serum creatinine (mmol/L)}}$$

        (4) Assess the impact of each medication on the patient's physical and mental functions, including appetite, gait, mood, memory, sexual performance, constipation, and incontinence (see Chapter 7).

2—Geriatric Assessment

ROSENBAUM POCKET VISION SCREENER

95

distance equivalent

$\frac{20}{800}$

874

Point   Jaeger $\frac{20}{400}$

2843

26   16 $\frac{20}{200}$

638   E Ш Ǝ   X O O   14   10 $\frac{20}{100}$

8 7 4 5   Ǝ m Ш   O X O   10   7 $\frac{20}{70}$

6 3 9 2 5   m E Ǝ   X O X   8   5 $\frac{20}{50}$

4 2 8 3 6 5   Ш E m   o x o   6   3 $\frac{20}{40}$

3 7 4 2 5 8   Ǝ Ш Ǝ   x x o   5   2 $\frac{20}{30}$

9 3 7 8 2 6   Ш m E   x o o   4   1 $\frac{20}{25}$

4 2 8 7 3 9   E Ш m   o o x   3   1+ $\frac{20}{20}$

Card is held in good light 14 inches from eye. Record vision for each eye separately with and without glasses. Presbyopic patients should read thru bifocal segment. Check myopes with glasses only.

DESIGN COURTESY J. G. ROSENBAUM, M.D.

PUPIL GAUGE (mm.)

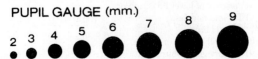

2   3   4   5   6   7   8   9

Figure 2-1 Rosenbaum chart for testing near vision. (From Ferri FF: *Practical guide to the care of the medical patient*, ed 6. St Louis, Mosby, 2004, p 4.)

4. Psychological data (see Appendix II for examples of functional assessment instruments).
   a. Cognitive function, including any episodes of acute confusion following medications, hospitalizations, surgery, or change in living situation.
   b. Emotional function, screen for depression, paranoia, anxiety, hallucinations, personality, and coping styles.
   c. Perceptive function, including vision, hearing, and speech.
5. Social data.
   a. Individual social skills, including marital history, issues of physical and emotional intimacy, need for control, acceptance of help, and presence of a confidant(e).
   b. Family support system, identifying primary contact. Include list of other potential caretakers and use of existing community resources.
   c. Feelings about medical treatments such as surgery, hospitalization, feeding tubes, ventilators, and cardiopulmonary resuscitation. Document existence of prior directives such as durable power of attorney, living will, do not resuscitate (DNR) order, and physician orders for scope of treatment (POST) (see Appendix III for an example).
6. Summary scales for function (see Appendix II for examples of functional assessment instruments).
   a. Basic activities of daily living (ADLs), such as dressing, bathing, getting out of bed, toileting, and feeding independently.
   b. Instrumental ADLs, such as shopping, using transportation, management of medications and one's finances independently.
   c. Performance Oriented Mobility Assessment (POMA), evaluating standing, sitting, and gait performance.
7. Physical examination.
   a. General.
      (1) Routine evaluation for orthostatic changes in pulse and blood pressure.
      (2) Examination of skin for malignant changes.
      (3) Observation of gait, mobility, and balance as patient enters room and gets in and out of a chair.
      (4) Observation of patient performing the basic or instrumental ADLs.
   b. Head, ears, eyes, nose, and throat.
      (1) Evaluation for evidence of recent trauma or fall.
      (2) Presence of cerumen in ear canals.
      (3) Any focal changes in extraocular or facial muscles.
      (4) Cataracts.
      (5) Presence of lower lid ectropion.
      (6) Thyroid nodules.
      (7) Carotid bruits.
      (8) Intraoral dryness or lesions.
      (9) Salivary gland obstruction.
   c. Upper body.
      (1) Full range of motion of the arms.

    (2) Full breast examination and routine cardiopulmonary, carotid, and peripheral vascular evaluation.

  d. Abdominal, rectal, and genital.

    (1) Evaluation for bladder or rectal prolapse.

    (2) Leakage of urine.

    (3) Femoral and inguinal hernias.

    (4) Full range of motion of the hips.

    (5) Routine palpation of abdomen.

  e. Neurologic.

    (1) Mini Mental State Exam,* recording the subcategories of orientation, registration, short-term memory, attention, and language; clock drawing; fast animal naming test (average normal is naming 33 in one minute).

    (2) Any focal changes in muscle strength and reflexes.

    (3) Balance.

    (4) Vibratory sensation and light touch sensation.

8. Laboratory evaluation.

  a. General.

    (1) Complete blood count with differential and platelets.

    (2) Electrolytes.

    (3) Blood urea nitrogen and creatinine.

    (4) Glucose, HbA1c.

    (5) Urinalysis.

  b. Nutrition.

    (1) Prealbumin, albumin.

    (2) Lipid profile.

    (3) Homocysteine.

  c. Cognition.

    (1) Calcium.

    (2) Triiodothyronine (T_3), thyroxine (T_4), and thyroid-stimulating hormone.

    (3) Folate, vitamin B_{12}.

    (4) Transaminase, alkaline phosphatase.

    (5) Blood levels of relevant medications.

STEP 2. ASSESSMENT

The assessment integrates patient data and organizes the problem list.

Overview

1. Nine areas of concern or attributes of the older patient, if systematically reviewed in preparing the care plan, lead to improved health outcomes and satisfaction with care.

2. The areas of concern can be used as a problem checklist to identify areas relevant to the individual patient.

---

*The Mini Mental State Examination, by Marshal Folstein and Susan Folstein, Copyright 1975, 1998, 2001 by Mini Mental LLC, Inc., is available from Psychological Assessment Resources, Inc., 16204 North Florida Avenue, Lutz, Florida 33549. Reproduction is prohibited without permission of PAR, Inc. The MMSE can be purchased from PAR, Inc. by calling (813) 968-3003.

3. The areas of concern can be used as the goals of care and the means for efficiently monitoring the progress of care.
4. The areas of concern are the critical variables that influence health outcomes in older patients.
   a. They provide a comprehensive view of the complexly ill patient.
   b. They help the physician provide accurate prognostic information to older patients and their families (see Appendix II).

Areas of Concern

1. Diagnosis.
   a. List diagnoses.
   b. Categorize each by severity, degree of reversibility, and impact on function (nutrition, defecation, continence, cognition, emotion, and mobility).
2. Medication.
   a. List all medications, including over-the-counter drugs.
   b. Categorize each by site of excretion (liver or kidney) and impact on function.
   c. Evaluate dosage; check blood levels when available.
3. Nutrition.
   a. Establish baseline for oral intake, weight, and prealbumin/albumin, homocysteine, folate, and vitamin B_{12}.
   b. If baseline is abnormal, list etiologic factors (e.g., diseases, medications, depression, impaction).
   c. Categorize etiologic factors by degree of reversibility.
4. Continence.
   a. Establish baseline for incontinent events (frequency, nocturia, daytime) and urinary retention.
   b. If applicable, list etiologic factors (diseases, medications, change in location, impaction).
   c. Categorize etiologic factors by degree of reversibility.
5. Defecation.
   a. Establish baseline for constipation, impaction, and diarrhea.
   b. If applicable, list etiologic factors (e.g., diseases, medications, immobility, depression).
   c. Categorize etiologic factors by degree of reversibility.
6. Cognition.
   a. Establish baseline for impairment of attention and short-term memory, hallucinations, paranoia.
   b. If applicable, list etiologic factors (e.g., disease, medications, change in location, depression, impaction).
   c. Categorize etiologic factors by degree of reversibility.
7. Emotion.
   a. Establish baseline for anxiety, agitation, depression, failure to thrive (sleep, appetite disturbance, energy disorder).
   b. If applicable, list etiologic factors (e.g., disease, medications, change in location, delirium, impaction).
   c. Categorize etiologic factors by degree of reversibility.
8. Mobility.
   a. Establish baseline for dependence in bed transfers, walking within and outside house, use of transportation.

   b. If applicable, list etiologic factors (e.g., disease, medications, depression, incontinence, lifestyle).
   c. Categorize etiologic factors by degree of reversibility.
9. Cooperation with care plan.
   a. Establish a baseline for capacity to cooperate with the care plan.
   b. If applicable, list obstructions (inappropriate care plan; physical, cognitive, or emotional; impaired patient or caretaker; medications).
   c. Categorize etiologic factors by degree of reversibility.
   d. Advance directives.

Prognosis

1. The prognosis focuses on medical and functional information.
2. The prognosis gives the physician a database for formulating accurate prognostic statements for the patient and family.
3. Patients and families can participate meaningfully in making decisions about medical care.

STEP 3. CARE PLAN

The care plan is the reconciliation between standards of medical practice and patient preference.

1. Reconciling standard medical practice and patient preference is the most critical step in creating an appropriate and successful care plan for patients.
2. Within each area of concern, assess and identify reversible or potentially treatable factors.
3. Make treatment recommendations consistent with standard medical practice for each problem listed in the areas of concern.
4. Reconcile or check the recommendation against the patient's preference for treatment.
   a. Older patients may request no hospitalization or surgery, no feeding tubes, no nursing home placement, no chemotherapy, for example.
   b. It is important to consider individual preferences in each area of concern.
5. Once recommendations have been reconciled with the patient's preferences, the patient and physician have common goals and treatment can proceed.

STEP 4. CHECKLIST

The checklist is used to monitor outcomes of care.

1. The nine areas of concern provide a comprehensive and convenient checklist (Table 2-1) by which the physician can monitor care:
   a. Outcomes of care plan recommendations.
   b. Reevaluation of the patient's current medical and functional status.
   c. Creation of up-to-date care plans that reflect new findings.
2. The CGA provides:
   a. A systematic approach to patient care.
   b. A framework for ongoing and objective inquiry into the human characteristics and behavior influencing health outcomes.
3. The comprehensive assessment allows the physician to see the multiple, complex biopsychosocial variables as predictable patterns rather than isolated events.

Table 2-1	**Outcomes of Care Checklist**
Areas of Concern	**Evaluation**
1. Diagnosis	Are diagnoses accurate and treatments
2. Medications	appropriate?
3. Nutrition	Are intake and output appropriate?
4. Continence	
5. Defecation	
6. Cognition	How is the patient thinking, feeling,
7. Emotion	and doing?
8. Mobility	
9. Cooperation with	Are all persons involved working
care plan	together?

4. The care plan focuses on everyday functions that are important to older patients and their families, and patients and physicians are more satisfied with care.

SUGGESTED READINGS

American Geriatric Society Public Policy Committee: Comprehensive geriatric assessment position statement. 2005 update. Available at http://www.americange-riatrics.org/products/positionpapers/cga.shtml (accessed January 20, 2007).

Applegate WB, Blass JP, Williams TF: Instruments for the functional assessment of older patients. *N Engl J Med* 322:1207-1214, 1990.

Boult C, Boult L, Morishita L, et al: Outpatient geriatric evaluation and management. *J Am Geriatr Soc* 46: 296-302, 1998.

Caplan GA, Williams AJ, Daly B, et al: A randomized, controlled trial of comprehensive geriatric assessment and multidisciplinary intervention after discharge of elderly from the emergency department—the DEED II study. *J Am Geriatr Soc* 52(9):1417-1423, 2004.

Rubenstein LZ, Stuck AE, Siu AL, Wieland D: Impacts of geriatric evaluation and management programs on defined outcomes: Overview of the evidence. *J Am Geriatr Soc* 39(9 Pt 2): 8S-16S, 1991.

Stuck AE, Siu AL, Wieland D, et al: Comprehensive geriatric assessment: A meta-analysis of controlled trials. *Lancet* 342:1032-1036, 1993.

Siu AL, Reuben DB, Moore AA: Comprehensive geriatric assessment. In Hazzard WR, Bierman EL (eds): *Principles of geriatric medicine and gerontology.* New York, McGraw-Hill, 1994.

Wieland D, Hirth V: Comprehensive geriatric assessment. *Cancer Control* 10(6): 454-462, 2003.

Health Maintenance in the Elderly

3

3.1 Preventive Medicine and Health Maintenance

Tom J. Wachtel and Cynthia Holzer

DEFINITION

Prevention refers to measures taken to avoid or postpone the occurrence of diseases and their complications.

1. Primary prevention: avoid or postpone occurrence of disease.
2. Secondary prevention: early detection (e.g., screening) of disease to enhance the treatment outcomes.
3. Tertiary prevention: treatment of chronic conditions (e.g., hypertension, diabetes mellitus, hyperlipidemia) to avoid or postpone complications.
4. The impact of preventive health measures should be judged by their effect on health status (quality or quantity of life), not by the potential to save health care costs because life prolongation might actually come with a price tag rather than savings. Nevertheless, if a limit of human life span exists, a strategy of postponement can lead to actual prevention (and cost savings), with people dying of "old age" without ever being ill or disabled (see Chapter 1). Much of the progress in life expectancy achieved for humanity during the 20th century can be attributed to community health interventions. The practicing physician also can provide substantial benefits to patients.

PRIMARY PREVENTION

1. Cardiovascular disease prevention.
   a. Smoking cessation.
   b. Reduction of serum cholesterol (also tertiary prevention).
   c. Treatment of hypertension (also tertiary prevention).
   d. Exercise (aerobic).
   e. Maintenance of ideal body weight.
   f. Prophylactic low-dose aspirin.
   g. Postmenopausal estrogen replacement therapy.
   h. Stress management or reduction.
2. Cancer prevention.
   a. Smoking cessation.
   b. Avoidance of occupational and environmental exposures (e.g., asbestos, radon, benzene).
   c. Avoidance of sun exposure.
   d. Diet (high fiber, low fat).

e. Certain cancer screening programs can provide primary prevention (e.g., detection and treatment of premalignant cervical conditions or colon polyps).
3. Injury prevention.
  a. Alcohol avoidance.
  b. Seat belt use.
  c. Motorcycle and bicycle helmet use.
  d. Occupational and home safety-enhancing actions (see Chapter 7).
  e. Fall prevention in the elderly.
  f. Firearm avoidance and gun legislation and enforcement.
  g. Domestic violence education and legislation and enforcement.
4. Chronic lung disease prevention: smoking cessation.
5. Osteoporosis prevention.
  a. Dietary calcium.
  b. Calcium supplements (calcium 1500 mg/d in postmenopausal women).
  c. Weight-bearing exercise (resistive, not aerobic).
  d. Postmenopausal estrogen replacement therapy.
    (1) Posthysterectomy patients: conjugated estrogen (Premarin) 0.3 mg qd to 0.625 mg qd.
    (2) Intact-uterus patients: conjugated estrogen (Premarin) 0.3 mg qd to 0.625 mg qd and medroxyprogesterone (Provera) 1.5 mg qd to 2.5 mg qd to prevent endometrial cancer risk increased by unopposed estrogen.
6. Infectious disease prevention.
  a. Safer sex.
  b. Immunizations.
    (1) Routine immunization in adults.
      (a) Tetanus.
        (i) Primary: tetanus toxoid, 0.5 mL three times (first and second 1 to 2 months apart, third 6 to 12 months later).
        (ii) Booster every 10 years or at age 65 years and stop.
      (b) Influenza: annual for adults over age 65, especially important in people with high-risk conditions (e.g., diabetes mellitus, chronic lung disease).
      (c) Pneumococcal polysaccharide, 0.5 mL once; same indications as influenza.
        (i) *Note:* Vaccinate those whose previous vaccination status is unknown.
        (ii) Booster after 5 to 10 years once.
    (2) Special recommendations for travelers: Immunizations depend on the travel plan; check with experts.
  c. Tuberculosis (TB).
    (1) Purified protein derivative (PPD).
      (a) Yearly for institutionalized elderly persons, alcoholics, and recent immigrants from high-prevalence countries.
      (b) Every 3 to 5 years for the general population.
      (c) Close contacts of infectious TB patients who share the same household or other enclosed environment.
    (2) A skin test reaction to tuberculin can be detected 2 to 10 weeks after the initial infection and persists indefinitely unless

anergy develops. The Mantoux test, rather than a multiple puncture test, should be used for PPD testing.

(a) The Mantoux test is performed by injecting 0.1 mL of PPD tuberculin containing 5 tuberculin units intradermally on the forearm. The injection should be made just beneath the surface of the skin, with the needle bevel facing upward to produce a discrete wheal. The test should be ready for evaluation 48 to 72 hours later, but positive reactions may be read up to 1 week after testing.

(b) The diameter of induration (not erythema) should be measured transversely to the long axis of the forearm.

(c) The result should be recorded as the number of millimeters of induration and not simply as positive or negative.

(d) Control skin test antigens may be used to test for anergy in patients with immunosuppressive disorders.

(3) The classification of tuberculin skin test results depends on the group being tested. The Centers for Disease Control and Prevention (CDC) has adopted the following classification system:

(a) A tuberculin reaction >5 mm is classified as positive in the following groups:

   (i) Persons who have had recent close contact with a patient with infectious TB.

   (ii) Persons who have chest radiographs with fibrotic lesions likely to represent old healed TB.

(b) A tuberculin reaction =10 mm is classified as positive in persons who do not meet the above criteria but who have other risk factors for TB.

   (i) Persons with medical risk factors.

   (ii) Foreign-born persons from high-prevalence areas.

   (iii) Medically underserved, low-income populations, including high-risk minorities.

(c) A tuberculin reaction =15 mm is classified as positive in all other persons.

(4) All persons with a positive PPD test result should have a chest x-ray study to evaluate for active tuberculosis before considering preventive therapy.

(5) Beware:

(a) A negative tuberculin skin test result does not rule out the diagnosis of TB or TB infection.

(b) There is a common misconception that the booster phenomenon indicates a false-positive tuberculin test result caused by sensitization from repeated tuberculin testing. In fact, repeated tuberculin testing of uninfected persons does not sensitize to tuberculin, and a positive result from a repeated test ("caused by" the booster phenomenon) is truly positive. In two-step testing (recommended for elderly debilitated persons), a second PPD test is placed 1 week after a first negative test result.

(c) Positive tuberculin reactions in bacille Calmette-Guérin–vaccinated persons usually indicate true infection with *Mycobacterium tuberculosis*.

Preventive Therapy for Tuberculosis

1. The goal of preventive therapy is to reduce the risk of developing active TB in persons who are infected. In considering a course of preventive therapy, one must weigh the known efficacy of this treatment against the toxicity of isoniazid 300 mg per day, which is the drug of choice. Because the risk of drug-induced hepatitis increases with age, chemoprophylaxis in the elderly is recommended only in persons who have:
   a. Recent skin conversion.
   b. Recent contact with an infectious person.
   c. Abnormal chest x-ray consistent with past TB.
   d. Diabetes.
   e. Long-term corticosteroid therapy.
2. Twelve months of continuous preventive therapy is recommended for persons with stable abnormal chest radiographs consistent with past TB. Other groups should receive a minimum of 6 continuous months of preventive therapy. Isoniazid can be given twice weekly in a dose of 15 mg/kg (up to 900 mg) when therapy must be directly observed and resources are inadequate for daily observed therapy.
3. Persons receiving preventive therapy should be monitored for:
   a. Symptoms of neurotoxicity such as paresthesias of the hands and feet (high risk: persons with diabetes, alcoholism); pyridoxine (50 mg/day) reduces the incidence.
   b. Signs consistent with hepatitis such as anorexia, nausea, vomiting, dark urine, jaundice, unexplained fever, right upper quadrant tenderness.
   c. Abnormalities of liver transaminases (10% to 20%), with higher risk of hepatotoxicity occurring among persons older than 35 years; if the alanine aminotransferase level is greater than three to five times the upper limit of normal, preventive therapy should be reconsidered.
   d. The emergence of multidrug-resistant TB is leading to new chemoprophylaxis regimens (e.g., rifampin). Please keep informed.
4. Persons with positive PPDs who do not receive chemoprophylaxis or who cannot complete a full course of it should have a chest x-ray every 1 to 2 years.

SECONDARY PREVENTION

1. Cancer.
   a. Cervical cancer: Pap smear every 1 to 3 years. Controversial in low-risk women over 65 previously screened or over 75 not previously screened. However, a pelvic exam should still be performed after those age thresholds to screen for endometrial and ovarian cancer. Not doing a Pap smear as part of a routine pelvic exam is difficult to justify except on the basis of its cost.
   b. Breast cancer: breast self-examination, monthly after menses; annual breast examination by physician after age 40 years; mammography (see Chapter 5) every 1 to 2 years after age 40.
   c. Colorectal cancer.
      (1) Rectal examination yearly in all adults after age 40 years.
      (2) Testing for fecal occult blood yearly (three pairs of specimens) or during rectal exam in all adults after age 50 years and in high-risk

persons (family history of adenocarcinoma, inflammatory bowel disease, or history of colorectal polyps) after age 40 years.

    (3) Endoscopy (sigmoidoscopy or colonoscopy) or double air contrast barium enema study in all adults after age 50 years (every 5 years) or preferentially in high-risk adults.

  d. Lung cancer: chest x-ray study and sputum cytology have marginal effectiveness even in high-risk persons (e.g., smokers, asbestos exposure).

  e. Endometrial cancer: endometrial biopsy is controversial without symptoms.

  f. Prostate cancer: annual digital rectal exam in men over 40 years; prostate-specific antigen (recommended by the American Cancer Society) annually between ages 50 and 70 years (see Chapter 5).

  g. Urologic cancers (renal cell and transitional): urinalysis for blood and urinary cytology is not proven effective.

  h. Ovarian cancer: annual pelvic exam after age 40 years, CA 125 not proven effective.

  i. Testicular.

    (1) Monthly self-examination.

    (2) Tumor markers (human chorionic gonadotropin [hCG], alpha fetoprotein) not indicated for screening.

  j. Hepatoma: alpha fetoprotein is not proven effective but may be considered in a patient with chronic active hepatitis B infection, cirrhosis, or hemochromatosis.

  k. Skin cancer: monthly skin self-examination, with special attention to pigmented lesions.

  l. All other cancers: physical examination with special attention to nasopharyngeal region, thyroid, liver, spleen, pelvic and genital organs, lymph node areas, and skin.

2. Total cholesterol every 3 to 5 years.

3. Routine use of blood chemistries, complete blood count (CBC), and urinalysis.

  a. No specific indication.

  b. Usual recommendation is one baseline set of complete blood count, urinalysis, fasting blood glucose, blood urea nitrogen (BUN), creatinine, calcium, aspartate aminotransferase, alkaline, phosphatase, total thyroxine (T_4).

4. Baseline electrocardiogram (ECG) (give copy to patient to help decision making in an emergency care setting in the event of chest pain).

5. Blood pressure measurement every 3 years before age 40 years and yearly thereafter.

6. Visual acuity and glaucoma screening every 1 to 3 years after age 50 years.

7. Hearing evaluation every 3 years after age 50 years.

8. Physical and mental function (cognitive and affective) assessment as needed in geriatric patients.

TERTIARY PREVENTION

The treatment of many chronic illnesses often has tertiary prevention as the single therapeutic goal (e.g., management of hypercholesterolemia) or as an added benefit to symptom relief (e.g., management of heart failure with angiotensin converting enzyme [ACE] inhibitors).

3—Health Maintenance

PREVENTION IMPLEMENTATION

1. Add "health maintenance" to the problem list in the medical record.
2. Use a prevention flow chart (Fig. 3-1). Without a flow chart (paper or computerized), compliance within health maintenance schedules is unlikely.
3. Physician reminders.
4. Patient reminders (by mail).
5. Educate patients so they request preventive services when they are due.

Health Maintenance—Flow Sheet															
Date:															
Assessment															
Height	× 1														
Weight	q visit														
Blood pressure	q visit														
Pulse	q visit														
Oxygen saturation	× 1														

Exams															
Breast self-exam	q month														
Pelvic exam	q 1–3 years														
Digital rectal exam	q year after 40														
Visual acuity	q year														
Hearing assessment	q year														
Testicular self-exam															
Intraocular pressure (over 65)	q year														
Dental exam by dentist	q year														

Health Risk (Yes or No)															
Smoking															
Alcohol/drugs															
Seat belts															
Safe sex															
Exercise															
Diet															

Figure 3-1   Health maintenance flow chart for the medical record.

Laboratory

Stool guaiac	q year after 40												
Pap smear	q 3 years												
Mammography	q 1–2 yrs after 40												
Cholesterol	q 3–5 years												
Bone density	q 5–10 yrs after 55												
Colonoscopy	q 10 yrs after 50												
PSA	q 1–2 yrs after 50												

Immunization—check if up to date

Flu vaccine	(over 65) q year												
Pneumovax	(over 65) × 1 and 1 booster after 5 yrs												
Tetanus booster	q 10 years												

Figure 3-1, cont'd   For legend see opposite page.

SUGGESTED READINGS

Bjelakovic G, Nikolova D, Gluud LL: Mortality in randomized trials of antioxidant supplements for primary and secondary prevention: Systematic review and meta-analysis. JAMA 297:842-857, 2007.

Boulware LE, Marinopoulos S, Phillips KA: Systematic review: The value of the periodic health evaluation. Ann Intern Med 146:289-300, 2007.

Davila RE, Rajan E, Baron TH, et al: ASGE guideline: Colorectal cancer screening and surveillance. Gastrointest Endosc 63:546-557, 2006.

Liu H, Bravata DM, Olkin I, et al: Systematic review: The safety and efficacy of growth hormone in the healthy elderly. Ann Intern Med 146:104-115, 2007.

MMWR Quick Guide: Recommended adult immunization schedule—United States, October 2006-September 2007. MMWR 55 Q1-Q4, 2006.

Sanders KM, Nicholson GC, Watts JJ: Half the burden of fragility fractures in the community occur in women without osteoporosis. When is fracture prevention cost-effective? Bone 38:694-700, 2006.

Siris ES, Chen YT, Abbott TA, et al: Bone mineral density thresholds for pharmacologic intervention to prevent fractures. Arch Intern Med 164:1108-1112, 2004.

3.2 Perioperative Medical Evaluation

Michael P. Gerardo

OVERVIEW

Older patients who undergo surgery are at significant risk for morbidity and mortality during the perioperative and postoperative period. Thus, geriatricians have an important role not only in preoperatively assessing the patient's cardiac, pulmonary, and cognitive status but also in suggesting methods for reducing risk during the perioperative period. Additionally, patients are likely to benefit from continued geriatric evaluation during the postoperative period.

PREOPERATIVE EVALUATION
Cardiac Assessment for Noncardiac Surgery

The factors listed in the first section determine which patients should undergo a cardiac assessment. The cardiac assessment itself includes three parameters that determine the risk of coronary events in the perioperative period: the clinical predictors, the surgical risk, and the functional capacity assessment. These terms are based on the 2002 American College of Cardiology/American Heart Association Task Force practice guidelines and should be taken into consideration when deciding which patients should undergo a coronary evaluation with standard imaging techniques such as exercise or pharmacologic treadmill stress test, exercise or pharmacologic echocardiogram, or nuclear perfusion imaging before surgery. The last section outlines special considerations for cardiac abnormalities related to carotid vascular disease, rhythm disturbance, and cardiac dysfunction.

Which Patients Should Undergo a Cardiac Assessment?

1. Urgency of the surgery.
   a. A cardiac assessment is warranted for all nonemergent surgeries. *Elective surgery* is a relative term; for example, hernia repair is more elective than a hemicolectomy for cancer. Every effort should be made to minimize the risk of coronary events following all nonemergent surgeries.
   b. If life-saving surgery is emergent, then the patient goes straight to the operating room.
2. Recent history of coronary revascularization.
   a. A cardiac assessment is indicated for patients who have had a coronary revascularization within the past 5 years and have had a recurrence of their angina.
   b. Any patient who has had a recent coronary revascularization (<5 years) and is free of angina may proceed to the operating room without a cardiac assessment.
3. Recent evaluation for ischemic heart disease: A patient with favorable result on a recent coronary evaluation (<2 years) and no change in symptoms may proceed to the operating room.

Risk of Coronary Events in the Perioperative Period

1. Determination of clinical predictors: As shown in Box 3-1, clinical predictors of an increased risk in perioperative cardiac events are categorized as major, intermediate, and minor clinical predictors.
   a. Whenever major clinical predictors are present, it is recommended that the patient undergo a modification of risk, and revascularization when appropriate, prior to surgery.
   b. A patient with minor or no clinical predictors (age older than 70 years is itself a minor clinical predictor) may proceed to the operating room if the surgery is of low or intermediate risk. It is recommended that all patients with minor or no clinical predictors undergoing a high-risk surgery have a functional capacity assessment.

BOX 3-1   Clinical Predictors of Increased Perioperative Cardiovascular Risk

Major Predictors

Recent myocardial infarction (in last 7 to 30 days)
Unstable angina
Decompensated congestive heart failure
Supraventricular arrhythmia with uncontrolled ventricular rate
Severe valvular disease

Intermediate Predictors

Stable angina
History of myocardial infarction
Compensated congestive heart failure
Diabetes mellitus

Minor Predictors

Advanced age
Left ventricular hypertrophy, left bundle branch block, or ST changes
  on resting ECG
History of cerebrovascular accident
Uncontrolled hypertension
Coronary artery bypass graft in last 6 months to 5 years

ECG, electrocardiogram.

2. The risk of surgery, shown in Box 3-2, is evaluated in all patients with intermediate clinical predictors.
   a. *High surgery risk* with *intermediate clinical predictors:* Patients who are undergoing a high-risk procedure with intermediate clinical predictors require a coronary evaluation before surgery.
   b. *Intermediate surgery risk* with *intermediate clinical predictors:* Those undergoing an intermediate-risk surgery require a functional capacity assessment.
   c. *Low surgery risk* with *intermediate clinical predictors:* Patients with intermediate clinical predictors and undergoing a low-risk surgery may proceed to the operating room.
3. Functional capacity assessment: A functional capacity assessment is indicated for two groups:
   a. Any patient with intermediate clinical predictors undergoing an intermediate-risk surgery.
   b. A patient with minor or no clinical predictors undergoing a high-risk surgery. Any patient who performs at less than 4 metabolic equivalents (METs) must have a coronary evaluation prior to surgery. Examples of tasks that require 4 METs include independence in activities of daily living, walking around the house, walking 2 blocks at 2 to 3 mph, or performing light housework such as dusting or washing dishes.

BOX 3-2   Risk of Myocardial Infarction or Cardiac
Death for Noncardiac Procedures

High Risk (>5%)

Aortic surgery
Prolonged procedures with large blood loss and/or fluid shifts
Peripheral vascular surgery

Intermediate Risk (1%-5%)

Intrathoracic and intraperitoneal surgery
Carotid endarterectomy
Head and neck surgery
Orthopedic surgery
Open prostatic surgery

Low Risk (<1%)

Endoscopic procedures
Cataract surgery
Breast biopsy

---

4. Determination of cardiac risk associated with noncardiac surgery. In the cardiac assessment, physicians should use standard cardiac-risk terminology when assessing risk of surgery. Patients are either at low risk, intermediate risk, or high risk for a cardiac event. Every patient carries the risk of experiencing a cardiac event, especially the older adult, and physicians should not use the term "no risk" or "cleared for surgery." Instead, the patient should be described as "average risk for surgery." If the surgery is low risk and the patient is lacking major clinical predictors, then the patient may proceed to the operating room.

Coronary Evaluation

All patients who require a coronary evaluation based on the cardiac assessment must undergo an evaluation with one of the following tests:

1. Exercise ECG is the most cost-effective method used to evaluate for heart disease. However, in the older population, comorbid illness, such as chronic obstructive pulmonary disease (COPD), arthritis, and deconditioning, is common. Such comorbid illness can preclude the use of exercise stress testing. For patients who cannot perform an exercise protocol, pharmacologic-based stress testing is achieved with dobutamine, adenosine, or Persantine.
2. Stress (exercise or pharmacologic-based) echocardiography and myocardial nuclear perfusion testing (scintigraphy) are both more costly than exercise ECG, but they provide additional information related to the location of lesion and left ventricular dysfunction. Myocardial scintigraphy distinguishes between ischemic and infarcted myocardium. Physicians should use these modalities when the baseline ECG is abnormal (i.e., resting ST depression, left bundle branch block, left ventricular hypertrophy with strain, paced rhythms).

3. Coronary angiogram should be considered for patients who have advanced heart disease (heart failure, unstable angina, arrhythmia with heart disease, severe valvular disease, recent myocardial infarction [MI], high-degree arteriovenous block).

Special Considerations

1. Arrhythmia: Cardiac rhythm disturbances in the absence of structural heart disease are unlikely to result in cardiac events. Physicians should investigate for structural heart disease in all patients with arrhythmias seen on the preoperative ECG. Patients who have an indication for a pacemaker should have one placed before surgery.
2. Heart failure: Patients with decompensated heart failure are at increased risk for cardiac events. Controlling the symptoms with diuretics and afterload-reducing therapies can reduce the risk of preoperative and postoperative cardiac events.
3. Carotid artery stenosis: In patients with an indication for endarterectomy, the endarterectomy should be performed before noncarotid surgery.

Pulmonary Assessment

1. The most common postoperative pulmonary complications are pneumonia and respiratory failure requiring mechanical ventilation. It is estimated that these complications occur in 2% to 19% of all surgical interventions.
2. Identifying risk factors for postoperative pulmonary complications is an important step in reducing the likelihood of postoperative pulmonary complications. Based on the risk factor assessment, recommendations can be made regarding preoperative, perioperative, and postoperative management.
3. Risk factors.
   a. General risk factors include:
      (1) Upper abdominal or cardiothoracic surgery.
      (2) Anesthetic time greater than 4 hours.
      (3) Morbid obesity.
      (4) COPD or asthma.
      (5) Greater than 20 pack-year smoking history.
      (6) History of stroke.
   b. The American College of Physicians also includes as risk factors for postoperative pulmonary complications:
      (1) Age older than 60 years.
      (2) Functional dependence.
      (3) Surgery longer than 3 hours.
      (4) Abdominal surgery, thoracic surgery, neurosurgery, head and neck surgery, vascular surgery, aortic aneurysm repair, or emergency surgery.
      (5) General anesthesia.
4. Pulmonary function testing is not recommended for patients undergoing non-lung resection surgery. Arterial blood gas is only used for patients suspected of having hypoxemia or hypercapnia.
5. Preoperative recommendations to reduce the risk of pulmonary complications include:
   a. Discontinue smoking 4 to 8 weeks before surgery (estimated 25% risk reduction in pulmonary complications).

b. Optimization of pulmonary function in COPD or asthma patients with bronchodilator therapy.
c. In patients with a respiratory infection, antibiotics should be administered, with a delay in surgery if respiratory symptoms persist (e.g., cough with purulent sputum).
d. Patients on theophylline should continue the medication through the perioperative and postoperative period. Intravenous (IV) administration may be necessary.
e. Incentive spirometry should be started 2 days prior to surgery and continued in the postoperative period.

Cognitive Assessment

1. Postoperative delirium is an independent predictor of morbidity and mortality. Such patients are at risk for pulmonary and cardiac complications, increased length of hospital stay, poor recovery, and death.
2. Risk factors for postoperative delirium include:
    a. Age greater than 70 years.
    b. History of alcohol abuse.
    c. Dementia.
    d. Impaired vision or hearing.
3. Regardless of the patient's risk, strategies to prevent delirium (see Postoperative Management below) have been shown to reduce the risk of postoperative delirium.
4. Mini Mental State Exam or other cognitive assessments (e.g., MiniCog) before surgery can be compared to repeat testing and thereby aid in the diagnosis and management of postoperative delirium.

End-of-Life Care

It is entirely appropriate for a person undergoing surgery to decline cardiopulmonary resuscitation and other lifesaving measures. Therefore, any preoperative evaluation should include a discussion of all end-of-life care issues, and advance directives should be documented in the patient's medical record.

PERIOPERATIVE RISK REDUCTION

β-Blocker Therapy

1. Persons with two or more of the following predictors of postoperative cardiac complications may benefit from prophylactic β-blocker therapy:
    a. Intrathoracic, intraperitoneal, or infrainguinal vascular surgery.
    b. Coronary artery disease.
    c. History of congestive heart failure.
    d. Use of insulin to manage hyperglycemia in diabetes mellitus.
    e. Chronic kidney disease (creatinine ≥2 mg/dL).
    f. History of stroke.
2. The following β-blockers have been studied:
    a. Atenolol 50 to 100 mg daily 3 to 30 days before surgery and continued for 1 week after surgery.
    b. Metoprolol 50 to 100 mg twice daily 3 to 30 days before surgery and continued for 1 week after surgery.
    c. Bisoprolol 5 to 10 mg daily 1 to 4 weeks before surgery and continued for 1 week after surgery.

3. Because bradycardia and hypotension are associated with this therapy in older patients, it is recommended that the patient be administered half the traditional starting dose and that the dose be titrated to the appropriate dose.

Lipid-Lowering Therapy

Limited research suggests that statin therapy can reduce the rates of nonfatal MI and cardiac death for patients with coronary artery disease (CAD). A randomized trial of atorvastatin 40 mg daily versus placebo in patients undergoing vascular surgery resulted in fewer cardiac deaths and nonfatal MIs. The dose was started 2 weeks before surgery and continued for 45 days after surgery.

Antibiotic Prophylaxis

Physicians should recommend the standard doses of antibiotic prophylaxis to prevent either surgical wound infections or endocarditis when appropriate.

POSTOPERATIVE MANAGEMENT

1. Delirium: Several strategies have demonstrated a reduction in the risk of postoperative delirium.
   a. Daily assessment of cognitive status is helpful for managing postoperative patients. Subtle changes in cognitive status may be easier to identify if the physician has frequent interaction with the patient.
   b. Avoid or minimize the use of anticholinergics, benzodiazepines, and antihistamines during the postoperative period. Each of these medications carries the risk of inducing delirium.
   c. Opioids can cause delirium. If narcotics are to be used, stool softeners should be coadministered. Delirium may be a clinical manifestation of poor bowel function.
   d. Urinary catheters should not be used routinely because the risk of infection-associated delirium is higher among patients with catheters.
   e. Delirium is reversible, although persons with dementia might not return completely to baseline functioning. The precipitant should be identified and removed. Common causes of postoperative delirium include drugs, electrolyte imbalances, anemia, dehydration, urinary tract infection, and pneumonia (DEAD-UP; Box 3-3).

BOX 3-3   Common Causes of Postoperative Delirium: DEAD-UP

Drugs
Electrolyte imbalances
Anemia
Dehydration
Urinary tract infection
Pneumonia

f. Trazodone, starting at 25 mg daily, can be very effective in alleviating agitation and other aggressive behavior.

g. If antipsychotic therapy is administered for aggression, agitation, or delusion, short-term treatment with haloperidol, starting at 0.25 mg at bedtime, may be appropriate.

h. Physicians should continually assess the need for antipsychotic therapy. One strategy is to slowly withdraw the medication once symptoms of delirium have been controlled and the precipitant treated. A subset of patients require prolonged use of antipsychotics. In patients with a slow recovery from delirium, atypical antipsychotics (risperidone, olanzapine, quetiapine, aripiprazole) may be the preferred form of therapy. However, limited data support the use of atypical antipsychotics over conventional therapies (haloperidol).

2. Deep venous thrombosis (DVT) and pulmonary embolism (PE).

   a. Risk factors for the development of DVT or PE include a history of venous thromboembolism, immobilization, malignancy, obesity, atrial fibrillation, heart failure, and hypercoagulable states.

   b. Early ambulation is recommended for persons younger than 40 years undergoing minor surgery (e.g., hernia repair).

   c. Thrombophylaxis is recommended to prevent DVT and PE for all other patients. Physicians should administer standard doses of low-dose unfractionated heparin or low molecular weight (LMW) heparin. In patients with these risk factors who are also older than 60 years, graded compression stockings or intermittent pneumatic compression should be used in conjunction with thrombophylactic therapy.

3. Pain should be adequately controlled and titrated to the minimal amount of medication required to control pain. Nonsteroidal antiinflammatory drugs (NSAIDs) and acetaminophen, when there is no contraindication, can reduce the amount of narcotic administered to the patient. All narcotics should be coadministered with stool softeners.

4. Bowel function should be assessed daily because many postoperative patients are on narcotics or are immobilized.

5. Infection: The most common postoperative infections are pneumonia and urinary tract infection. Prompt evaluation and management with antibiotics can reduce postoperative morbidity and mortality.

TRANSITIONS OF CARE

Older patients might require some rehabilitative period either at a skilled nursing facility (SNF) or with home care services. It is important to address these issues before surgery so that the case manager can find a bed at an acceptable nursing home or have home services prepared for the day of discharge. Direct communication between the acute-care team and SNF team can reduce medical errors and improve both adherence to care plans and patient and family satisfaction with care.

PRIMARY CARE FOLLOW-UP

The primary care physician should follow up with the patient after discharge from the hospital. Follow-up can be at the SNF or after the patient has been discharged from the SNF unit.

1. Patients who have fractured a hip in a fall might benefit from a fall risk assessment. A fall risk assessment includes a gait assessment, home safety evaluation, and physical therapy when appropriate.
2. All patients who have experienced a fracture should have dual energy x-ray absorptiometry (DEXA) to assess for the presence of osteoporosis. Patients with a low-impact fracture could be treated for osteoporosis without DEXA, because a low-impact fracture is an osteoporosis-defining event.
3. Postoperative delirium warrants close observation for dementia. Patients who have experienced postoperative delirium are at increased risk for dementia.

OTHER CONSIDERATIONS

1. Diabetes: Hyperglycemia impairs the function of the immune system. In post-MI patients, tight glycemic control has resulted in better outcomes.
   a. Target glucose levels are:
      (1) Intensive care unit (ICU) patients: 100 mg/dL.
      (2) Non-ICU patients:
         (a) 110 mg/dL preprandial.
         (b) 180 mg/dL postprandial.
   b. The American College of Endocrinology recommends insulin infusion for patients who are fasting for longer than 12 hours, for critically ill patients, and for patients undergoing major surgery.
   c. Oral hypoglycemics should be withheld on the morning of surgery, and glucose should be monitored with sliding-scale (regular insulin) coverage.
   d. Patients on insulin should be given half their AM insulin dose preoperatively and then receive an infusion of 5% dextrose containing 5 to 15 units of insulin per liter at a rate of 100 mL/h. Glucose levels should be checked hourly until they stabilize.
2. Adrenal insufficiency.
   a. All patients who have been on steroids for prolonged periods or who have known adrenal suppression should be given appropriate dosages of hydrocortisone.
   b. Most patients require 100 mg hydrocortisone every 8 hours beginning the morning of surgery and continued for 2 days after surgery.
   c. Patients undergoing more stressful procedures (coronary artery bypass graft, abdominal surgery) might require higher doses of glucocorticoid during the perioperative period.
3. Thyroid disease.
   a. Hypothyroid patients should receive their thyroid hormone replacement preoperatively.
   b. Hyperthyroid patients should be given antithyroid medications and β-blockade and should be monitored for the possibility of thyroid storm (delirium, severe tachycardia, vomiting, diarrhea, dehydration, high fever).
4. Renal disease.
   a. Risk factors for developing acute renal failure (ARF) include chronic kidney disease, aortic surgery, cardiac surgery, peripheral vascular disease, imaging contrast dye, decompensated heart failure, preoperative jaundice, age greater than 70 years, and diabetes.

3—Health Maintenance

b. All patients with chronic kidney disease are at increased risk for electrolyte imbalances and ARF and are more susceptible to the toxic effects of renally excreted medications. Therefore, all medications should be renally adjusted when appropriate. Monitoring of electrolytes, renal function, and fluid balance is appropriate in those at risk of ARF.

5. Hematologic: The hematocrit should be maintained above 30. Thrombocytopenia will impair surgical hemostasis if the platelet level is below 50,000.

6. Liver.

a. Patients with normal liver function (albumin, cholesterol, partial thromboplastin time) and no signs of liver failure (ascites or jaundice) are at minimal risk for hepatic decompensation.

b. The surgical risk increases with cirrhosis (ascites, encephalopathy, or liver test abnormalities). Preoperative assessment should aim for control of coagulopathy, ascites, and encephalopathy.

SUGGESTED READINGS

American College of Cardiology; American Heart Association Task Force on Practice Guidelines; American Society of Echocardiography; et al: ACC/AHA 2006 guideline update on perioperative cardiovascular evaluation for noncardiac surgery: Focused update on perioperative β-blocker therapy. J Am Coll Cardiol 47:2343-2355, 2006.

Axelrod L: Perioperative management of patients treated with glucocorticoids. Endocrinol Metab Clin North Am 32:367-383, 2003.

Eagle KA, Berger PB, Calkins H, et al: ACC/AHA guideline update for perioperative cardiovascular evaluation for noncardiac surgery—executive summary: A report of the American College of Cardiology/American Heart Association Task Force on Practice Guidelines (Committee to Update the 1996 Guidelines on Perioperative Cardiovascular Evaluation for Noncardiac Surgery) J Am Coll Cardiol 39:542-553, 2002.

Garber AJ, Moghissi ES, Bransome ED Jr, et al: American College of Endocrinology position statement on inpatient diabetes and metabolic control. Endocr Pract 10:77-82, 2004.

Lindenauer PK, Pekow P, Wang K, et al: Perioperative β-blocker therapy and mortality after major noncardiac surgery. N Engl J Med 353:349-361, 2005.

Lindenauer PK, Pekow P, Wang K, et al: Lipid-lowering therapy and in-hospital mortality following major noncardiac surgery. JAMA 291:2092-2099, 2004.

Qaseem A, Snow V, Fitterman N, et al: Risk assessment for and strategies to reduce perioperative pulmonary complications for patients undergoing noncardiothoracic surgery: A guideline from the American College of Physicians. Ann Int Med 144:575-580, 2006.

Smetana G, Lawrence VA, Cornell JE; American College of Physicians: Preoperative pulmonary risk stratification for noncardiothoracic surgery: Systematic review for the American College of Physicians. Ann Int Med 144:581-595, 2006.

Wang PS, Schneeweiss S, Avorn L, et al: Risk of death in elderly users of conventional vs. atypical antipsychotic medications. N Engl J Med 353(22):2335-2341, 2005.

3.3 Menopause

George T. Danakas, Fred F. Ferri, and Tom J. Wachtel

DEFINITION

Menopause (change of life) is the cessation of menstrual periods for 1 year after age 40 years resulting from the permanent loss of ovarian activity.

3—Health Maintenance

EPIDEMIOLOGY

1. Average age of menopause in the United States is 51 years.
2. Age at which menopause occurs is genetically determined.
3. More than one third of a woman's life is spent after menopause.

CLINICAL FINDINGS

1. Atrophic vaginitis can cause burning, itching, bleeding, dyspareunia. Vaginal dryness usually begins several years after menopause and can worsen with time; approximately 25% of women experience this effect by 5 years after menopause.
2. Onset of menopause can be either complete cessation of menses or a period of irregular cycles and diminished or heavier bleeding.
3. Psychological dysfunction.
   a. Anxiety.
   b. Depression.
   c. Insomnia.
   d. Nervousness.
   e. Irritability.
   f. Inability to concentrate.
   g. Decreased libido.
4. Urinary incontinence.
   a. Stress incontinence is related to relaxation of pelvic ligaments.
   b. Urge or mixed incontinence can also occur.
5. Vasomotor symptoms (hot flashes, flushes).
   a. Night sweats.
      (1) Hot flushes affect 75% of postmenopausal women.
      (2) Most hot flushes begin 1 to 2 years before menopause and resolve after 2 years.
   b. Fifteen percent of women report duration of hot flushes longer than 15 years.
   c. Hot flushes can occur in men and are associated with testicular failure or castration.
6. Headaches, tiredness and fatigue.
7. Associated conditions.
   a. Osteoporosis.
   b. CAD.

ETIOLOGY

1. Physiologic (most common etiology).
2. Surgical castration.

WORK-UP

Work-up is not needed in geriatric women, but assess for CAD, osteoporosis, cigarette smoking, personal history of breast cancer, liver disease, active coagulation disorder, or any unexplained vaginal bleeding.

LABORATORY TESTS

Follicle-stimulating hormone (FSH), luteinizing hormone (LH), and estrogen levels; a markedly elevated FSH and a markedly depressed estrogen level support the diagnosis of ovarian failure. These tests are rarely performed.

IMAGING STUDIES

1. Mammogram (routine).
2. Pelvic ultrasound to check endometrial stripe in selected cases or in any woman with postmenopausal vaginal bleeding (see Chapter 5).

TREATMENT

1. Hot flushes.
   a. Estrogen replacement therapy (ERT).
      (1) Reduces hot flushes by 80% to 90%.
      (2) Estrogen therapy is contraindicated in many women, and others are fearful of its use. Potential risks and side effects should be considered before using estrogen in any patient.
      (3) Formulation and dosing.
         (a) It is best to use a low-dose formulation, such as conjugated equine estrogen 0.45 mg or 0.3 mg plus medroxyprogesterone 1.5 mg (Prempro).
         (b) Femring is an intravaginal ring that is changed every 3 months and approved to treat vasomotor symptoms in women who have had a hysterectomy. It provides both local and systemic estrogen.
         (c) Many other estrogen and progesterone preparations and formulations are available.
      (4) Hormone replacement therapy should be used only for short-term symptom control.
   b. Results of the Women's Health Initiative study for every 10,000 women taking hormone replacement therapy (HRT) for 1 year (10,000 person-years) compared with women taking placebo.
      (1) Adverse events: 7 more women would have coronary events, 8 more would have strokes, 8 more would have PEs, and 8 more would develop early breast cancer.
      (2) Benefits: 6 fewer cases of colorectal cancer and 5 fewer hip fractures per 10,000 women.
   c. HRT should not be initiated or continued for primary or secondary prevention of coronary heart disease or osteoporosis.
   d. Megestrol acetate, a progestational agent, is a safer alternative to estrogen in women with a history of breast or uterine cancer and in men receiving androgen ablation therapy for prostate cancer. Usual dose is 20 mg bid.
   e. Venlafaxine (Effexor) has been reported to be 60% effective in reducing hot flushes and represents an alternative treatment modality in women unable or unwilling to use estrogens. Starting dose is Effexor XR 37.5 mg qd, increased as tolerated up to a maximum of 300 mg/day.
   f. Selective serotonin reuptake inhibitors (SSRIs) (e.g., fluoxetine, paroxetine) are also used to treat hot flushes but are probably less effective than venfaxine. A trial showed that paroxetine is an effective agent for diminishing hot flushes in men receiving androgen ablation therapy.
   g. Gabapentin (300 to 1200 mg/day) can be used alone or in combination with venlafaxine to treat hot flushes.

h. Clonidine is effective in reducing the frequency of hot flushes. Adverse effects include dry mouth, sedation, and dizziness.

i. Soy protein is often used; soy extracts contain plant-derived estrogens (phytoestrogens); however, clinical trials have not shown clear efficacy, and dosing is imprecise.

j. Tibolone improves vasomotor symptoms, libido, and vaginal lubrication; it is not currently available in the United States.

k. Several herbal remedies are available to patients and are commonly used without significant benefit. Commonly used agents are *Cimicifuga racemosa* (aka black cohosh, snakeroot, or bugbane), *angelica sinensis*, and evening primrose (evening star).

l. Balanced diet low in fat, with total fat intake being less than 30% of calories, and total calories sufficient to maintain body weight or to produce weight loss if that is needed.

m. Avoidance of smoking, excessive alcohol intake, or excessive caffeine intake.

n. Change in the ambient temperature might ameliorate hot flushes and reduce night sweats.

o. Behavioral interventions such as relaxation training and paced respiration have been reported effective in reducing symptoms in some women.

2. Treatment of other menopausal problems.

 a. Evaluate for osteoporosis (e.g., DXA) and consider treatment or prevention with:
 (1) Calcium.
 (2) Vitamin D.
 (3) Weight-bearing exercise.
 (4) Bisphosphonate.
 (5) Raloxifene.

 b. Address vaginal atrophy (sexual and urinary function).
 (1) Kegel exercises for strengthening the pelvic floor.
 (2) Vaginal lubricants to help with dyspareunia secondary to vaginal dryness (e.g., Replens, K-Y Jelly, Zestra, or Gyne-Moistrin cream).

 c. Patient education materials can be obtained through the American College of Obstetricians and Gynecologists, 409 12th Street SW, Washington, DC 20024; and Menopause News, 2074 Union Street, San Francisco, CA 94123; phone: 1-800-241-MENO. Patient educational brochures are produced by many pharmaceutical companies.

SUGGESTED READINGS

Fitzpatrick LA, Santen RJ: Hot flashes: The old and the new, what is really true? *Mayo Clin Proc* 77:1155-1158, 2002.

Gambrell RD: The Women's Health Initiative reports: Critical review of the findings. *The Female Patient* 29(11):23-30, 2004. PDF available at http://www.femalepatient.com/html/arc/sel/gamb/029110023.pdf (accessed January 14, 2007).

Loprinzi CL, Barton DL, Carpenter LA, et al: Pilot evaluation of paroxetine for treating hot flashes in men, *Mayo Clin Proc* 79:1247-1251, 2004.

Loprinzi CL, Barton DL, Sloan JA, et al: Pilot evaluation of gabapentin for treating hot flashes. *Mayo Clin Proc* 77:1159-1163, 2002.

Nelson HD, Humphrey LL, Hygren P, et al: Postmenopausal hormone replacement therapy. *JAMA* 288:872-881, 2002.

Nelson HD, Vesco KK, Haney E, et al: Nonhormonal therapies for menopausal hot flashes: Systematic review and meta-analysis. *JAMA* 295:2057-2071, 2006.

Rossouw JE, Anderson GL, Prentice RL, et al: Writing Group for the Women's Health Initiative Investigators: Risks and benefits of estrogen plus progestin in healthy postmenopausal women: Principal results from the Women's Health Initiative randomized controlled trial. *JAMA* 288:321-333, 2002.

Santoro N: The menopause transition: An update. *Hum Reprod Update* 8:155-160, 2002.

Shanafelt TD, Barton DL, Adjei AA, Loprinzi CL: Pathophysiology and treatment of hot flashes. *Mayo Clin Proc* 77:1207-1218, 2002.

Sikon A, Thacker HL: Treatment options for menopausal hot flashes. *Cleveland Clinic J Med* 71:578-582, 2004.

Warren MP: Historical perspectives in postmenopausal hormone therapy: Defining the right dose and duration. *Mayo Clin Proc* 82:219-226, 2007.

3.4 Exercise and Aging

Marsha D. Fretwell and Deborah Adams Wingate

BACKGROUND

1. Aging, disease, and disuse.
   a. Some of the physical and mental decline and loss of functional reserve blamed on aging alone can be more accurately attributed to a complex interaction among genetic aging, disease, and disuse.
   b. Older women with chronically elevated inflammatory markers such as C-reactive protein have a higher risk of developing muscle weakness and physical disability.
   c. Disuse exacerbates the decline in endurance, strength, and flexibility related to the true changes of aging and/or disease.
   d. Societal norms about aging reduce expectations of both mental and physical performance and promote inactivity and disuse.
2. Epidemiology.
   a. Three fourths of older adults do not currently exercise at recommended levels.
   b. Fifty percent of persons older than 60 years describe themselves as sedentary.
   c. Twenty percent reductions in endurance (aerobic) exercise capacity, 50% reductions in muscle strength, and 23% reductions in lean body or muscle mass are routinely noted in cross-sectional and longitudinal studies including persons between the ages of 20 and 90 years.
   d. Approximately 50% of persons older than 60 years have signs of osteoarthritis on knee films and 20% of older adults are using a prescription NSAID, suggesting that joint pain and stiffness are significant problems.
   e. Persons age 70 years or older (average age, 83 years) can improve muscle strength, balance, perceived health status, overall physical function, and oxygen consumption following a 9-month multidimensional high-intensity exercise program.
3. Health benefits of physical activity for older adults are listed in Box 3-4.

BOX 3-4 Health Benefits of Physical Activity for Older Adults

Cardiovascular Health

Improves myocardial performance
Increases peak diastolic filling
Increases heart muscle contractility
Reduces premature ventricular contractions
Improves blood lipid profiles
Increases aerobic capacity
Reduces systolic blood pressure
Improves diastolic blood pressure
Improves endurance
Improves muscle capillary blood flow

Body Composition

Decreases abdominal adipose tissue
Increases muscle mass

Metabolism

Increases total energy expenditure
Improves protein synthesis rate and amino acid uptake into skeletal muscle
Reduces low-density lipoproteins
Reduces very low-density lipoproteins
Reduces triglycerides
Increases high-density lipoproteins
Increases glucose tolerance

Bone Health

Slows decline in bone mineral density
Increases total body calcium and nitrogen

Psychological Well-being

Improves perceived well-being and happiness
Decreases levels of stress-related hormones
Improves attention span
Improves cognitive processing speed
Increases slow-wave and rapid-eye-movement (REM) sleep
Provides sense of accomplishment
Decreases anxiety and improves overall mood

Muscle Weakness

Reduces risk of musculoskeletal disability
Improves functional capacity
Improves strength and flexibility
Reduces risk of falls
Improves dynamic balance
Improves physical functional performance

Falls and Fear of Falling

Decreases falls and fear of falling

Adapted from Resnick B: Across the aging continuum: Motivating older adults to exercise. *Adv Nurse Pract* 13(9):37-40, 2005.

DELIBERATE EXERCISE PRESCRIPTIONS

1. Definition: A deliberate exercise prescription is a planned exercise program designed to:
   a. Improve endurance, aerobic exercise capacity, muscle strength, joint flexibility, and overall functional ability.
   b. Reduce cardiovascular risk factors such as excess weight, dyslipidemia, hypertension, and elevated pulse rate.
2. Target patients who have:
   a. Increased cardiovascular risk factors.
   b. The metabolic syndrome.
   c. Arthritis or decrease in joint range of motion.
   d. History of falls.
   e. Loss of muscle mass, strength, and endurance.
   f. Gait disorders.
   g. Decreased aerobic capacity.
   h. Osteoporosis.
   i. Depression.
3. Deliberate exercise as a treatment plan.
   a. Any increase in activity level is better than no exercise at all.
   b. Each prescription should address:
      (1) Muscular strength.
      (2) Muscular endurance.
      (3) Cardiorespiratory endurance.
      (4) Flexibility and coordination.
      (5) Prevention of relapse.
   c. The starting point for deliberate exercise is an activity that is both tolerated well and enjoyed by the older adult. Most people quit exercise within the first 6 weeks because it is too intense. Walking is an appropriate start-up activity.
   d. Consider the following factors to determine the appropriate level of intensity:
      (1) Is the patient on medications that influence heart rate?
      (2) Is the patient at risk for cardiovascular or orthopedic injury?
      (3) What is the patient's current level of fitness?
      (4) What is the patient's recent exercise experience?
      (5) What are the patient's preferences for exercise modality?
      (6) What are the targeted goals or objectives of the patient and physician?
   e. After the patient has demonstrated an understanding of the activity and a tolerance for regular activity, other components can be slowly added but never to the point where past consistency or gains are compromised. This is to be a lifetime program; do not do too much too soon.
   f. Relapse prevention.
      (1) Regular follow-up and modification are critical to the long-term success of any exercise program.
      (2) The physician should understand and emphasize the specific benefits to the patient.
      (3) The physician should outline clearly the commitment required of the patient.
      (4) The physician should provide both group and individual support.

PRESCRIPTION PRINCIPLES AND SUGGESTIONS
Principles

Every exercise program should include a warm-up period, an activity phase, and a cool-down period.

1. Warm-up period:.
   a. Warm up is usually 5 to 10 minutes.
   b. The warm-up period can consist of gentle stretching, light calisthenics, or an activity done at low intensity (e.g., walking or stationary bicycling at less than target heart rate).
   c. This is an important transition phase that allows the musculoskeletal and cardiorespiratory systems to prepare for physical activity.
2. Activity phase: This is the cardiorespiratory or aerobic part of the workout. The basic recommendations for a cardiorespiratory program are easily recalled by the mnemonic FITT (frequency, intensity, type, time) (Box 3-5).
   a. Frequency.
      (1) At least 3 days/week.
      (2) Encourage the patient to make this a habit, similar to brushing teeth.
      (3) Choose a time of day that is convenient.
      (4) Schedule exercise as any appointment.
      (5) When weight reduction is a major goal, daily exercise can be extremely helpful.
   b. Intensity.
      (1) The intensity depends on the patient's age and the presence or absence of cardiovascular disease or risk factors.
      (2) Light to moderate intensity (<70% of maximum heart rate for age).
      (3) Vigorous intensity (>70% of maximum heart rate for age).
      (4) Moderate intensity allows the participant to comfortably carry on a conversation.
   c. Type (mode) of physical activity.
      (1) Aerobic activity is a sustained, rhythmic activity using large muscle groups.
      (2) Ask the patient to choose an activity that is enjoyable. This increases success in making this lifestyle change.
      (3) Suggest several different types of exercise to increase enjoyment and improve compliance.

BOX 3-5   Basic Cardiorespiratory Program: FITT

Frequency
Intensity
Type
Time

(4) Discourage the patient from beginning an unrealistic activity—one that is too strenuous or incompatible with lifestyle.

d. Time (duration) of physical activity.
   (1) The goal of 20 to 60 minutes per session is recommended.
   (2) For weight reduction, recommend low-intensity exercise for a longer duration, at least 30 minutes.
   (3) A sedentary patient might need to start slowly with 5- to 10-minute sessions.
   (4) Some patients may prefer (or better tolerate) two or three brief sessions per day rather than a single session. This builds self-confidence and compliance.

3. Cool-down period.
   a. Cool down is usually 5 to 10 minutes.
   b. As with the warm-up period, a low-intensity activity, such as walking or stretching, should be performed.
   c. This period is important to prevent hypotension that can occur at the sudden cessation of exercise.

Prescriptions

1. Healthy older adults.
   a. For aerobic exercise capacity.
      (1) Overload gradually by increasing duration of the exercise until the patient can complete 20 minutes of continuous cardiorespiratory activity.
      (2) At this point, add to intensity.
   b. For muscular strength.
      (1) Begin with a resistance that allows completion of 8 to 10 repetitions with moderate exertion for one set only, using all the major muscle groups. Do this at least two times per week with at least 48 hours of rest between sessions.
      (2) Add one set after 3 or 4 weeks as opposed to adding weight. After completion of 10 repetitions on the second set, the patient may add 5% weight to increase intensity every 3 weeks.
   c. For muscular endurance.
      (1) Use the same progression principles but with half the resistance that is used for muscular strength.
      (2) Sets should include 15 repetitions and can add one session per week to the muscle-strengthening program.
   d. For resistance training (to preserve bone mass).
      (1) Form in resistance training means moving the weight both in the concentric and eccentric contraction in a slow, controlled manner without using jerking or momentum.
      (2) In general, it is safer to use weight machines than free weights.
      (3) Proper form for resistance training allows normal breathing (no breath-holding allowed).
   e. For flexibility.
      (1) Optimal functional ability requires an adequate range of motion in all joints.
      (2) Flexibility in lower back, hamstring, and shoulder regions is critical.

    (3) All exercise programs should emphasize proper stretching in the upper and lower trunk, neck, and hip regions.

    (4) Static stretching is done by slowly stretching the muscle to a point of mild discomfort, taking and releasing a deep breath, and holding the stretch for a period of time (begin with 10 seconds and gradually build up to 30 seconds).

    (5) This progression will slowly increase the range of motion over several weeks.

    (6) For the very frail and deconditioned older adult, static stretching might be an appropriate start to an exercise program and be all the intensity that can be tolerated.

2. Cardiac patients.

   a. After a cardiac event, patients should exercise in an established cardiac rehabilitation program under a physician's supervision for phases 1 and 2.

   b. Phase 3 exercise should remain under the physician's supervision, but the physician can use ACCN* and ACSM's *Guidelines for Exercise Testing and Prescription* for individualized exercise prescriptions.

   c. The patient should not begin resistance training until 4 to 6 weeks of supervised cardiorespiratory endurance exercise have been completed.

3. Pulmonary patients.

   a. Choose exercise intensity by one of the following methods:

    (1) Exercise at 50% VO_2peak.

    (2) Exercise at near maximal intensity (drastically limits the duration of the exercise time).

    (3) Exercise at an intensity that is above the anaerobic threshold.

    (4) Use dyspnea ratings to set intensity. Moderate-intensity exercise corresponds to a 3 dyspnea rating (50% VO_2peak); vigorous intensity corresponds to a 6 dyspnea rating (85% VO_2peak).

   b. Frequent short exercise sessions may be needed in the initial stages of the exercise program.

   c. The goal remains to work up to 20 to 30 minutes of continuous cardiorespiratory activity.

   d. The patient should maintain SaO_2 >88%.

4. Diabetic patients.

   a. This disease responds best to a program of a minimum of 5 d/wk, with an endurance component on each day.

   b. Blood glucose should be monitored before and after exercise.

   c. Intensity should be very low at the beginning and build up gradually. This allows patients to adjust their diet to the exercise program and glucose stabilization.

   d. Begin the program with several short exercise times and work up to 20 to 30 minutes of continuous activity. The last 15 minutes of continuous activity are the most beneficial in improving glucose tolerance.

5. Obese patients.

   a. Choose an activity that maximizes caloric expenditure (<70% VO_2peak), minimizes stress on joints, and monitors orthopedic concerns.

*American College of Cardiac Nurses

b. At first, set daily caloric expenditure for exercise at 200 to 300 kcal.

c. Cross-training with some non–weight-bearing activities should be included.

d. Posture and body mechanics should be emphasized. Proper attention to engaging the lower abdominal and gluteal muscles to stabilize the lower back are critical to safer functional activity and activities of daily living.

ROLE OF THE PHYSICIAN

1. The physician plays a critical role in the success of any exercise program.

2. The patient must truly believe that the physician's philosophy toward good health includes exercise as a major component equal to all other factors that determine good health.

3. The physician must serve as an example, a role model, if the treatment plan is to achieve maximum outcomes.

4. A positive attitude is critical to the success of the program.

SUGGESTED READINGS

American College of Sports Medicine: *Resource Manual for Guidelines for Exercise Testing and Prescription*, ed 4. Philadelphia, Lea & Febiger, 1991.

American College of Sports Medicine: *Guidelines for Exercise Testing and Prescription*, ed 6. Philadelphia, Williams & Wilkins, 2000.

Binder E, Schechtman K, Ehsani A, et al: Effects of exercise training on frailty in community-dwelling older adults: Results of a randomized, controlled trial. *J Am Geriatr Soc* 50:1921-1928, 2002.

Bruunsgaard H, Bjerregaard E, Schroll M, Pedersen B: Muscle strength after resistance training is inversely correlated with baseline levels of soluble tumor necrosis factor receptors in the oldest old. *J Am Geriatr Soc* 52:237-241, 2004.

Colbert L, Visser M, Simonsick E, et al: Physical activity, exercise, and inflammatory markers in older adults: Findings from the Health, Aging, and Body Composition Study. *J Am Geriatr Soc* 52:1098-1104, 2004.

Ferrucci L, Penninx B, Volpato S, et al: Change in muscle strength explains accelerated decline of physical function in older women with high interleukin-6 serum levels. *J Am Geriatr Soc* 50:1947-1954, 2002.

Fiatarone MA, et al: Exercise training and nutritional supplementation for physical frailty in very elderly people. *N Engl J Med* 330:1769, 1994.

Heath J, Stuart M: Prescribing exercise for frail elders. *J Am Board Fam Pract* 15(3):218-228, 2002.

Neid R, Franklin B: Promoting and prescribing exercise for the elderly. *Am Fam Physician* 65(3): 419-426, 2002.

Penninx B, Kritchevsky S, Newman A, et al: Inflammatory markers and incident mobility limitation in the elderly. *J Am Geriatr Soc* 52:1105-1113, 2004.

Resnick B: Across the aging continuum: Motivating older adults to exercise. *Adv Nurse Pract* 13(9):37-40, 2005.

Schwartz RS, Kohrt WM: Exercise in the elderly: Physiologic and functional effects. In Hazzard WR, Glass JP, Halter JB, et al (eds): *Principles of Geriatric Medicine and Gerontology*, ed 5. New York, McGraw-Hill, 2003, 931-946.

Selected Functional Syndromes

4

4.1 Nutrition

Marsha D. Fretwell and Deborah Adams Wingate

OBESITY

1. Definition: *Obesity* refers to an excess of body fat.
   a. Clinically useful measures of obesity include:
      (1) A body weight more than 30% above the age-, height-, and sex-specific population average.
      (2) Body mass index (BMI).
         (a) A person with a BMI 25 to 29.9 kg/m^2 is considered overweight.
         (b) A person with a BMI 30 or greater is considered obese.
      (3) A waist-to-hip ratio of >1.0 for male patients and >0.85 for female patients.
   b. The two major types of obesity are central (or abdominal) and peripheral (or lower body).
2. Epidemiology: The prevalence of obesity is greater among persons aged 65 to 74 years than among people age 75 and older.
   a. Thirty-two percent of men 65 to 74 years are obese, compared with 18% of men 75 years and older.
   b. Thirty-nine percent of women 65 to 74 years are obese, compared with 24% of women aged 75 and over.
3. Significance
   a. Central or abdominal obesity is highly correlated with increased morbidity and mortality. Based on scientific evidence, persons with obesity are at risk for developing one or more serious medical conditions, which include:
      (1) Hyperinsulinemia.
      (2) Non–insulin-dependent diabetes mellitus.
      (3) Hypertension.
      (4) Cardiovascular disease.
      (5) Hypercholesterolemia.
      (6) Hypertriglyceridemia.
      (7) Reduced high-density lipoprotein (HDL) cholesterol levels.
      (8) Sleep apnea.
   b. All obesity is associated with increased morbidity from:
      (1) Cholelithiasis.
      (2) Endometrial, colon, and postmenopausal breast cancer.

      (3) Osteoarthritis, especially of the knee, including the hand, hip, and back.

      (4) Asthma and other respiratory disease.

4. Diagnosis

  a. Measurement of height and weight to calculate BMI:

$$BMI = \frac{\text{weight in pounds} \times 703}{\text{height in inches}}$$

$$BMI = \frac{\text{weight in kilograms}}{\text{height in meters}^2}$$

  b. Measurement of waist and hip to calculate waist-to-hip ratio (WHR):

$$WHR = \frac{\text{waist measurement}}{\text{hip measurement}}$$

      (1) Waist is measured at the narrowest point between the rib cage and iliac crests.

      (2) Hip is measured at the maximal point for the buttocks.

5. Causes: The cause of obesity is not fully understood.

  a. Overweight and obesity result from an imbalance involving excessive calorie consumption and/or inadequate physical activity.

  b. Body weight is the result of a combination of genetic, metabolic, behavioral, environmental, cultural, and socioeconomic influences.

6. Treatment. To date, obesity has resisted our best therapeutic efforts. In theory the treatment is simple: increase physical activity and reduce caloric intake. In reality, although many achieve short-term weight loss, over the years the results are dismal.

  a. Approaches include:

      (1) Diet.

      (2) Behavioral therapy.

      (3) Exercise.

      (4) Medications.

      (5) Surgery.

  b. It has been suggested that obesity should be treated like hypertension or diabetes, as a chronic physiologically based disorder that requires ongoing medication therapy to reduce the excessive morbidity and mortality associated with the disorder. Bupropion and fluoxetine are medications for weight loss that also appear safe for use in older adults.

  c. Weight loss is most successful when there is interdisciplinary support by physicians, psychologists, nutritionists, and exercise physiologists.

ANOREXIA

Forty-three percent of independent elderly persons consume less than 1500 calories per day and 16% to 18% consume less than 1000 calories.

1. Definition.
   a. Physiologic decreases in the older person's food intake are referred to as *anorexia*.
   b. Anorexia leads to protein malnutrition and weight loss, both of which are risk factors for increased morbidity and mortality.
2. Physiologic changes of aging that predispose to anorexia.
   a. Decrease in opioid feeding drive.
   b. Increase in concentration of satiety hormone cholecystokinin.
   c. Reduction in nitric oxide can lead to gastric retention and early satiety.
   d. Decreased testosterone leads to increased leptin. Activin, a testicular hormone, is increased in men. These changes lead to a greater decrease in food intake in men.
   e. Increased leptin hormone decreases the desire for food and increases energy metabolism.
   f. Elevated cytokines, associated with infections and inflammation, decrease food intake.
   g. Other factors include poor dentition, dysphagia, decreased saliva production, constipation, decreased sense of smell, and decreased sense of taste.
      (1) Some drugs have a significant effect on taste (Box 4-1).
      (2) Depression is the most commonly diagnosed cause of pathologic weight loss in older persons.
3. Diagnosis: Anorexia is multifactorial. The comprehensive geriatric assessment process described in Chapter 2 is useful in guiding the identification of causes of anorexia.
4. Treatment.
   a. Nonpharmacologic interventions.
      (1) Social dining experiences.
      (2) Palatability and presentation of meals.
      (3) Time of day that meals are served.
      (4) Dietary supplements.
      (5) Enhanced foods.
   b. Pharmacologic interventions.
      (1) Antidepressants.
         (a) Mirtazapine is a noradrenergic and specific serotoninergic antidepressant with H_1 receptor antagonism and $5\text{-}HT_2$ and $5\text{-}HT_3$ receptor antagonism, which may explain some aspects of sedation (antihistamine) and weight gain.
         (b) The dose is 7.5 to 15 mg hs to optimize the usefulness of this medication.
      (2) Cannabinoids.
         (a) Dronabinol was found in small studies to increase body weight and reduce disruptive behavior.
         (b) Dose 2.5 mg bid before lunch and supper. May titrate to a maximum of 10 mg/day.

BOX 4-1   Drugs with Potentially Anorexiant Effects in the Elderly

Amlodipine (Norvasc)
Aspirin
Cholestyramine (Questran)
Ciprofloxacin (Cipro)
Conjugated equine estrogens
   (Premarin)
Digoxin (Lanoxin)
Enalapril (Vasotec)
Famotidine (Pepcid)
Fentanyl transdermal
   (Duragesic)
Fluoxetine (Prozac)
Furosemide (Lasix)
Hydralazine (Apresoline)
Levothyroxine sodium
   (Synthroid)
Nifedipine (Procardia)

Nizatidine (Axid)
Omeprazole (Prilosec)
Paroxetine (Paxil)
Phenytoin (Dilantin)
Potassium replacement
   (K-Dur)
Propoxyphene plus
   acetaminophen
   (Darvocet, Propacet)
Quinidine (Quinagulate
   Duratabs)
Ranitidine (Zantac)
Risperidone (Risperdal)
Sertraline (Zoloft)
Theophylline
Vitamin A
Warfarin (Coumadin)

Data from Endoy, MP: Anorexia among older adults. *Am J Nurse Pract* 9(5):31-37, 2005.

   (3) Progestogens.
      (a) Studies of megestrol acetate in older persons are sparse.
      (b) Megestrol acetate should be used cautiously in non–weight bearing persons at risk for venous thromboembolism.
      (c) Mechanism of action may be related to reduction of inflammatory cytokines.
      (d) The dose is 800 mg/day.

PROTEIN-CALORIE MALNUTRITION

1. Definition.
   a. A serum albumin level less than 3.5 g/dL reflects visceral protein depletion.
   b. A serum prealbumin level less than 15.0 mg/dL is the preferred marker for malnutrition.
2. Epidemiology: Twenty to sixty percent of older patients in hospitals and nursing homes suffer from inadequate nutrition and/or protein-calorie malnutrition.
3. Significance in medical care of older patients.
   a. The prealbumin level is the earliest laboratory indicator of nutritional status and correlates with patient outcomes in a wide variety of clinical conditions.
   b. Adequate protein nutrition is critical for maintenance of skin integrity, healing of surgical wounds, and effective functioning of the immune system for host defense against infections.

    c. The stress of acute illness and inflammation and the use of glucose as the primary source of nutrition during the early stages of hospital care accelerate nitrogen wasting and protein malnutrition.

    d. Nourishing patients is perceived by caretakers as a central feature of excellent care; malnourishment during the process of care may be seen as a failure of caretaking.

4. Diagnosis.

    a. History of weight loss.

    b. Measurement of height and weight.

    c. Serum albumin level (<3.5 g/dL equals visceral protein depletion).

    d. Serum prealbumin level (<15.0 mg/dL is preferred marker for malnutrition).

5. Treatable causes: Remember, older patients are likely to have multiple causes.

    a. Functional limitations such as tremors and physical limitations.

    b. Depression, delirium, and failure-to-thrive syndromes.

    c. Drugs (e.g., digoxin, fluoxetine, hydralazine, psychoactives); see Box 4-1.

      (1) Drugs causing malabsorption (e.g., sorbitol in theophylline, cholestyramine).

      (2) Withdrawal from drugs (e.g., alcohol, anxiolytics, psychoactives).

    d. Chronic obstructive pulmonary disease (COPD), congestive heart failure (CHF).

    e. Intestinal ischemia.

    f. Metabolic causes (hyperthyroidism).

    g. Zinc deficiency (secondary to diuretics).

    h. Malabsorption syndromes (celiac disease, pancreatic insufficiency).

    i. Chronic impaction.

    j. Social factors (isolation, poverty, manipulation of caretaker to regain locus of control).

6. Treatment: All etiologic factors must be treated. Diet consultation is useful to confirm diagnosis, plan appropriate diet supplementation, and educate the patient and family.

    a. Remove all offending drugs (see Chapter 7).

    b. Remove impaction.

    c. Supplement intake of protein, vitamins, trace elements, fats, and carbohydrates.

    d. Use adaptive utensils.

    e. Treat depression, delirium, and failure-to-thrive syndrome (see later).

    f. Maintain optimal pulmonary and cardiac function.

    g. Treat intestinal ischemia with nitrates or calcium channel blockers.

    h. Treat metabolic or malabsorption syndromes.

    i. Obtain social services consultation.

WEIGHT LOSS

1. Unintentional weight loss.

    a. Encountered in 8% of all adult outpatients.

    b. Occurs in 27% of frail people 65 years and older.

    c. Associated with increased mortality from 9% to as high as 38% within 1 to 2.5 years after the weight loss has occurred.

    d. Can reflect disease severity or undiagnosed illness.

    e. Weight loss of 4% to 5% or more of body weight within 1 year or 10% or more over 5 to 10 years is associated with increased mortality, morbidity, or both.

2. Unintentional weight loss in ambulatory patients: A review of unexplained weight loss in older ambulatory patients found these final diagnoses:

    a. Cancer (lung, colon, breast, pancreas, prostate): 16% to 36%.

    b. Psychiatric disorder (especially depression): 9% to 42%.

    c. Gastrointestinal (GI) disorder other than cancer (occult ulcers, achalasia, hepatitis): 6% to 19%.

    d. Endocrine (hyperthyroidism): 4% to 11%.

    e. Cardiovascular disease: 2% to 9%.

    f. Nutritional disorders: 4% to 8%.

    g. Chronic infection: 2% to 5%.

    h. Medications (e.g., procainamide, theophylline, thyroxine, nitrofurantoin): ~2%.

    i. Other (tuberculosis, poor intake, cholesterol phobia): 6%.

    j. Unknown etiology: 10% to 36%.

3. No obvious cause of weight loss.

    a. A very gradual loss of weight is often noted over the last 6 months of life in persons who have no observable medical illnesses.

    b. A number of age-associated changes might lead to a reduced caloric intake and weight loss in persons older than 85 years. These include:

       (1) Decreased demand (lower metabolic rate and reduced physical activity).

       (2) Decreased sensory input (taste, smell, vision).

       (3) Decreased feeding drive (neurotransmitters).

       (4) Increased activity of satiety factors (cholecystokinin).

REFUSAL OF FOOD AND THE PLACEMENT OF FEEDING TUBES

1. The lowest level of function measured on Katz's Activities of Daily Living is the ability to feed oneself. Persons who are unable to feed themselves because of cognitive or physical disabilities are usually hand-fed by caretakers.

2. When an older person refuses to be fed, one additional cause should be considered: preparation for death.

3. There is no evidence that percutaneous endoscopic gastrostomy prolongs survival in patients with dementia.

4. Evaluation of the patient should include:

    a. Comprehensive geriatric assessment to provide physician, patient, and family with complete and accurate prognostic information.

    b. Careful focus on the treatable causes of weight loss and protein malnutrition, especially depression and impaction.

   c. Respect for the patient's preferences about tube feedings, both current and historic (see Chapter 10 for discussion of competency and proxy decision making).

   d. Continued support and care (including offerings of food) for those who refuse hand or tube feedings.

DEHYDRATION

With aging, there is slow, chronic dehydration.

1. Risk factors.
   a. Age-associated changes such as decreased thirst perception, abnormal vasopressin responses to osmotic stimuli, and decreased ability of renal tubules to reabsorb water.
   b. Fear of urinary incontinence.
   c. Fear of dysphagia and aspiration.
   d. Administration of diuretics.
   e. Physiologic changes leading to anorexia.
   f. Decreased water access as a result of immobility, poor visual acuity, and altered mental status.
   g. Acute medical illnesses with increased insensible losses from fever, diaphoresis, tachypnea, emesis, or diarrhea.

2. Assessment.
   a. Weight loss, orthostatic blood pressure, skin turgor, fever.
   b. Electrolytes, blood urea nitrogen (BUN), glucose, urinalysis (specific gravity).
   c. Charting of intake and output, including insensible loss.

3. Treatment.
   a. Address underlying acute and chronic illness (e.g., infections).
   b. Calculate free water deficit (FWD):

$$FWD = \text{Weight (kg)} \times 0.45 - (140/\text{serum Na}) \times \text{Weight (kg)} \times 0.45$$

   c. Replace FWD at a rate of 25%/day.

   d. Monitor for signs of fluid overload.

   e. Monitor electrolytes and BUN.

   f. Address chronic risk factors (e.g., diuretics, fear of incontinence, immobility, confusion, dysphagia).

SUGGESTED READINGS

Alibhai SM, Greenwood C, Payette H: An approach to the management of unintentional weight loss in elderly people. *CMAJ* 172(6):773-780, 2005.

Aoyama L, Weintraub N, Reuben DB: Is weight loss in the nursing home a reversible problem? *J Am Med Dir Assoc* 7(3 suppl):S66-S72, 65, 2005.

Center for the Advancement of Health: Weighing the data: Obesity affects elderly, too. *Facts of Life: Issue Briefings for Health Reporters* 9(12):1,2004.

Endoy MP: Anorexia among older adults. *Am J Nurse Pract* 9(5):31-38, 2005.

Huffman GB: Evaluating and treating unintentional weight loss in the elderly. *Am Fam Physician* 65(4):640-650, 2002.

Lewko M, Chamseddin A, Zaky M, Birrer RB: Weight loss in the elderly: What's normal and what's not. P+T Community. http://www.ptcommunity.com/ptjournal/index.cfm?page=guidelines.

Li Z, Maglione M, Tu W, et al: Meta-Analysis: Pharmacologic treatment of obesity. *Ann Int Med* 142(7):532-546, 2005.

Murphy LM, Lipman TO: Percutaneous endoscopic gastrostomy does not prolong survival in patients with dementia. *Arch Intern Med* 163:1351-1353, 2003.

4.2 Urinary Incontinence

Marsha D. Fretwell and Deborah Adams Wingate

OVERVIEW

1. Epidemiology.
   a. Prevalence.
      (1) The prevalence of urinary incontinence increases with age. It is 11% in men and 17% in women older than 65 years and increases to more than 20% after age 80 years.
      (2) The prevalence also varies with the location of the patient. It is 15% to 30% in elderly living in the community, 33% in acute-care hospitals, and 50% to 84% in the institutionalized elderly.
   b. Costs.
      (1) The economic cost of incontinence exceeds $12 billion to $15 billion annually.
      (2) The direct cost of caring for incontinence in nursing facility patients is $5.2 billion.
      (3) The average cost for supplies and laundry alone exceeds $1000/year for each incontinent person living in the community.
      (4) The cost in social terms is even more impressive: social isolation, interference with domestic life and activities of daily living (ADLs), scorn and derision by society in general, institutionalization of the patient.
   c. Physicians in general have a low awareness of incontinence. Less than one third of community physicians document incontinence on patient problem lists. A study revealed that 24% of incontinent patients believed that the physician or nurse with whom they had discussed their problem was either embarrassed or unsympathetic, and nearly 40% of patients assumed that their urinary incontinence was a result of their age.
2. Physiology of micturition. Understanding incontinence requires knowledge of the fundamentals of the complex physiology of micturition. Figure 4-1 illustrates the three major components involved in urine storage and release.
   a. Central nervous system (CNS).
      (1) Inhibition from the cortical (frontal lobe) micturition center permits bladder relaxation and filling and sphincter closure to prevent leakage of urine.
      (2) When cortical inhibition ceases (e.g., the patient wants to urinate), the brainstem (pontine) micturition center sends impulses down the spinal cord to the detrusor muscle, resulting in muscle contraction.
   b. Bladder.
      (1) Increase in bladder volume stimulates proprioception receptors in the bladder wall and results in transmission of sensory impulses through the sacral nerves (S2-S4 roots) to trigger bladder contraction.
      (2) This stimulus for bladder contraction is under inhibitory control by the central inhibitory center.

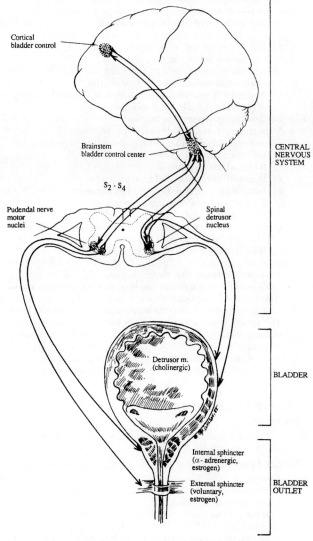

Figure 4-1 Simplified diagram of neurologic bladder control. (Redrawn from Lavizzo-Mourey R, Day SC, Diserens D, Grisso JA (eds): *Practicing prevention for the elderly*. Philadelphia, Hanley & Belfus, 1989.)

(3) Cholinergic stimulation (e.g., bethanechol, urecholine) results in bladder contraction.
  c. Bladder outlet: The two major factors in maintaining urethral pressure are the internal and external urethral sphincters.
    (1) Internal sphincter: α-Adrenergic stimulation causes muscle contraction, preventing flow of urine.
    (2) External sphincter consists of striated muscle under voluntary control. Contraction prevents flow of urine.
    (3) Estrogen deficiency in women can result in decreased competence of the internal and external sphincters.
3. Age-related changes in urologic function.
  a. Normal aging does not cause urinary incontinence.
  b. The following changes can, however, contribute to incontinence:
    (1) Decreased bladder capacity.
    (2) Increased residual urine.
    (3) Increased uninhibited bladder contractions.
    (4) Increased nocturnal sodium and fluid excretion.
    (5) Decreased urethral resistance in women, associated with decrease in estrogen.
    (6) Increased urethral resistance in men, associated with enlargement of the prostate gland.
    (7) Weakness of pelvic floor muscles in women.
4. Types of incontinence
  a. Stress incontinence: The patient is aware but involuntarily loses small amounts of urine with increases in intraabdominal pressure (e.g., laughing, coughing, sneezing, exercising).
  b. Urge incontinence: This is the most common type of incontinence. The patient is aware but leaks large volumes of urine because of inability to delay voiding after the sensation of bladder fullness is perceived.
  c. Overflow incontinence: The patient is not aware of small volumes of urine being continually leaked as a result of the mechanical forces on an overextended bladder.

EVALUATION AND TREATMENT
Mnemonics
Mnemonics and acronyms to evaluate the most common causes of acute, reversible incontinence are given in Box 4-2.

Clinical Evaluation
1. History.
  a. Type (stress, urge, overflow, or mixed).
  b. Timing (new onset, persistent).
  c. Flow pattern (large infrequent flow, small intermittent flow, time of day or night).
  d. Associated symptoms (straining to void, dripping, dysuria, incomplete emptying).
  e. Pertinent associated diagnoses (cancer, diabetes, acute illness, neurologic disease, lower urinary tract surgery).
  f. Medications, including over-the-counter (OTC) drugs.

BOX 4-2   Mnemonics for Evaluating Incontinence

These acronyms can be used to evaluate the most common causes of acute, reversible incontinence.

DIAPPERS

Delirium and dementia
Infections
Atrophic vaginitis, atrophic urethritis, atonic bladder
Psychological causes (e.g., depression), prostatism
Pharmacologic agents
Endocrine abnormalities (diabetes, hypercalcemia, hypothyroidism)
Restricted mobility (severe degenerative joint disease, restraints, postural hypotension)
Stool impaction (causes up to 10% of incontinence in nursing homes)

DRIP

Delirium
Restricted mobility, retention
Infection, inflammation
Polyuria, pharmaceuticals

2. Physical examination.
   a. Abdominal assessment.
      (1) Masses.
      (2) Bladder distention.
   b. Stress test for urine leakage with full bladder.
   c. Palpation for bladder distention after voiding.
   d. Pelvic exam.
      (1) Atrophic vaginitis or urethritis.
      (2) Prolapse or pelvic mass.
   e. Rectal exam.
      (1) Resting tone and voluntary control of anal sphincter.
      (2) Prostate nodules.
      (3) Fecal impaction.
   f. Neurologic exam.
      (1) Cognitive function.
      (2) Sacral reflexes.
      (3) Perineal sensation.
3. Laboratory investigation.
   a. Electrolytes, calcium, glucose, BUN.
   b. Urine analysis and culture.
   c. Chart of incontinence pattern.
   d. Postvoid measurement of residual volume.
4. Figure 4-2 illustrates the suggested diagnostic flow diagram.

New Onset of Transient Urinary Incontinence

1. Causes: Many older patients are best described as "compensated incontinent," and any disruption of their carefully maintained compensation

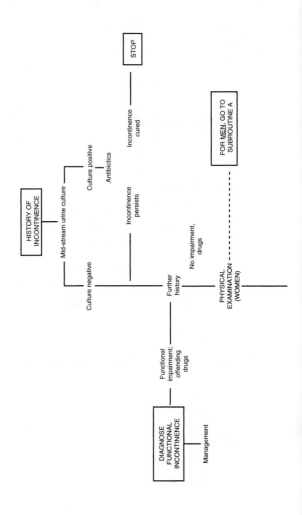

Figure 4-2 Flow diagram for evaluating urinary incontinence. PVR, postvoid residual. (Redrawn from Lavizzo-Mourey R, Day SC, Diserens D, Grisso JA (eds): *Practicing prevention for the elderly.* Philadelphia, Hanley & Belfus, 1989.)

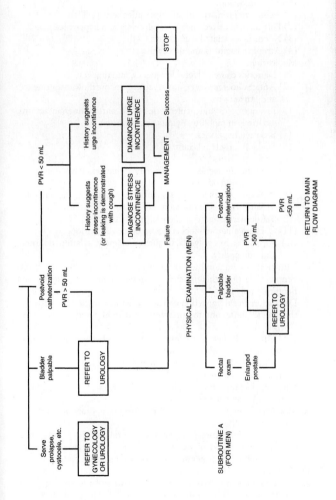

Figure 4-2, cont'd   For legend see opposite page.

strategies (e.g., an acute illness, hospitalization, a change in location, introduction of new medications) can precipitate the acute onset of incontinence.

a. Illness or infection.

(1) Acute symptomatic urinary tract infections (UTIs).

(2) Polyuria associated with hyperglycemia and hypercalcemia.

(3) Nocturia associated with occult CHF.

(4) Atrophic vaginitis and urethritis.

b. Medication.

(1) Diuretics cause polyuria, frequency, and urgency.

(2) Anticholinergics cause urinary retention, overflow incontinence, and impaction.

(3) Psychotropics and neuroleptics cause anticholinergic actions, sedation, immobility, rigidity, and delirium.

(4) Sedative/hypnotics.

(5) Skeletal muscle relaxants.

(6) Sympatholytics.

(7) Narcotic analgesics cause urinary retention, fecal impaction, sedation, and delirium.

(8) α-Adrenergic blockers cause incompetent urethral sphincter.

(9) α-Adrenergic agonists cause urinary retention.

(10) β-Adrenergic agonists cause urinary retention.

(11) Calcium channel blockers cause urinary retention.

(12) Alcohol causes polyuria, frequency, urgency, sedation, delirium, and immobility.

c. Nutrition: In immobilized older hospital patients, 24-hour intravenous (IV) fluid therapy can precipitate urgency, frequency, and nocturnal polyuria.

d. Defecation: Fecal impaction can lead to a mechanical obstruction of the bladder outlet and to urinary retention and overflow.

e. Cognition.

(1) Delirium disrupts the central cortical inhibiting influence over the sacral micturition center.

(2) Delirium leads to a restriction in mobility by physical or chemical restraints (see later).

f. Emotion: Depression and failure-to-thrive syndromes reduce motivation to be continent.

g. Mobility: Immobility of any cause disrupts appropriate toileting behavior.

h. Cooperation with care plan: Lack of information about the nurse call bell or location of the toilet, urinal, or bedpan reduces the patient's ability to cooperate with a continence care plan.

2. Prognosis.

a. The prognosis of new-onset urinary incontinence in the setting of hospitalization for acute illness is very good if appropriate interventions of the causes of transient urinary incontinence are applied. More than 75% of these patients will be cured by this approach.

b. If after discharge and resolution of the acute illness the patient has persistent incontinence, further evaluation and intervention are always indicated.

Persistent Urinary Incontinence

1. Causes.
   a. Neurologic causes: Normal micturition requires coordination of both the central and peripheral nervous systems.
      (1) The cerebral cortex exerts a predominantly inhibitory influence on the sacral spinal cord reflex. Diseases such as dementia, delirium, stroke, and parkinsonism lead to an *urge incontinence without awareness*.
      (2) The brainstem, cerebellum, and suprasacral spinal cord exert a predominantly facilitatory and coordinating influence. Diseases such as stroke and multiple sclerosis lead to an *overflow incontinence without awareness*, referred to as *neurogenic* or *detrusor–sphincter dyssynergy*.
      (3) The sacral spinal cord reflexly controls bladder filling and emptying.
         (a) Local irritations in the bladder and outflow obstructions lead to *urge incontinence with awareness*.
         (b) Injuries to the sacral cord, persistent outlet obstruction, and diabetes mellitus lead to an acontractile bladder and *overflow incontinence without awareness*
   b. Urologic causes: Normal micturition requires that the bladder and lower genitourinary tract appropriately perform their storage and emptying functions.
      (1) Failure to store urine may be caused by:
         (a) A hyperactive or poorly compliant bladder (secondary to cystitis, stones, tumor, or diverticuli) leading to *urge incontinence*.
         (b) Diminished outflow tract resistance (secondary to laxity of pelvic floor muscles, bladder outlet, or sphincter weakness) leading to *stress incontinence*.
      (2) Failure to empty the bladder may be caused by:
         (a) A poorly contractile bladder (secondary to diabetes mellitus) leading to *overflow incontinence*.
         (b) Increased outflow resistance (secondary to anatomic obstruction by prostate, stricture, or cystocele) leading to chronic urinary retention and *overflow incontinence*.
   c. Mixed types of incontinence.
      (1) Often more than one type of incontinence is present simultaneously. The most common example is the development of urge incontinence in a woman with a typical history of stress incontinence.
      (2) In all patients, the goal of the evaluation and treatment is continence; if that is not achieved by treatment of the most obvious cause of incontinence, multiple etiologic factors must be considered.
2. Management.
   a. Complete clinical evaluation.
      (1) General examination if indicated.
         (a) Look for conditions such as edema that can contribute to nocturia and nocturnal urinary incontinence.

      (b) Look for neurologic abnormalities that suggest multiple sclerosis, stroke, spinal cord compression, or other neurologic conditions.

      (c) Assess mobility, cognition, and manual dexterity related to toileting skills.

  (2) Abdominal examination.

      (a) Check for organomegaly, masses, peritonitis, fluid collections, and so on.

      (b) Abnormality of abdominal contents can influence intra-abdominal pressure and detrusor physiology.

  (3) Rectal examination to test for:

      (a) Perineal sensation.

      (b) Sphincter tone (resting and active).

      (c) Fecal impaction or rectal mass.

  (4) Pelvic examination in women.

      (a) Assess perineal skin condition, genital atrophy, pelvic organ prolapse (cystocele, rectocele, uterine prolapse), pelvic mass, paravaginal muscle tone, or other abnormalities.

      (b) Palpation of the anterior vaginal wall and urethra might elicit urethral discharge or tenderness that suggests urethral diverticula or inflammatory condition of the urethra.

      (c) Pelvic organ prolapse might not relate to urinary symptoms, especially in the elderly.

  (5) Direct observation of urine loss using the cough stress test.

      (a) Observation of urine loss can be performed by having the patient cough vigorously while the examiner observes for urine loss from the urethra.

      (b) In women who are being evaluated for specific treatments for stress incontinence, this test is important for objective demonstration of urine loss and identification of provoking factors.

b. Specific treatments.

  (1) For *new-onset incontinence* during acute hospitalization, proceed with assessment and treatment of the causes of transient incontinence as outlined above.

  (2) For a *postvoid residual volume* >100 mL, urologic consultation is recommended. Postvoid residual volume >100 mL is most often seen in older men.

  (3) For a *urinary infection*, sterilize the urine.

  (4) Urologic, gynecologic, or urodynamic consultation is recommended for any of the following:

      (a) Recent history of lower urinary tract or pelvic surgery or irradiation.

      (b) Recurrent symptomatic UTIs.

      (c) Symptomatic pelvic prolapse.

      (d) Marked prostatic enlargement or nodules.

      (e) Severe hesitancy, straining, or interrupted stream.

      (f) Hematuria without infection.

  (5) For *stress incontinence*, one or more of the following treatments should be attempted:

      (a) Pelvic floor or Kegel exercises.

(b) α-Adrenergic agonists (imipramine, pseudoephedrine).

(c) Estrogen (oral or topical).

(d) Biofeedback, behavior training.

(e) Surgical bladder neck suspension.

(f) Diet and fluid modification: Eliminate bladder irritants including caffeine, spicy foods, carbonated drinks, citrus fruit or juices, smoking, and alcohol.

(6) For *urge incontinence*, one or more of the following treatments should be attempted:

(a) Bladder relaxants (Box 4-3).

(b) Estrogen (if vaginal cell atrophy is present).

(c) Biofeedback, behavior therapy including timed or scheduled toileting, bladder retraining, and pelvic floor exercises (Box 4-4).

(d) Surgical removal of bladder irritants or outlet obstruction.

(e) Diet and fluid modification: Eliminate bladder irritants including caffeine, spicy foods, carbonated drinks, citrus fruit or juices, smoking, and alcohol.

(7) For *overflow incontinence:*

(a) Attempt to decompress the bladder with short-term (10 days) indwelling or intermittent catheterization.

(b) Remove the obstruction surgically.

(c) Use an α-adrenergic blocker (prazosin).

(d) Perform intermittent catheterization as maintenance.

(e) Insert an indwelling catheter.

c. Management of the patient who is still incontinent after appropriate treatment.

(1) Consider mixed incontinence of multiple etiologies.

(2) Consider referral to an incontinence specialist (geriatric nurse or physician, urologist, or gynecologist).

(3) Train the caretaker(s).

(4) Use external collection devices and incontinence undergarments and pads.

Indications for Using Foley Catheters

1. Short-term use.

a. Monitoring volume status in acute illness (should not exceed 3 or 4 days).

BOX 4-3   Long-Acting Bladder Relaxants

Intermediate-release tolterodine (Detrol) 2 mg bid
Extended-release tolterodine (Detrol LA) 4 mg daily
Extended-release oxybutynin (Ditropan XL) 5-30 mg daily
Oxybutynin transdermal delivery system (Oxytrol) twice weekly
Solifenacin succinate (VESIcare) 5-10 mg daily
Extended-release darifenacin (Enablex) 7.5-15 mg daily

BOX 4-4   Bladder Training and Kegel Exercises

The following methods are used to strengthen the muscle of your pelvic floor:

Bladder Training

Bladder training involves urinating on a schedule, whether you feel a need to go or not, and waiting in between until the next scheduled time.

Kegel Exercises

1. Contract the pelvic floor muscles for 10 seconds.
2. Relax them for 10 seconds.

Repeat 10 times. Do these exercises three times per day.

---

    b. Bladder decompression in overflow incontinence (10 to 14 days).
    c. Patients with skin breakdown and pressure sores. This patient group has the highest risk of nosocomial UTIs. Every effort should be made to improve nutrition and mobility and remove the catheter.

2. Long-term use.
    a. Care of terminally ill patient.
    b. Management of urinary retention that cannot be managed medically or surgically and is causing renal disease, UTIs, or persistent overflow incontinence.

SUGGESTED READINGS

DuBeau CE, Bent AE, Dmochowski RR, et al: Addressing the unmet needs of geriatric patients with overactive bladder: Challenges and controversies. *Clin Geriatr* 11(12):16-28, 2003.

Holroyd-Leduc JM, Straus SE: Management of urinary incontinence in women: Clinical applications. *JAMA* 291:996-999, 2004.

Jumadilova Z, Zyczynski T, Paul B, Narayanan S: Urinary incontinence in the nursing home: resident characteristics and prevalence of drug treatment. *Am J Managed Care* 11(4 suppl):S112-S120, 2005.

Ouslander JG: Management of overactive bladder. *N Engl J Med* 350:786-799, 2004.

Scientific Committee of the First International Consultation on Incontinence: Assessment and treatment of urinary incontinence. *Lancet* 355(9221):2153-2158, 2000.

Thakar R, Addison R, Sultan A: Management of urinary incontinence in the older female patient. *Clin Geriatr* 13(1):44-54, 2005.

Weiss BD: Diagnostic evaluation of urinary incontinence in geriatric patients. *Am Fam Physician* 57:2675-2684, 1998.

4.3 Defecation

Marsha D. Fretwell, Deborah Adams Wingate, E. Gordon Margolin, and Tom J. Wachtel

1. There are two types of colonic motility: shuttling and mass peristalsis.
    a. Shuttling of the fecal bolus between the haustra of the bowel is continuous, although it is decreased at night and increased after meals. Its function is to promote absorption of water from the fecal bolus.

   b. Mass peristalsis occurs two or three times a day and is stimulated
      by the gastrocolic reflex and physical mobility. It moves the fecal
      bolus from the transverse colon to the rectum and creates the urge
      to defecate.
2. Frequency of defecation and transit time are unchanged in active,
   older persons.
   a. The normal range of frequency of defecation is from three times a
      day to three times a week.
   b. Transit time is markedly slowed by sedentary lifestyle and low-
      fiber diet.

CONSTIPATION AND IMPACTION

1. Definitions.
   a. Constipation is a change in bowel function consisting of diminished
      frequency of defecation and often increased difficulty with defeca-
      tion.
   b. Impaction is the end result of prolonged exposure of accumulated
      stool to the absorptive forces of the colon and rectum.
2. Etiology in older persons.
   a. Decreased physical mobility and low-fiber diets leading to prolonged
      colon transit time.
   b. Systemic diseases (e.g., hypothyroidism, uremia, hypercalcemia,
      depression, or neurologic disorders such as parkinsonism, cerebrovas-
      cular accidents, and diabetes).
   c. Hypokalemia, hypomagnesemia.
   d. Medications such as anticholinergics, codeine, aluminum hydroxide,
      calcium channel blockers, nonsteroidal antiinflammatory drugs,
      and iron.
   e. Diseases of the colon such as irritable bowel syndrome or diverticulitis.
   f. Dyschezia or the failure of the defecation mechanism.
3. Presentation.
   a. Complaints about a change in frequency.
   b. Secondary fecal incontinence.
   c. Refusal to eat.
   d. Urinary retention or incontinence.
   e. Refusing or resistance to taking new medication.
4. Clinical evaluation.
   a. History: Focus on patient's perception of change in daily bowel
      habits and on the symptoms relating to the etiologic factors
      (e.g., diseases, depression, new drugs) listed earlier, particularly those
      of localized abdominal pain or rectal bleeding.
   b. Physical examination: Focus on possible underlying systemic
      diseases and careful abdominal and rectal exams, including a guaiac
      test of the stool.
      (1) Rectum full of stool suggests dyschezia.
      (2) Rectum empty suggests decreased motility of the entire colon.
   c. Laboratory or special studies.
      (1) Glucose, thyroid function, calcium, electrolytes, magnesium,
         and BUN.
      (2) Sigmoidoscopy and colonoscopy as indicated.

5. Management.
    a. Acute impaction.
        (1) Impaction must be reversed immediately, using local maneuvers such as:
            (a) Manual removal of hard fecal masses.
            (b) Stimulant suppositories.
            (c) Enemas.
        (2) Work closely with the family or nursing staff, with the goal of resolving the impaction within 48 hours.
    b. Constipation.
        (1) Treat all underlying systemic diseases, especially depression.
        (2) Replace potassium and magnesium.
        (3) Remove or replace all offending medication.
        (4) Train the bowel by using timing of the postprandial gastrocolic reflex along with glycerin suppositories.
        (5) Increase patient mobility.
        (6) Increase daily intake of fluids and dietary fiber.
        (7) Use laxatives as shown in Table 4-1.
    c. Prevention: once constipation or impaction has been successfully treated, steps should be taken to ensure that it does not recur.
        (1) Encourage continuation of exercise and increase in dietary fiber.

Table 4-1 Laxatives

Agent	Dosage
Bulk-Forming Agents	
Calcium polycarbophil (Fibercon)	2 tab qd-qid with 8 oz of liquid after each dose
High-fiber supplement (Fibermed)	2 biscuits qd
Psyllium hydrophilic mucilloid (Metamucil)	1 tbsp or packet qd-tid with 8 oz of liquid with each dose
Psyllium, senna (Perdiem)	1 tbsp qd-bid with 8 oz of liquid with each dose
Osmotic Agents	
Lactulose (Chronulac, Cephulac)	1-2 tbsp qd-bid
Sorbitol (30%-70%)	30 mL qd
Glycerin suppository	1-2 PR qd
Stimulants	
Castor oil	30-60 mL qd
Bisacodyl (Dulcolax)	5-15 mg PO qd
Emollients	
Casanthranol docusate sodium (Pericolace)	100 mg PO bid
Salts	
Milk of magnesia	30 mL qd
Magnesium citrate	30 mL qd

From Ferri FF: *Practical guide to the care of the medical patient*, 3rd ed, St. Louis, Mosby, 1995.

(2) Encourage a regular bowel pattern.
(3) Anticipate constipation when initiating any additional medications by choosing a less-constipating alternative or by adding a laxative.
(4) Monitor bowel function at every visit.
(5) Educate caretakers.

6. Complications in institutionalized older patients.
   a. History: When very old or cognitively impaired patients are admitted to the hospital or nursing home, they are often unable to give histories or volunteer other complaints. Because of chronic illnesses, ongoing medications, and immobility, many of these persons are already constipated and have impending or existing fecal impactions. This state is usually not addressed and has serious consequences for the patient.
   b. Complications and management.
      (1) Refusal of food or feedings: It is normal to resist food or feedings when one is unable to evacuate the bowel.
      (2) Aspiration of food or feedings: This is caused by the well-intended attempts of caretakers to nourish patients.
      (3) Avoid aspiration pneumonia as a complication by evaluating and reversing all fecal impactions within the first 48 hours of care.

FECAL INCONTINENCE

1. Definition
   a. Fecal incontinence is the involuntary loss of stool through the anal canal.
   b. It can range from inadvertent escape of flatus and undergarment soiling to the involuntary excretion of feces.
2. Epidemiology.
   a. Prevalence is extremely variable depending on definition, site, and mode of data collection.
      (1) Average range: 10% to 15%.
      (2) U.S. nursing homes report: 47%.
   b. Frequency (in U.S. study).
      (1) Daily: 2.7% of patients.
      (2) Weekly: 4.5%.
      (3) Monthly or less: 7.1%.
   c. Demographics.
      (1) Older than 65 years: 30%.
      (2) Female: 63%.
      (3) Notable with advanced age, severe debility, and multiple comorbidities.
   d. Risk factors.
      (1) Constipation and diarrhea.
      (2) Age older than 80 years.
      (3) Urinary incontinence.
      (4) Impaired mobility.
      (5) Dementia.
      (6) Neurologic disease.

e. Physiology: The process of normal defecation is complex and involves a sequence of events that are initiated by the entry of stool into the rectum.

3. Clinical findings.

   a. Uncontrolled loss of fecal matter or staining of underclothes.

      (1) Often is not reported to physicians or is reported as "pruritis," "diarrhea," or "urgency."

      (2) Can cause complications, such as pressure sores and urinary infections.

      (3) Can lead to isolation, avoidance of normal activities, and depression.

   b. Abdominal exam for masses and bladder distension.

   c. Inspection of anal area for deformed perineal body, scar formation, skin breakdown, gaping of anus.

   d. Digital rectal exam to evaluate anal tone and to identify fecal impaction.

   e. Evaluation of perineal sensation and anal wink reflex.

4. Etiology

   a. Anatomic.

   b. Sphincter disrupted by vaginal deliveries, anorectal surgery, radiation, and trauma.

   c. Pelvic floor neuropathy with rectal prolapse, chronic straining at stool, and pelvic floor descent.

   d. Isolated degeneration of internal anal sphincter.

   e. Neurologic.

   f. CNS damage or malfunction, including dementia.

   g. Diabetes mellitus, multiple sclerosis, and other specific entities.

   h. Functional.

   i. Fecal impaction.

   j. Abnormal GI function with excessive stool volume and rapid gut transport.

   k. Laxative abuse.

5. Work-up.

   a. Colonoscopy for masses and inflammatory conditions when pathology is suspected.

   b. Anorectal physiology testing: imaging, manometry, and electromyogram.

   c. Laboratory tests.

      (1) Thyroid-stimulating hormone, calcium, magnesium, glucose, BUN, creatinine, electrolytes.

      (2) Urinalysis.

   d. Imaging studies.

      (1) Abdominal x-ray.

      (2) Postvoid residual.

6. Treatment

   a. Nonpharmacologic therapy.

      (1) Diet changes.

         (a) Avoid food stimulants (e.g., lactose).

         (b) Add fiber.

      (2) Habit training.

      (3) Barrier creams to protect skin.

      (4) Biofeedback by trained personnel.

b. Pharmacologic therapy consists of antidiarrheal meds such as loperamide, diphenoxylate, and bile-acid binders.

SUGGESTED READINGS

Borum ML, Prather CM, Wald, A: Constipation, diarrhea, and fecal incontinence. In Beers MH, Berkow R (eds): *The Merck manual of geriatrics*. Rahway, NJ, Merck Sharp & Dohme, 2000, pp 1080-1094.

Hazzard WR: Colonic disorders. In Hazzard WR, Blass JR, Ettinger WH, et al (eds): *Principles of geriatric medicine and gerontology*. New York, McGraw-Hill, 1999, pp 881-888.

Madoff RD, Parker SC, Varma MG, Lowry AC: Fecal incontinence in adults. *Lancet* 364:621-632, 2004.

4.4 Cognitive Dysfunction

Marsha D. Fretwell and Deborah Adams Wingate

DELIRIUM

Background

1. Delirium is a transient global cognitive disorder commonly seen in frail older patients, especially those with dementia.
2. In hospitalized older patients, it is associated with increased morbidity, mortality, and lengths of stays.
3. Delirium is often the cardinal presenting symptom for serious physical illness or drug intoxication.
4. Early recognition and appropriate management of delirium substantially improves the medical and functional outcomes of the frail older patient.

Definition and Diagnostic Criteria

1. Delirium is characterized by:
   a. Global cognitive impairment.
   b. Disturbances of attention.
   c. Reduced level of consciousness.
   d. Reduced or increased psychomotor activity.
   e. Disorganized sleep-wake cycle.
   f. Acute onset, fluctuating course, and a relatively brief duration.
2. The confusion assessment method (CAM) diagnostic algorithm is shown in Box 4-5.
3. Incidence and importance.
   a. Delirium occurs in 13% of community-dwelling persons older than 65 years who have dementia.
   b. Delirium increases the risk of permanent institutionalization.
   c. Delirium occurs in more than 50% of hospitalized adults older than 70 years.
   d. Approximately 70% of delirious patients are delirious at admission, and 30% become delirious while in the hospital.
   e. Delirium goes unrecognized in more than 43.3% of patients seen by physicians in the emergency department.
   f. Delirium is often the presenting feature of an acute physical illness or adverse drug reaction. If it is unrecognized, the medical condition will also go unrecognized and untreated.
   g. Delirium has an associated 1-year mortality of 62%.

BOX 4-5   The Confusion Assessment Method (CAM) Diagnostic Algorithm

Diagnosis of delirium by CAM requires the presence of features 1 and 2 plus either feature 3 or feature 4.

Feature 1. Acute Onset and Fluctuating Course

This feature is usually obtained from a family member or nurse and is shown by positive responses to the following questions:
Is there evidence of an acute change in mental status from the patient's baseline?
Did the (abnormal) behavior fluctuate during the day, i.e., tend to come and go, or increase and decrease in severity?

Feature 2. Inattention

This feature is shown by a positive response to the following questions:
Did the patient have difficulty focusing attention? Was the patient easily distractible, or have difficulty keeping track of what was being said?

Feature 3. Disorganized Thinking

This feature is shown by a positive response to the following questions:
Was the patient's thinking disorganized or incoherent? Did the patient have rambling or irrelevant conversation, unclear or illogical flow of ideas, or unpredictable switching from subject to subject?

Feature 4. Altered Level of Consciousness

This feature is shown by any answer other than "alert" to the following questions:
Overall, how would you rate this patient's level of consciousness? Was the patient alert (normal), vigilant (hyperalert), lethargic (drowsy, easily aroused), in a stupor (difficult to arouse) or in a coma (unarousable)?

Adapted from Inouye SK: The dilemma of delirium: Clinical and research controversies regarding diagnosis and evaluation of delirium in hospitalized elderly medical patients. *Am J Med* 97:278-288, 1994.

4. Etiology and predictors.
   a. The etiology of delirium is multifactorial and commonly reversible.
      (1) Predisposing nonreversible factors.
         (a) Age greater than 65 years.
         (b) Brain damage, e.g., cerebral vascular accident.
         (c) Alzheimer's disease and other dementias.
      (2) Facilitating factors.
         (a) Psychological stress, e.g., change in environment, placement of urinary catheters and physical restraints.
         (b) Sleep loss.
         (c) Sensory deprivation or overload.
      (3) Precipitating factors.
         (a) Primary cerebral diseases.

    (b) Systemic illnesses affecting the brain secondarily, e.g., metabolic encephalopathies, neoplasms, infections, and cardiovascular and collagen diseases.

    (c) Fecal impaction and urinary retention.

    (d) Intoxication with exogenous substances, including medical and recreational drugs, and poisons.

    (e) Withdrawal from substances such as alcohol or sedative-hypnotics.

b. In older patients, often more than one factor is present.

c. Intoxication with medications, particularly anticholinergics and opioids, is probably the most common cause of delirium in the hospitalized older patient (Box 4-6).

d. The metabolic abnormalities, medical diseases, and surgical procedures most frequently associated with delirium are:

    (1) Hypoxia.

    (2) Hypoglycemia.

    (3) Hyponatremia, hypokalemia, uremia, and hypoalbuminemia.

    (4) CHF.

BOX 4-6   Medications Associated with Delirium

Antiarrhythmics (quinidine, disopyramide)
Antibiotics (aminoglycosides, penicillins, cephalosporins, sulfonamides)
Anticholinergics
Anticonvulsants
Antihistamines (diphenhydramine, hydroxyzine)
Antihypertensives (propranolol, methyldopa, reserpine, clonidine)
Antiparkinsonian agents (benztropine, trihexyphenidyl)
Antispasmodics (belladonna, diphenoxylate, oxybutynin)
Atypical antipsychotics (olanzapine, quetiapine, clozapine)
Benzodiazepines (flurazepam, diazepam)
Barbiturates
Cardiac (digitalis, lidocaine, amiodarone)
Cimetidine
Levodopa
Lithium
Metoclopramide
Narcotics
Nonsteroidal antiinflammatory drugs
Phenothiazines (haloperidol, thorazine, thioridazine)
Salicylates
Sleeping medications (chloral hydrate)
Steroids
Tricyclic antidepressants (amitriptyline, imipramine, doxepin)

Data from Inouye SK: The dilemma of delirium: Clinical and research controversies regarding diagnosis and evaluation of delirium in hospitalized elderly medical patients. *Am J Med* 97:278-288, 1994.

(5) Infections such as urinary tract and pneumonia.

(6) Fever or hypothermia.

(7) Repair of hip fractures and open heart surgery.

5. Diagnosis.

   a. The diagnosis of delirium is made on clinical grounds and has two crucial steps:

     (1) Recognition of delirium on the basis of history from nurses, family members, and the essential clinical features.

     (2) Identification of its etiologies, reversible and irreversible.

     (3) The comprehensive geriatric assessment process described in Chapter 2 is useful in guiding the diagnosis and identifying causes.

   b. Database.

     (1) Chief complaint.

       (a) Families and caretakers bring the patient to medical attention because of acute onset of confusion, restlessness, difficulty in thinking coherently, insomnia, disturbing dreams, or frank hallucinations.

       (b) Information about time of onset and duration of symptoms is critical.

       (c) Hallucinations are often the focus of concern to caretakers.

       (d) Patients might appear either somnolent or hyperactive with delirium. Somnolence is often associated with delayed recognition of delirium in older patients.

     (2) Initial screen of vision, hearing, and cognition.

       (a) Patient might have difficulty remaining awake or might be easily distracted.

       (b) Patient is unable to count backward from 10 to 1 or to name days of the week in reverse order.

       (c) Patients with very low scores on the Mini Mental State Examination* should be evaluated for delirium *before* the problem is diagnosed as dementia.

     (3) Biomedical, psychological, social, and functional history should focus on etiologic factors discussed earlier.

     (4) Review medication list.

       (a) Discontinue all psychoactive medication or substitute less toxic alternatives.

       (b) Review side effects of all medications.

     (5) Physical examination.

       (a) Fever, hypothermia, low cardiac output, dehydration, hyperthyroidism or hypothyroidism, signs of pneumonia, and/or UTI should be evaluated and corrected.

       (b) Evaluation of cognitive function generally reveals an inability to attend, rambling thoughts, somnolence, or agitation.

       (c) Usually there is an absence of new focal neurologic changes.

---

*The Mini Mental State Examination, by Marshal Folstein and Susan Folstein, Copyright 1975, 1998, 2001 by Mini Mental LLC, Inc., is available from Psychological Assessment Resources, Inc., 16204 North Florida Avenue, Lutz, Florida 33549. Reproduction is prohibited without permission of PAR, Inc. The MMSE can be purchased from PAR, Inc. by calling (813) 968-3003.

      (6) Targeted laboratory evaluation.
- (a) Electrolytes.
- (b) BUN, creatinine.
- (c) Brain natriuretic peptide.
- (d) Complete blood count (CBC) with differential.
- (e) Glucose, calcium, and phosphate.
- (f) Liver enzyme tests.
- (g) Blood level of all medications.

      (7) Search for occult infections.
- (a) Chest x-ray.
- (b) Urine, sputum, and blood cultures.

      (8) When no obvious cause is identified by the history, physical examination, and laboratory evaluation, consider the following in selected patients:
- (a) Laboratory tests: magnesium, thyroid function, vitamin B_{12} level, toxicology screen, ammonia level.
- (b) Arterial blood gas in patients with dyspnea, tachypnea, acute pulmonary process, or history of significant respiratory disease.
- (c) Electrocardiogram (ECG) in patients with chest pain, shortness of breath, or cardiac disease history.
- (d) Cerebrospinal fluid examination in febrile patients where meningitis is suspected.
- (e) Computed tomography (CT) or magnetic resonance imaging (MRI) in patients with new focal neurologic signs or with a history or signs of head injury.
- (f) Electroencephalogram (EEG) in patients where occult seizure disorder is suspected and delirium must be differentiated from functional psychiatric disorders.

6. Assessment and management.
  a. Treatment of the underlying causes.
     (1) The causative factors listed earlier should be pursued, treated, and/or reversed whenever possible. Management of organ system abnormalities and medical diagnoses are covered in Chapter 5. Issues relating to the optimal use of medications are outlined in Chapter 7.
     (2) Two studies in hospital settings used multifactorial interventions (educated existing staff and reduced benzodiazepines, antihistamines, and opiate) and demonstrated reductions in the duration of delirium, the length of hospitalization, and mortality in delirious patients.

  b. Symptomatic treatment.
     (1) Treat agitation with high-potency, low-anticholinergic antipsychotics, such as resperidone orally or ziprasidone parenterally.
- (a) Start resperidone at 0.25 to 1.0 mg PO bid, maximum 2 mg /day.
- (b) If parenteral delivery is required, give ziprasidone 10 mg q2h until a moderate level of sedation is achieved.
- (c) Maximum dose of ziprasidone is 40 mg daily, and it cannot be used longer than 3 days.

     (2) If the patient was not on an antipsychotic medication before hospitalization, it is unlikely that he or she will need to be discharged on it.

(3) Most toxicity associated with antipsychotic medications occurs during long-term use, not while it is being used to control acute agitation.

c. New functional impairments that inevitably accompany delirium in older patients (e.g., malnutrition, incontinence, fecal impactions, falling, and disruptive or uncooperative behavior) should be anticipated and prevented, if possible. Management of each is covered in detail later.

DEMENTIA

Definition

1. Dementia is a syndrome characterized by:
   a. Impairment in memory functions and one or more areas of intellectual or cognitive function despite a state of clear consciousness.
   b. Gradual deterioration of previously acquired intellectual abilities that interferes with social, occupational, and self-care functions.
2. The persistent and stable nature of the impairment distinguishes dementia from the altered consciousness and fluctuating deficits of delirium.

Epidemiology

1. The prevalence of dementia in the community-dwelling population older than 65 years is 10% to 50%, and the percentage doubles with every 5 years over age 65 years.
2. In the nursing home population, more than 50% of the patients carry the diagnosis of a dementing disorder.
3. The three most common dementias are Alzheimer's disease (60%), vascular dementia (20%), and Lewy body dementia (15%).

Classification of Dementia Syndromes

1. History.
   a. Original classifications of dementia syndromes began with clinical patterns demonstrated by patients with various dementias.
   b. Neuropathologic and structural imaging studies began to show that this system was not anatomically accurate.
   c. Neuropsychological studies of patients with focal brain lesions, neuroanatomic studies in humans and animals, experiments in animals, positron-emission tomography, functional MRI, and event-related potentials have refined and improved our understanding and classification of dementing disorders.
2. Clinical diagnostic classification. The clinical diagnostic criteria of the American Psychiatric Association classify the dementias in the following schema. Notably, dementia of the Lewy body type, characterized by visual hallucinations, falls, parkinsonian motor disturbances, and intermittent lucidity, is not mentioned in the *Diagnostic and Statistical Manual of Mental Disorders*, 4th edition, *Text Revision* (DSM-IV-TR) classification system.
   a. Dementia of the Alzheimer's type.
   b. Vascular dementia.
   c. Dementia caused by other general medical conditions.
      (1) Human immunodeficiency virus (HIV).
      (2) Head trauma.
      (3) Parkinson's disease.
      (4) Huntington's disease.

    (5) Pick's disease.

    (6) Creutzfeldt–Jakob disease (CJD).

    (7) Normal-pressure hydrocephalus.

    (8) Hypothyroidism.

    (9) Vitamin B_{12} deficiency.

  d. Substance-induced persisting dementia.

    (1) Alcohol.

    (2) Inhalants.

    (3) Sedative, hypnotic, or anxiolytic medications.

  e. Dementia of multiple etiologies.

    (1) Alzheimer's and vascular.

    (2) Vascular and alcohol.

    (3) Head trauma and alcohol.

3. Neuropathologic classifications.

  a. Alzheimer's disease.

    (1) Amyloid plaques are present in the association areas of the frontal, temporal, and parietal lobes and in the amygdala, the hippocampus, and the piriform cortex.

    (2) Neurofibrillary tangles are seen mostly in the neocortex, hippocampus, amygdala, nucleus basalis of Meynert, locus ceruleus, dorsal raphe, and other brainstem nuclei.

  b. Vascular dementia.

    (1) Multiple areas of focal ischemic changes.

    (2) Lacunae are tiny deep infarctions resulting from small arteries in subcortical structures, such as basal ganglia, thalamus, and internal capsule.

  c. Lewy body dementia: Inclusion bodies of α-synuclein (Lewy bodies) are present in the cell bodies of neurons in the cortex and substantia nigra.

  d. Pick's disease.

    (1) Swollen neurons (Pick's cells) and intraneuronal inclusions (Pick's bodies) are seen mostly in frontal temporal lobes.

    (2) May be accompanied by demyelination and gliosis of the frontal lobe white matter.

  e. Frontal lobe dementia.

    (1) No plaques or tangles.

    (2) Marked frontal gliosis and neuronal loss.

  f. Parkinson's disease.

    (1) Predominant degeneration of dopaminergic cells in the substantia nigra, globus pallidus, putamen, and caudate.

    (2) Overlaps lesions seen in Alzheimer's disease and Lewy body dementia.

  g. Syphilis: Diffuse degeneration with marked lymphocytic infiltration throughout.

  h. Creutzfeldt-Jakob disease (CJD).

    (1) Spongiform neuronal degeneration and gliosis throughout the cortical and subcortical gray matter.

    (2) White matter is spared.

  i. Huntington's disease: Disruption of the corticostriatothalamocortical relays.

4. Functional neuroimaging classification.
   a. Single-photon emission computed tomography (SPECT) was used in one study for clinical evaluation, and autopsy diagnosis was made of 27 consecutive dementia patients seen at a university clinic.[1]
   b. Four different types of brain hypoperfusion were seen on SPECT.
      (1) Bilateral posterior temporal and parietal lobes (17/27 patients).
         (a) Nine patients had Alzheimer's disease pathologic findings.
         (b) One patient had Alzheimer's and Parkinson's.
         (c) One patient had atypical Alzheimer's disease (diffuse).
         (d) Two patients had a Lewy body variant of Alzheimer's disease.
         (e) Two patients had Alzheimer's disease and ischemic foci.
         (f) One patient had Parkinson's disease pathologic findings.
         (g) One patient had diffuse cortical Lewy bodies.
      (2) Bilateral frontal lobes (7/27 patients).
         (a) Four patients had frontal gliosis and neuronal loss.
         (b) Three patients had Pick's bodies.
      (3) Mottled: Two of 27 patients had CJD pathologic findings.
      (4) Focal (2/27 patients).
         (a) One patient had Alzheimer's disease and ischemic foci (noted above).
         (b) One patient had focal laminar necrosis in the right posterior region.
5. Memory system classification.
   a. Memory is now understood to be a collection of mental abilities that depend on several systems within the brain.
   b. The four memory systems that are of clinical relevance (Table 4-2) include:
      (1) Episodic memory.
      (2) Semantic memory.
      (3) Procedural memory.
      (4) Working memory.

Diagnosis

1. Chief complaint: Families often bring the patient to medical attention because of memory problems (e.g., repetitive questions, misplacement of items, missed appointments, getting lost away from home), hallucinations, disruptive behavior, insomnia, and anxiety/depression disorders.
2. General cognitive screening for detection of dementia: Perform Mini Mental State Exam (see footnote, page 76).
   a. Orientation to time and space.
      (1) Based on intact registration and recall (short-term memory).
      (2) Orientation to space is preserved longer than orientation to time.
   b. Registration.
      (1) Depends on hearing and paying attention.
      (2) If the patient is unable to complete the task, consider the diagnosis of delirium (see above).
   c. Attention and calculation.
      (1) To avoid educational bias, use simple tasks such as saying the days of the week forward and backward or counting backward from 20 to 0.

Table 4-2 **Selected Memory Systems**

Memory Type	Major Anatomic	Length of Storage	Type of Awareness	Examples
Episodic	Medial temporal lobes, anterior thalamic nucleus, mamillary body, fornix, prefrontal cortex	Minutes to years	Explicit, declarative	Remembering a short story, what you had for dinner last night, and what you did on your last birthday
Semantic	Inferolateral temporal lobes	Minutes to years	Explicit, declarative	Knowing who was the first president of the United States, the color of a lion, how a fork differs from a comb
Procedural	Basal ganglia, cerebellum supplementary motor area	Minutes to years	Explicit or implicit, nondeclarative	Driving a car with a standard transmission (explicit) and learning the sequence of numbers on a touch-tone phone without trying (implicit)
Working	Phonologic: prefrontal cortex, Broca's area Spatial: prefrontal cortex, visual association areas	Seconds to minutes; information actively rehearsed or manipulated	Explicit, declarative	Phonologic: Keeping a phone number in your head before dialing Spatial: Mentally following a route or rotating an object in your mind

From Budson AE, Price BH: *N Engl J Med* 352; 7: 692, 2005. Copyright © 2005 Massachusetts Medical Society. All rights reserved.

        (2) Because this function is preserved very late in Alzheimer's, if the patient us unable to complete the task, consider a frontal lobe dementia such as Pick's disease and/or delirium.

   d. Recall.

       (1) Patients with early stages of dementia make their first errors in this function, often with no other errors in the examination.

       (2) Errors in orientation follow next.

3. Other cognitive screening options.

   a. Clock drawing to assess loss of visual spatial memory in early Alzheimer's.

   b. Fast Naming Animal Test (average normal is naming 33 in one minute).

4. Consider neuropsychiatric tests, particularly those emphasizing memory function, by a qualified neuropsychologist to confirm screening mental status testing. This testing can help differentiate parietal-temporal dementias (Alzheimer's or Parkinson's) from frontal-temporal dementias, such as Pick's, or focal dementias, such as vascular dementia.

5. Medical history: Review treatable causes of dementia.

   a. Metabolic disorders (e.g., glucose, calcium, thyroid, renal, hypoxia).

   b. CNS infections (e.g., HIV, syphilis, viral encephalitis).

   c. Medication (see Chapter 7).

   d. Nutrition (vitamin B_{12}, folate, thiamine).

   e. Depression.

6. Neurologic history: The onset and course of neurologic symptoms provide clues to the etiology.

   a. Sudden onset suggests a stroke.

   b. Subacute course over weeks and months suggests a tumor or CJD.

   c. Early appearance of a spastic-like gait with urinary incontinence suggests hydrocephalus.

   d. Rigidity and bradykinesis suggest Parkinson's disease.

   e. A recent fall suggests subdural hematoma; multiple falls suggest Lewy body dementia.

   f. Insidious onset and progression in the absence of early motor signs suggest Alzheimer's.

   g. Personality changes such as disinhibition, lack of insight, difficulty with concentration that outweighs memory problems suggest frontal lobe dementia.

   h. Early onset of hallucinations suggests Lewy body dementia.

7. Physical examination.

   a. Fever, atrial fibrillation, low cardiac output, dehydration, hyperthyroidism or hypothyroidism, and signs of infection are evaluated.

   b. Asymmetric motor signs, abnormal involuntary movements, bradykinesis, and gait disorders suggest a neurologic etiology.

8. Laboratory evaluation.

   a. Electrolytes, BUN, creatinine, calcium, glucose, magnesium, thyroid function tests, CBC with differential, vitamin B_{12}, folate, Venereal Disease Research Laboratory tests, blood levels of ethanol, any current medications.

   b. Structural neuroimaging with a noncontrast CT scan or MRI is appropriate in the routine initial evaluation of patients and can

detect cerebrovascular accidents, hematomas, hydrocephalus, tumor, or other focal lesions.
c. Functional imaging with proton-emission tomography (PET) and SPECT, which reveal specific location of hypometabolism in different dementias, is not recommended for routine use. Currently, these studies are available as research instruments in large academic programs.
d. Genetic testing for suspected Alzheimer's, dementia with Lewy bodies, and CJD is not recommended.
e. Cerebrospinal fluid or other biomarkers are not recommended in Alzheimer's.
f. Cerebrospinal fluid 14-3-3 is recommended for confirming or rejecting the diagnosis in CJD.

Management

1. Pharmacologic treatment of cognitive and functional symptoms of dementia (Tables 4-3 and 4-4).
   a. Cholinesterase inhibitors.
      (1) Characteristics.
         (a) Increase the availability of acetylcholine.
         (b) Have demonstrated benefit for cognition, mood, behavioral symptoms and daily functions.
         (c) Can delay nursing home placement.
      (2) Drugs and dosing.
         (a) Donepezil (Aricept) 5 mg hs for 4 weeks, then increase to 10 mg hs.
         (b) Galantamine (Razadyne) 8mg qd for at least 4 weeks, then 16 mg qd for at least 4 weeks, then increase to 24 mg qd.
         (c) Rivastigmine (Exelon) 1.5 mg bid for 2 weeks, then increase by 3 mg as tolerated. Maximum dosage is 6 mg bid.
   b. N-methyl-D-aspartate (NMDA).
      (1) Characteristics.
         (a) A subtype of glutamate receptor antagonist.
         (b) Reduces the effect of excessive glutamate of Alzheimer's on the NMDA receptor.
         (c) Might enhance new learning.
      (2) Memantine (Namenda).
         (a) Give 5 mg qd for 1 week, then increase by 5 mg each week.
         (b) Maximum dose is 10 mg bid.
         (c) Doses >10 mg should be divided bid.
2. Pharmacologic treatment of noncognitive features of dementia (Tables 4-5 and 4-6).
   a. Antidepressants.
      (1) Selective serotonin reuptake inhibitor (SSRI) treats depression, long-term anxiety, insomnia, pain.
      (2) Serotonin–norepinephrine reuptake inhibitor (SNRI) treats depression and pain and maintains circadian rhythm.
      (3) Tricyclic antidepressant (TCA) (nortriptyline [Pamelor]) treats depression, anxiety, and pain and maintains circadian rhythm.
      (4) Tetracyclic antidepressant (mirtazapine [Remeron]) treats anorexia and insomnia.

Table 4-3 **Management of Dementia**		
Type of Dementia	**Preferred Treatment**	**Also Consider**
Alzheimer's	NMDA antagonist plus Cholinesterase inhibitor	Cholinesterase inhibitor alone NMDA antagonist (Namenda) alone Control of hypertension and diabetes Cholinesterase inhibitor plus vitamin E
Vascular	Control of hypertension and diabetes Aspirin Cholinesterase inhibitor alone Lipid-lowering agents	NMDA antagonist plus cholinesterase inhibitor
Mixed Alzheimer's and vascular	Control of hypertension and diabetes NMDA antagonist plus cholinesterase inhibitor	Cholinesterase inhibitor alone Aspirin NMDA antagonist (Namenda) alone Cholinesterase inhibitor plus vitamin E Lipid-lowering agent
Frontotemporal	—	Control of hypertension and diabetes
Lewy body	Cholinesterase inhibitor alone	NMDA antagonist plus cholinesterase inhibitor Cholinesterase inhibitor plus vitamin E Lipid-lowering agent

NMDA, *N*-methyl-D-aspartate.
Data from Alexopoulos GS, Jeste DV, Chung H, et al: *Postgrad Med* Spec No 6-22, 2005.

     (5) Serotonin antagonist and reuptake inhibitor (SARI) (trazodone [Desyrel]) treats insomnia and anxiety.
  b. Atypical antipsychotics (Tables 4-7 and 4-8).
    (1) Serotonin dopamine antagonists.
      (a) Treat agitation, delirium, and psychosis.
      (b) Examples include olanzapine (Zyprexa), quetiapine (Seroquel), risperidone (Risperdal), and ziprasidone (Geodon).

Table 4-4 Choice of Cholinesterase Inhibitors

Type of Dementia	Preferred Treatment	Also Consider
Alzheimer's	Donepezil 10 mg/day Galantamine 16 mg/day	Rivastigmine 6-12 mg/day bid
Vascular	Donepezil 10 mg/day	Galantamine 16-24 mg/day
Mixed Alzheimer's and Vascular	Donepezil 10 mg/day Galantamine 16-24 mg/day	Rivastigmine 6-12 mg/day bid
Frontotemporal	—	Donepezil 10 mg/day
Lewy body	Rivastigmine 6-12 mg/day bid	Galantamine 16 mg/day

Data from Alexopoulos GS, Jeste DV, Chung H, et al: *Postgrad Med* Spec No 6-22, 2005.

Table 4-5 Management of Depression in Dementia

Type of Depression	Preferred Treatment	Also Consider
Nonpsychotic	Antidepressant alone	Antidepressant plus cholinesterase inhibitor Antidepressant plus psychotherapy
Psychotic	Antidepressant plus antipsychotic	

Data from Alexopoulos GS, Jeste DV, Chung H, et al: *Postgrad Med* Spec No 6-22, 2005.

Table 4-6 Medications for Depression in Dementia

Medication Class	Preferred First Line	Also Consider	Other
Antidepressants	Citalopram Sertraline Escitalopram	Venlafaxine Mirtzapine	Paroxetine Bupropion
Antipsychotics for use in combination with an antidepressant for psychotic depression	Risperidone	Quetiapine Olanzapine	Aripiprazole

Data from Alexopoulos GS, Jeste DV, Chung H, et al: *Postgrad Med* Spec No 6-22, 2005.

Table 4-7 **Management of Psychosis**			
Medication Class	**Preferred Treatment**	**Also Consider**	**Other**
Short-term PRN	Risperidone 0.2-2.0 mg/day Quetiapine 50-100 mg/day	Olanzapine 5.0-20 mg/day	Aripiprazole 5-15 mg/day
Long term	Risperidone 0.2-2.0 mg/day Quetiapine 50-200 mg/day	Aripiprazole 5.0-15 mg/day Olanzapine 2.5-10 mg	None
Ongoing use in Parkinson's	Quetiapine 50-200 mg/day	None	Aripiprazole 5.0-15 mg/day

Data from Alexopoulos GS, Jeste DV, Chung H, et al: *Postgrad Med* Spec No 6-22, 2005.

(2) Dopamine partial antagonist/agonist and serotonin antagonist/agonist (aripiprazole [Abilify]) treats agitation, psychosis, and delirium.
  c. Anticonvulsants (Table 4-9).
    (1) Voltage-sensitive sodium-channel modulator (valproate [Depakote]) treats agitation, delirium, psychosis, and aggression.
    (2) $\alpha_2\delta$ Ligand at voltage-sensitive calcium channels (gabapentin [Neurontin]) treats pain.
    (3) Voltage-sensitive sodium channel antagonist (lamotrigine [Lamictal]) treats agitation, delirium, psychosis, aggression, and pain.
  d. Anxiolytics (Table 4-10).
    (1) SARI: Trazodone (Desyrel) treats insomnia and anxiety.
    (2) TCA: Nortriptyline (Pamelor) treats depression, anxiety, and pain and maintains circadian rhythm.
    (3) SSRI treats depression, long-term anxiety, insomnia, and pain.
    (4) Serotonin–dopamine antagonists.
      (a) Treat anxiety, agitation, psychosis, and delirium.
      (b) Examples include olanzapine (Zyprexa), quetiapine (Seroquel), risperidone (Risperdal), and ziprasidone (Geodon).
    (5) Dopamine partial antagonist–agonist and serotonin antagonist–agonist (aripiprazole [Abilify]) treats anxiety, agitation, psychosis, and delirium.
    (6) Serotonin type 1A partial agonist (buspirone [BuSpar]) treats anxiety and agitation.
    (7) Benzodiazepine (lorazepam [Ativan]) for acute treatment only treats anxiety and agitation.

Table 4-8 Management of Delirium in Dementia

Medical Issue	Preferred First Line	Also Consider	Other
Benzodiazepine withdrawal	Benzodiazepine with short life (Lorazepam)	Lower the dose and taper slowly	None
Medication toxicity or interaction	Reduce or stop the offending medication	None	None
Diabetes	None	Risperidone 0.25-2.0 mg/day	Quetiapine 50-200 mg/day
Congestive heart failure; COPD or pneumonia; dehydration or electrolyte imbalance; infection (URI, UTI)	Risperidone 0.25-2.0 mg/day	Quetiapine 50-200 mg/day	Olanzapine 2.5-20 mg/day

URI, upper respiratory infection; UTI, urinary tract infection.
Data from Alexopoulos GS, Jeste DV, Chung H, et al: *Postgrad Med* Spec No 6-22, 2005.

Table 4-9 **Comparison of Anticonvulsants in Managing Agitation in Dementia**

Drug	Starting Dose	Dosage	Therapeutic Range	Baseline Labs	Monitoring Labs
Carbamazepine	100 mg bid	100-1200 mg	4-12 μg/mL	CBC, LFTs	TDM, sodium
Lamotrigine	25 mg hs	25-250 mg	Not determined	CBC, LFTs	Not determined
Oxcarbazepine	150 mg bid	150-1200 mg	Not determined	CBC, LFTs	TDM, sodium
Valproic acid	125 mg bid	250-2000 mg	50-100 μg/mL	CBC, LFTs	TDM, amylase

CBC, complete blood count; LFT, liver function test; TDM, therapeutic drug monitoring.
Data from Espinoza RT, Eslami MS: Update on treatment for Alzheimer's disease—Part II: Management of noncognitive, psychiatric, and behavioral complications. *Clin Geriatr* 12(1): 45-53, 2004.

Table 4-10 Comparative Receptor Affinities and Pharmacologic Properties of Atypical Antipsychotics

Receptor	Effect	Drug					
		Aripiprazole	Clozapine	Olanzapine	Quetiapine	Risperidone	Ziprasidone
α_1-Adrenergic	Orthostatic hypotension, sedation, weight gain	Low-moderate	High	Low-moderate	Low-moderate	High	Low-moderate
D_2	Decreased psychotic symptoms, EPS, elevated prolactin	High-partial antagonist/agonist	Low	Moderate	Low	High	High
H_1-histaminergic	Sedation, weight gain	Low-moderate	High	High	High	Low-moderate	Low-moderate
5-HT_{1a}	Anxiolytic and antidepressant effect	High	Low	Negligible	Low	Low	High
5-HT_{2a} 5-HT_{2c}	Decreased EPS Decreased psychosis, weight gain	High High	High Low	High High	Low Negligible	High High	High Low
M_1-muscarinic	Cognitive impairment, urinary retention, constipation, dry mouth, decreased EPS	Negligible	Excess saliva production is usually a problem rather than dry mouth	High	Low-moderate	Negligible	Negligible

EPS, extrapyramidal symptoms; 5-HT, serotonin.
Data from Keys MA, DeWald C: *Annals of Long-Term Care* 13(2):25-32, 2005.

3. Nonpharmacologic management of symptoms (wandering, pacing, poor social skills, willfulness, demandingness, hoarding, repetitive actions).
   a. Caregiver education is the treatment of choice.
   b. Reduce caregiver burden.
      (1) Offer psychotherapy for the caregiver.
      (2) Refer the patient to a day treatment program.
      (3) Offer respite care on a regular basis.
   c. Optimize patient function.
      (1) Scheduled toileting.
      (2) Prompted voiding.
      (3) Physical therapy and exercise programs.
      (4) Positive reinforcement.
   d. Problem behavior management.
      (1) Develop positive communication skills.
      (2) Maintain a calm environment.
      (3) Encourage socialization and meaningful activities.
         (a) Music.
         (b) Simulated presence therapy.
         (c) Massage.
         (d) Pet therapy.
         (e) Cognitive remediation.

Educational Interventions for Families of Patients with Dementia

1. Educate the patient and caretakers about increased susceptibility to delirium from medications, environmental changes, and stressors.
2. Encourage the family to create calm, caretaking environment by structuring daily and weekly activities.
3. Educate the family about the need to assist the patient in regular toileting every 2 to 3 hours to prevent incontinence. Easy on and off clothing is recommended
4. Educate the patient and caretakers about the nature of amnesia, aphasia, apraxia, and agnosia and the disabilities they cause.
   a. Emphasize that the patient's feelings are quite intact despite loss of cognitive function.
   b. Help caretakers relate to the fear and/or frustration that the patient is experiencing
5. Encourage the patient and family to discuss the diagnosis openly and to make out a durable power of attorney for health care and financial decision making.
6. Encourage the patient and family to take advantage of community resources for the care of those with dementing disorders.
   a. Senior citizens and daycare centers.
   b. Alzheimer's disease support groups (1-800-272-3900).
   c. Respite programs.
   d. Geriatric assessment and care centers.

REFERENCE

1. Read SL, Miller BL, Mena I, et al: SPECT in dementia: Clinical and pathological correlation. *J Am Geriatr Soc* 43:1243-1247, 1995.

SUGGESTED READINGS

Alexopoulos GS, Jeste DV, Chung H, et al: Treatment of dementia and its behavioral disturbances. *Postgrad Med* Spec No 6-22, 2005.

American Geriatric Society Clinical Practice Committee: Guidelines abstracted from the American Academy of Neurology's Dementia Guidelines for Early Detection, Diagnosis, and Management of Dementia. *J Am Geriatr Soc* 51(6): 869-873, 2003.

Budson AE, Price BH: Memory dysfunction. *N Engl J Med* 352(7):692-699, 2005.

Caine ED, Lyness JM: Delirium, dementia, and amnestic and other cognitive disorders. In Sadock BJ, Sadock VA (eds): *Comprehensive textbook of psychiatry*, ed 7. Philadelphia, Lippincott, Williams & Wilkins, 2000, pp 854-923.

Espinoza RT, Eslami MS: Update on treatment for Alzheimer's disease—Part II: Management of noncognitive, psychiatric, and behavioral complications. *Clin Geriatr* 12(1): 45-53, 2004.

Fick DM, Agostini JV, Inouye SK: Delirium superimposed on dementia: A systematic review. *J Am Geriatr Soc* 50: 1723-1732, 2002.

Fick DM, Kolanowski AM, Waller JL, et al: Delirium superimposed on dementia in a community-dwelling managed care population: A 3-year retrospective study of occurrence, costs, and utilization. *J Gerontal A Biol Sci Med Sci* 60(6): 748-753, 2005.

Folstein MF, Folstein SE, McHugh PR: "Mini-mental state": A practical method for grading the cognitive state of patients for the clinician, *J Psychiatr Res* 12: 189-198, 1975.

Francis J, Martin D, Kapoor WN: A prospective study of delirium in hospitalized elderly. JAMA 263:1097-1101, 1990.

Hachinski V: Preventable senility: A call for action against the vascular dementias. *Lancet* 340:645-648, 1992.

Inouye SK: The dilemma of delirium: Clinical and research controversies regarding diagnosis and evaluation of delirium in hospitalized elderly medical patients. *Am J Med* 97:278-288, 1994.

Keys MA, DeWald C: Clinical perspectives on choice of antipsychotics in elderly patients with dementia, part I. *Annals of Long-Term Care* 13(2): 25-32, 2005.

Leslie DL, Zhang Y, Holford TR, et al: Premature death associated with delirium at 1-year follow-up. *Arch Intern Med*. 165(14): 1657-1662, 2005.

Tune LE: Delirium. In Hazzard WR, Blass JP, Ettinger WH, et al (eds): *Principles of geriatric medicine and gerontology*. New York, McGraw-Hill, 1999, pp 1229-1237.

Lundström M, Edlund A, Karlsson S, et al: A multifactorial intervention program reduces the duration of delirium, length of hospitalization, and mortality in delirious patients. *J Am Geriatr Soc* 53,4: 622-628, 2005.

Solomon PR, Budson AE: Alzheimer's disease. *Clinical Symposia*. 54:1-40, 2003.

4.5 Emotion

Marsha D. Fretwell and Deborah Adams Wingate

OVERVIEW

A spectrum of disorders fall under the domain of emotional function. These syndromes often include a mixture of cognitive, emotional, and physical dysfunction. Therefore, an optimal outcome might involve treatment with an antidepressant, antipsychotic, and/or cognitive enhancer, as well as nonpharmacologic interventions.

1. General anxiety disorder (GAD).
2. Specific anxiety disorders.
   a. Phobic disorder.
   b. Obsessive compulsive disorder (OCD).
   c. Panic disorder.
   d. Posttraumatic stress disorder (PTSD).
3. Major depressive disorder.
4. Failure to thrive.
5. Bipolar disorder.
6. Psychosis.
   a. Hallucinations.
      (1) Dementia (sundowning).
      (2) Delirium.
      (3) Psychotic depression.
      (4) Loss of vision.
      (5) Extreme old age.
      (6) Social isolation.
   b. Delusions.
      (1) Paranoia.
      (2) Schizophrenia.
7. Sleep disorder.
8. Disruptive behavior.

DIAGNOSIS

A comprehensive geriatric assessment (see Chapter 2) is particularly useful in clarifying the diagnosis and implementing treatment in this difficult group of patients.

1. Database.
   a. Chief complaint.
      (1) Primary: symptoms of anxiety, depressed mood, anorexia, insomnia, low energy, hallucinations, obsessions, delusions.
      (2) Secondary: failure to resolve medical problem despite best efforts of primary care and specialty physicians.
   b. Initial screen of vision, hearing, and cognition: Mild impairments in short-term memory may be promoting symptoms and/or interfering with cooperation with care plan.
   c. Biomedical history.
      (1) Hypothyroidism and hyperthyroidism.
      (2) Occult pulmonary emboli or metastases.
      (3) Carcinoma.
      (4) Vitamin deficiency.
      (5) Arrhythmias.
      (6) Anemia
      (7) Hypercalcemia
      (8) Hypoglycemia
      (9) Drug withdrawal or toxicity.
   d. Psychosocial history.
      (1) Focus on current and past history of anxiety, depression, use of drugs and alcohol, paranoia, hallucinations, and suicidal thoughts.

(2) Evaluate social skills and support system.

(3) Evaluate family history of anxiety, depression, suicide, and abuse.

  e. Physical examination: Focus carefully on the areas of health and symptoms of greatest concern to the patient.

  f. Laboratory and diagnostic evaluation.

(1) Obtain and review all old records to update the laboratory and diagnostic database.

(2) Repeat only the necessary tests, because anxious, depressed older patients often experience unintentional adverse effects from diagnostic work-ups (e.g, GI work-ups).

2. Assessment: Patient data are integrated and organized in the problem list (Table 4-11).

3. Care plan.

  a. Within each area of concern, assess and identify reversible or potentially treatable etiologic factors.

  b. Make treatment recommendations consistent with standard medical practice for each problem listed.

  c. Reconcile recommendations with patient's preference for treatment.

DISORDERS

Anxiety

General Anxiety Disorder

1. Definition: Excessive anxiety and worry accompanied by motor tension and hypervigilance.

  a. Anxiety disorders are defined by persistence (>6 months) of the following symptoms:

(1) Motor tension: Shakiness, jumpiness, trembling, inability to relax.

(2) Autonomic hyperactivity: Sweating, palpitations, dry mouth, dizziness, hot or cold spells, frequent urination, diarrhea.

(3) Apprehensive expectation: Constant worry or anticipation of personal or family misfortune.

(4) Vigilance and scanning: Distractibility, poor concentration, insomnia, edginess.

  b. Most primary anxiety disorders in late life have persisted from earlier years.

  c. New-onset anxiety in the elderly person is commonly associated with:

(1) Depression.

(2) Medical illness.

(3) Medication side effects.

  d. Drug withdrawal.

2. Epidemiology

  a. Anxiety disorders are common in later life, and more than 5% of community-dwelling older persons meet the DSM-IV-TR criteria.

  b. Because anxiety is associated with many medical diseases, with adverse drug reactions, and with delirium and dementia, as many as *half of the patients* in physicians' offices, acute care hospitals, and nursing homes have one or more symptoms of anxiety.

Table 4-11   Evaluation for Anxiety, Depression, and Failure to Thrive

Areas of Concern	Focus of Evaluation
Diagnosis	Acute: Delirium, myocardial infarction, paroxysmal atrial tachycardia, anemia, hypoglycemia, hypercalcemia, hypothyroidism or hyperthyroidism, metastases to lung, central nervous system tumor or metastases, cerebrovascular event
	Chronic: Dementia, pulmonary disease, mitral valve prolapse, irritable bowel syndrome, lower back or other intractable pain syndromes
Medications	Drug toxicity
	Anticholinergics, digoxin, prednisone, antihypertensive side effects, OTC cold drugs, theophylline
	Withdrawal of sedative-hypnotics (Xanax) and alcohol
Nutrition	Caffeine, vitamin deficiencies
	Difficulty swallowing
Continence	Increased frequency
	Fear of urge incontinence might underlie nocturnal arousal and anxiety
Defecation	Might experience constipation or diarrhea
Cognition	Impairment in short-term memory often underlies emergence of anxiety or depressive disorder in a susceptible person
Emotion	Check for the mood and vegetative (e.g., sleep, energy, appetite) signs of depression, hallucinations, paranoia, and delusions
	Ask about suicide
Mobility	Check for a reduction in personal and social mobility
	Review diagnoses carefully to rule out physical etiologies such as Parkinson's disease or a cerebrovascular accident
	Look for fear of falling
Cooperation with care plan	Consider anxiety, depression, or failure-to-thrive syndromes whenever physical symptoms or reduced physical function persists despite a careful review of history, physical exam, and laboratory evaluation

OTC, over the counter.

3. Classification of anxiety disorders.
   a. A traditional classification of anxiety disorders is based on patterns of behavior and symptoms demonstrated by community epidemiological studies.
   b. A neurologic theory organizes the disorders by three specific neurocircuits within the brain:
      (1) Amygdala-centered circuit underlies the symptoms of *fear* (phobic disorder, panic disorder).
      (2) Cortico-striatal-thalamic-cortical circuit underlies the symptoms of *worry* (GAD, OCD).
      (3) Hippocampal stimulation of the amygdala circuit underlies the symptoms of *flashback* (PTSD).

Specific Anxiety Disorders

1. Phobic disorder.
   a. Persistent, irrational fear of a situation, object, or activity that results in a compelling desire to avoid the phobic stimulus.
   b. Examples include agoraphobia occurring after traumatic events such as physical illness, falls, muggings, or strokes.
   c. Prevalence rate is 0% to 10 %
2. OCD.
   a. Obsessions are recurrent ideas, thoughts, or impulses that are experienced as senseless, intrusive, and persistent despite attempts to suppress them.
   b. Compulsions are repetitive, purposeful behavior performed in response to an obsession with the goal to reduce stress.
   c. The presentation of illness does not change as people grow older.
   d. Prevalence rate is 0% to 1.5%.
3. Panic disorder.
   a. Discrete period of intense fear or discomfort.
   b. The patient presents with somatic symptoms that develop abruptly and peak within 10 minutes.
   c. Prevalence rate is 0.1% to 1.0%.
4. PTSD: Symptoms of re-experienced trauma including distressing recollections, dreams, and flashbacks.

Significance in Medical Care of Older Patients

1. Anxiety disorders often underlie recurrent episodes of acute medical illness that appear resistant to best therapeutic efforts. These include patients with:
   a. Somatization.
   b. Hypochondriasis.
   c. Functional decline unexplained by medical illness.
   d. Recurrent episodes of shortness of breath (SOB) and chest pain.
   e. Hypertension.
   f. Peptic ulcer symptoms.
   g. Irritable bowel syndrome.
2. Other complications of anxiety disorders include:
   a. Alcohol abuse.
   b. Insomnia.
   c. Increased mortality of cardiovascular origin.

d. Depression.

e. Suicide.

Assessment

1. Start with a comprehensive geriatric assessment, looking especially for somatic complaints unsupported by medical illness (chest pain, SOB, insomnia, generalized pain).
2. It is important for the physician to validate the patient's perception of the symptoms.
3. The physician interviews the patient. The interview itself begins the treatment process. The physician:
   a. Phrases questions to define the patient's personality (Are you a worrier? Do you ruminate?).
   b. Obtains a developmental history outlining childhood stressors such as traumatic events, or abuse.
   c. Identifies current stressors such as recent losses or accumulated illnesses.

Treatment

1. Nonpharmacologic.
   a. Exposure therapy is the psychological treatment of choice for phobias and the rituals of OCD.
      (1) Encourages the patient to face the feared situation or object.
      (2) Occurs over a period of several weeks.
      (3) Takes place in real life and is practiced by the patient with self-exposure homework.
      (4) Allows withdrawal of any unnecessary support by family.
   b. Cognitive therapy is effective in patients with panic disorder, PTSD, OCD, and GAD.
      (1) Helps the person change expectations and interpretations of events causing the anxiety.
      (2) Identifies, evaluates, controls, and modifies negative thoughts and cognitive distortions and attributions.
      (3) Is brief (5 to 20 sessions) and highly structured.
      (4) Is carried out by a psychiatrist or psychologist trained in the procedure.
2. Pharmacologic (Table 4-12).
   a. Antidepressants are the preferred agents for managing anxiety because they are effective and they lack side effects that affect function.
      (1) TCAs: Nortriptyline 10 to 50 mg daily in single or divided doses.
      (2) SSRI: Sertraline 50 to 150 mg daily.
      (3) SNRI.
         (a) Venlafaxine 37.5 to 150 mg daily (in the morning).
         (b) Duloxetine 20 to 40 mg daily; divide doses for 40 mg.
   b. Anxiolytics.
      (1) Benzodiazepines.
         (a) Use for short term only.
         (b) Use a low dose to resolve initial symptoms pending the antidepressant effect.
         (c) Example: Lorazepam 0.5 mg to 1 mg q4-6 h.

Table 4-12 **Pharmacologic Treatment of Anxiety Disorders: Results of Controlled Studies**

Disorder	Drug					
	Benz	Busp	MAOI	Other Ant	SSRI	TCA
Generalized anxiety disorder	✓	✓		✓	✓	✓
Obsessive-compulsive disorder					✓	✓
Panic disorder	✓		✓		✓	✓
Posttraumatic stress disorder			✓		✓	✓
Social phobia	✓		✓		✓	

✓, Established efficacy; Benz, benzodiazepine; Busp, buspirone; MAOI, monoamine oxidase inhibitor; Other Ant, other antidepressants (trazodone, venlafaxine); SSRI, selective setotonin reuptake inhibitor; TCA, tricyclic antidepressant.
Data from Flint AJ: *Clin Geriatr* 9(11):21-30, 2001.

    (2) Azapirone.
        (a) Often given as augmenting agent to SSRI and SNRI.
        (b) Example: Buspirone 20 to 30 mg qd.

Major Depressive Disorder

Definition

1. Depression is a disorder of mood, a syndrome that includes a cluster of symptoms:
   a. Vegetative: Sleep, appetite, weight, sex drive.
   b. Cognitive: Attention span, frustration tolerance, memory, negative distortions.
   c. Impulse control: Suicide, homicide.
   d. Behavior: Motivation, pleasure, interest, fatigability.
   e. Somatic: Headaches, stomach aches, muscle tension.
2. In medical practice this translates into three major clinical presentations associated with depression in older patients.
   a. Community-dwelling persons who have recently experienced a significant loss and whose initial presentation is one of depressed mood and loss of pleasure, accompanied by vegetative symptoms.
   b. Recently ill or hospitalized persons whose initial presentation is primarily a failure-to-thrive or vegetative state (loss of appetite, energy, and sleep–wake rhythm) without clear symptoms of depressed mood. This group is best identified by a decline in physical and cognitive function that is out of proportion to or unexplained by the recent episode of illness (see "Failure-to-Thrive Disorder").
   c. A recent onset of delusions, hallucinations, or disruptive behavior might represent an initial presentation of depressed mood and/or a failure-to-thrive syndrome (see "Psychosis").

Epidemiology

The prevalence of depressive symptoms varies among the sites of care and residence.

1. Prevalence of significant depressive symptoms.
   a. From 8% to 15% of community-dwelling older persons.
   b. About 30% of institutionalized persons.
2. Prevalence of major depressive disorder.
   a. About 3% in community-dwelling older persons.
   b. About 11% in hospitalized older patients.
   c. About 12% in older patients in long-term care facilities.

Significance in Medical Care

1. Depression promotes the loss of physical, cognitive, and social function in older patients and prevents older persons from regaining their physical and cognitive function following treatment of acute medical illnesses. An example is poststroke depression, because patients with depression following stroke have greater impairment of activities of daily living and cognitive function and an increased risk of death.
2. Despite appropriate treatment of medical and surgical diseases, undiagnosed and/or untreated depression leads to poor patient outcomes.

Symptoms

DSM-IV-TR lists the following symptoms as diagnostic criteria for major depression in older persons:

1. Depressed mood and/or loss of interest or pleasure plus four additional criteria.
2. Additional criteria.
   a. Weight loss or gain.
   b. Insomnia or hypersomnia.
   c. Psychomotor retardation or agitation.
   d. Loss of energy.
   e. Feelings of worthlessness.
   f. Difficulty concentrating.
   g. Recurrent thoughts of death or suicide.

Treatment

1. Treatment issues.
   a. Any loss incurred by an older person can precipitate the onset of major depressive disorder.
      (1) Financial loss.
      (2) Loss of a loved one or pet.
      (3) Transition to a nursing home.
      (4) Loss of physical independence from amputation, medical illness, and loss of vision.
   b. Unstable medical illnesses must be treated in parallel with the major depression for optimal outcome.
   c. Exacerbation or relapses are typically resistant to treatment as a result of multiple comorbid illnesses. Therefore, maintenance therapy should be continued indefinitely.
   d. Common mistakes made in pharmacotherapy include:
      (1) Dose too low.

    (2) Treatment too short.

    (3) Settling for a partial response to therapy instead of complete resolution of symptoms. Careful and frequent follow-up is important.

  e. Many patients present with a mixture of cognitive, emotional, and physical dysfunction. Therefore, an optimal outcome might involve treatment with not only an antidepressant but also an antipsychotic and/or cognitive enhancer.

2. Nonpharmacologic treatment.

  a. Social support to reduce isolation, including referrals to senior centers or adult daycare.

  b. Psychotherapy, including cognitive-behavior therapy, interpersonal therapy, or group therapy.

  c. Family counseling.

  d. Substance-abuse interventions as indicated.

  e. Bereavement counseling.

  f. Health promotion and maintenance, including good nutrition, light physical exercise, attention to chronic medical conditions, and a regular daily routine.

3. Pharmacologic treatment (Table 4-13).

  a. Antidepressants.

    (1) SSRI: Sertraline, citalopram, escitalopram, paroxetine, fluoxetine.

    (2) SNRI: Venlafaxine, duloxetine.

    (3) Norepinephrine dopamine reuptake inhibitor (NDRI): Bupropione.

    (4) Combination SSRI/SNRI: Mirtazapine.

    (5) TCA: Nortriptyline, desipramine.

    (6) SARI: Trazodone, nefazodone.

  b. Psychostimulants including methylphenidate or modafinil.

Major Depressive Disorder with Psychosis

1. Psychotic symptoms associated with depression are treated by adding an atypical antipsychotic medication to the antidepressant therapy.

  a. Using both medications at the lowest effective-dose prevents additive side effects.

  b. Atypical antipsychotics.

    (1) Serotonin dopamine antagonists.

      (a) Treat agitation, delirium, psychosis.

      (b) Examples include olanzapine (Zyprexa), quetiapine (Seroquel), risperidone (Risperdal), and ziprasidone (Geodon).

    (2) Dopamine partial antagonist–agonist and serotonin antagonist–agonist (aripiprazole [Abilify]) treat agitation, psychosis, and delirium (see Table 4-7 for dosing).

2. Patients with pervasive symptoms of psychomotor retardation, anorexia, and insomnia despite appropriate pharmacologic therapy, may be referred to a geropsychiatrist, an in-patient psychiatric treatment unit, electroconvulsive therapy, and/or vagus nerve stimulation. These are appropriate next steps when counseling and antidepressant medications have not been effective in controlling symptoms. Patients who experience multiple adverse reactions to low doses of several types of antidepressants may also benefit from a referral.

Table 4-13 **Medications Useful in Treating Depression**

Medication	Dose Range	Indications	Precautions
Selective Serotonin Reuptake Inhibitors			
Citalopram	10-40 mg/day	} Depression, dysthymia, anxiety	GI upset, nausea, vomiting, insomnia
Fluoxetine	10-40 mg/day		
Paroxetine	10-40 mg/day		
Sertraline	25-150 mg/day	When sedation is desirable	Sedation, falls, hypotension
Trazodone	25-200 mg/day		
Tricyclic Antidepressants			
Desipramine	10-50 mg/day	Adjunctive pain management, neuropathic pain	Anticholinergic effects, hypotension, sedation, cardiac arrhythmias
Nortriptyline	10-50 mg/day	Highly effective for depression if patient can tolerate side effects	Anticholinergic effects, hypotension, sedation, cardiac arrhythmias
Other Agents			
Bupropion	75-225 mg/day	More activating, lack of cardiac effects	Irritability, insomnia
Cymbalta	20-40 mg/day	Adjunctive pain management, neuropathic pain	Dizziness, somnolence
Mirtazapine	7.5-30 mg/day	Useful for insomnia	Sedation, hypotension
Nefazodone	50-200 mg/day	Useful for insomnia	Sedation, hypotension. Do not use in liver disease
Venlafaxine	37.5-150 mg/day	Useful in severe depression	Hypertension may be a problem, insomnia
Psychostimulants			
Methylphenidate	2.5-20 mg/day	Often rapid onset augments antidepressant	Tachycardia, irritability, tremor, excitation, insomnia

Data from Lantz MS: *Clin Geriatr* 10(10):18-24, 2002.

3. Depressed patients with cognitive impairment might require treatment with acetylcholinesterase inhibitors as well as antidepressants.
   a. Cholinesterase inhibitors.
      (1) Donepezil (Aricept) 5 mg at bedtime for four weeks, then increase to 10 mg at bedtime.
      (2) Galantamine (Razadyne) 8 mg daily for at least four weeks, then 16 mg for at least 4 weeks, then increasing to 24 mg daily.
      (3) Rivastigmine (Exelon) 1.5 mg twice daily for two weeks, increase by 3 mg as tolerated, maximum dosage is 6 mg twice daily.
   b. NMDA subtype of glutamate receptor antagonist.
      (1) Memantine (Namenda) 5 mg daily for 1 week, then increase by 5 mg each week.
      (2) Maximum dose is 10 mg bid.
      (3) Doses >10 mg should be divided bid.

Suicide

1. Epidemiology
   a. One-fifth of all successful suicides are committed by persons older than 65 years.
   b. Men older than 69 years have the highest rate of completed suicides.
   c. The rate of completed suicides for persons age 80 to 84 years is double that of the general population.
   d. More than 75% of older persons who successfully committed suicide had been recently seen by their primary care physician, who diagnosed the first episode of major depression.[1]).
2. Patient characteristics that help to identify those at risk for committing suicide include:
   a. Male sex.
   b. Presence of painful or disabling physical illness; think particularly of impotence and incontinence following prostate surgery.
   c. Solitary living situation.
   d. Depression, especially associated with agitation, excessive guilt, self-reproach, and insomnia.
   e. Bereavement.
   f. History of previous attempt or psychiatric illness.

Failure-to-Thrive Disorder

Definition

1. Failure to thrive is a significant decline in multiple areas of functioning (cognitive, emotional, and physical) often accompanied by weight loss and loss of interest.
2. This state often follows an acute event or illness, such as hospitalization, pneumonia, chest pain, multiple falls, or fracture (Table 4-14).

Epidemiology

1. Failure to thrive affects:
   a. About 5% to 35% of community-dwelling older adults.
   b. About 25% to 40% of nursing home residents.
   c. About 50% to 60% of hospitalized veterans.
2. Lantz[2] found that the in-hospital mortality rate in patients with failure to thrive was 15.9%.

Table 4-14 **Key Domains of Failure to Thrive in Older Adults**

Domain	Features	Contributing Factors
Cognitive impairment	Apathy Behavioral disturbances Loss of functional status Loss of language skills Loss of recognition Memory loss	Dementia Medications Superimposed delirium Treatable medical conditions
Depressive features	Apathy/loss of interest Guilt Sadness/tearfulness Unhappiness Withdrawal Worthlessness	Grief and bereavement Lack of social support Isolation Multiple medications Multiple medical problems Multiple stressors Prior history of depression
Impaired physical function	Decline in activities of daily living Loss of instrumental activities of living	Acute medical problems Caregiver problems/burden Chronic medical conditions Environmental barriers Medication problems Musculoskeletal problems Sensory loss
Malnutrition	Overweight, but poor diet Weight loss	Abuse/neglect Denture problems Economic problems Medication factors Sensory loss Social stressors Swallowing disorders

Adapted from Lantz MS: *Clin Geriatr* 13(3):20-23, 2005.

Management

Establish the diagnosis by ruling out all disease or medication etiologies that might underlie the unexplained loss of physical and cognitive function.

1. Nonpharmacologic.
   a. Work with nurses, dietitian, social worker, physical therapist, and family to create an integrated care plan that addresses the

malnutrition, incontinence, constipation, confusion, immobility, and difficulty with discharge planning.
b. Initiate dietary supplements, laxatives, physical therapy, and bladder training.
c. Discuss the prognosis with the patient and family.
    (1) These patients often think they are dying, and if they are not treated, they might actually die.
    (2) They respond well to hearing that there is a treatable diagnosis.
    (3) They might respond with an increase in physical function simply by being given an accurate prognostic statement.
2. Pharmacologic: The combinations of depressive and vegetative symptoms require the use of a tricyclic, an SNRI, or an SSRI with a psychostimulant.
    a. TCAs:
        (1) Patient with anxious affect: Nortriptyline 10 to 50 mg/day.
        (2) Patient with flat affect: Desipramine 10 to 50 mg/day.
    b. SNRI antidepressants.
        (1) Patient with anxious affect: Venlafaxine 37.5 to 150 mg daily (in the morning).
        (2) Patient with flat affect: Duloxetine 20 to 40 mg daily (divided dosing for 40 mg).
    c. SSRI antidepressant and psychostimulant.
        (1) Sertraline 50 mg to 150 mg daily.
        (2) Methylphenidate 10 mg at 6:30 and 11:30 AM.
    d. Therapeutic response (improved energy, appetite, and sleep) may be seen within 3 days of achieving therapeutic level.
    e. Once the patient is stabilized (4 to 6 weeks), medication may be discontinued if all symptoms have resolved.

Bipolar Disorder

Definition

1. A lifetime history of at least one episode of mania, hypomania, or mixed mania and hypomania.
    a. Mania is a distinct period of abnormally elevated or irritable mood lasting at least 1 week. The disturbance is severe enough to impair social function and might include psychotic features.
    b. Hypomania is a distinct period of persistently elevated, expansive, or irritable mood lasting at least 4 days but with no impairment of social functioning and no psychosis.
    c. In the mixed state, the criteria for a manic episode and a major depressive disorder are met simultaneously, nearly every day, for at least 1 week. Severe social and psychotic features may be present.
2. Depressive symptoms are typical but not required. Bipolar depression, in contrast to unipolar depression, includes hypersomnia, hyperphagia, carbohydrate craving, weight gain, low energy, leaden paralysis, and mood inactivity.

Epidemiology

1. There are no prevalence data for manic symptoms in the general population of older adults.

2. Manic symptoms occur in 5% to 19% of older adults presenting to inpatient or outpatient mood disorder clinics.
3. Many people do not receive the diagnosis until late in life. Eight percent of patients with a diagnosis of bipolar disorder made their first visit to a mental health service after the age of 65 years.

Classifications

1. Bipolar I disorder is a lifetime history of at least one manic or mixed episode.
2. Bipolar II disorder is a lifetime history of a hypomanic episode but no manic episodes.
3. Cyclothymia is many episodes of depressed mood (no major depression) and episodes of hypomania occurring over 2 years.

Significance in Medical Care of Older Patients

1. Bipolar disorder is often misdiagnosed, and treatment delays can drive poor outcomes.
2. Bipolar disorder may be misdiagnosed as unipolar depression, psychosis, or disruptive behavior, and therefore there is either no response to antidepressants or there is an increase in manic symptoms.
3. Persistent irritability in family relationships can lead to early nursing home placement.
4. Incidence of alcohol and substance abuse is higher in patients with bipolar disorder and is associated with less compliance, poor response to treatment, more hospitalization, and poor psychosocial outcomes.
5. In these patients, the lifetime prevalence of anxiety disorders is 50%, and this is associated with worse outcome.

Common Substances Associated with Manic Symptoms

1. Alprazolam.
2. Anabolic steroids.
3. Antiparkinsonian medications.
4. Cocaine.
5. Corticosteroids.
6. Dextroamphetamine.
7. Hallucinogens.
8. *Hypericum perforatum* (St. John's wort).
9. Methylphenidate.
10. Opiates.

Symptoms

1. Irritability.
2. Insomnia.
3. Distractibility.
4. Grandiosity.
5. Flight of ideas.
6. Pressured speech.
7. Decreased inhibition.

Treatment

Develop a trusting and supportive relationship. The clinician must be able to deal with the patient's lack of insight and tendency to minimize the severity of symptoms.

1. Nonpharmacologic.
   a. Identify significant others who can provide timely and appropriate information.
   b. Educate the patient and family about bipolar disorder.
   c. Focus on adherence to medication regimens.
   d. Center attention on health maintenance, exercise, and diet.
   e. Offer psychosocial therapy.
2. Pharmacologic.
   a. Mood stabilizer for mania, bipolar depression, and mixed episodes (Table 4-15).
      (1) Valproic acid.
      (2) Lithium.
      (3) Lamotrigine.
   b. Atypical antipsychotic for mania, bipolar depression, and mixed episodes (Table 4-16).
      (1) Olanzapine.
      (2) Risperidone.
      (3) Quetiapine.
      (4) Aripiprazole.
   c. Antidepressant for bipolar depression (Table 4-17).
      (1) SSRI/SNRI: Use to augment lithium.
      (2) Bupropion: Mixed results in studies.
      (3) TCA: Might increase cycling to mania.

Psychosis

Definition

1. Psychosis is a syndrome, a mixture of symptoms that can be associated with many different psychotic disorders.
2. It is not a specific disorder itself. *Psychosis*, which means having delusions and/or hallucinations, generally includes symptoms such as disorganized speech, disorganized behavior, and gross distortion of reality testing.
3. Understanding the response to certain medications has led to a description of four dopamine pathways in the brain.
   a. The nigrostrial dopamine pathway is part of the extrapyramidal nervous system. Depletion leads to movement disorders, such as decreased mobility and postural changes (leaning to the left).
   b. The mesolimbic dopamine pathway relates to pleasurable sensations, delusions, and hallucinations.
   c. The mesocortical dopamine pathway mediates negative and cognitive symptoms of schizophrenia.
   d. The tuberoinfundibular dopamine pathway controls prolactin secretion.

Hallucinations

1. Hallucinations are perceptions in the visual, auditory, olfactory, or touch realms that are experienced as very real by the patient but are not experienced by the observer.
2. New onset of hallucinations occurs most often in older patients who are experiencing:
   a. Delirium and dementia.
   b. Anxiety and depression.

Table 4-15 **Mood Stabilizers for the Treatment of Bipolar Disorder**

Drug	Geriatric Dose Range	Geriatric Therapeutic Range	Side Effects	Comments
Carbamazepine	200-1000 mg/day	4-12 μg/mL	Nausea, fatigue, ataxia, blurred vision, hyponatremia	Poor tolerability in older adults Must monitor CBC, LFTs, electrolytes every 2 weeks for first 2 months, then every 3 months
Lamotrigine	25-200 mg/day Must titrate slowly, 25 mg per week	Not known	Headache, nausea, infections, rash	Little geriatric data May be useful for bipolar depression
Lithium*	150-1200 mg/day	0.5-1.0 mEq/L	Nausea, vomiting, tremor, confusion, leukocytosis	Poor tolerability in older adults Toxicity at low serum levels Monitor thyroid and renal function
Valproate*	250-2000 mg/day	40-100 μg/mL	Nausea, GI upset, ataxia, sedation	Requires monitoring CBC, platelets, LFTs at baseline and every 6 months

*Food and Drug Administration approved for treatment of bipolar disorder.
CBC, complete blood count; GI, gastrointestinal; LFTs, liver function tests.
Adapted from Lantz MS: *Clin Geriatr* 11(7):19-22, 2003.

Table 4-16 Antipsychotic Agents for Treating Bipolar Disorder

Drug	Geriatric Dose Range	Side Effects	Comments
Aripiprazole	5-15 mg/day	Mild sedation, mild hypotension	Newest agent Well tolerated Few studies with geriatric patients
Olanzapine	2.5-10 mg/day	Sedation, falls, gait disturbance	FDA approved for acute mania
Quetiapine	25-300 mg/day	Sedation, hypotension	FDA approved for acute mania
Risperidone	0.5-2 mg/day	EPS, sedation, hypotension	Warning regarding cerebrovascular events in patients with dementia

EPS, extrapyramidal side effects; FDA, U.S. Food and Drug Administration.
Adapted from Lantz MS: *Clin Geriatr* 11(7):19-22, 2003.

Table 4-17 Antidepressants for Treating Bipolar Disorder

Medication	Dose Range	Indications	Precautions
Selective Serotonin Reuptake Inhibitors			
Citalopram	10-40 mg/day	Depression, dysthymia, anxiety	GI upset, nausea, vomiting, insomnia
Fluoxetine	10-40 mg/day		
Paroxetine	10-40 mg/day		
Sertraline	25-150 mg/day		
Trazodone	25-200 mg/day	When sedation is desirable	Sedation, falls, hypotension
Tricyclic Antidepressants			
Desipramine	10-50 mg/day	Adjunctive pain management, neuropathic pain	Anticholinergic effects, hypotension, sedation, cardiac arrhythmias
Nortriptyline	10-50 mg/day	High efficacy for depression if patient can tolerate side effects	Anticholinergic effects, hypotension, sedation, cardiac arrhythmias
Other Agents			
Bupropion	75-225 mg/day	More activating, lack of cardiac effects	Irritability, insomnia
Cymbalta	20-40 mg/day	Adjunctive pain management, neuropathic pain	
Mirtazapine	7.5-30 mg/day	Useful for insomnia	Sedation, hypotension
Nefazodone	50-200 mg/day	Useful for insomnia	Sedation, hypotension
Venlafaxine	37.5-150 mg/day	Useful in severe depression	Do not use in liver disease; Hypertension may be a problem; Insomnia

Data from Lantz MS: *Clin Geriatr* 11(7):19-22, 2003.

    c. Loss of vision (Charles Bonnet syndrome) and hearing.

    d. Extreme old age.

    e. Social isolation.

3. Diagnosis.

    a. Assessment for dementia and delirium (see earlier).

    b. Assessment for offending medications (see Chapter 7).

    c. Assessment for anxiety and depression (see earlier).

    d. In cognitively intact persons, assess for social isolation, anxiety, extreme age, and loss of vision and hearing.

    e. Ask about inadequate lighting.

    f. Given the multiple etiologies and the anxiety that hallucinations provoke in patients and caregivers, comprehensive geriatric assessment is suggested for patients who present with hallucinations (see Chapter 2).

4. Treatment issues.

    a. General.

      (1) Whenever hallucinations are frightening or lead to disruption in the behavior of the patient, treatment is indicated.

      (2) Patients appear truly unable to discern any difference between their hallucinatory and real perceptions.

      (3) Reassurance should be focused on the experienced feeling (e.g., fear), not on the patient's distortion of time and space.

      (4) Particularly in patients without delirium, failure to validate their reality often frustrates and angers them. In this situation, it is appropriate and helpful to validate feelings without correcting the time-space orientation.

      (5) Time-space orientation is more useful as a long-term environmental strategy to structure daily activities for cognitively impaired persons.

    b. Delirium.

      (1) The hallucinations that accompany the agitation of delirium should resolve with:

        (a) Appropriate treatment of the underlying systemic disorder.

        (b) Removal of the offending medications.

        (c) Short-term treatment with an atypical antipsychotic (see earlier).

      (2) If the hallucinations do not resolve, the patient should be carefully evaluated for more long-term causes of hallucinations (dementia, loss of hearing and vision, extreme old age).

    c. Dementia: The most common hallucinatory syndrome of dementia is referred to as *sundowning* because of its onset between 4 and 6 PM.

      (1) The most accepted theory of the cause of sundowning is centered on the dysfunction of circadian rhythm.

      (2) Prevalence of sundowning ranges between 2.4% and 66% in institutionalized dementia patients.

      (3) It is more common in the winter, in new and stressful situations, and in patients with concurrent anxiety and depression.

      (4) It is important to note that a patient may be alert and reasonably coherent on morning rounds and completely out of control at sundown; trust the family and nurses.

(5) Patients are often unable to articulate the content of the hallucinations and often wander aimlessly or appear agitated.

(6) Nonpharmacologic treatment.

    (a) Provide bright light during the late morning hours between 9:30 and 11:30 AM significantly lowers patients' agitation during the evening.

    (b) Provide low lights at bedtime.

    (c) No daytime napping.

(7) Pharmacologic treatment.

    (a) There are mixed reviews on the use of melatonin (6 mg hs).

    (b) Regular treatment with low doses of atypical antipsychotics in early afternoon.

    (c) Regular treatment with low doses of valproic acid in the early afternoon.

    (d) Acetylcholinesterase inhibitors improve cognitive function, increase daytime activity, and reduce evening agitation.

d. Loss of hearing and vision.

    (1) In otherwise healthy and cognitively intact patients, these hallucinations are not frightening and do not have to be treated with medication.

    (2) Every attempt should be made to optimize vision and hearing by medical referrals and by changes in the person's home environment (e.g., improved lighting and telephones with volume controls).

    (3) Social isolation exacerbates these hallucinations.

e. Extreme old age.

    (1) In otherwise healthy and cognitively intact persons, hallucinations can occur, especially in times of stress or with social isolation.

    (2) These hallucinations often involve visions of people who have already died, such as parents or spouse, and have the characteristics of a dream state, except the older person feels that the visions are really happening.

    (3) These patients are also particularly susceptible to drug-induced delirium with hallucinations.

    (4) Medication with methylphenidate 5 to 10 mg/day sometimes helps the patient to keep these dreamlike hallucinations from impinging on their waking state.

f. Social isolation.

    (1) Isolation often exacerbates hallucinations in persons with other predisposing problems.

    (2) Patients with cognitive, vision, or hearing impairments are often isolated from human interaction despite living in nursing homes or with others.

    (3) The stimulation of caring human interaction is often the safest and most effective therapy for these hallucinations.

Paranoia

1. Definition.

    a. Paranoia is a state of abnormal suspiciousness that can evolve into a delusional state under the stress of aging, acute illness, dementia, and social isolation.

b. A person may have vague complaints of external forces plotting against him or her. This usually begins in early adulthood. As the paranoid person grows older, the degree of paranoia can increase and grow into a delusional disorder.

c. Under the perception of a loss of control, these beliefs become a focus and are often directed at adult children.

d. With memory loss, an inability to find one's personal belongings or way in a familiar setting is often the trigger for suspecting others of plotting against one.

2. Epidemiology.

a. Between 2% and 5% of community-dwelling older persons exhibit abnormal suspiciousness.

b. The prevalence of delusions and hallucinations in older persons is 4% to 5%.

c. Paraphrenia is often associated with female sex, social isolation, and a past history of difficult social interactions.

3. Diagnosis.

a. Patients with paraphrenia or paranoid delusions are usually willing to discuss them with a sympathetic clinician.

b. One question often serves to identify patients who are paranoid: "Is anyone trying to harm you?"

4. Assessment: Whenever an older person experiences persistent delusional thinking or hallucinations, an assessment for dementia, delirium (see earlier), offending medications (see Chapter 7), depression, or an anxiety disorder (see above) should be completed.

5. Treatment.

a. A trusting and supportive relationship.

(1) The clinician is willing to listen to complaints and fears but must not deceive the patient by pretending to agree with paranoid beliefs.

(2) Responding to and validating the emotional affect of the complaints and hallucinations are important.

b. Atypical antipsychotics (see Tables 4-7 and 4-9).

(1) Paranoid patients often require long-term therapy and must be monitored carefully for extrapyramidal side effects, increased sedation, hyperprolactinemia, and cognitive impairment.

(2) Although 1.5% of patients may be at increased risk for cardiovascular disease, previously used antipsychotics such as haloperidol carry a risk of 4.5%. These risks should be discussed with patients and their families.

(a) Serotonin dopamine antagonists, such as olanzapine (Zyprexa), quetiapine (Seroquel), risperidone (Risperdal), ziprasidone (Geodon).

(b) Dopamine partial antagonist–agonist and serotonin antagonist–agonist (aripiprazole [Abilify]).

c. Cooperation with treatment depends on the level of trust. Assuring the older patient that the medication will help improve sleep and decrease anxiety and working with the family will help ensure initial compliance.

Sleep Disorders

Definition

Disordered sleep includes difficulty falling asleep, not being able to stay asleep, and not feeling restored by sleep.

Epidemiology

1. Thirty percent of people in the general population complain of sleep difficulties.
2. This fraction increases to approximately 50% for those older than 65 years.
3. Forty-three percent have difficulty initiating or maintaining sleep; 30% have nocturnal wakening; 13% awake without feeling rested.
4. The highest prevalence appears to be in older people in poor health (Table 4-18).

Consequences

1. Fatigue, malaise, and impairment of social and vocational function.
2. Loss of motivation, energy, and initiative.
3. Somatic symptoms such as headaches and GI dysfunction.
4. Cognitive impairment, including decreased attention, slow response time, and impairment in memory.

Table 4-18 Epidemiology of Sleep Disorders by ASD Classification

Clinical Problem	Estimated Incidence
Disorders of Initiating and Maintaining Sleep	
Psychiatric problem	18%-47%
Sleep apnea	16%-18%
Nocturnal myoclonus	0%-33%
Psychophysiologic problem	21%-31%
Drugs and alcohol	21%
Restless legs	5%
Symptoms of organic disease (e.g., arthritic pain, nocturia, nocturnal dyspnea, chronic brain syndrome)	Common; exact incidence unknown
Disorders of Excessive Sleepiness	
Sleep apnea	28%-71%
Nocturnal myoclonus	16%
Narcolepsy	11%-29%
Drugs	Common
Miscellaneous (e.g., postinfection fatigue, chronic brain syndrome)	?Common
Disrupted Sleep–Wake Cycle	
Early morning arousal, evening drowsiness	?Common
Parasomnias	?Less common
Abnormal sleep behavior (e.g., nocturnal confusion, wandering, seizures)	?Less common

ASD, Association of Sleep Disorders.

5. Impairment of driving skills and increased risk of falls.
6. Increased mortality (two times higher) from heart disease, stroke, and suicide.

Causes

1. Age-related changes.
   a. Reduction in time spent in deeper levels of sleep, stages 3 and 4. This results in lighter sleep and increased awakening.
   b. Circadian rhythm disturbances such as advanced sleep phase syndrome. This results in sleepiness in the early evening and waking up at 3 or 4 AM. Loss of neurons in the suprachiasmatic nucleus of the hypothalamus might account for this finding.
2. Primary sleep disorders.
   a. Periodic limb movement in sleep.
   b. Restless legs syndrome (RLS).
   c. Sleep disorder breathing.
   d. Rapid eye movement (REM) sleep behavior disorder.
3. Medical psychiatric illnesses.
4. Medications.
5. Psychosocial factors.

Diagnosis

1. Database.
   a. Chief complaint.
      (1) Patients have difficulty falling asleep, staying awake during the day, or staying asleep for the entire night.
      (2) They complain that they do not feel refreshed by the hours that they do sleep.
      (3) Demented patients are often brought by the family or nursing home caretakers.
      (4) Sleep apnea patients are also most often identified by family.
   b. Initial screen of hearing, vision, and cognitive function because short-term memory impairments often underlie sleep disorders.
   c. Biomedical and psychosocial history.
      (1) Table 4-14 outlines the many interacting biomedical and psychosocial factors that can underlie a sleep disorder in an older person.
      (2) Nocturia, leg twitches, SOB, or nightmares can awaken.
      (3) Worrying can prevent initiation of sleep.
      (4) Early morning awakening or extended morning sleep suggests depression.
   d. Physical exam: Focus on signs of the primary and secondary diseases that can underlie a sleep disorder, such as obesity and hypertension in sleep apnea or occult CHF.
   e. Laboratory and diagnostic evaluation.
      (1) Blood alcohol levels.
      (2) Blood levels of medications.
      (3) Oxygen levels or degree of oxygen saturation.
      (4) Electrolytes.
2. Assessment: Patient data are integrated and organized in the problem list (Table 4-19).

Table 4-19 **Assessment of Sleep Disorders**

Area of Concern	Focus of Assessment
Diagnosis	Primary: Sleep apnea syndrome, periodic leg movements, restless legs syndrome, sleep disorder breathing, REM sleep behavior disorder
	Secondary: Arthritis and other pain syndromes; respiratory or cardiac diseases
Medications	Timing of medications such as sympathomimetics or diuretics
	Long-term use of alcohol or sedative-hypnotics
	Nightmares initiated by propranolol, levodopa, reserpine, or withdrawal of benzodiazepines or alcohol
Nutrition	Timing or excessive use of coffee, tea, and soft drinks containing caffeine before bedtime
Continence	Fear of or actual urge-type incontinence in an aware patient
Defecation	Fear of or actual fecal incontinence
Cognition	Delirium
	Dementia
Emotion	Anxiety disorders with arousal
	Depression
	Nightmares (dream anxiety)
	Paranoid ideation
Mobility	Immobility secondary to illness or sedentary lifestyle
Cooperation with care plan	Alcohol use
	Learned behavior incompatible with sleep

REM, rapid eye movement.

3. Care plan.
   a. Within each area of concern listed in Table 4-19, assess and identify the reversible or potentially treatable etiologic factors underlying the sleep disorder.
   b. Make treatment recommendations consistent with the standard of medical practice for each problem listed.
   c. Reconcile recommendations against the patient's preference for treatment.

Treatment

1. Approach.
   a. If the etiologic factors are assessed and appropriately treated, older patients will achieve an adequate amount of sleep to maintain their quality of life and ADLs.
   b. Anxiety disorders and depression are the most common causes of sleep disorders in older patients.

    c. If no clear-cut diagnostic factor is apparent and the older patient is still symptomatic, consider bedtime medication, which may be effective in reestablishing a normal sleep-wake rhythm or cycle.

    d. Bright lighting (300 to 500 watts halogen) from 4 to 9 PM, especially from September to March, can help regulate the diurnal rhythm and improve nighttime sleep.

    e. The basic elements of therapy of sleep disturbances are summarized in Table 4-20.

2. Nonpharmacologic.
    a. Bright light therapy.
    b. Relaxation therapy.
    c. Sleep restriction (curtail hours in bed).
    d. Sleep hygiene education (reduced noise and light).

Table 4-20 Treatment of Sleep Disorders in Older Patients

Area of Concern	Recommendation
Primary Area: Sleep Disorders	
Periodic leg movement	Dopamine agonist (Requip) 1 mg in evening
Sleep apnea syndrome	Weight loss, nasal oxygen, tracheostomy, referral to sleep disorder center
Secondary Area: Diseases	
Pain	Acetaminophen 650 -1000 mg q4h scheduled
Shortness of breath	Optimize respiratory and cardiac function
Medications	Discontinue or replace offending drugs; introduce others
	Initiate alcohol withdrawal and treatment program
Nutrition	Minimize or alter timing of stimulants (coffee, tea, soda)
	Initiate alcohol treatment program
Continence	Evaluate and treat urinary incontinence
Defecation	Evaluate and treat constipation, impaction, or fecal incontinence
Cognition	Evaluate and treat delirium
	Evaluate and treat dementia
Emotion	Treat anxiety, depression, and paranoia
	Introduce relaxation therapy
Mobility	Advise patient that daytime activities such as social involvement, and regular physical exercise can improve sleep
Cooperation with care plan	Encourage patient to regularize and curtail hours in bed and be physically and socially active during the daytime
	Encourage patient to create an optimal environment for sleep (reduced noise and light)

3. Pharmacologic.
   a. Herbal sleep inducers: California poppy, hops, Jamaican dogwood, passion flower, valerian, chamomile, lime blossom, red clover (drink as a tea or soak in a bath).
   b. Hormonal or naturopathic: Melatonin 3 to 6 mg hs.
   c. Sedating antidepressants: Trazadone 50 to 200 mg hs.
   d. Hypnotics: Ambien (Zolpidem) 5 to 10 mg hs.
   e. Dopamine agonists: Requip 0.5 to 1 mg in the evening.

Disruptive Behavior

Definition

As people age and become dependent on their families and other caretakers, certain kinds of behavior can emerge that is disruptive to the caretaking relationship.

1. Disruptive behavior is any activity of a patient perceived by nurses or family caretakers to be physically or emotionally harmful to the patient, other patients in proximity, or the caretakers themselves.
2. Disruptive behavior can include:
   a. Disturbed physical behavior, including striking out, physical abuse of others, self-destructive behavior, throwing objects around the room, and restless agitation.
   b. Resistance to restriction: Patient removes Foley catheter or IV lines, wanders out of the house or off the unit, enters others' rooms.
   c. Resistance to physical care: Patient spits out or refuses medications, spits out food, resists assistance with ADLs.
   d. Disturbed verbal behavior including screams and yells, verbal abuse or threats, repetitive vocalizations.
   e. Disturbed social behavior: Patient urinates/defecates in inappropriate places, takes others' belongings, hoards items, behaves sexually inappropriately.

Factors Influencing Disruptive Behavior

1. Patient characteristics include cognitive impairment, hallucinations, delusions, physical health status, immobility, and incontinence.
2. Characteristics of the physical and social environment include noise level, inadequate lighting, relocation from familiar to unfamiliar places, physical restraints, and family malfunctioning.
3. Characteristics of caretakers include expectations or tolerance of certain behavior, educational experience, ethnic background, and stress or frustration tolerance levels.

Epidemiology

1. The prevalence of disruptive behavior in nursing home patients is 25% to 30%.
2. Eighty percent of patients who exhibit disruptive behavior have cognitive impairments.
3. Disruptive patients with cognitive impairments are more likely to also have hallucinations.

Significance in Medical and Long-Term Care

1. Disruptive behavior can become a major obstacle to diagnosis and treatment of medical diseases and the provision of long-term care.

Table 4-21 **Management of the Disruptive Older Patient**	
Area of Concern	**Recommendations**
Diagnosis	Treat all active medical diseases
Medications	Remove or replace medications that can adversely affect patient
Nutrition	Respect patient's preferences for types of food and eating site
Continence	Evaluate and treat incontinence
	Place commode near bed
Defecation	Initiate bowel program to structure appropriate behavior
Cognition	Evaluate and treat delirium and any hallucinations
	Document degree of cognitive impairment
Emotion	Target pharmacologic treatments to specific states
	Anxiety, agitation
	Depression
	Paranoia
	Delusions
Mobility	Optimize patient's mobility
Cooperation with care plan	Understand premorbid personality and family function and structure care appropriately

2. Attempts to manage disruptive behavior with physical and chemical restraints often lead to progressive declines in patients' physical, cognitive, and emotional function and an increased susceptibility to falls and infections.

Diagnosis

1. Disruptive behavior is not a diagnostic term, and many different factors can interact to promote it in each patient.
2. Comprehensive geriatric assessment (see Chapter 2) is useful in systematically documenting and treating the various etiologic factors.

Management

Table 4-21 outlines the steps in the management of disruptive patients.

REFERENCES

1. Hall RCW, Hall RCW, Chapman MJ: Identifying geriatric patients at risk for suicide and depression. *Clin Geriatr* 11(10):36-44, 2003.
2. Lantz MS: Failure to thrive. *Clin Geriatr* 13(3):20-23, 2005.

SUGGESTED READINGS

Al Jurdi R, Pulakhandam S, Kunik ME, Marangell L: Late-life mania: Assessment and treatment of late-life manic symptoms. *Geriatrics* 60(10):18-20, 22-23, 2005.
Flint AJ: Anxiety disorders. *Clin Geriatr* 9(11):21-30, 2001.
Khouzam HR, Battista MA, Emes R, Ahles S: Psychoses in late life: Evaluation and management of disorders seen in primary care. *Geriatrics* 60(3):26-33, 2005.
Kim P, Louis C, Muralee S, Tampi RR: Sundowning syndrome in the older patient. *Clin Geriatr* 15(4):32-36, 2005.

Lantz MS: Bipolar disorder in the older adult. *Clin Geriatr* 11(7):19-22, 2003.

Lantz MS: Depression in the elderly: Recognition and treatment. *Clin Geriatr* 10(10):18-24, 2002.

Lantz MS: Failure to thrive. *Clin Geriatr* 13(3):20-23, 2005.

Mathews M, Mathews M, Budur K, et al: Post-stroke depression. *Clin Geriatr* 12(10):35-38, 2004.

McCall WV: Diagnosis and management of insomnia in older people. *J Am Geriatr Soc* 53(7 suppl):S272-S277, 2005.

Stahl SM: Essential Psychopharmacology: Neuroscientific Basis and Practical Applications, 2nd ed. Cambridge, Cambridge University Press, 2000.

St. John D: Bipolar affective disorder: Diagnosis and current treatments. *Clinician Reviews* 15(6):44-49, 2005.

4.6 Mobility

Marsha D. Fretwell and Deborah Adams Wingate

OVERVIEW

1. The ability to move freely in the home environment and the larger community environment is critical to the physical and emotional independence that is valued by many older patients.
2. Older patients with profound slowness or an abnormal pattern of ambulation have a gait disorder.
3. Gait velocity remains stable until age 70 years, then declines by 15% per decade.
4. Walking without assistance requires the effective coordination of adequate sensation, musculoskeletal and motor control, and attention.

Gait Disorders

1. Diagnoses common in persons with gait disorders.
   a. Neurologic diseases.
      (1) Cerebrovascular accidents (CVAs).
      (2) Parkinson's disease.
      (3) Normal-pressure hydrocephalus.
      (4) Peripheral neuropathy.
      (5) Cerebellar ataxia.
      (6) Subdural hematoma.
      (7) Vitamin B_{12} deficiency.
      (8) Cervical tumors and spondylosis.
      (9) Progressive supranuclear palsy.
      (10) Spinal stenosis and pseudoclaudication syndrome.
      (11) Chronic pain.
   b. Other diseases.
      (1) Hypothyroidism.
      (2) Hyperthyroidism.
      (3) Unsuspected fractures.
      (4) Osteoarthritis.
      (5) Osteoporosis with kyphosis.
2. Medications.
   a. Review all medications, including over-the-counter medication.
   b. Consider stopping any medication that causes hypotension, dopamine depletion, proximal muscle weakness, or oversedation (see Chapter 7).

3. Nutrition.
   a. Folate, thiamine, pyridoxine, vitamin B_{12} deficiencies, vitamin D deficiency.
   b. Protein malnutrition.
   c. Alcohol abuse.
   d. Obesity.
4. Cognition.
   a. Delirium.
   b. Dementia (especially frontotemporal and Lewy body).
5. Emotion.
   a. Fear of falling or physically expressed anxiety disorder.
   b. Depression and failure-to-thrive syndromes at the end of hospitalization for acute illness.
6. Cooperation with care plan.
   a. Sedentary lifestyle.
   b. Environmental and social barriers.

Falls

1. Falls are common in older adults.
   a. About 30% to 40% of community-dwelling older persons fall each year.
   b. About 50% of nursing home residents fall each year.
2. Falls and fractures.
   a. Most falls are not associated with fractures, but more than 90% of hip fractures are the result of a fall.
   b. Fear of falling causes as many as 50% of older patients to limit their activities in some way to avoid falls.
   c. The most common factors associated with falls as a cause of hip fracture include:
      (1) Diagnoses.
         (a) Parkinson's disease.
         (b) CVA.
         (c) Visual impairment.
         (d) Lower-body weakness.
      (2) Medications, especially taking four or more or taking any psychoactive medication.
         (a) Sedative-hypnotics: Short-acting and long-acting benzodiazepines.
         (b) Anticholinergics.
         (c) Long-acting barbiturates.
         (d) Antidepressants: TCAs.
         (e) Antihypertensive drugs: α-adrenergics.
      (3) Nutrition.
         (a) Low body mass index.
         (b) Postprandial orthostatic hypotension.

DIAGNOSIS

1. Database (Table 4-22 lists predisposing risk factors and potential intervention).
   a. Chief complaint: History of a fall, problems with balance, a gradual reduction in mobility, or no complaints are the usual presentation for an older person who has a gait disorder.

Table 4-22 Predisposing Risk Factors and Potential Interventions

Risk Factor	Potential Interventions
Sensory	
Hearing	Cerumen removal; hearing aid
Vestibular: drugs, previous infections, surgery, benign positional vertigo	Avoid toxic drugs; surgery; balance exercises; good lighting
Vision: close-range and distance perception, dark adaptation	Appropriate refraction, surgery, medications, good lighting
Proprioceptive	
Cervical: arthritis, spondylosis	Balance exercises; surgery
Peripheral nerves, spinal cord	Treatment of underlying disease; good lighting; appropriate walking aid and footwear
Central Nervous System	
Any central nervous system disease impairing problem solving and judgment	Treatment of underlying disease; supervised, structured, safe environment
Musculoskeletal	
Arthritides, especially lower extremities	Medical and possibly surgical treatment of underlying disease
Foot disorders: bunions, calluses, deformities	Podiatry; appropriate footwear
Muscle weakness, contractures	Strengthening exercises; balance and gait training; appropriate adaptive devices
Systemic Diseases	
Cardiac, respiratory, metabolic diseases	Treatment of underlying diseases
Postural hypotension	Hydration; lowest effective dosage of necessary medications; reconditioning exercises; elevation of head of bed; stockings
Other	
Depression	Carefully consider risk-to-benefit ratio of antidepressant medication
Environment	Environmental hazard checklist; appropriate adaptations and manipulations
Medications: all, but especially sedating medications	Lowest effective dosage of essential medications, starting low and increasing slowly

Adapted from Coogler CE, Wolf SL: Falls. In Hazzard WR, Blass JP, Ettinger WH, et al (eds): *Principles of geriatric medicine and gerontology.* New York, McGraw-Hill, 1999, pp 1535-1546.

   b. Initial screen of vision, hearing, and cognition: Difficulty with distance vision and a mild impairment in short-term memory may be present.
   c. Medical history: Review the treatable causes of a gait disorder.
      (1) Delirium.
      (2) Hypothyroidism and hyperthyroidism.
      (3) Parkinson's disease.
      (4) A series of small CVAs.
      (5) Medications that can influence balance, blood pressure, and alertness.
      (6) Symptoms of vitamin deficiencies.
      (7) Weight loss.
   d. Psychosocial history: Check for anxiety about:
      (1) Ambulation.
      (2) Depression.
      (3) Dependent personality.
      (4) Physical and social barriers to ambulation outside the home.
   e. Physical exam to detect deficits in motor, balance, and/or skeletal and joint function.
      (1) Orthostatic hypotension.
      (2) Arrhythmia.
      (3) Carotid or vertebrobasilar artery involvement.
      (4) Decreased vision.
      (5) Loss of balance and increased sway.
      (6) Deforming arthritis.
      (7) Limitation of joint range of motion.
      (8) Bradykinesia.
      (9) Tremor.
      (10) Decreased vibratory sense.
      (11) Asymmetric motor signs.
   f. Table 4-23 shows the performance-oriented evaluation of balance and gait.
2. Laboratory evaluation.
   a. Electrolytes, BUN, calcium, magnesium, glucose, thyroid function, CBC, folate, vitamin B_{12}, vitamin D, blood levels of ethanol and current medications.
   b. CT or MRI for patients with motor signs, gait apraxia of frontal origins, or ataxia of cerebellar origin.
   c. Cervical spine films for those with bilateral long-tract signs.
   d. Neurophysiologic studies in patients with sensory abnormalities.
      (1) Electromyography.
      (2) Nerve-conduction studies.
      (3) Testing of evoked potentials.

MANAGEMENT OF GAIT DISORDERS AND PREVENTION OF FALLS

1. Establish cause of gait disorder and/or fall. Causes may be multifactorial.
2. Treat specific causes.
   a. Diagnoses.
      (1) Parkinson's disease.
      (2) Vitamin B_{12} deficiency.

Table 4-23   Performance-Oriented Evaluation of Balance and Gait

Abnormal Maneuver	Possible Causes[a]	Possible Therapeutic or Rehabilitative Measures[b]	Possible Preventive or Adaptive Measures[b]
Difficulty rising from chair	Proximal muscle weakness (many causes) Arthritides (especially involving hips and knees) Parkinson's disease Hemiparesis or paraparesis Deconditioning	Treatment of specific disease states (e.g., with steroids, L-dopa) Hip and quadriceps exercises Transfer training	High, firm chair with arms Raised toilet seats Ejection chairs
Instability on first standing	Postural hypotension Cerebellar disease Multisensory deficits Lower-extremity weakness or pain Foot pain causing reduced weight bearing	Treatment of specific diseases (e.g., adequate salt and fluid status, fludrocortisone)	Slow rising Head of bed on blocks Supportive aid (e.g., walker, quadcane)
Instability with nudge on sternum or pull test	Parkinson's syndrome Back problems Normal-pressure hydrocephalus ?Peripheral neuropathy Deconditioning	Treatment of specific diseases (e.g., with L-dopa, shunt) ?Back exercises Analgesia ?Balance exercises (e.g., Frankel's)	Obstacle-free environment Appropriate walking aid (cane, walker) Night-lights (less likely to fall or bump into an object) Close observation with acute illness (high risk of falling) Avoidance of slippers

Instability with eyes closed (stable with eyes open)	Multisensory deficits, Reduced proprioception, position sense (e.g., B_{12} deficiency, diabetes mellitus)	Treatment of specific diseases (e.g., B_{12} deficiency), Correction of visual, hearing problems	Bright lights, Night-lights, Cane
Instability on neck turning or extension	Cervical arthritis, Cervical spondylosis, Vertebral-basilar insufficiency	?Balance exercises, ?Antiarthritic medication, ?Cervical collar, ?Neck exercises	Avoidance of quick turns, Turning of body, not just head, Storage of objects in home low enough to avoid need to look up, Appropriate walking aid, Obstacle-free environment, Properly fitting shoes
Instability on turning	Cerebellar disease, Hemiparesis, Visual field cut, Reduced proprioception, Mild ataxia	Gait training, ?Proprioceptive exercises	
Unsafeness on sitting down (misjudges distance or falls into chair)	Reduced vision, Proximal myopathies, Apraxia	Treatment of specific diseases, ?Coordination training, Leg-strengthening exercises	High, firm chairs with arms, in good repair, Transfer training

*This is not an exhaustive list.
†Most of these measures have not been subjected to clinical trials; evidence for effectiveness is usually anecdotal at best.
‡Patients often have a flexed posture with all of these conditions.
Adapted from Coogler CE, Wolf SL: Falls. In Hazzard WR, Blass JP, Ettinger WH, et al (eds): *Principles of geriatric medicine and gerontology.* New York, McGraw-Hill, 1999, pp 1535-1546.

Continued

Table 4-23 **Performance-Oriented Evaluation of Balance and Gait—cont'd**

Abnormal Maneuver	Possible Causes	Possible Therapeutic or Rehabilitative Measures	Possible Preventive or Adaptive Measures
Decreased step height and length (bilateral)‡	Parkinson's syndrome Pseudobulbar palsy Myelopathy (usually spastic gait) Normal-pressure hydrocephalus Advanced Alzheimer's disease (frontal lobe gait) Compensation for reduced vision or proprioception Fear of falling Habit	Treatment of specific diseases (e.g., with L-dopa) Vision correction Gait training (correct problems, suggest compensations, increase confidence)	Avoidance of throw rugs Good lighting Proper footwear (good fit, not too much friction or slipperiness) Appropriate walking aid

(3) Vitamin D deficiency.
(4) Cervical spondylosis.
(5) Control of arthritis pain.
(6) Syncope (see Chapter 5).

b. Medications.
   (1) Remove or replace all medications that interfere with motor, balance, or joint functioning.
   (2) Acetaminophen 650 to 1000 mg every 4 to 6 hours while awake is an excellent strategy for pain management of arthritis.

c. Nutrition.
   (1) Make sure the patient is replete with vitamin D, vitamin B_{12}, and protein.
   (2) Instruct the patient to rise slowly after meals.

d. Continence.
   (1) Evaluate and modify the bathroom with nonslip tiles, grab bars, and an elevated toilet seat.
   (2) Treat urge incontinence.

e. Cognition: treat delirium or metabolic encephalopathy.

f. Emotion.
   (1) Treat fear of falling as any other chronic and debilitating anxiety disorder (see "Anxiety" earlier).
   (2) Treat failure-to-thrive syndromes (see "Failure-to-Thrive Disorder" earlier).

g. Mobility.
   (1) Physical therapy.
       (a) Gait training and recommendations for ongoing muscle-strengthening exercises.
       (b) Focus on increasing lower-body strength and improving balance.
   (2) Evaluate the home environment.
       (a) Remove loose throw rugs.
       (b) Secure all handrails.
       (c) Clear clutter in stairways.
       (d) Tack down loose carpet edges.
   (3) Provide opportunities for socialization and encouragement. Tai chi is a proven resource.[1]

h. Cooperation with care plan.
   (1) Educate the patient and family on the importance of all factors leading to gait disorders, immobility, and falling.
   (2) Emphasize the importance of daily physical exercise, motivation to change long-standing health behavior, and reorganization of the home.

REFERENCES

1. Li F, Harmer P, Fisher KH, et al: Tai chi and fall reductions in older adults: A randomized controlled trial. *J Gerontol Biol Sci Med Sci* 60:187-194, 2005.

SUGGESTED READINGS

Flicker L, MacInnis RJ, Stein MS, et al: Should older people in residential care receive vitamin D to prevent falls? Results of a randomized trial. *J Am Geriatr Soc* 53:1881-1888, 2005.

King MB, Tinetti ME: A multifactorial approach to reducing injurious falls. *Clin Geriatric Med* 12:745-759, 1996

Li F, Harmer P, Fisher KH, et al: Tai chi and fall reductions in older adults: A randomized controlled trial. *J Gerontol Biol Sci Med Sci* 60:187-194, 2005.

Sudarsky L: Geriatrics: Gait disorders in the elderly, *N Engl J Med* 322:1441-1446, 1990.

Tromp AM, Pluijm SM, Smit JH, et al: Fall-risk screening test: A prospective study on predictors for falls in the community-dwelling elderly. *Clin Epid* 54: 837-844, 2001.

4.7 Sexuality and Aging

Tom J. Wachtel

SEXUAL ACTIVITY IN OLDER ADULTS

1. Overview.
   a. Human sexual expression is a multifactorial end point, which to date has been studied inadequately in the aged.
   b. Lopsided demographics combined with older male spouses in the majority of married couples, societal norms and expectations (current and, perhaps more relevant, from the early 20th century), environmental and functional limitations, comorbidities, and physiologic changes of sexual function can all interplay and contribute to decreased sexual activity in older adults.
2. Demographics.
   a. Women outlive men in the U.S. population (1987); they have a 7-year longer life expectancy.
   b. Elderly women are more likely to be widowed because they outlive men (Table 4-24).
      (1) Women have longer life expectancy.
      (2) Women outlive their husbands because they are typically younger than their husbands.
3. Societal norms and expectations.
   a. Religious beliefs: sex as a means to procreate only.
   b. Linkage of sexual desirability to youthful appearance.
   c. Less permissive sexuality among older cohorts, thereby linking sex to marriage at a time when widowhood increases exponentially.
   d. Unwillingness by adult children to accept or support new intimate relationships for their widowed parent.

Table 4-24 **Marital Status**

Age (y)	Marital Status		
	Married	**Widowed**	**Other**
Men			
65-74	79.5%	9.3%	11.2%
75+	68.6%	22.7%	8.7%
Women			
65-75	49.9%	38.9%	11.3%
75+	23.4%	67.7%	8.9%

    e. Societal attitudes regarding sex in general and sex in the elderly in particular.
4. External barriers to sexual activity.
    a. Social isolation related to living arrangements (Table 4-25).
    b. Lack of opportunity for social interactions.
    c. Lack of opportunity for intimacy in many institutional settings.
5. Nonsexual personal barriers to sexual activity or performance.
    a. Functional limitations.
      (1) Physical.
        (a) Instrumental ADLs: transportation or communication problems.
        (b) ADLs.
        (c) Continence.
      (2) Mental (dementia).
    b. Debilitating illness.
    c. Neurologic, muscular, and skeletal illness limiting movement or causing pain with movement.
    d. Psychological issues.
      (1) Depression.
      (2) Anxiety, stress.
      (3) Body image self-perception.
      (4) Performance anxiety (men).
    e. Medications.
      (1) Antihypertensives.
      (2) Antipsychotics.
      (3) Antidepressants (tricyclics and SSRIs).
      (4) Narcotics.
      (5) Anticholinergics.
      (6) Anxiolytics and sedatives.
      (7) Antiandrogens and estrogens in men.
      (8) Antiestrogens and progesterone in women.
      (9) Other medications can have sexual side effects.
    f. Alcohol and drug abuse.

GENITAL AND SEXUAL PROBLEMS ASSOCIATED WITH AGING

Women

1. Current evidence suggests an independent epidemiologic association between menopause and sexual decline, although the effects of

Table 4-25 **Living Arrangements**			
Age	**Live Alone**	**Live with Spouse**	**Other**
Men			
65-75	12.0%	78.9%	8.8%
75+	19.9%	67.4%	12.8%
Women			
65-75	35.0%	49.1%	15.9%
75+	49.9%	22.8%	27.3%

menopause and estrogen deficiency are difficult to separate from other interacting factors.
2. Our understanding of sexual physiology is further complicated by individual variation. Some women experience enhanced sexual activity or satisfaction after menopause.
3. The impact of estrogen deficiency is genital atrophy.
   a. Atrophic vaginitis (with irritation and dyspareunia)
   b. Clitoral and labial atrophy.
   c. Decreased vaginal lubrication.
   d. Decreased clitoral tumescence during intercourse.
4. Prevention and treatment of genital atrophy.
   a. Genital atrophy can be prevented or postponed by treatment with topical or oral estrogens.
   b. Genital atrophy, once established, can be treated with estrogens. Since the publication of the Women's Health Initiative Study results, the use of oral estrogens has fallen out of favor, because risks appear to outweigh benefits.
   c. In addition, particularly in women who will not or cannot use estrogens, a water-based lubricating jelly (e.g., K-Y) should be recommended.

Men

Definitions

1. Impotence is defined as the sustained inability to achieve or maintain an erection of sufficient quality to permit penetration and ejaculation.
2. Loss of libido is not impotence but might accompany it.

Etiology

1. Arterial insufficiency (large or small vessel disease).
2. Neuropathy.
   a. Autonomic neuropathy (e.g., in diabetes).
   b. Spinal cord injury or other cord pathologic condition.
   c. Brain pathologic condition (vascular, neoplastic, multiple sclerosis).
3. Toxic substances.
   a. Alcohol.
   b. Opiates.
   c. Prescription drugs (e.g., antihypertensives, TCAs).
4. Endocrine.
   a. Primary hypogonadism.
      (1) Surgical or medical castration.
      (2) Genetic disorders.
      (3) Trauma.
      (4) Infection.
      (5) Metabolic, such as hemochromatosis.
      (6) Toxic substances, such as alcohol..
   b. Thyroid dysfunction.
   c. Adrenal dysfunction.
   d. Secondary hypogonadism.
      (1) Pituitary tumors.
      (2) Pathologic conditions.

5. Pelvic surgery such as cystectomy, abdominopelvic bowel resection, or prostatectomy.
6. Abnormal penile anatomy.
   a. Congenital (chordee).
   b. Acquired (Peyronie's disease).
7. Any condition that causes painful intercourse.
   a. Urethritis, prostatitis, epididymitis.
   b. Penile skin infections (herpes, *Candida*).
   c. Lower back and hip arthropathies.
8. Chronic debilitating illness.
9. Psychogenic.
   a. Stressful life situations.
   b. Depression.
   c. Anxiety.
   d. Preoccupation about successful sexual performance can lead to loss of arousal.

Evaluation

1. History.
   a. Duration.
   b. Absolute versus relative impotence.
   c. Loss of libido suggests a psychogenic cause or contribution or an endocrine cause.
   d. Presence of morning erection suggests psychogenic cause.
2. Examination.
   a. Vascular exam.
   b. Neurologic exam.
   c. Exam of genitalia.
   d. Signs of endocrine disease.
3. Diagnostic procedures.
   a. Urinalysis.
   b. Fasting blood glucose.
   c. Testosterone, luteinizing hormone, follicle stimulating hormone, prolactin levels.
   d. Thyroid function tests.
   e. Nocturnal penile tumescence test at home or in a sleep lab.
   f. Noninvasive vascular testing.
   g. Nerve conduction velocity.
   h. Cystometrics for autonomic neuropathy.

Treatment

1. Absolute impotence.
   a. Eliminate impotence-causing drugs.
   b. Testosterone replacement therapy should be used only in documented hypogonadism.
   c. Papaverine injection into the corpora cavernosa.
      (1) Should be prescribed and monitored by a urologist.
      (2) Sometimes combined with phentolamine or prostaglandin.
      (3) About 3% have priapism as a complication.
   d. Negative-pressure suction devices.

    e. Implantable penile prosthesis.
      (1) Inflatable type.
      (2) Permanently stiff type.
    f. Phosphodiesterase inhibitors: Sildenafil, vardenafil, and tadalafil.
2. Relative impotence and other disorders.
    a. Ejaculatory control "improves" with aging.
    b. Lubricating jelly can help a man with borderline erectile function achieve penetration.
    c. Treat any underlying reversible organic cause, such as vascular reconstructive surgery.

COUPLES ISSUES AND SEXUAL COUNSELING

1. Some older couples are no longer engaging in sexual activities and have no interest in discussing the issue.
    a. Before laying sexuality to rest, the physician should ascertain the lack of interest or the unwillingness to discuss it with each partner separately if both partners are the physician's patients.
    b. Book references for laypeople should be offered.
    c. In many cases, even when patients do not volunteer concerns with sex in the course of the visits, they acknowledge concern during a sexual history.
    d. Assuming that the work-up and management of treatable conditions have been addressed and intercourse will not be possible, the physician should explore with the patient modes of sexual expression that might not involve actual coitus.
2. Marital discord in elderly couples who have remained together often leads to acceptable compromises that should not be disrupted. In such situations, one or both partners may be interested in self-stimulation for sexual release and pleasure and should be reassured if necessary that masturbation is safe at any age.
3. Counseling for couples who are interested in intimacy.
    a. Couples should be advised that sexual satisfaction with or without an orgasmic end point can be achieved in one or both partners without penetration.
    b. Such counseling sessions should begin by asking patients what currently happens during sexual encounters, as well as what used to happen before performance became impaired, in order to build from a starting point.
    c. This information is best acquired from each partner separately, although considerable tact may be needed when partners ask the physician to keep some points secret about the other partner.
4. Single and widowed patients might need specific advice to increase social contacts.
5. Occasionally, adult children may need counseling when they object to a surviving parent's engaging in a new intimate relationship.

SUGGESTED READINGS

Gott M, Hinchli S: Barriers to seeking treatment for sexual problems in primary care: A qualitative study with older people. *Fam Prac* 20:690-695, 2003.
Miller TA: Diagnostic evaluation of erectile dysfunction. *Am Fam Physician* 61: 95-104, 2000.

4.8 Wound Care

Laura Trice and Tom J. Wachtel

1. Definitions.
   a. Pressure ulcer is a localized area of tissue necrosis that develops when soft tissue is compressed between a bony prominence and an external surface for a prolonged period.
   b. Arterial ulcer is an area of arteriosclerosis that leads to insufficient oxygenation of the skin and underlying tissues.
   c. Diabetic ulcer is a chronic ulcer in a diabetic patient due to extrinsic factors (e.g., trauma, injury) and/or intrinsic factors (e.g., neuropathy, microvascular disease).
   d. Venous ulcer is a discontinuity of the epidermis occurring as a result of venous hypertension and venous insufficiency.
2. Epidemiology.
   a. The incidence of pressure ulcers in acute care facilities has ranged from 2.7% to 29.5%.
   b. Prevalence has varied from 3.5% to 29.5%.
   c. High-risk populations include:
      (1) Quadriplegic patients (60% prevalence).
      (2) Elderly patients admitted for femoral fracture (66% incidence).
      (3) Critical care patients (33% incidence).
   d. Risk factors.
      (1) Pressure ulcers
         (a) Altered sensation or response to discomfort.
         (b) Altered mobility.
         (c) Significant changes in weight.
         (d) Bowel or bladder incontinence.
      (2) Arterial ulcers.
         (a) Arterial insufficiency.
         (b) Tobacco abuse.
      (3) Diabetic ulcers.
         (a) Diabetic neuropathy.
         (b) Structural foot deformity.
         (c) Peripheral arterial occlusive disease.
      (4) Venous ulcers.
         (a) Venous insufficiency.
         (b) History of leg injury, obesity, phlebitis, varicose vein surgery.
         (c) History of prolonged sitting or standing.
3. Clinical findings: Pressure ulcers usually occur over bony prominences and are graded or staged to classify the degree of tissue damage observed.
   a. Stage 1: Nonblanchable erythema of intact skin.
   b. Stage II: Partial-thickness skin loss involving the epidermis or dermis, or both.
   c. Stage III: Full-thickness skin loss involving damage or necrosis of subcutaneous tissue that can extend down to, but not through, underlying fascia or muscle.
   d. Stage IV: Full thickness skin loss with extensive destruction and tissue damage to muscle, bone, or supporting structures.

4. Etiology.
   a. Prolonged unrelieved pressure often associated with impaired or restricted mobility.
   b. Friction or shearing forces on skin.
   c. Presence of risk factors.
5. Work-up.
   a. Many pressure ulcers are preventable when a comprehensive risk assessment is in place.
   b. Risk assessment.
      (1) Consider all bedridden or chair-bound persons, or those whose ability to reposition is impaired, to be at risk for pressure ulcers.
      (2) Select and use a method of risk assessment, such as the Norton Scale or Braden Scale, that ensures systematic evaluation of individual risk factors.
      (3) Assess all at-risk patients at the time of admission to health care facilities and at regular intervals thereafter.
      (4) Identify all individual risk factors (decreased mental status, moisture, incontinence, nutritional deficits) to direct specific preventive treatments. Modify care according to the individual factors.
      (5) All ulcers should have a description of:
         (a) The ulcer's stage, location, and size.
         (b) The wound bed, including epithelialization, granulation tissue, necrotic tissue, and eschar.
         (c) The presence of any exudates, which includes type and amount.
         (d) The wound edges, including undermining, sinus tracts, tunneling, or fistulas.
         (e) Signs of infection.
         (f) Pain.
      (6) Laboratory testing when infection is suspected.
         (a) CBC.
         (b) Sedimentation rate.
         (c) Imaging studies when osteomyelitis is suspected.
         (d) X-ray.
6. Treatment.
   a. Pressure ulcers.
      (1) Managing tissue loads.
         (a) Reduce skin pressure through repositioning and pressure-reducing devices.
         (b) Positioning devices should be used to raise the ulcer off the support surface.
         (c) Prevent shear injury by maintaining the head of the bed at the lowest level of elevation and for the shortest period of time that is consistent with medical conditions and other restrictions.
      (2) Ulcer care.
         (a) Any necrotic tissue observed during initial or subsequent assessments should be debrided. The clinician should select the debridement method (sharp, mechanical enzymatic,

or autolytic) most appropriate to the patient's condition and goals.

(b) Ulcer wounds should be cleansed (preferably with normal saline) at each dressing change, using a minimum amount of mechanical force.

(c) Select a dressing that will keep the ulcer bed continuously moist while allowing the surrounding intact skin to remain dry.

(d) Consider whirlpool therapy for cleansing pressure ulcers that contain thick exudates, slough, or necrotic tissue.

(3) Managing bacterial colonization and infection.

(a) All stage II, III, and IV pressure ulcers are colonized with bacteria. Effective cleansing and debridement will minimize colonization. More frequent cleansing and debridement may be needed if purulence or a foul odor develops.

(b) A topical antibiotic should be considered if a clean ulcer continues to have exudates despite optimal care for 2 to 4 weeks. Topical antiseptics should not be used.

(c) Swab cultures have no diagnostic value; however, if the ulcer does not respond to topical antibiotic therapy, quantitative bacterial cultures, preferably by means of tissue biopsy, should be obtained to evaluate for osteomyelitis.

(d) Systemic antibiotics should be given to patients with bacteremia, sepsis, advancing cellulitis, or osteomyelitis.

(4) Operative repair.

(a) Operative procedures should be considered for clean stage III or IV ulcers that do not respond to optimal care and include:

   i. Direct closure.

   ii. Skin grafting.

   iii. Skin flaps, musculocutaneous flaps, and free flaps.

(b) Quality of life, patient preferences, treatment goals, risk of recurrence, and anticipated rehabilitative outcomes should be considered.

(5) Education and quality improvement.

(a) Institutions and health care agencies are responsible for developing and implementing pressure ulcer prevention and treatment programs for patients, families, and caregivers.

(b) In addition, a quality improvement program should be established.

b. Arterial ulcers.

(1) Restore adequate vascular supply whenever possible.

(2) Manage underlying medical issues such as hypertension and diabetes.

(3) Maintain a moderate level of exercise.

(4) Quit smoking.

(5) Avoid caffeine, cold temperatures, and constrictive garments.

(6) Keep wounds clean.

(7) Use nonocclusive moist wound dressings.

(8) Manage local infection.

(9) Treatment failure can lead to amputation.

   c. Diabetic ulcers.
      (1) Offload mechanical stress.
      (2) Perform sharp wound debridement.
      (3) Perform revascularization.
      (4) Use a moist wound dressing.
      (5) Manage local infection.
      (6) Treatment failure can lead to amputation.
   d. Venous ulcers.
      (1) Use a compression bandage system.
      (2) Manage local infection.
      (3) Moist wound dressing.
      (4) Use bioengineered skin appropriately.

SUGGESTED READINGS

National Pressure Ulcer Advisory Panel: Statement on Pressure Ulcer Prevention (1992). Available at http://www.npuap.org/positn1.html (accessed January 19, 2006).

Thomas D: Wound care: Prevention, management, and nursing care. American Medical Director's Association Annual Symposium, Phoenix, Arizona, 2004.

U.S. Agency for Health Care Policy and Research: Treatment of pressure ulcers. Clinical Guideline Number 15. Available at http://www.ncbi.nlm.nih.gov/books/bv.fcgi?rid=hstat2.chapter.5124 (accessed January 19, 2006).

4.9 Cooperation with Care Plan

Marsha D. Fretwell and Deborah Adams Wingate

Critical to successful care of all patients is a cooperative relationship between the providers and recipients of the care. In the case of older patients, the barriers that may interfere with accomplishing the care plan can be related to the three groups involved in the care: clinicians; the older patient; and spouses, children, or other caretakers.

1. The role of the physician in successful care plans.
   a. Make accurate diagnoses and prognoses.
   b. Educate the patient and/or family about the appropriate treatments.
   c. Respect the personal preferences of the patient about the treatments.
   d. Monitor the outcomes of treatments undertaken..
   e. Listen fully to the patient so that a treatment or care plan can be directed at the issues of most concern. Failure to do so is a major barrier to a patient's cooperation with a care plan. An inappropriate care plan will fail.
   f. Educate the patient about the potential risks and benefits of new medications and other types of treatment. Lack of understanding of medications often impairs the patient's and the family's ability to cooperate.
2. The role of the older patient in successful care plans.
   a. Several attributes of an older patient can lead to active or passive uncooperativeness with a care plan.
      (1) Personality traits.
         (a) The characteristic emotional, interpersonal, experiential, and motivational styles that are stable over a person's life span.
         (b) Form the basic elements of the personality.

(2) A cluster of personality traits—or in their extreme, personality disorders—can interfere with cooperation with an appropriate care plan.

(a) Eccentric, or odd, group.

　　i. Paranoid type is mistrustful of others.

　　ii. Schizoid type is indifferent to social relationships.

(b) Dramatic, emotional, or erratic group.

　　i. The patient with antisocial personality disorder is unable to conform to social norms and rules.

　　ii. The patient with histrionic personality disorder is emotionally labile and self-centered and has many minor complaints.

　　iii. The patient with narcissistic personality disorder has an extreme sense of self-importance with entitlement.

(c) Anxious group.

　　i. The patient with avoidant personality disorder is extremely shy.

　　ii. The patient with dependent personality disorder is unable to make decisions or take responsibility for his or her role in the care plan.

　　iii. The patient with obsessive-compulsive personality disorder is characterized by perfectionism and a focus on details.

　　iv. The patient with passive-aggressive personality disorder appears to understand the care plan but then covertly does not follow through with recommendations.

b. Change in personality: On the whole, personality traits do not change over one's life span.

(1) A review of past emotional, interpersonal, and motivational styles in an older person can provide valuable prognostic information about response to the stress of the current situation.

(2) If a patient experiences a change in personality, think first about the diseases, medications, changes in sites of care, or overwhelming personal losses that might underlie the change.

3. The role of spouses, children, and other family caretakers in successful care plans: When an appropriate care plan is not succeeding, it is important to examine the cognitive and emotional capacities of the spouse (most often the primary caretaker) and the overall functioning of the family support network.

a. Spouse.

(1) The spouse of an older patient is often also older and subject to the same diseases, difficulties with hearing and vision, and barriers to communication as the patient is.

(2) Brief screening examinations for vision, hearing, cognition, and anxiety or depression are indicated, especially if the patient has a dementia and no progress is being made in the care plan.

b. Children and other family caretakers.

(1) "What goes around comes around" is a phrase that succinctly captures how children and other family caretakers can become a barrier to a successful care plan.

(2) Because adult children are often the most critical element for a successful care plan, it is important to recognize and address the problem.

(3) In some families the critical step of the parent-child relationship—separation and individuation of the child—has not been successfully navigated. Many years later, when the child is called on to take care of the parents, two responses can interfere with a successful care plan.

    (a) The overly connected family.

        i. The child is often unable to set limits on the parent's behavior that are necessary to appropriate and safe care. This is particularly difficult if the parent has a dementia but it might also be true for physically impaired patients who are demanding and abusive to caretakers.

        ii. It is critical to recognize and obtain counseling and support for these children caretakers.

        iii. It is also crucial to obtain prior directives from these older patients while they are cognitively intact, because the children may be emotionally unable to function as a proxy for substituted judgment (see Chapter 10).

    (b) The disconnected family.

        i. The physician might become the target of unresolved anger at the parent/authority figure.

        ii. The child might have inappropriate expectations of the physician's responsibility for the well-being of the parent.

        iii. It is important for the physician to set limits, identify responsible family members, and clarify roles and responsibilities early in the course of the care plan.

        iv. Obtaining prior directives from the patient or from the parent while parent is cognitively intact greatly helps in implementing the successful care plan.

SUGGESTED READINGS

Fenton, WS: Schizophrenia and related disorders. In Abrams WB, Berkow R, editors: *The Merck manual of geriatrics*, Whitehouse Station, NJ, Merck, 2006, pp 1721-1732.

Costa PT, McCrae RR: Personality and aging. In Hazzard WR, Bierman EL (eds): *Principles of geriatric medicine and gerontology.* New York, McGraw-Hill, 1994, pp 107-113.

Holroyd S, Rabins PV: Personality disorders. In Hazzard WR, Bierman EL (eds): *Principles of geriatric medicine and gerontology.* New York, McGraw-Hill, 1994, pp 1131-1135.

Laitman LB, Davis KL: Paraphrenias and other psychosis. In Hazzard WR, Bierman EL (eds): *Principles of geriatric medicine and gerontology.* New York, McGraw-Hill, 1994, pp 1111-1117.

Selected Organ System Abnormalities

5

5.1 Neurologic Disorders

DYSTONIA

Lynn McNicoll and Mark J. Fagan

Definitions

1. Dystonia is characterized by involuntary muscle contractions (sustained or spasmodic) that lead to abnormal body movements or postures.
2. Dystonia is usually focal but it can be generalized.

Epidemiology

1. Prevalence.
   a. Estimated at 1 in 3000 persons.
   b. Female preponderance is 3:2.
2. Genetics.
   a. Hereditary forms can have an onset in childhood or adulthood.
   b. Autosomal dominant, autosomal recessive, and X-linked forms of dystonia have been identified.

Clinical Findings

1. Focal dystonias produce abnormal sustained muscle contractions in an area of the body.
   a. Neck (torticollis).
      (1) A commonly affected site.
      (2) There is a tendency for the head to turn to one side.
   b. Eyelids (blepharospasm): Involuntary repetitive closures of the eyelids.
   c. Mouth (oromandibular dystonia): Involuntary contraction of muscles of the mouth, tongue, or face.
   d. Hand (writer's cramp): Patient may be unable to hold a pen or form written words.
2. Generalized dystonia.
   a. Affects multiple areas of the body.
   b. Can lead to marked joint deformities.

Etiology

1. Primary dystonia.
   a. Postulated mechanism is a reduced and abnormal pattern of neuronal activity in the basal ganglia, which results in disinhibition of the motor thalamus and cortex, which leads to abnormal movement.

137

    b. Hereditary forms have been described, including the severe progressive form, dystonia musculorum deformans.

    c. Sporadic or idiopathic forms occur.

2. Secondary dystonia.

    a. Dystonia can occur secondary to other diseases such as central nervous system (CNS) disease, hypoxia, Huntington's disease, Wilson's disease, and Parkinson's syndrome.

    b. Acute dystonia can occur following treatment with drugs that block dopamine receptors, such as phenothiazines or butyrophenones.

    c. Tardive dyskinesia or dystonia can result from:

      (1) Long-term treatment with antipsychotic drugs such as phenothiazines or butyrophenones (e.g., haloperidol).

      (2) Treatment with levodopa, metoclopramide, anticonvulsants, or ergots.

Differential Diagnosis

1. Parkinson's disease.
2. Progressive supranuclear palsy.
3. Wilson's disease.
4. Huntington's disease.
5. Drug effects.

Work-up

1. History.
    a. Family history.
    b. Birth history.
    c. Medication use.
2. Physical examination.
3. Laboratory tests and imaging are usually not helpful for establishing a diagnosis.

Treatment

1. Heat, massage, physical therapy to relieve pain.
2. Splints to prevent or delay contractures.
3. For acute dystonic reactions to phenothiazines or butyrophenones, use diphenhydramine 50 mg intravenous (IV) or benztropine 2 mg IV.
4. Slowly withdraw potentially offending agents.
5. Diazepam, baclofen, or carbamazepine may be effective.
6. Trihexyphenidyl may be helpful in tardive dyskinesia or dystonia.
7. Injections of botulinum toxin into the affected muscles can be used for refractory cases of focal dystonias.
8. Surgical procedures for severe, refractory cases.
    a. Myectomy.
    b. Rhizotomy.
    c. Thalamotomy.
    d. Deep brain stimulation.

SUGGESTED READING

Tan NC, Chan LL, Tan EK: Hemifacial spasm and involuntary facial movements. QJM 95:493-500, 2002.

GUILLAIN-BARRÉ SYNDROME

Eroboghene E. Ubogu and Tom J. Wachtel

Definition

Guillain-Barré syndrome is an acute immune-mediated polyradiculoneuropathy (affects nerve roots and peripheral nerves), with predominant motor involvement.

Epidemiology

1. Incidence.
   a. There are 0.6 to 1.9 cases/100,000 persons annually without geographic variation.
   b. Incidence increases with age.
   c. A slight male preponderance (1.25:1) also exists.
2. Predisposing factors.
   a. Viral infections.
      (1) Human immunodeficiency virus (HIV).
      (2) Cytomegalovirus.
      (3) Epstein–Barr virus.
      (4) Influenza.
   b. Bacterial infections.
      (1) *Campylobacter jejuni*.
      (2) *Mycoplasma pneumonia*.
   c. Systemic illness.
      (1) Hodgkin's lymphoma.
      (2) Immunizations.

Clinical Findings

1. Symmetric weakness.
   a. Initially involves proximal muscles, subsequently involves both proximal and distal muscles.
   b. Difficulty in ambulating, getting up from a chair, or climbing stairs.
   c. Maximal clinical weakness occurs within 4 weeks of disease onset.
2. Depressed or absent reflexes bilaterally.
3. Minimal to moderate glove-and-stocking paresthesias, dysesthesia, anesthesia, and/or back pain.
4. Pain (caused by involvement of posterior nerve roots) may be prominent.
5. Autonomic abnormalities.
   a. Brady- or tachyarrhythmias.
   b. Hypo- or hypertension.
6. Respiratory insufficiency caused by weakness of bulbar or intercostal muscles.
7. Facial paresis, ophthalmoparesis, dysphagia secondary to cranial nerve involvement.

Etiology

1. Unknown.
2. Preceding infectious illness 1 to 4 weeks before disease onset in 66% of patients.

3. Humoral and cell-mediated immune attack of peripheral nerve myelin and Schwann cells, sometimes with axonal involvement.

Differential Diagnosis

1. Toxic peripheral neuropathies.
   a. Heavy metal poisoning (lead, thallium, arsenic).
   b. Medications (vincristine, disulfiram).
   c. Organophosphate poisoning.
   d. Hexacarbon (glue sniffer's neuropathy).
2. Nontoxic peripheral neuropathies.
   a. Acute intermittent porphyria.
   b. Vasculitic polyneuropathy.
   c. Infectious neuropathies, such as poliomyelitis, diphtheria, or Lyme disease.
   d. Tick paralysis.
3. Neuromuscular junction disorders.
   a. Myasthenia gravis.
   b. Botulism.
   c. Snake envenomation.
4. Myopathies.
   a. Polymyositis.
   b. Acute necrotizing myopathies caused by drugs (e.g., statins).
5. Metabolic derangements.
   a. Hypermagnesemia.
   b. Hypokalemia.
   c. Hypophosphatemia.
6. Acute CNS disorders.
   a. Basilar artery thrombosis with brainstem infarction.
   b. Brainstem encephalomyelitis.
   c. Transverse myelitis.
   d. Spinal cord compression.
7. Hysterical paralysis or malingering.

Work-up

1. Complete blood count (CBC) might reveal early leukocytosis with left shift.
2. Electrolytes to exclude metabolic causes.
3. Heavy metal testing, urine porphyria screen, creatine kinase, HIV titers.
4. Neuroimaging of the brain and spinal cord if diagnosis is uncertain.
5. Lumbar puncture (may be normal in the first 1 or 2 weeks of the illness).
   a. Typical findings include elevated cerebrospinal fluid (CSF) protein with few mononuclear leukocytes (albuminocytologic dissociation) in 80% to 90% of patients.
   b. Elevated CSF cell counts is an expected feature in cases associated with HIV seroconversion.
6. Electromyogram/nerve conduction studies (EMG/NCS).
   a. May be normal in the first 10 to 14 days of the disease.
   b. The earliest electrodiagnostic abnormality is prolongation or absence of H-reflexes.

Treatment

Nonpharmacologic Therapy

1. Close monitoring of respiratory function because respiratory failure is the major complication in Guillain-Barré syndrome. Frequent measurements of:
   a. Vital capacity.
   b. Negative inspiratory force.
   c. Pulmonary toilet.
2. Ventilatory support may be necessary in 10% to 20% of patients.
3. Adequate fluid/electrolyte support and nutrition, especially in patients with dysautonomia or bulbar dysfunction.
4. Aggressive nursing care to prevent decubitus ulcers, infections, fecal impactions, and pressure nerve palsies.
5. Monitoring and treatment of autonomic dysfunction.
   a. Bradyarrhythmias or tachyarrhythmias.
   b. Orthostatic hypotension.
   c. Systemic hypertension.
   d. Altered sweating.
6. Treatment of back pain and dysesthesia with low-dose tricyclics, gabapentin, etc.
7. Stress ulcer prevention in patients receiving ventilator support.
8. Prevention of thromboembolism.
   a. Antithrombotic stockings.
   b. Subcutaneous heparin 5000 U q12h in nonambulatory patients.
9. Emotional support and social counseling.

Pharmacologic Treatment

1. Infusion of IV immunoglobulins (IVIg).
   a. Infuse IVIg 0.4 g/kg/day for 5 days.
   b. Always check serum immunoglobulin A (IgA) levels before infusion to prevent anaphylaxis in deficient patients.
2. Early therapeutic plasma exchange (TPE) or plasmapheresis.
   a. Exchange of 200 to 250 mL/kg over 5 sessions qod, started within 7 days of onset of symptoms, is beneficial in preventing paralytic complications in patients with rapidly progressive disease. Plasmapheresis is contraindicated in patients with cardiovascular disease (recent myocardial infarction, unstable angina), active sepsis, and autonomic dysfunction.

Prognosis

1. Mortality is approximately 5% to 10%.
2. One study showed 62% complete recovery, 14% mild weakness, 9% moderate weakness, 4% bed-bound or ventilated, and 8% dead at 1 year.
3. Predictors for poor recovery (inability to walk independently at 1 year).
   a. Age >60 years.
   b. Preceding diarrheal illness.
   c. Recent cytomegalovirus infection.
   d. Fulminant or rapidly progressing course.
   e. Ventilator dependence.
   f. Reduced motor amplitudes (<20% normal) or inexcitable nerves on NCS.

SUGGESTED READINGS

Gorson KC, Ropper AH: Guillain-Barré syndrome (acute inflammatory demyelinating neuropathy) and related disorders. In Katirji B, Kaminski HJ, Preston DC, et al (eds): *Neuromuscular disorders in clinical practice.* Boston, Butterworth-Heinemann, 2002, pp 544-566.
Kuwabara S: Guillain-Barré syndrome: Epidemiology, pathophysiology and management. *Drugs* 64:597-610, 2004.

HEADACHE

Tom J. Wachtel

Epidemiology

1. Headache is a very common complaint; more than 90% of all people acknowledge some experience with it.
2. Demographics.
   a. Older patients are more likely than their younger counterparts to visit a physician when they experience headache.
   b. Women are more likely than men to seek medical care for headache.
   c. Women are more likely to report a longer duration of the problem.
3. Type.
   a. Lay people often misuse the term *migraine* as synonymous with headache.
   b. Migraine is the second most common cause of chronic headaches.
   c. Only 5% of all headaches are migraine.
   d. About 80% of all headaches are tension headaches.
4. Care.
   a. Many people with headache rely on self-care with over-the-counter medications.
   b. Headaches account for 2% to 4% of all primary care office visits.

Etiology

1. Tension headaches (muscle contraction headache or stress headache).
2. Vascular headaches.
   a. Idiopathic or primary.
      (1) Migraine (classic or common).
      (2) Cluster headache.
   b. Secondary or associated with vascular disorders.
      (1) Temporal arteritis (giant cell arteritis).
      (2) Other vasculitis.
      (3) Hypertension.
3. Mixed tension/vascular headaches.
4. Headaches associated with opththalmologic, otolaryngologic, facial, or dental diseases.
   a. Eye.
      (1) Refraction errors.
      (2) Acute glaucoma.
      (3) Red eye (conjunctivitis, keratitis, iritis, uveitis).
      (4) Miscellaneous painful eye conditions.
   b. Nose and sinuses (rhinitis/sinusitis).
      (1) Bacterial infection.
      (2) Viral infection.

    (3) Allergic rhinitis.

    (4) Nasopharyngeal carcinoma.

  c. Ear (e.g., otitis).

  d. Oral cavity.

    (1) Dental and gingival problems.

    (2) Oropharyngeal malignancies.

    (3) Oropharyngeal infections (e.g., pharyngitis, tonsillitis, abscess).

  e. Temporomandibular joint disease.

  f. Bruxism (teeth grinding).

5. Cranial neuralgias (e.g., trigeminal neuralgia or tic douloureux).

6. Associated with head trauma.

7. Cervical spine and neck diseases.

  a. Arthritis (degenerative or inflammatory).

  b. Cervical disk disease.

  c. Whiplash injuries.

  d. Torticollis (stiff neck).

  e. Odynophagia and other referred pain resulting from laryngeal or upper esophageal problems, usually malignancies, or rarely from cervical lymphadenopathy or thyroid enlargement.

8. Meningitis or meningoencephalitis. *Note:* Pure encephalitis does not cause a headache in the absence of cerebral edema.

9. Associated with distant infection or fever (probably a variant of tension headache).

10. Spinal headache following a lumbar puncture or spinal anesthesia.

11. Medication-induced headache: Many prescription and over-the-counter drugs can cause headache as an adverse reaction, some more frequently than others (e.g., nitrates).

12. Associated with substance abuse or withdrawal.

  a. Alcohol.

  b. Caffeine.

  c. Recreational (illicit) drugs.

13. Intracranial mass lesions.

  a. Hematoma.

    (1) Epidural.

    (2) Subdural.

    (3) Subarachnoid.

    (4) Intracerebral.

  b. Tumor.

    (1) Primary (e.g., astrocytoma, meningioma).

    (2) Metastatic.

  c. Abscess.

    (1) Protozoan (toxoplasmosis).

    (2) Bacterial.

14. Pseudotumor cerebri (benign intracranial hypertension); rare in the elderly.

15. Malingering.

Work-up

Table 5-1 lists clinical characteristics of some types of headaches.

1. History.

  a. Location, especially unilateral versus bilateral.

Table 5-1 Clinical Characteristics of Selected Headaches

Pain	Tension	Migraine	Sinusitis	Mass Lesion
Location	Bilateral (frontal, occipital, bandlike)	Unilateral (but not always on same side)	Bifrontal (may be unilateral)	Unilateral (always on same side) or bilateral
Character	Pressure	Throbbing	Pressure	Pressure
Severity	Mild to moderate	Moderate to severe	Moderate	Progressively worse as mass expands
Time of occurrence	Late in day or any time	Morning or any time	Worse in morning	Constant (may be intermittent early in course)
Frequency	Several times per week	Less than weekly	Daily until resolved	Constant
Aura	No	Sometimes	No	No
Precipitants	Stress	Bright lights, menstruation, alcohol (see text)	None	None but pain aggravated by Valsalva type of provocation (coughing, sneezing, defecation)
Alleviating factors	Relaxation or sleep	Reclining in dark room Migraine-specific drugs	Decongestants, antihistamines, antibiotics	None
Associated symptoms	None or stress related	Vomiting, photophobia	Nasal stuffiness or dripping, epistaxis	Projectile vomiting, neurologic symptoms, may have known primary cancer
Age at onset	Any age	10-30 y	Any age	Any age for primary brain tumor, older for metastatic brain tumor
Gender	Both	Majority female	Both	Both
Family history	Sometimes	Often	No	No
Chronicity	Several months to years	Several months to years	Acute except in allergic rhinitis (may be seasonal)	Progressive

   b. Temporal features.
      (1) Overall duration of the pain (days, months, years).
      (2) Duration of each episode if recurrent.
      (3) Circadian rhythm (e.g., does it begin in the morning or in the evening?).
   c. Character of the pain (e.g., pounding vs. constant ache).
   d. Severity (e.g., on a scale from 1 to 10).
   e. Precipitating factors.
   f. Aggravating factors.
   g. Alleviating factors.
   h. Associated symptoms (e.g., prodromal or during the headache).
   i. Prior evaluation.
   j. Psychosocial background (e.g., family situation, occupational history, drug use).
   k. Functional impact (e.g., disability).
2. Physical examination.
   a. A complete physical exam is obviously desirable.
   b. Minimum.
      (1) Evaluate vital signs.
      (2) Thorough head, eyes, ears, nose, oral, throat, and neck exams.
      (3) Neurologic exam.
         (a) Reflexes.
         (b) Cranial nerves.
         (c) Motor, sensory, and cerebellar functions.
      (4) Mental status.
3. Ancillary tests: Most patients can be managed without any labs or imaging.
   a. Laboratory.
      (1) Erythrocyte sedimentation rate (ESR) if temporal arteritis is suspected.
      (2) Lumbar puncture (following brain imaging) for abrupt onset of severe headaches or meningeal signs.
   b. Imaging.
      (1) The most difficult decision is when to perform a head computed tomography (CT) scan or magnetic resonance imaging (MRI) to rule out an intracranial mass lesion. Because most patients have tension headache or migraine, it is usually reasonable to initiate treatment based on a clinical impression and defer a decision regarding further work-up based on the patient's response during follow-up.
      (2) If a high-probability etiologic diagnosis can be made at the first visit (e.g., sinusitis), further diagnostic tests for other causes of headache are not indicated initially.
      (3) Caution and a low threshold for imaging procedures are advisable when the symptoms are of very recent onset and unusually severe.
      (4) Imaging is required if the neurologic exam reveals new abnormalities.
      (5) Failure to improve with a treatment targeted at the most likely etiologic diagnosis often indicates cerebral imaging.

Most Common Headaches

Tension Headaches

1. Presentation.
   a. Tension headaches can manifest as mild intermittent headaches or severe continuous daily headaches.
      (1) Mild, intermittent tension headaches are usually associated with usual life stresses.
      (2) Severe, continuous tension headaches are more likely found in patients with depression or anxiety.
      (3) In either case, the pathophysiology is presumed to be contraction of facial expression muscles, scalp muscles, or neck muscles.
   b. See Table 5-1 for the clinical description.
2. Treatment.
   a. Nonpharmacologic management.
      (1) Information and reassurance.
      (2) Stress reduction and relaxation.
      (3) Psychotherapy for depression or anxiety if present.
      (4) Scalp massage or acupressure.
      (5) Transcutaneous electrical nerve stimulation.
      (6) Physical therapy including stretching exercises, massage, and ultrasound.
      (7) Environment modification, family counseling.
   b. Pharmacologic options.
      (1) Aspirin or acetaminophen.
      (2) NSAIDs.
      (3) Narcotic agents should not be used.
      (4) Propoxyphene (Darvon) or aspirin–caffeine–butalbital combinations (Fiorinal) may be used reluctantly for short courses only, because of their addictive potential and the risk of delirium.
      (5) Consider a trial of muscle relaxants (e.g., metaxalone [Skelaxin] 400-800 mg tid) if headache is related to cervical muscle spasm.
      (6) Treatment with antidepressant or anxiolytic drugs may be used when underlying depression or anxiety is present.

Migraine

1. Presentation.
   a. Migraine headache.
      (1) Classic migraine (with aura) is less common.
         (a) Prodromal symptoms.
             i. Vague malaise.
             ii. Visual phenomena (usually scotomas).
             iii. Olfactory or auditory perceptions.
             iv. Focal neurologic symptoms.
      (2) Common migraine (no aura) is more common.
2. Pathogenesis.
   a. Unknown, but the most widely accepted hypothesis (albeit unproven) is a primary neuronal event resulting in a trigeminovascular reflex causing neurogenic inflammation.
   b. Serotonin, nitric oxide, and calcitonin gene–related peptide also play a role, but the exact mechanism is unknown.

    c. Cortical spreading depression is responsible for the aura.

    d. An alternative mechanism is an episode of intracranial or extracranial vasoconstriction contemporary with the aura (when present), followed by vasodilation resulting in a unilateral throbbing headache, often associated with nausea, vomiting, diarrhea, and photophobia.

    e. Age of onset of migraine is usually before 40 years, but many patients have a lifelong course of illness requiring knowledge of the condition by geriatricians.

    f. See Table 5-1 for a complete clinical description. Note that a migraine headache can lead to a tension headache or a mixed syndrome.

3. Treatment of acute attack (Table 5-2).

    a. Mild attacks are treated the same as tension headache (together with lying down in a dark, quiet room).

    b. Severe attacks.

      (1) Migraine-specific agents: Early administration improves effectiveness.

        (a) Sumatriptan (Imitrex).

          i. A single SC injection of sumatriptan 6 mg can be administered by the patient at home or by a physician. A second identical dose may be administered after 30 minutes if a partial response is obtained. If no response is achieved after the first dose, a second dose will not be successful.

          ii. Sumatriptan may also be given orally at a dose of 25 to 100 mg followed, if needed, by another 25 to 100 mg tablet after 2 hours for incomplete response.

          iii. Sumatriptan is also available as a nasal spray 5 to 20 mg once; may repeat after 2 hours if needed.

          iv. Sumatriptan is contraindicated in patients with known occlusive arterial disease and therefore should be used with caution in anyone older than 40 years.

        (b) Table 5-2 gives a list of other available triptans.

      (2) If migraine-specific treatment is not effective or not tolerated, narcotic analgesic agents should be used.

      (3) Antiemetics (prochlorperazine, metoclopramide, domperidone): Acute dystonic reactions and akathisia are rare side effects.

4. Prophylaxis.

    a. Nonpharmacologic.

      (1) Avoidance of triggering factors.

        (a) Drugs such as NSAIDs and vasodilators.

        (b) Stress.

        (c) Coffee.

        (d) Identifiable dietary components.

        (e) Bright lights.

        (f) Sleep deprivation.

        (g) Alcohol.

      (2) Relaxation training and biofeedback.

    b. Pharmacologic.

      (1) Many medications can reduce the frequency and severity of migraine attacks. None are better than 50% effective. Therefore,

Table 5-2 Abortive and Analgesic Therapy for Migraine		
Drug	**Dose**	**Route**
Triptans (Serotonin Agonists)		
Sumatriptan	6 mg, repeat in 2 h (max 2 doses/day)	SC
	25 mg, 50 mg, repeat in 2 h (max 200 mg/day)	Oral
	5 mg and 20 mg, repeat in 2 h (max 40 mg/day)	Nasal spray
Zolmitriptan	1.25 mg, 2.5 mg, repeat in 4 h (max 10 mg/day)	Oral
	5 mg, repeat in 2 h (max 10 mg/day)	Nasal spray
	2.5 mg, 5 mg, repeat in 2 h (max 10 mg/day)	OD tab
Naratriptan	1 mg, 2.5 mg, repeat in 4 h (max 5 mg/day)	Oral
Rizatriptan	5 mg, 10 mg, repeat in 2 h (max 30 mg/day)	Oral
Almotriptan	6.25 mg, 12.5 mg, may repeat in 2 h (max 25 mg/day)	Oral
Eletriptan	20 mg, 40 mg, may repeat in 2 h (max 80 mg/day)	Oral
Frovatriptan	2.5 mg, may repeat in 2 h (max 7.5 mg/day)	Oral
Ergotamine Preparations		
Ergotamine and caffeine	2 tablets, may repeat 1 tab q30min (max 6/day)	Oral
	1 suppository, repeat in 1 h (max 2/day)	Rectal
Ergotaminel	1 tablet, repeat in 1 h (max 2/day)	Sublingual
Dihydroergotamine	0.5–1.0 mg, repeat twice at 1-h intervals (max 3 mg/attack)	IM
Sympathomimetics (with or without Barbiturates or Codeine)		
Isometheptene + dichloralphenazone + acetaminophen	1 or 2 capsules, repeat in 4 h (max 8/day)	Oral

Nonsteroidal Antiinflammatory Drugs

Acetaminophen + aspirin + caffeine	2 tablets, repeat in 6 h (max 8/day)	Oral
Naproxen	550-750 mg, repeat in 1 h (max 3 times/wk)	Oral
Meclofenamate	100-200 mg, repeat in 1 h (max 3 times/wk)	Oral
Flurbiprofen	50-100 mg, repeat in 1 h (max 3 times/wk)	Oral
Ibuprofen	200-300 mg, repeat in 1 h (max 3 times/wk)	Oral

Antiemetics

Promethazine	50-125 mg	Oral, IM
Prochlorperazine	1-25 mg	Oral
	2.5-25 mg (suppository)	Rectal
	5-10 mg	IM
Chlorpromazine	10-25 mg	Oral
	50-100 mg (suppository)	Rectal
	Up to 35 mg	IV
Trimethobenzamide	250 mg	Oral
	200 mg	Rectal
Metoclopramide	5-10 mg	Oral
	10 mg	IM
	5-10 mg	IV
Dimenhydrinate	50 mg	Oral

max, maximum; OD, orally disintegrating; tab, tablet.
Data from Wiederholt WC: *Neurology for non-neurologists*, ed 4. Philadelphia, WB Saunders, 2000.

treatment should be reserved for patients with more than six severe attacks per year or when symptomatic treatments are ineffective or contraindicated.

(2) Medications are most effective when initiated during a headache-free period.

(3) All prophylaxis should be maintained for at least 3 months before deeming medication a failure.

(4) Patients should be instructed to keep a pretreatment and treatment migraine diary to evaluate effectiveness of any prescribed medication.

(5) Medications.

    (a) β-Blockers (e.g., propranolol 40 to 320 mg/day).

    (b) Calcium channel blockers (CCBs) (e.g., nifedipine 20 to 60 mg/day).

    (c) Amitriptyline 10 to 175 mg/day.

    (d) Carbamazepine 400 to 800 mg/day (monitor drug levels) and other antiepileptic drugs (valproate, gabapentin, topiramate).

    (e) Selective serotonin reuptake inhibitors (SSRIs).

SUGGESTED READINGS

Dodick DW: The chronic daily headache. *N Eng J Med* 354:158-165, 2006.

Friedman BW, Corbo J, Lipton RB, et al: A trial of metoclopramide vs sumatriptan for the emergency department treatment of migraines. *Neurology* 64:463-468, 2005.

Goadsby PJ, Lipton RB, Ferrari MD: Migraine-current understanding and treatment. *N Engl J Med* 346:257-270, 2002.

Headache Classification Committee of the International Headache Society: The international Classification of Headache Disorders. *Cephalgia* 24(suppl 1):1-151, 2004. PDF available at http://216.25.100.131/ihscommon/guidelines/pdfs/ihc_II_main_no_print.pdf (accessed January 29, 2007).

Holroyd KA, O'Donnell FJ, Stesland M, et al: Management of chronic tension-type headache with tricyclic antidepressant medication, stress management therapy, and their combination: A randomized controlled trial. *JAMA* 285:2208-2215, 2001.

Lipton RB, Bigal ME, Steiner TJ, et al: Classification of primary headaches. *Neurology* 63:427-435, 2004.

Millea P, Brodie J: Tension-type headache. *Am Fam Physician* 66:797-804, 2002.

Silberstein SD, Rosenberg J: Multispecialty consensus on diagnosis and treatment of headache. *Neurology* 54:1553, 2000.

Silberstein SD, for the US Headache Consortium: Practice parameter: Evidence-based guidelines for migraine headache (an evidence-based review). Report of the Quality Standards Subcommittee of the American Academy of Neurology. *Neurology* 55:754-762, 2000.

Silberstein SD, Freitag FG, Rozen TD, et al: Tramadol/acetaminophen for the treatment of acute migraine pain: Findings of a randomized, placebo-controlled trial. *Headache* 45:1317-1327, 2005.

Smith TR, Sunshine A, Stark SR, et al: Sumatriptan and naproxen sodium for the acute treatment of migraine. *Headache* 45:983-991, 2005.

INSOMNIA
Clifford Milo Singer, with revisions by Tom J. Wachtel

Definitions
1. Insomnia is a disturbance of initiating or maintaining sleep.
2. Restless, nonrestorative sleep may also be described as insomnia.
3. The disturbance may be subjective, without daytime sequelae, but still a cause of distress, or it may be objectively measurable, with poor sleep efficiency and daytime consequences of sleepiness and functional impairment.

Epidemiology
1. Incidence (in United States): 30% to 45% of adults experience insomnia per year.
2. Prevalence (in United States).
   a. From 1% to 15% of all adults develop persistent insomnia.
   b. About 25% of older adults have persistent insomnia.
   c. Insomnia is more common in women.
3. Predominant age.
   a. Transient insomnia is common at any age.
   b. Persistent insomnia is more common in those older than 60 years.
   c. Younger adults usually complain of sleep-onset insomnia.
   d. Older adults usually have more difficulty maintaining sleep.

Clinical Findings
1. Complaints of:
   a. Difficulty falling asleep.
   b. Difficulty staying asleep.
   c. Early morning awakening.
   d. Restless or nonrestorative sleep.
   e. Difficulty sleeping at desired times.
2. Patients might or might not complain of daytime sleepiness or fatigue.
3. Chronicity.
   a. Acute and self-limited.
   b. Chronic but intermittent.
   c. Chronic and frequent.

Etiology
1. Transient insomnia.
   a. Stress.
   b. Illness.
   c. Travel (jet lag).
   d. Environmental disruptions (e.g., noise, heat, cold, poor bedding, unfamiliar surroundings).
2. Persistent insomnia.
   a. Mood disorders (depression, bipolar illness).
   b. Primary (with or without poor sleep hygiene).
   c. Sleep-related breathing disorders (e.g., obstructive sleep apnea).

      d. Chronobiologic disorder or circadian rhythm problem.
        (1) Delayed sleep phase syndrome.
        (2) Advanced sleep phase syndrome.
        (3) Shift work.
      e. Drug and alcohol abuse.
      f. Restless legs syndrome.
      g. Periodic leg movements.
      h. Neurodegenerative disorder (e.g., Alzheimer's disease, Parkinson's disease).
      i. Medical problem (e.g., pain, gastroesophageal reflux disease (GERD), nocturia, orthopnea, medications).

Work-up

1. History (with bed partner interview, if possible).
2. Sleep diary.
    a. The patient should keep a sleep diary for 2 weeks to document:
      (1) Severity.
      (2) Frequency.
      (3) Daytime function and distress.
    b. A sample sleep diary can be downloaded from the National Sleep Foundation Web site: http://www.sleepfoundation.org.
3. Primary insomnia is a diagnosis of exclusion in elderly patients. Make every effort to exclude depression, especially in the nursing home population.
4. Laboratory tests.
    a. Evaluate for:
      (1) Iron deficiency and uremia (for restless legs).
      (2) Anemia.
      (3) Thyroid function (if other signs are present).
    b. Sleep study: Polysomnography (in home or in sleep lab) for symptoms suggesting something other than primary insomnia.
      (1) Daytime sleepiness: obstructive sleep apnea, narcolepsy.
      (2) Nonrestorative sleep: periodic leg movements.
      (3) Sleep behavior suggesting parasomnia: somnambulism, rapid eye movement sleep behavior.

Treatment

Treatment of insomnia should focus on reducing daytime sleepiness and improving daytime function rather than attempting to achieve uninterrupted nighttime sleep.

1. Sleep hygiene measures (Box 5-1).
2. Cognitive behavior therapy to address anxiety and insomnia-perpetuating behavior.
3. Bright light exposure timed to correct a circadian phase disturbance can be helpful for insomnia secondary to delayed or advanced sleep phase, jet lag, or shift work.
4. Avoid alcohol.
5. Benzodiazepine sedative-hypnotics (e.g., temazepam 7.5 to 30 mg, triazolam 0.125 to 0.25 mg, estazolam 1 to 2 mg). Not generally a first-line choice.
6. Benzodiazepine receptor agonists.
    a. For sleep-onset and maintenance insomnia: zolpidem [Ambien] 5 to 10 mg hs or Ambien CR 6.25 to 12.2 mg hs.

BOX 5-1   Sleep Hygiene

The following sleep habits (sleep hygiene measures) might relieve insomnia.

- Reduce caffeine, alcohol, or tobacco late in the day or evening.
- Avoid heavy meals at night.
- Increase daytime activity.
- Increase daytime exposure to natural light.
- Take a warm bath as part of the bedtime ritual.
- Restrict the bed to sleep and sex.
- Get out of bed if not asleep after 30 minutes and return when drowsy. Repeat this if awakened during the night.
- Maintain regular sleep and wake times.
- Go to bed with calm mind; resolve arguments or deal with problems earlier in the day.

---

    b. For sleep-onset insomnia: zaleplon [Sonata] 5 to 10 mg hs.

    c. For sleep-onset difficulty: eszopiclone [Lunesta] 1 mg hs.

    c. For sleep-maintenance problem: eszopiclone 2 mg hs.

7. Ramelteon (Rozerem) 8 mg qhs is a melatonin agonist.

8. Do not use antihistamines (e.g., diphenhydramine) in geriatric patients because of the high risk of delirium.

9. Some evidence exists that benzodiazepines and benzodiazepine receptor agonists can be used for chronic insomnia either intermittently or nightly with only moderate risk of tolerance and dependence and low risk of addiction.

10. Zolpidem extended release (Ambien CR), eszopiclone, and ramelteon are approved by the Food and Drug Administration (FDA) for long-term use.

11. Sedating antidepressants (e.g., trazodone 25 to 150 mg, mirtazapine 7.5 to 30 mg).

    a. These are in widespread use but have limited data on safety and efficacy for insomnia.

    b. They are the treatments of choice for comorbid depression or anxiety.

    c. Amitriptyline should be avoided in older adults.

12. Sedating antipsychotics (e.g., quetiapine 25 to 200 mg, olanzapine 2.5 to 10 mg) for severe mood or psychotic disorders associated with insomnia.

13. Melatonin.

    a. Melatonin has been studied in controlled trials.

    b. It may shorten sleep-onset latency in some patients.

    c. Melatonin can be very effective for insomnia caused by circadian rhythm disturbances if it is scheduled to correct the underlying circadian phase disturbance.

SUGGESTED READINGS

Doghramji K: The epidemiology and diagnosis of insomnia. *Am J Manag Care* 12:S214-S220, 2006.

Jacobs GD et al: Cognitive behavior therapy and pharmacotherapy for insomnia: A randomized controlled trial and direct comparison. *Arch Int Med* 164(17): 1888-1896, 2004.

Krystal AD: The changing perspective on chronic insomnia management. *J Clin Psychiatry* 65(Suppl 8):20-25, 2004.

Morin AK: Strategies for treating chronic insomnia. *Am J Manag Care* 12:S230-S245, 2000.

Ringdahl EN, Pereira SL, Delzell JE: Treatment of primary insomnia. *J Am Board Fam Pract* 17(3):212-219, 2004.

Smith MT, Perlis ML, Park A, et al: Comparative meta-analysis of pharmacotherapy and behavior therapy for persistent insomnia. *Am J Psychiatry* 159:5-11, 2002.

PARKINSON'S DISEASE

Fred F. Ferri and Tom J. Wachtel

Definition

1. Idiopathic Parkinson's disease is a progressive, neurodegenerative disorder characterized clinically by rigidity, tremor, and bradykinesia.
   a. The major manifestations of the disease are due to loss of dopamine in the substantia nigra pars compacta.
   b. Its pathological hallmark is the Lewy body, which is a cytoplasmic eosinophilic inclusion body.

Epidemiology

1. Affects more than 1 million people in North America.
2. In persons younger than 40 years, fewer than 5/100,000 are affected.
3. In those older than 70 years, 700/100,000 are affected.
4. Highest incidence is in whites, lowest incidence is in Asians and Africans.

Physical Findings and Clinical Presentation

1. Tremor.
   a. Typically, a resting tremor with a frequency of 4 to 6 Hz that is often first noted in the hand as a pill-rolling tremor (thumb and forefinger). Can also involve the leg and lip.
   b. Tremor improves with purposeful movement.
   c. Tremor usually starts asymmetrically but can eventually involve the other hemibody.
   d. Tremor is absent in one fourth of the patients.
2. Rigidity (increased muscle tone).
   a. Rigidity is usually asymmetric in onset, involving the arm, leg, or both.
   b. It is resistance that persists throughout the range of passive movement of a joint.
3. Akinesia/bradykinesia (slowness in initiating movement).
4. Mask facies.
   a. Face seems expressionless, giving the appearance of depression.
   b. Decreased blink.
   c. Often there is excess drooling.
5. Gait disturbance.
   a. In the elderly, falls (particularly backwards) may be the first sign of Parkinson's, particularly in those with comorbid fall risk.

b. Stooped posture and decreased arm swing.
c. Difficulty initiating the first step.
d. Small shuffling steps that increase in speed (festinating gait) as if the patient is chasing his or her center of gravity (steps become progressively faster and shorter while the trunk inclines farther forward).

6. Other complaints and findings early on include:
   a. Micrographia: Handwriting becomes smaller.
   b. Hypophonia: Voice becomes softer.

7. Postural instability. Tested by the pull test.
   (1) Ask the patient to stand in place with the back to the examiner.
   (2) The examiner pulls the patient back by the shoulders.
   (3) Proper response is to take no steps back or very few steps back without falling.
   (4) Retropulsion is a positive test, as is falling straight back. This is not usually severe early on.

Treatment

Therapeutic Approach

1. General principles.
   a. Physical therapy.
   b. Encouragement and reassurance.
   c. Treatment of possible associated conditions (e.g., depression).

2. Avoidance of drugs that can induce or worsen Parkinson's.
   a. Neuroleptic agents (especially haloperidol).
   b. Certain antiemetics (e.g., prochlorperazine, trimethobenzamide); these drugs block dopamine receptors.
   c. Metoclopramide (Reglan) and cisapride (Propulsid).
   d. Nonselective monoamine oxidase (MAO) inhibitors (can induce hypertensive crisis).
   e. Certain antihypertensives (reserpine, methyldopa).

3. Pharmacologic therapy.
   a. Principles.
      (1) Drug therapy should be initiated when symptoms significantly limit patient's daily activities, but not before, because tolerance and side effects to antiparkinsonian agents are common. Deprenyl may have some early benefit.
      (2) Whether L-dopa or dopamine agonists should be the initial treatment is controversial, but treatment with these is the prevailing practice in the United States.
      (3) Pharmacotherapy should be initiated when required by symptoms. The prior practice of waiting for limitation of activities of daily living is now outdated.
      (4) Motor complications that develop during the course of the disease reflect the combination of disease progression and side effects of dopaminergic medications.
   b. Levodopa therapy.
      (1) Cornerstone of therapy should be L-dopa with a peripheral dopa decarboxylase inhibitor (carbidopa) to minimize side effects

(nausea, mood changes, postural hypotension). The combination of the two drugs is marketed under the trade name Sinemet.

(2) Usual dose is 25/100 mg (carbidopa/levodopa) tid 1 hour before meals.

(3) Controlled-release preparations (Sinemet CR) are available.

    (a) Levodopa/carbidopa 200 mg/50 mg.

    (b) Levodopa/carbidopa 100 mg/25 mg.

(4) Entacapone (Comtan) is a reversible inhibitor of catechol-O-methyl transferase.

    (a) It is used as an adjunct to levodopa/carbidopa.

    (b) Side effects include orthostatic hypotension, diarrhea, hallucinations.

    (c) Not to be used with any nonselective MAO inhibitor.

    (d) Dosage is 200 mg tid given with each dose of Sinemet.

    (e) Do not use as monotherapy.

c. Dopamine receptor agonists (ropinirole, pramipexole, pergolide, and bromocriptine).

(1) These are not as potent as levodopa, but they are often used as initial treatment in younger patients to attempt to delay the onset of complications (dyskinesias, motor fluctuations) associated with levodopa therapy.

(2) These medications are more expensive than levodopa.

(3) In general, they cause more side effects than levodopa. These include nausea, vomiting, lightheadedness, peripheral edema, confusion, and somnolence.

(4) Dosing.

    (a) Ropinirole (Requip): Initial dose is 0.25 mg tid; may titrate to 8 mg tid.

    (b) Pramipexole (Mirapex): Initial dose is 0.125 mg tid; may titrate to 1.5 mg tid.

    (c) Pergolide (Permax).

        (i) Initial dose is 0.05 mg for first 2 days, increased by 0.1 mg every third day over next 12 days to 1 mg tid.

        (ii) There have been cases of restrictive valvulopathy, most commonly in the tricuspid valve, associated with Permax use. All patients on this medication need a clinical cardiac examination, and if there is any concern, an echocardiogram.

    (d) Bromocriptine (Parlodel): Initial dose, 1.25 mg qhs; may titrate to 30 mg tid.

d. Selegiline (Deprenyl), an inhibitor of MAOB.

(1) Can be used early as initial therapy in those with mild disease or as adjunctive therapy.

(2) Selegiline was once advocated as early, first-line therapy because of proposed neuroprotective effects; however, those benefits are probably less robust than once thought.

(3) Usual dose is 5 mg bid with breakfast and lunch.

(4) It can be useful in treating the fatigue that is commonly associated with Parkinson's.

(5) Concurrent use of stimulants and sympathomimetics should be avoided.

   e. Amantadine (Symmetrel).
      (1) Amantadine is an antiviral agent that augments release and decreases reuptake of dopamine.
      (2) It can be used alone early in the disease or in combination with levodopa.
      (3) Dosage is 100 mg tid; titrate every week from 100 mg qd.
      (4) Must adjust for renal impairment.
      (5) Most notable side effect, especially in the elderly, is confusion.
   f. Anticholinergic agents.
      (1) These drugs are helpful in treating the tremor and drooling.
      (2) Anticholinergics can be used alone or in combination with levodopa.
      (3) Potential side effects include constipation, urinary retention, memory impairment, and hallucinations.
      (4) They should generally be avoided in the elderly.
      (5) Drugs and dosing.
         (a) Trihexyphenidyl (Artane): Initial dose, 1 mg tid.
         (b) Benztropine (Cogentin): Usual dose, 0.5 to 1 mg qd or bid.

Symptom Management

 1. To improve activities of daily living and to prevent frozen shoulder and falls: Physical therapy.
 2. Low-volume speech: Speech therapy.
 3. Dysarthria: Clonazepam 0.5 to 1 mg tid.
 4. Spastic bladder: Oxybutynin 5 to 10 mg tid.
 5. Constipation: High-fiber diet, fiber supplements (psyllium seed husks [Metamucil]), stool softeners (docusate [Colace]).
 6. Action tremor (often coexists with Parkinson's: Propranolol 40 to 80 mg tid.
 7. Painful dystonia of limbs: Baclofen 5 to 10 mg tid.
 8. Paroxysmal drenching sweats: β-blockers.
 9. Depression: Selective serotonin receptor inhibitors, electroconvulsive treatment (rarely).
10. Coexisting dementia can represent diffuse Lewy body disease or can be a late complication of Parkinson's.
    a. An acetylcholinesterase inhibitor trial should be prescribed.
    b. Delirium and hallucinations.
       (1) Management of delirium and hallucinations is often difficult because most antipsychotic drugs have extrapyramidal side effects, which worsen parkinsonian symptoms.
       (2) The atypical antipsychotic drugs of choice are clozaril (watch for agranulocytosis) and quetiapine.
11. Walkers, if prescribed, should always have wheels. Parkinson's patients risk falling backward when lifting a nonwheeled walker.

Surgical Options

 1. Pallidal (globus pallidus internal) and subthalamic deep brain stimulation are currently the surgical options of choice.
 2. Thalamic deep brain stimulation may be useful for refractory tremor.
 3. Surgery is limited to patients with disabling, medically refractory problems, and patients must still have a good response to L-dopa to undergo surgery.

4. Deep brain stimulation results in decreased dyskinesias, fluctuations, rigidity, and tremor.

Parkinson's-plus

Parkinson's-plus refers to symptoms and signs of parkinsonism occurring in association with other multisystem degenerative diseases.

1. Progressive supranuclear palsy.
   a. Usual onset at end of sixth or beginning of seventh decade.
   b. Characterized by parkinsonian symptoms plus:
      (1) Supranuclear gaze palsies (vertical > horizontal, downward > upward).
      (2) Subcortical dementia, depression.
      (3) Pseudobulbar palsy: dysphagia, dysarthria.
      (4) Axial rigidity: increased truncal and neck tone.
   c. Prognosis is poor.
      (1) Disease follows a rapid course, with significant incapacity within 2 to 4 years.
      (2) Mean survival is 6 years.
2. Olivopontocerebellar atrophy.
   a. Parkinsonian symptoms.
   b. Cerebellar signs: Scanning speech, ataxia, tremor of trunk and head.
   c. Mild dementia.
3. Shy–Drager syndrome (multiple systems atrophy).
   a. Parkinsonian features.
   b. Orthostatic hypotension (see "Syncope" in Section 5.6).
   c. Dizziness, unsteady gait.
4. Diffuse Lewy body disease.
   a. Parkinsonism with concomitant dementia.
   b. Patients often have early hallucinations and fluctuations in level of alertness and mental status.

SUGGESTED READINGS

Ahlskog JE: Parkinson's disease: Medical and surgical treatment. *Neurol Clin* 19(3): 579-605, 2001.

Lang AE, Lozano AM: Parkinson's disease. First of two parts. *N Engl J Med* 339(15): 1044-1053, 1998.

Lang AE, Lozano AM: Parkinson's disease. Second of two parts. *N Engl J Med* 339(16):1130-1143, 1998.

Nutt JG, Wooten GF: Diagnosis and initial management of Parkinson's disease. *N Engl J Med* 353:1021-1027, 2005.

Siderowf A: Parkinson's disease: Clinical features, epidemiology and genetics. *Neurol Clin* 19(3):565-578, 2001.

PERIPHERAL NEUROPATHY

Tom J. Wachtel

Definitions

Diseases of the peripheral nervous system can be distinguished from CNS disorders by the distribution of the neurologic abnormalities. Motor system involvement is characterized by flaccidity and eventually atrophy of involved muscles and areflexia. Peripheral neuropathies can affect all sensory modalities as well.

1. Anatomic classifications are shown in Figures 5-1 and 5-2 and in Tables 5-3 and 5-4.
   a. Radiculopathies are diseases of the nerve roots.
      (1) Monoradiculopathy involves a single dermatome.
      (2) Polyradiculopathy involves multiple dermatomes.
   b. Mononeuropathy is a single nerve dysfunction.
   c. Mononeuropathy multiplex or multifocal mononeuropathies.
      (1) Several nerves are dysfunctional concurrently or sequentially.
      (2) Usually not symmetric.
   d. Polyneuropathy has symmetric, distal, and graded distribution (stocking and glove).
   e. Autonomic neuropathy.
      (1) Manifests by orthostatic hypotension, gastroparesis, hypoperistalsis, incontinence, impotence.
      (2) Often associated with polyneuropathy.
2. Pathophysiologic classification.
   a. Axonal neuropathy (dying-back neuropathy) is usually a toxic polyneuropathy most commonly seen in chronic alcohol abuse or diabetes mellitus and is predominantly sensory.
   b. Demyelinating neuropathy.
      (1) Motor involvement is more likely and may predominate.
      (2) Subjective sensory complaints may be out of proportion to the objective findings, such as is seen in Guillain-Barré syndrome.
   c. Mixed axonal and demyelinating neuropathy is often seen in diabetes.

Clinical Features

1. Onset: acute vs. chronic.
2. Distribution of deficits: dermatome vs. peripheral nerve.
3. History.
   a. Past medical history.
   b. Family history.
   c. Occupational history.
   d. Medications and drugs, including alcohol.
4. Ancillary tests.
   a. Blood work.
      (1) In all cases: CBC, sedimentation rate, serum creatinine, urinalysis, fasting blood glucose, transaminase, vitamin B_{12} level, folate level, chest x-ray.
      (2) In selected cases: Watson-Schwartz test for acute intermittent porphyria, serum protein electrophoresis for multiple myeloma, heavy metals (lead, mercury, arsenic), B vitamins, HIV test, antinuclear antibody, screening for occult cancer.
   b. EMG looking for evidence of denervation.
   c. Nerve conduction studies.
      (1) Mild slowing in axonopathies: 40 m/sec.
      (2) Marked slowing in demyelinating neuropathies: 10 to 15 m/sec.
   d. Nerve biopsy.

Classification

1. Radiculopathies.
   a. Acute polyradiculopathy (Guillain-Barré syndrome).

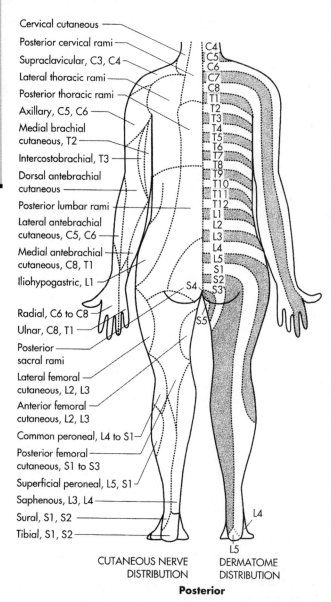

CUTANEOUS NERVE
DISTRIBUTION

DERMATOME
DISTRIBUTION

Posterior

Figure 5-1 Cutaneous sensation on the posterior aspect of the body. (From DeGowin EL, DeGowin RL: *Bedside diagnostic examination*, ed 4. New York, Macmillan, 1981.)

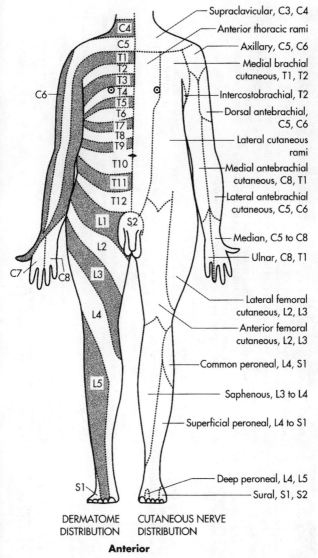

Figure 5-2 Cutaneous sensation on the anterior aspect of the body. (From DeGowin EL, DeGowin RL: *Bedside diagnostic examination*, ed 4. New York, Macmillan, 1981.)

Table 5-3   Common Mononeuropathies

Nerve	Clinical Presentation	Causes
Spinal accessory	Shoulder pain, droop, and weakness of abduction; trapezius wasting	Nerve trauma
Long thoracic	Winging of scapula	Backpacking, idiopathic
Axillary	Deltoid weakness, sensory loss over lateral upper arm	Trauma
Radial at spiral groove (Saturday night palsy)	Wrist and finger drop, weakness and areflexia of brachioradialis, sensory loss over dorsum of first web space	Acute compression
Musculocutaneous	Weakness of elbow flexion, sensory loss over radial aspect of forearm	Trauma, elbow hyperextension
Ulnar at elbow	Wasting, weakness of interossei; sensory loss over palmar and dorsal surface of ulnar aspect of hand	Chronic compression
Radial in forearm (posterior interosseous palsy)	Forearm pain, finger drop, radial deviation of extended wrist	Mass lesion, trauma, idiopathic
Median at wrist (carpal tunnel syndrome)	Nocturnal hand tingling; weakness, wasting of abductor pollicis brevis; sensory loss over volar aspect of fingers 1-3	Chronic compression
Ulnar at wrist	Weakness, wasting of interossei; variable sensory loss over fourth and fifth fingers	Occupational trauma
Femoral	Hip, groin pain; knee buckling; knee extensor weakness; absent knee jerk; sensory loss over anteromedial thigh and medial calf	Diabetes, retroperitoneal hemorrhage or tumor, postsurgical
Lateral femoral cutaneous at inguinal ligament	Thigh pain; sensory loss over lateral thigh; Tinel's sign in lateral inguinal ligament	Chronic compression
Sciatic	Weakness of dorsiflexion and plantar flexion; foot eversion and inversion; sensory loss over dorsum and sole of foot	Hip surgery, prolonged bed rest
Peroneal at fibular head (peroneal palsy)	Tripping; foot drop; sensory loss over lateral calf and dorsum of foot; normal foot eversion and inversion	Acute compression (i.e., leg crossing)
Posterior tibial at ankle (tarsal tunnel syndrome)	Nocturnal foot pain and tingling; Tinel's sign posterior to medial malleolus	Chronic compression, trauma

Table 5-4 Spinal Root Signs and Symptoms

Spinal Root	Distribution of Pain, Paresthesias, or Sensory Loss	Weak Muscles	Diminished Reflexes
C5	Shoulder, anterolateral arm, forearm	Deltoids, infraspinatus and supraspinatus, biceps	Pectoralis, biceps
C6	Shoulder, radial forearm, thumb	Biceps and brachioradialis, pronator teres	Biceps, brachioradialis
C7	Pectoral area, axilla, posterolateral forearm, second and third digits	Triceps, wrist extensors	Triceps
C8	Axilla, posteromedial arm, fourth and fifth digits	Hand interossei (ulnar nerve), abductor pollicis brevis (median nerve)	Finger flexors
L4	Hip, anterior thigh, anteromedial leg, great toe	Knee extensors, hip flexors	Knee
L5	Hip, posterolateral thigh, anterolateral leg, middle of foot	Foot extensors, great toe extensors, knee flexors	Medial hamstring
S1	Gluteal area, posterior thigh and leg, lateral foot	Foot flexors	Ankle
S2	Posterior thigh and leg	Toe flexors	—
S3-5	Sacral area	Sphincters	Bulbocavernosus, anal wink

C, cervical; L, lumbar; S, sacral.
Data from Stein J (ed): *Internal medicine*, ed 4. St Louis, Mosby, 1994.

(1) Signs and symptoms.
  (a) Patient presents with generalized weakness (sometimes ascending) associated with sensory complaints (subjective and objective) that progress over several days to weeks, following an infectious illness.
  (b) Weakness begins proximally; cranial nerves and respiratory muscles may be involved.
  (c) Autonomic neuropathy may also be present (e.g., sphincter dysfunction).
  (d) Cerebrospinal fluid characteristically shows an elevated protein with few or no cells.
(2) Treatment.
  (a) Mainly supportive because the disease is self-limited in most cases (90%).
  (b) If the disease is severe, plasmapheresis and IVIg may be effective.
  b. Chronic polyradiculopathy may be idiopathic or associated with malignancies (e.g., multiple myeloma).
  c. Monoradiculopathy.
    (1) Cervical disk hernation.
    (2) Lumbar disk herniation (sciatica).
    (3) Herpes zoster (shingles).
2. Mononeuropathies (distribution of the deficits is a single nerve).
  a. Chronic compression (entrapment neuropathies).
    (1) Medial nerve (carpal tunnel syndrome).
    (2) Ulnar nerve (compression at elbow).
    (3) Lateral femoral cutaneous nerve (tight belt).
  b. Acute compression.
    (1) Radial nerve (compression at spiral groove of humerus by someone's head during sleep).
    (2) Peroneal nerve at fibular head (leg crossing).
  c. Trauma.
3. Mononeuropathy multiplex (distribution of deficits is several nerves; etiology is usually a vasculitis).
  a. Polyarteritis nodosa.
  b. Vasculitides associated with other collagen vascular diseases.
  c. Diabetes.
  d. Sarcoidosis.
  e. Leprosy.
4. Polyneuropathies.
  a. Axonal.
    (1) Vitamin deficiencies.
      (a) B_1 (beriberi).
      (b) B_6.
      (c) B_{12}.
      (d) Niacin (pellagra).
    (2) Metabolic diseases.
      (a) Diabetes mellitus.
      (b) Uremia.
      (c) Thyroid dysfunction.

(3) Infections.
  (a) HIV.
  (b) Lyme disease.
(4) Paraneoplastic neuropathies.
(5) Neuropathies associated with connective tissue diseases.
(6) Hereditary neuropathies.
  (a) Neuropathy associated with Friedreich's ataxia and variants.
  (b) Ataxia-telangiectasia.
(7) Neuropathies associated with dysproteinemias and amyloidosis.
(8) Neuropathies induced by drugs (amiodarone, dapsone, dideoxyinosine, fluoxetine, hydralazine, isoniazid, nitrofurantoin, phenytoin, vincristine).
(9) Neuropathies induced by toxins (acrylamide, arsenic, cyanide, hexacarbons, mercury, methylbromide, organophosphorous esters).
  b. Demyelinating neuropathies. In clinical practice, demyelinating neuropathies are very difficult to distinguish from polyradiculopathies.
    (1) Lead toxicity.
    (2) Dysproteinemia.
    (3) Hereditary (Charcot-Marie-Tooth disease).

Neuropathic Pain

1. Neuropathic pain is defined as the sensation derived from the abnormal discharges of impaired or injured neural structures in either the peripheral or central nervous system, including receptors, axons, and cell bodies.
  a. Hyperalgesia is extreme sensitivity to painful stimuli or reduced threshold to feel pain.
  b. Hypalgesia is decreased sensitivity to pain or increased threshold to feel pain.
  c. Hyperesthesia is abnormal acuteness of sensitivity to touch, pain, or other sensory stimuli.
  d. Hypesthesia is diminished sensitivity to stimulation.
  e. Allodynia is feeling pain from a nonpainful stimulus.
2. Neuropathic pain is not a disease. It is a symptom, or at most a syndrome, that can result from any of several illnesses.
3. Neuropathic pain should prompt a search for its cause.
4. Neuropathic pain affects 1.5% of the U.S. population, but this is likely an underestimate.

Treatment

1. Antiepileptics.
  a. Gabapentin (Neurontin).
    (1) Initial dose: 300 mg PO qd, advance to 300 mg PO tid by the end of the first week.
    (2) Effective dose is higher than 1600 mg/day.
    (3) Maximum dose is 1500 mg PO tid.
  b. Pregebalin (Lyrica).
    (1) Initial dose: 50 mg tid.
    (2) May increase to 100 mg bid or 150 mg bid.

    c. Topiramate (Topamax).
      (1) Initial dose: 25 mg PO qd.
      (2) Increase by 25 mg/week up to the maximum effective dose of 400 to 800 mg/day.
    d. Lamotrigine (Lamictal).
      (1) Initial dose: 25 mg PO bid.
      (2) Increase slowly (by 100 mg every 2 weeks) to maximum effective dose of 200 to 300 mg PO bid.
      (3) Risk: Stevens-Johnson syndrome.
    e. Carbamazepine (Tegretol): Especially for trigeminal neuralgia.
      (1) Initial dose: 400 mg PO bid.
      (2) Increase to tid if necessary.
      (3) Side effects and/or drug levels should determine safe increase in dosing.
      (4) Risk: Aplastic anemia.
  2. Antidepressants.
    a. Tricyclic antidepressants: Use nortriptyline rather than amitriptyline (fewer anticholinergic side effects).
      (1) Initial dose: 10 mg PO pq in elderly.
      (2) Can increase by 25 mg every week to usual maximal effective dose of 150 mg/day.
      (3) The older the patient, the more caution should be used because of the anticholinergic activity of this class of drug.
      (4) Avoid in demented patients.
    b. SSRIs.
      (1) Paroxetine.
        (a) Initial dose: 10 mg PO qd.
        (b) Increase by 10 mg/week.
        (c) Maximum dose 60 mg PO qd.
          (i) Sertraline: 25 to 200 mg qd.
          (ii) Citalopram: 10 to 40 mg qd.
    c. Serotonin and norepinephrine reuptake inhibitors (SNRIs).
      (1) Duloxetine (Cymbalta): 30 to 60 mg qd.
      (2) Venlafaxine (Effexor XR): 37.5 to 150 mg qd.
  3. Analgesics.
    a. Tramadol.
      (1) Initial dose: 150 mg/day (50 mg tid).
      (2) Increase by 50 mg/week.
      (3) Maximum 200 to 400 mg/day.
    b. Morphine (oral).
      (1) Initial dose: 15 to 30 mg q8h.
      (2) Maximum 90 to 360 mg/day.
    c. Oxycodone (Oxycontin).
      (1) Initial dose: 20 mg q12h.
      (2) Increase by 10 mg/week.
      (3) Maximum 40 to 160 mg/day.
    d. See "Palliative Care" in Chapter 7.
  4. Topical anesthetics.
    a. A 5% lidocaine patch may be applied to the area of pain; maximum three patches in 12 hours.

   b. Capsaicin 0.075% lotion, cream, or stick is inconsistent in its ability to relieve pain and can exacerbate it.

5. Procedures.
   a. Nerve blocks.
   b. Spinal cord stimulator.

6. Counseling should be considered to address psychologic issues exacerbating physiologic pain.

RESTLESS LEGS SYNDROME

Tom J. Wachtel

Definitions

1. Restless legs syndrome (RLS) is a primary neurologic disorder of unknown cause.
2. It manifests with both sensory and motor symptoms usually involving the lower extremities and disrupting sleep.
3. It is possibly related to dopaminergic dysregulation at the level of the spinal cord or higher in the CNS.

Epidemiology

1. About 10% of patients up to age 79 years, but only 1% to 2% find it bothersome enough to warrant treatment.
2. About 19% of patients age 80 years and older.
3. Prevalence increases with age (might explain the slight female overrepresentation).
4. Symptoms worsen with age.
5. Primary RLS has an autosomal dominant mode of inheritance and follows a female-to-male ratio of 6:4.
6. Probably underdiagnosed in most practices because patients do not report it (unable or embarrassed).

Clinical Findings

1. Sensory nocturnal complaints usually affect both lower extremities.
   a. Crawly feeling or fizzle under the skin.
   b. Itching under the skin.
   c. Pain or ache.
   d. Electric shocks.
   e. Irresistible urge to move the symptomatic leg.
   f. Other words used by patients to describe the leg symptoms: creeping, burning, searing, tugging, pulling, drawing, like water flowing, worms or bugs under the skin, restless, weird, indescribable.
   g. Occasionally, these symptoms are misinterpreted as psychotic (e.g., in patients with dementia, the "bugs" are diagnosed as hallucinations) and are incorrectly treated with neuroleptic drugs.
2. Leg movements during sleep can occur but are not the prevailing complaint (unlike the urge to move). These movements are short bursts lasting less than 5 seconds.
3. Rarely progresses to upper extremities.
4. Effects include sleep disruption, occasional daytime somnolence.
5. Patients obtain consistent symptom relief or improvement with leg movement or walking, rubbing, pressure, or heating pad.

Etiology

Primary RLS is found in 50% to 60% of RLS patients. Causes include:
1. Iron deficiency.
2. End-stage renal failure.
3. Peripheral neuropathy or radiculopathy.
4. Rheumatologic conditions such as rheumatoid arthritis or fibromyalgia.
5. Medications such as SSRIs.

Differential Diagnosis

1. Periodic limb movement disorder occurring during sleep.
   a. Repetitive limb movements (lower extremities > upper extremities).
   b. Associated with arousals from sleep and with daytime sleeping.
   c. Patient is typically unaware of the limb movements, but the bed partner reports restlessness or kicking during sleep.
   d. Periodic limb movement is often associated with RLS.
2. Peripheral neuropathy and radiculopathy.
3. Anxiety and mood disorders.
4. Chronic fatigue.
5. Other sleep disorders.
6. Neuroleptic-induced akathisia.
7. Dyskinesias while awake.
8. Nocturnal leg cramps with or without peripheral artery disease.

Work-up

1. History is typically diagnostic, with sensitivity and specificity both >90%.
2. Family history of RLS or "night walking."
3. Polysomnography leads.
4. Ambulatory recording of leg activity over several nights with sleep logs.
5. Serum iron studies including CBC, iron level and total iron binding capacity (TIBC), or ferritin.
6. EMG for neuropathy, radiculopathy, or myelopathy, if suspected.
7. CNS MRI for myelopathy or stroke, if suspected.

Treatment

1. Dopaminergic drugs are first line. Dose may be divided bid or tid as needed.
   a. Pramipexole (Mirapex).
      (1) Initial dose: 0.125 mg hs.
      (2) Typical dose: 0.375 mg per day hs.
      (3) Maximum dose: 0.75 mg hs.
   b. Ropinirole (Requip).
      (1) Initial dose: 0.25 mg hs.
      (2) Typical dose: 2 mg hs.
      (3) Maximum dose: 4 mg hs.
   c. Levodopa/carbidopa (Sinemet).
      (1) Initial dose: 25/100 hs.
      (2) Maximum 3 to 4 doses per day.
2. Antiepileptics.
   a. Gabapentin (Neurotin).
      (1) Initial dose: 300 mg hs.
      (2) Maximum dose: 3600 mg/day (divided tid).

b. Carbamazepine (Carbatrol).
  (1) Initial dose: 200 mg.
  (2) Maximum dose: 1200 mg/day (divided bid).
c. Topiramate (Topamax).
  (1) Initial dose: 25 mg.
  (2) Maximum dose: 200 mg/day (divided bid).
3. Benzodiazepines.
4. Trazodone.
5. Opioids.

SUGGESTED READINGS

Allen RP, Picchietti D, Hening WA, et al: Restless legs syndrome: diagnostic criteria, special considerations, and epidemiology. A report from the restless legs syndrome diagnosis and epidemiology workshop at the National Institutes of Health. *Sleep Med* 4:101-119, 2003.

Avecillas JF, Golish JA, Giannini C, Yataco JC: Restless legs syndrome: Keys to recognition and treatment. *Cleve Clin J Med* 72:769-770, 773-774, 776 passim, 2005.

Bogan RK, Fry JM, Schmidt MH, et al: Ropinirole in the treatment of patients with restless legs syndrome: A US-based, double blind, placebo-controlled clinical trial. *Mayo Clin Proc* 81:17-27, 2006.

Earley CJ: Clinical practice. Restless legs syndrome. *N Engl J Med* 348:2103-2109, 2003.

Happe S, Trenkwalder C: Role of dopamine receptor agonists in the treatment of restless legs syndrome. *CNS Drugs* 18:27-36, 2004.

National Heart, Lung, and Blood Institute Working Group on Restless Legs Syndrome: Restless legs syndrome: Detection and management in primary care. *Am Fam Physician* 62:108-114, 2000.

Phillips B, Young T, Finn L, et al: Epidemiology of restless legs symptoms in adults. *Arch Intern Med* 160:2137-2141, 2000.

SEIZURE DISORDERS

John E. Croom and Tom J. Wachtel

Definitions

1. Generalized tonic–clonic seizures.
   a. Marked by paroxysmal hypersynchronous neuronal activity involving both cerebral hemispheres and resulting in loss of consciousness.
   b. Tonic muscle contraction is followed by rhythmic clonic contractions.
   c. The seizure can start focally in one region or hemisphere of the brain and develop subsequent secondary generalization.
2. Partial seizures.
   a. The onset of abnormal electrical activity originates in a focal region or lobe of the brain.
   b. Clinical manifestations can involve sensory, motor, autonomic, or psychic symptoms.
   c. Consciousness may be preserved (simple partial seizures) or impaired (complex partial seizures).

Epidemiology and Demographics

1. Incidence in the United States is 100 cases/100,000 persons per year.
2. Prevalence in the United States is approximately 6.5 cases/1000 persons for all types of epilepsy.
3. Predominance: Male slightly higher than female.
4. Genetic predisposition exists for the idiopathic generalized epilepsies.

Clinical Findings

The hallmark for a seizure is typically its unpredictable occurrence as a spell.

1. Generalized tonic-clonic seizure (described as *grand mal seizure* in now-outdated texts).
   a. Sequence of motor events during the seizure typically includes widespread tonic muscle contraction evolving to clonic jerking.
   b. Typically associated with postictal confusion lasting up to several hours.
   c. May be associated with tongue, cheek, or lip biting and/or urinary incontinence.
   d. Generally normal neurologic examination.
      (1) Focal deficits may be found in patients with an underlying lesion causing the seizures.
      (2) Rarely, postictal neurologic deficits are seen in the absence of specific brain lesions; they resolve in less than 48 hours.
   e. Postictal fever usually resolves in 24 to 48 hours if there is no comorbid infection.
   f. Aspiration pneumonitis is more common in the elderly as a complication.
2. Partial seizure.
   a. Clinical presentation is varied and depends on the site of origin of the abnormal electrical discharges.
   b. Simple partial seizure symptoms can include:
      (1) Focal motor or sensory symptoms.
      (2) Language disturbance.
      (3) Olfactory, visual, or auditory hallucinations.
      (4) Visceral sensations.
      (5) Fear or panic.
   c. Complex partial seizure symptoms can include:
      (1) Loss or reduction of awareness, which may be preceded by an aura.
      (2) There may be associated automatisms or alterations in behavior.
   d. There may be a march or progression of symptoms over seconds to minutes as the ictal focus spreads along the cortex.
   e. Neurologic examination ranges from normal to focal neurologic deficits, depending on the underlying cause.

Etiology

1. Seizures are not a disease, they are a symptom of an underlying abnormality affecting the CNS.
2. Etiology of seizures can be divided into idiopathic, symptomatic, or cryptogenic.
3. With idiopathic generalized tonic-clonic seizures, there is a postulated inherited basis for the disorder. They can continue over the patient's lifetime.
4. Symptomatic generalized tonic-clonic seizures and most partial seizures result from an underlying cause such as:
   a. Metabolic or toxic abnormalities (including medications).
   b. Stroke.

    c. Vascular malformations.
    d. CNS infection.
    e. Brain tumor.
    f. Trauma.
5. Cryptogenic seizures are those without a clear underlying cause (rare onset in the elderly).

Work-up

1. Laboratory.
    a. Glucose, BUN, creatinine, electrolytes.
    b. CBC.
    c. Alanine aminotransferase (ALT), alkaline phosphatase.
    d. Calcium, phosphorus, magnesium.
    e. Oxygen saturation.
    f. Alcohol level and toxicology screen when appropriate.
2. Lumbar puncture as indicated by history and physical examination.
3. Electroencephalogram (EEG).
    a. EEG is the most valuable diagnostic tool for identifying seizure type and predicting the likelihood of recurrence.
    b. EEG is normal in as many as 50% of patients; thus, diagnosis is made primarily by history.
4. MRI with contrast is the modality of choice because of its high sensitivity for stroke, tumor, abscess, atrophy, and vascular malformations.
5. CT scan without contrast if hemorrhage is suspected.
6. When a seizure is not witnessed, the work-up should also consider the possibility of syncope.

Treatment

1. Nonpharmacologic therapy: Avoid sleep deprivation or environmental precipitants (e.g., photosensitive epilepsy).
2. Pharmacologic therapy (Table 5-5).
    a. Generalized tonic-clonic seizures.
       (1) Sodium valproate and phenytoin are appropriate first-line therapeutic agents.

Table 5-5 Drug of Choice in Treatment of Epilepsy

Seizure Type	Drug of Choice
Standard Drugs	
Generalized tonic-clonic, simple, and complex partial	Phenytoin, valproic acid, carbamazepine phenobarbital, levetiracetam, zonisamide
Absence	Ethosuximide, valproic acid
Temporal epilepsy	Phenytoin, gabapentin
Newer Drugs	
Generalized tonic-clonic, simple, partial, and complex partial	Lamotrigine, tigabine, topiramate, zonisamide, oxcarbazepine, levetiracetam, gabapentin

(2) Newer agents such as lamotrigine and topiramate may be better tolerated.

(3) For each patient, anticonvulsant choice is influenced by factors such as effectiveness, cost, adverse effects, ease of administration, and type of epilepsy syndrome if present.

(4) A single seizure with an identifiable and easily correctable provoking factor (e.g., hyponatremia) does not warrant long-term use of anticonvulsants.

b. Partial seizures.

(1) Carbamazepine or phenytoin are common first-line therapeutic agents.

(2) Sodium valproate may also be effective.

(3) Newer agents such as lamotrigine or oxcarbazepine may be better tolerated, but they are more expensive.

c. Usually a single seizure is not treated with chronic anticonvulsants.

d. Status epilepticus.

(1) Defined as continuous seizure activity for longer than 30 minutes or sequential seizures with full recovery of consciousness between seizures.

(2) Treatment.

(a) Maintain and protect the airway.

(b) Give oxygen.

(c) Monitor and maintain vital signs.

(d) Gain IV access.

i. Lorazepam 0.1 mg/kg IV at 2 mg/min.

ii. If lorazepam is ineffective, give phosphenytoin 20 mg/kg IV at 150 mg/min or phenytoin at 50 mg/min.

iii. If phosphenytoin or phenytoin is ineffective, use phenobarbital 20 mg/kg IV at 100 mg/min.

iv. Thiamine and hypertonic glucose, both IV, are usually also administered.

SUGGESTED READINGS

Browne TR, Holmes GL: Epilepsy. N Engl J Med 344:1145-1151, 2001.

Chabolla DR: Characteristics of the epilepsies. Mayo Clin Proc 77:981-990, 2002.

Torres MR, Ahern GL, Labiner DM. Seizures and epilepsy: An approach to diagnosis and management. J Clin Outcomes Manage 12:103-115, 2005.

Wiebe S, Blume WT, Girvin JP, et al: A randomized, controlled trial of surgery for temporal-lobe epilepsy. N Engl J Med 345:311-318, 2001.

STROKE

Richard S. Isaacson and Tom J. Wachtel

Definition

Stroke, or cerebrovascular accident, is an acute brain injury caused by decreased blood supply or hemorrhage.

Epidemiology

1. Incidence is 10 to 20/100,000 persons older than 65 years.
2. Peak incidence is 80 to 84 years.
3. Prevalence in the United States is estimated at 2 million persons.
4. Predominance is 30% higher in men than in women.

Clinical Findings

1. Motor and/or sensory and/or cognitive deficits, depending on distribution and extent of involved vascular territory.
   a. Transient ischemic attack (TIA).
      (1) Precedes stroke in more than 50% of cases.
      (2) Carotid artery TIA.
         (a) Monocular loss of vision (amaurosis fugax).
         (b) Unilateral limb or face paresis or paresthesias.
         (c) Transient aphasia.
         (d) Unilateral headache.
         (e) Carotid bruit.
      (3) Vertebrobasilar artery TIA.
         (a) Binocular visual disturbances, diplopia.
         (b) Vertigo, nausea, vomiting.
         (c) Cerebellar dysfunction (ataxia, gait disturbance).
         (d) Loss of postural tone (drop attack)—rare.
   b. Stroke: mode of onset depends on etiology.
      (1) Progressive in thrombotic stroke.
      (2) Sudden onset in embolic stroke.
      (3) Variable onset in hemorrhagic stroke.
2. Manifestations (Table 5-6).
   a. Contralateral motor weakness or sensory loss.
   b. Language difficulties (aphasia; predominantly left-sided lesions).
   c. Visuospatial/neglect phenomena (predominantly right-sided lesions).

Etiology

1. About 70% to 80% are caused by ischemic infarcts.
2. About 20% to 30% are hemorrhagic-ischemic strokes or cerebral infarction. These are caused by the following:
   a. Large-vessel atheromatous disease (most common).
   b. Lacunar infarcts.
   c. Cardiogenic embolism usually associated with atrial fibrillation.
   d. Migrainous stroke.
   e. Vasculitis.
3. Hemorrhagic strokes or intracranial hemorrhage.
   a. Subarachnoid hemorrhage.
      (1) Berry aneurysm.
      (2) Arteriovenous malformation.
      (3) Vasculitis, endocarditis, coagulopathy.
      (4) Unknown.
   b. Intracerebral hemorrhage.
      (1) Usually secondary to hypertension.
      (2) Less common causes are arteriovenous malformations, tumors, coagulopathy, amyloid angiopathy.
      (3) Ischemic strokes can become hemorrhagic, particularly in anticoagulated patients.

Differential Diagnosis

1. TIA.
   a. Traditionally defined as focal neurologic deficits lasting less than 24 hours.
   b. TIAs usually last less than 60 minutes.

Table 5-6　Neurologic Signs Associated with Cerebrovascular Accident by Location

Artery	Function	Neurologic Signs
Internal carotid artery	Supplies the cerebral hemispheres and diencephalon by the ophthalmic and ipsilateral hemisphere arteries	Occasional unilateral blindness Severe contralateral hemiplegia, hemianesthesia, and hemianopia
Middle cerebral artery	Supplies structures of higher cerebral processes of communication; language interpretation; perception and interpretation of space, sensation, form, and voluntary movement	Profound aphasia if left hemisphere is involved Alterations in communication, cognition, mobility, and sensation Homonymous hemianopia Contralateral hemiplegia or hemiparesis
Anterior cerebral artery	Supplies medial surfaces and upper convexities of frontal and parietal lobes and medial surface of hemisphere, which includes motor and somesthetic cortex serving the legs	Emotional lability Confusion, amnesia, personality changes Urinary incontinence Impaired mobility, with weakness greater in lower extremities than in upper
Posterior cerebral artery	Supplies medial and inferior temporal lobes, medial occipital lobe, thalamus, posterior hypothalamus, and visual receptive area	Homonymous hemianopia Hemianesthesia Cortical blindness Memory deficits
Vertebral or basilar arteries	Supply the brainstem and cerebellum	*Incomplete occlusion* Drop attacks Unilateral and bilateral weakness of extremities Diplopia, homonymous hemianopia Nausea, vertigo, tinnitus, syncope Dysphagia Dysarthria Sometimes confusion and drowsiness

		Anterior portion of pons Locked-in syndrome—no movement except eyelids; sensation and consciousness preserved *Complete occlusion or hemorrhage* Coma Miotic pupils Decerebrate rigidity Respiratory and circulatory abnormalities Death
Posterior inferior cerebellar artery	Supplies the lateral and posterior portion of the medulla	Wallenberg's syndrome Dysphagia, dysphonia Ipsilateral anesthesia of face and cornea for pain and temperature (touch preserved) Ipsilateral Horner's syndrome Contralateral loss of pain and temperature sensation in trunk and extremities Ipsilateral decompensation of movement (cerebellar signs)
Anterior inferior and superior cerebellar arteries	Supply the cerebellum	Difficulty in articulation, swallowing, gross movements of limbs; nystagmus (cerebellar signs)
Anterior spinal artery	Supplies the anterior spinal cord	Flaccid paralysis, below level of lesion Loss of pain, touch, temperature sensation (proprioception preserved, sensory level)
Posterior spinal artery	Supplies the posterior spinal cord	Sensory loss, particularly proprioception, vibration, touch, and pressure (movement preserved)

Adapted from Seidel HM (ed): *Mosby's guide to physical examination,* ed 4. St Louis, Mosby, 1999.

2. Migraine (can cause a stroke).
3. Seizure.
   a. Postictal state can mimic stroke.
   b. Seizure can result from cerebrovascular disease.
4. Mass lesion.
   a. Tumor.
   b. Abscess.
   c. Subdural hematoma.
5. Amyotrophic lateral sclerosis (may begin unilaterally).
6. Multiple sclerosis.

Work-up

1. Laboratory tests.
   a. CBC.
   b. Platelet count.
   c. Prothrombin time (PT) (international normalized ratio [INR]).
   d. Partial thromboplastin time (PTT).
   e. Blood urea nitrogen (BUN), creatinine.
   f. Lipid panel.
   g. Glucose.
   h. Electrolytes.
   i. Urinalysis.
   j. Additional tests, depending on suspected etiology.
2. Imaging studies.
   a. CT scan without contrast to distinguish hemorrhage from infarct.
   b. MRI.
      (1) MRI is superior to CT in identifying abnormalities in the poste-
          rior fossa and, in particular, lacunar (small vessel) infarcts.
      (2) Diffusion weighted imaging is best to determine hyperacute
          ischemia (positive within 15 to 30 min of symptom onset).
      (3) Magnetic resonance angiography (MRA) is recommended to
          help identify vascular pathology (e.g., extent of intracranial
          atherosclerosis or vascular distribution of ischemia).
   c. In select cases (e.g., hemorrhagic stroke), conventional angiography
      can identify aneurysms or other vascular malformations.
   d. Carotid Doppler should be performed in cases of ischemic stroke to
      anterior or middle cerebral artery territory.
   e. Cardiac evaluation is warranted especially in suspected embolic strokes.
      (1) Electrocardiogram (ECG) and cardiac enzymes in selected cases.
      (2) Telemetry.
      (3) Two-dimensional echocardiography.
      (4) Holter monitor or loop recorder if paroxysmal atrial fibrillation
          is suspected.

Treatment

1. Initial management is shown in Box 5-2.
2. Control of blood pressure (BP).
   a. In patients with chronic hypertension, the area of infarction can be
      extended if the BP is lowered into the "normal" range.
   b. It is best not to lower BP too aggressively in the acute setting unless
      it is very markedly elevated.

BOX 5-2   Initial Considerations for Patients with Strokes

Initial Care

- Stabilize the patient, secure the airway, and provide adequate oxygenation
- Assess level of consciousness, language, visual fields, eye movements, and pupillary movements
- Obtain history and perform physical examination
- Perform CT of head without contrast
- Obtain CBC with platelets and differential, electrolytes, creatinine, BUN, glucose, PT/PTT, arterial blood gas, or oxygen saturation
- Consider a toxicology screen
- Consider special coagulation studies such as antiphospholipid antibodies, factor V Leiden assay, protein C and protein S, antithrombin III, ANA, fibrinogen, RPR, homocysteine, serum protein electrophoresis

Acute Intervention

- Consider acute intervention with t-PA if the symptoms have occurred for less than 3 h.

Admission

Consider the following with admission orders:
- Transthoracic echocardiogram; consider transesophageal echocardiogram if the transthoracic echocardiogram is equivocal or there is a high suspicion of cardiogenic thromboembolism
- Carotid duplex ultrasonography
- Telemetry
- Supplemental oxygen and appropriate oxygen saturation monitoring
- Antiplatelet therapy
- Fluid restriction if the infarct is large, to reduce cerebral edema
- Close monitoring of intake and output
- Regular determinations of blood glucose levels to avoid hyperglycemia
- NPO if there are concerns about the pharyngeal reflex pending swallowing evaluation
- Elevate the head of the bed 20 to 30 degrees to reduce cerebral edema
- Bed rest for the first 24 h with fall precautions, then advance as appropriate
- Vital signs and neurologic checks every 2 h four times or until stable
- Prophylaxis for DVT if immobile (elastic stockings at a minimum)
- Speech therapy consultation to evaluate swallowing
- Neurology, physical therapy, occupational therapy, nutrition, and social services consultations

ANA, Antinuclear antibodies; BUN, blood urea nitrogen; CBC, complete blood count; CT, computed tomography; DVT, deep venous thrombosis; NPO, nothing by mouth; PT/PTT, prothrombin time/partial thromboplastin time; RPR, rapid plasma reagin; t-PA, tissue plasminogen activator.
From Rakel RE (ed): *Textbook of Family Medicine,* ed 7. Philadelphia, Saunders Elsevier, 2007, p 1292.

    c. Adequate hydration and bed rest.
      (1) Head of bed down in pressure-dependent ischemia.
      (2) Head of bed up if patient has aspiration risk.
3. Tight glycemic control is recommended (e.g., insulin sliding scale).
4. Patients presenting less than 3 hours after onset of a nonhemorrhagic stroke.
    a. Thrombolytic therapy in a specialized stroke center is beneficial in selected populations.
    b. In some patients presenting at more than 3 hours but less than 6 hours after onset, an interventional neuroradiologist or neurosurgeon may be able to offer either direct injection of a clot-busting agent (such as intraarterial tPA) or direct extraction of the clot (e.g., FDA-approved Merci Retrieval System). However, this remains investigational and has yet to be well studied in a controlled trial.
    c. Intracranial angioplasty/stenting may also be a consideration.
5. Anticoagulation.
    a. If atrial fibrillation and/or a cardiac mural thrombus are found on echocardiography, heparin may be considered.
    b. Warfarin is appropriate for patients with cardioembolic stroke as well as for patients with atrial fibrillation, in the absence of contraindications.
6. Antiplatelet therapy reduces the risk of subsequent stroke.
    a. Medications.
      (1) Aspirin.
      (2) Dipyridamole/aspirin (Aggrenox).
      (3) Clopidogrel (Plavix).
      (4) Rarely ticlopidine.
    b. Approach.
      (1) If the patient presents with a first TIA/stroke and was on no prior antiplatelet agent, aspirin 325 mg or 81 mg daily is usually chosen initially.
      (2) If a TIA occurs while the patient is on aspirin, the patient should be switched to dipyridamole/aspirin or clopidogrel.
7. Perform a swallowing evaluation in patients with absent gag reflex or patients who cough or choke during meals in the aftermath of a stroke.
8. If a subarachnoid or intracerebral hemorrhage is found on CT:
    a. MRA and/or cerebral angiography may be indicated to identify an aneurysm.
    b. If no aneurysm is found and the clot is expanding, neurosurgical evacuation of the clot may be attempted, but outcomes are generally poor.
9. Modification of risk factors (e.g., smoking cessation, exercise, diet).
10. Carotid endarterectomy is recommended in patients with carotid artery TIA or stroke associated with 70% to 99% ipsilateral carotid stenosis. Carotid endarterectomy should be performed by an experienced surgeon who has demonstrated low morbidity and mortality.
11. A polymodality physical medicine and rehabilitative approach is an integral part of poststroke recovery. This includes physical, occupational, and speech therapy individualized depending on deficits (see Chapter 8).

Prognosis

1. Prognosis depends on severity of deficits, etiology, and other concurrent medical and surgical illness.
2. Most functional recovery can be expected to occur during the first 6 months following a completed stroke.

SUGGESTED READINGS

Benavente D, Hart RG: Stroke: Part II. Management of acute ischemic stroke. *Am Fam Physician* 59:2828-2834, 1999.

Diener HC, Bogousslavsky J, Brass LM, et al: Aspirin and clopidogrel compared with clopidogrel alone after recent ischaemic stroke or transient ischaemic attack in high-risk patients (MATCH): Randomized, double-blind, placebo-controlled trial. *Lancet* 364(9431):331-337, 2004.

Goldstein LB, Adams R, Alberts MJ, et al: Primary prevention of ischemic stroke: A Guideline from the American Heart Association/American Stroke Association Stroke Council. *Stroke* 37:1583-1633, 2006. PDF available for download at http://stroke.ahajournals.org/cgi/reprint/37/6/1583 (accessed February 1, 2007).

Meschia JF, Miller DA, Brott TG: Thrombolytic treatment of acute ischemic stroke. *Mayo Clin Proc* 77:542-551, 2002.

Straus SE, Majumdar SR, McAlister FA: New evidence for stroke prevention: Scientific review. *JAMA* 288:1388-1395, 2002.

SUBDURAL HEMATOMA

Daniel T. Mattson, with revisions by Tom J. Wachtel

Definition

A subdural hematoma is bleeding into the subdural space, caused by rupture of bridging veins between the brain and venous sinuses.

Epidemiology

1. Nearly all cases are caused by trauma, although the trauma may be quite trivial and easily overlooked.
2. Victims are often very old.
3. Coagulation abnormalities, especially use of anticoagulation in the elderly, is a significant risk factor, particularly in patients with a history of falls.

Clinical Findings

1. Recent head injury, usually during fall.
   a. Loss of consciousness is not necessary.
   b. Injury is often described as minimal brain trauma.
2. Vague headache, often worse in morning than evening.
3. Some apathy, confusion, and clouding of consciousness are common.
   a. Frank coma can complicate late cases.
   b. Chronic subdural hematomas can cause a dementia picture.
4. Neurologic symptoms may be transient, simulating TIA.
5. Almost any sign of cortical dysfunction may occur, including hemiparesis, sensory deficits, or language abnormalities, depending on which part of the cortex the hematoma presses on.
6. New-onset seizures should raise the index of suspicion.

Etiology

Traumatic rupture of cortical bridging veins, especially where stretched by underlying cerebral atrophy.

Differential Diagnosis

1. Epidural hematoma.
   a. Usually results from more substantial trauma.
   b. May be associated with a skull fracture.
2. Subarachnoid hemorrhage.
3. Mass lesion (e.g., tumor).
4. Ischemic stroke.
5. Intraparenchymal hemorrhage.

Work-up

1. CT scan is sensitive for diagnosis and should be performed in a timely fashion.
   a. Any head trauma in a patient on anticoagulant therapy should lead to a head CT scan.
   b. Any trauma substantial enough to cause a scalp or face hematoma or an ecchymosis should lead to a head CT scan, even in the absence of anticoagulation.
   c. Caution should be taken in interpreting CT findings in the subacute stage where blood appears as isodense to brain, and therefore the distance from the cortical sulci to the skull needs to be evaluated.
2. Coagulation values should be checked routinely.
   a. Hemoglobin (Hb).
   b. Platelet count.
   c. PTT and PT/INR.

Treatment

1. Small subdural hematomas may be left untreated and the patient observed, but if there is an underlying cause, such as anticoagulation, this should be rapidly corrected to prevent further accumulation of blood.
2. Neurosurgical drainage of blood from subdural space via burr hole is the definitive procedure, although it is common for the hematoma to reaccumulate, sometimes requiring a drain for a few days.
3. Risk of seizures is increased, and they should be treated appropriately if they arise.

SUGGESTED READINGS

Andrews M, Bruns J: Mild traumatic brain injury: Early evaluation and management. *Consultant* 45:1271-1276, 2005.

Chen JC, Levy ML: Causes, epidemiology, and risk factors of chronic subdural hematoma. *Neurosurg Clin N Am* 11(3):399-406, 2000.

Esselman PC, Uomoto JM: Classification of the spectrum of mild traumatic head injury. *Brain Inj* 9:417-424, 1995.

Haydel MJ, Preston CA, Mills TJ, et al: Indications for computed tomography in patients with minor head injury. *N Engl J Med* 343:100-105, 2000.

Hofman PA, Nelemans P, Kemerink GJ, Wilmink JT: Value of radiological diagnosis of skull fracture in the management of mild head injury: meta-analysis. *J Neurol Neurosurg Psychiatry* 68:416-422, 2000.

Jagoda AS, Cantrill SV, Wears RL, et al: Clinical policy: neuroimaging and decision making in adult mild traumatic brain injury in the acute setting. *Ann Emerg Med* 40:231-249, 2002.

Miller EC, Derlet RW, Kinser D: Minor head trauma: Is computed tomography always necessary? *Ann Emerg Med* 27:290-294, 1996.

Stiell IG, Wells GA, Vandemheen K: The Canadian CT Head Rule for patients with minor head injury. *Lancet* 357:1391-1396, 2001.

Stuss D: A sensible approach to mild traumatic brain injury. *Neurology* 45;1251-1252, 1995.

Voelker JL: Nonoperative treatment of chronic subdural hematoma. *Neurosurg Clin N Am* 11(3):507-513, 2000.

TARDIVE DYSKINESIA

Mitchell D. Feldman, with revisions by Tom J. Wachtel

Definitions

1. Tardive dyskinesia (TD) is a syndrome of involuntary movements associated with the long-term use of antipsychotic medication, particularly dopamine-blocking neuroleptics.
2. Patients usually exhibit rapid, repetitive, stereotypic movements mostly involving the oral, buccal, and lingual areas.
3. Some drugs for nausea (such as metoclopramide and prochlorperazine) and depression (such as amoxapine) can also cause TD.

Epidemiology

1. The disorder is caused by dopamine-blocking neuroleptics (e.g., haloperidol [Haldol]).
2. At least 20% of patients treated with standard neuroleptic drugs are affected with TD, and approximately 5% are expected to develop TD with each year of neuroleptic treatment.
3. The risk is greatest in the early years of exposure.
4. Higher incidence and lower remission rates are seen in older persons.
5. The incidence is declining with the use of newer-generation antipsychotics.

Clinical Findings

1. TD primarily involves the tongue, lips, and the jaw.
   a. Movements include tongue twisting and protrusion, lip smacking and puckering, and chewing.
   b. Movements are repetitive and stereotypic.
2. Some patients have slow, writhing movements of the arms and legs.
3. TD often appears with the reduction or withdrawal of the antipsychotics.
4. Relief or suppression of symptoms.
   a. Symptoms can subside when the antipsychotic is reintroduced.
   b. The involuntary mouth movements in TD may be voluntarily suppressed by patients.
   c. Movements are also suppressed by voluntary actions such as putting food in the mouth or talking.

Differential Diagnosis

1. Huntington's chorea.
2. Excessive treatment with L-dopa.

Work-up

1. Complete neuropsychiatric history (including medication history) and examination.

2. If presentation is atypical, consider laboratory evaluation.
   a. CBC.
   b. Serum electrolytes.
   c. Thyroid function tests.
   d. Serum ceruloplasmin.
   e. Connective tissue disease screen.
3. Brain imaging is normal in TD.

Treatment

1. Treatment is predicated on prevention.
   a. Limit the indications for neuroleptics.
   b. Use the lowest effective dose and withdraw the drug as quickly as feasible.
2. Use atypical antipsychotics if possible.
   a. Clozapine and quetiapine have the lowest reported incidence of TD.
   b. The safety of this class of drugs has not been established for geriatric patients.
3. Benzodiazepines and vitamin E may be helpful, but controlled trial evidence is weak.
4. Clozapine, olanzapine, and amisulpride may be of symptomatic help, but long-term efficacy and safety are unproven.
5. Only as a last resort for persistent, disabling, and treatment-resistant TD should neuroleptics be resumed to treat TD in the absence of active psychosis.

SUGGESTED READINGS

Bai YM, Yu SC, Chen JY, et al. Risperidone for pre-existing severe tardive dyskinesia: A 48-week prospective follow-up study. *Int Clin Psychopharmacol* 20:79-85, 2005.

Casey DE: Pathophysiology of antipsychotic drug–induced movement disorders. *J Clin Psychiatry* 65(suppl 9):25-28, 2004.

Fernandez HH, Friedman JH: Classification and treatment of tardive syndromes. *Neurologist* 9(1):16-27, 2003.

Jeste DV, Okamoto A, Napolitano J, et al: Low incidence of persistent tardive dyskinesia in elderly patients with dementia treated with risperidone. *Am J Psychiatry* 157:1150-1155, 2000.

Louza MR, Bassitt DP: Maintenance treatment of severe tardive dyskinesia with clozapine: 5 years' follow-up. *J Clin Psychopharmacol* 25:180-182, 2005.

McGrath JJ, Soares KV: Miscellaneous treatments for neuroleptic-induced tardive dyskinesia. *Cochrane Database Syst Rev* (2):CD000208, 2003.

Soares KV, McGrath JJ: The treatment of tardive dyskinesia—a systematic review and meta-analysis. *Schizophr Res* 39:1-16, 1999.

Woerner MG, Alvir JM, Saltz BL, et al: Prospective study of tardive dyskinesia in the elderly: Rates and risk factors. *Am J Psychiatry* 155:1521-1528, 1998.

TREMORS

Fred F. Ferri

Definition

Tremors are characterized by rhythmic oscillations, usually involving distal parts of the body.

Etiology

1. Metabolic abnormalities.
   a. Liver failure.
   b. Uremia.

2. Endocrine disorders.
   a. Hypoglycemia.
   b. Pheochromocytoma.
   c. Thyrotoxicosis.
3. Drugs.
   a. β-Agonists.
   b. Alcohol.
   c. Amiodarone.
   d. Amphetamines.
   e. Bronchodilators.
   f. Caffeine.
   g. Lithium.
   h. Metoclopramide.
   i. Nifedipine.
   j. Theophylline.
   k. Tricyclics.
   l. Valproic acid.
4. Cerebellar disorders.
5. Huntington's disease.
6. Cerebrovascular disease.
7. Other.
   a. Alcohol withdrawal.
   b. Anxiety.
   c. Benzodiazepine withdrawal.
   d. Exercise.
   e. Fatigue.

Classification

1. Behavioral situation.
   a. Rest tremor occurs in the absence of voluntary muscle activity (e.g., Parkinson's disease).
   b. Movement tremor is provoked by any movement (e.g., essential tremor, brain stem disorders, cerebellar disease).
   c. Postural tremor occurs with maintenance of posture (e.g., physiologic tremor, drug-induced tremor, essential tremor, postural tremor of parkinsonism).
2. Disease process: Table 5-7 describes the major distinguishing characteristics of the various conditions causing tremor.

5.2 Endocrine and Metabolic Disorders

DIABETES MELLITUS
Fred F. Ferri and Tom J. Wachtel

Definitions
General

1. Diabetes mellitus (DM) is a syndrome of hyperglycemia resulting from many different causes (see Etiology).
2. It can be classified into type 1 (T1DM) and type 2 (T2DM). Table 5-8 provides a general comparison of the two most common types of DM.
   a. Patients with T1DM require insulin.

Table 5-7 Characteristics of Tremor in Selected Conditions

Type of Tremor	Frequency (Hz)	Characteristics	Therapy
Parkinsonism	4-7.5	See text	See text
Essential senile tremor	8-12	Commonly affects hands and head Usually begins asymmetrically and tends to remain asymmetric Initially not present at rest Suppressed by alcohol, worsened by fatigue and emotional factors	Propranolol 20 mg tid initially is effective in approximately 50% of patients Primidone 25 mg tid initially may be effective in patients refractory to propranolol (max 250 mg tid)
Cerebellar	3-5	Tremor is evident when patient holds arms outstretched Tremor is accentuated by targeting (e.g., finger-to-nose testing) (intention tremor)	No effective therapy
Alcohol withdrawal	Variable	Rapid and coarse Involves entire body Abolished by alcohol intake	Abstinence from alcohol
Hysterical tremor	Variable	Variable frequency from moment to moment Can be rest, movement, or postural tremor Can affect any part of the body Usually diminished when patient is distracted	Psychotherapy

Table 5-8 **General Comparison of the Two Most Common Types of Diabetes Mellitus**

Feature	Type 1	Type 2
Previous terminology	Insulin-dependent diabetes mellitus (IDDM), type I, juvenile-onset diabetes	Non-insulin-dependent diabetes mellitus, type II, adult-onset diabetes
Age of onset	Usually < 30 y, particularly childhood and adolescence, but any age	Usually >40 y, but any age
Genetic predisposition	Moderate; environmental factors required for expression; 35%-50% concordance in monozygotic twins; several candidate genes proposed	Strong; 60%-90% concordance in monozygotic twins; many candidate genes proposed; some genes identified in maturity-onset diabetes of the young
Human leukocyte antigen associations	Linkage to DQA and DQB, influenced by DRB (3 and 4) (DR2 protective)	None known
Other associations	Autoimmune; Graves' disease, Hashimoto's thyroiditis, vitiligo, Addison's disease, pernicious anemia	Heterogeneous group, ongoing subclassification based on identification of specific pathogenic processes and genetic defects
Precipitating and risk factors	Largely unknown; microbial, chemical, dietary, other	Age, obesity (central), sedentary lifestyle, previous gestational diabetes
Findings at diagnosis	85%-90% of patients have one and usually more autoantibodies to ICA512, IA-2, IA-2β, GAD$_{65}$, insulin (IAA)	Possibly complications (microvascular and macrovascular) caused by significant preceding asymptomatic period
Endogenous insulin levels	Low or absent	Usually present (relative deficiency), early hyperinsulinemia
Insulin resistance	Only with hyperglycemia	Mostly present
Prolonged fast	Hyperglycemia, ketoacidosis	Euglycemia
Stress, withdrawal of insulin	Ketoacidosis	Nonketotic hyperglycemia, occasionally ketoacidosis

GAD, glutamic acid decarboxylase; IA-2/IA-2β, tyrosine phosphatases; IAA, insulin autoantibodies; ICA, islet cell antibody; ICA512, islet cell autoantigen 512 (fragment of IA-2).
From Andreoli TE (ed): *Cecil essentials of medicine*, ed 5. Philadelphia, WB Saunders, 2001.

b. Most patients with T2DM do not require insulin.
c. When a type 2 diabetic patient needs insulin, he or she becomes classified as type 2, requiring insulin.

Clinical

1. The American Diabetes Association (ADA) defines DM on one of the following criteria:
   a. A fasting plasma glucose ≥126 mg/dL.
   b. A nonfasting plasma glucose ≥ 200 mg/dL.
   c. An oral glucose tolerance test (OGTT) ≥200 mg/dL in the 2-hour sample.
2. The ADA also defines a value of 110 mg/dL on fasting blood sugar as the upper limit of normal for glucose.
3. Impaired fasting glucose.
   a. A fasting glucose between 110 mg/dL and 126 mg/dL.
4. Results of the oral glucose test between 110 mg/dL and 200 mg/dL.

Clinical Findings

1. Symptomless: discovered on routine examination (screening).
2. Acute or subacute onset.
   a. Progressive loss of weight despite hyperphagia.
   b. Polyuria and polydipsia.
   c. Diabetic ketoacidosis (rare in T2DM).
   d. Diabetic hyperosmolar state.
   e. Postprandial hypoglycemia.
3. Gradual onset.
   a. Pruritus, generalized, or perigenital.
   b. Recurrent infections.
   c. Polyuria and polydipsia.
   d. Blurring of vision.
4. Late manifestations.
   a. Neuropathic.
      (1) Peripheral polyneuropathy (lower limbs).
      (2) Mononeuropathy.
         (a) Vascular (e.g., oculomotor).
         (b) Compression (e.g., carpal tunnel syndrome).
      (3) Autonomic neuropathy.
      (4) Amyotrophy.
   b. Vascular.
      (1) Premature large vessel disease (atherosclerosis).
      (2) Small vessel disease (microangiopathy).
   c. Renal: glomerulosclerosis (nephrotic syndrome and uremia).
   d. Ophthalmic.
      (1) Diabetic retinopathy.
      (2) Cataract.
      (3) Glaucoma.
   e. Dermatologic.
      (1) Necrobiosis lipoidica.
      (2) Foot ulcer.

Etiology

1. Hypoinsulinemic causes.
   a. T1DM (sometimes called *insulin-dependent DM, juvenile-onset DM, ketosis-prone diabetes, brittle diabetes*).
      (1) Onset is rare in the elderly.
      (2) Most elderly patients with T1DM have had T1DM since childhood or young adulthood.
   b. Pancreatic disease.
      (1) Pancreatitis.
      (2) Pancreatic cancer.
      (3) Cystic fibrosis.
      (4) Hemochromatosis.
   c. Drugs.
      (1) Diuretics.
         (a) Thiazides.
         (b) Diazoxide.
         (c) Furosemide.
         (d) Ethacrynic acid.
      (2) Psychoactive agents.
         (a) Lithium carbonate.
         (b) Neuroleptics.
         (c) Tricyclic antidepressants.
         (d) Marijuana.
      (3) Antineoplastic agents.
         (a) Streptozocin.
         (b) Cyclophosphamide (Cytoxan).
      (4) Miscellaneous medications.
         (a) Phenytoin.
         (b) Propranolol (Inderal).
         (c) Isoniazid.
         (d) Nicotinic acid.
         (e) Cimetidine.
         (f) Pentamidine.
   d. T2DM can lead to pancreatic beta cell burnout, making patients insulin dependent.
2. Hyperinsulinemic causes.
   a. T2DM (also called *adult-onset DM, non–insulin-dependent DM, maturity-onset diabetes, ketosis-resistant diabetes*).
   b. Insulin receptor abnormalities (rare).
      (1) Hereditary defect in insulin receptor.
      (2) Congenital lipodystrophy associated with virilization or acanthosis nigricans.
      (3) Antibody to insulin receptor–associated immune disorders.
      (4) Ataxia–telangiectasia.
      (5) Myotonic dystrophy.
   c. Hormone disorders.
      (1) Glucocorticoids (Cushing's syndrome or exogenous).
      (2) Progestins and estrogens.
      (3) Growth hormone (acromegaly).

(4) Glucagon (glucagonoma).

(5) Epinephrine (pheochromocytoma).

Initial Evaluation

Medical History

1. Symptoms and previous laboratory test results related to diagnosis of diabetes.
2. Dietary habits, nutritional status, and weight history.
3. Details of previous treatment programs, including diabetes education.
4. Current treatment of diabetes.
   a. Medications.
   b. Diet.
   c. Results of glucose monitoring.
5. Exercise history.
6. Frequency, severity, and cause of acute complications such as ketoacidosis and hyperosmolar syndrome.
7. Prior or current infections.
   a. Skin.
   b. Foot.
   c. Dental.
   d. Genitourinary.
8. Symptoms and treatment of chronic complications associated with diabetes.
   a. Eyes.
   b. Heart.
   c. Kidney.
   d. Nerve.
   e. Sexual function.
   f. Peripheral vascular.
   g. Cerebrovascular.
9. Medications that can affect carbohydrate metabolism (see list under Etiology).
10. Risk factors for atherosclerosis.
    a. Smoking.
    b. Hypertension.
    c. Obesity.
    d. Hyperlipidemia.
    e. Family history.
11. Psychosocial and economic factors that might influence management of diabetes.
12. Family history.
13. Gestation history.

Physical Examination

1. Height and weight measurement.
2. BP determination (with orthostatic measurements).
3. Ophthalmoscopic examination, if possible with dilation.
4. Thyroid palpation.
5. Cardiac examination.
6. Evaluation of pulses (and arterial auscultation).
7. Foot examination.

8. Skin examination (including insulin-injection sites).
9. Neurologic examination.
10. Dental and periodontal examination.

Laboratory Evaluation

1. Fasting plasma glucose.
   a. Initial in the office, and then at home for blood glucose monitoring.
   b. Glucose oxidase strips are used in conjunction with a meter to give a digital reading.
   c. Timing.
      (1) The testing can be done once a day, but the time should be varied each day.
      (2) Variable timing allows the serum glucose level before meals and at bedtime to be assessed frequently without pricking the patient's fingers four times daily.
2. Glycosylated hemoglobin (HbA$_{1c}$) initial and every 6 months.
3. Fasting lipid profile initial and then yearly.
   a. Total cholesterol.
   b. High-density lipoprotein (HDL) cholesterol.
   c. Low-density lipoprotein (LDL) cholesterol.
   d. Triglycerides.
4. Serum creatinine initial and yearly.
5. Urinalysis.
   a. Ketones.
   b. Glucose.
   c. Protein, microscopic if indicated.
6. Urine for microalbumin (unless proteinuria on urinalysis) initial and yearly.
7. Urine culture if microscopic exam is abnormal or if urinary symptoms are present.
8. Thyroid function tests (thyroid stimulating hormone [TSH]) initial and episodically.
9. CBC initially.
10. ECG initial and every 3 years.

Treatment

Nonpharmacologic Therapy

1. Diet.
   a. Calories.
      (1) Daily intake.
         (a) The diabetic patient can be started on 15 calories/lb of ideal body weight.
         (b) An active person can be started on 20 calories/lb.
         (c) If the patient does heavy physical labor, start with 25 calories/lb.
      (2) The calories should be distributed as:
         (a) Carbohydrate 55% to 60%.
         (b) Fat 25% to 35%.
         (c) Protein 15% to 20%.
      (3) The emphasis should be on complex carbohydrates rather than simple and refined starches and on polyunsaturated instead of saturated fats.

b. The ADA's exchange diet.
  (1) Categories include protein, bread, fruit, milk, and low- and intermediate-carbohydrate vegetables.
  (2) The name of each exchange is meant to be all inclusive (e.g., cereal, muffins, spaghetti, potatoes, rice are in the bread group; meats, fish, eggs, cheese, peanut butter are in the protein group).
c. Fiber.
  (1) Insoluble fiber (bran, celery) and soluble globular fiber (pectin in fruit) delay glucose absorption and attenuate the postprandial serum glucose peak.
  (2) Fiber also appears to lower the elevated triglyceride level often present in patients with uncontrolled diabetes.
d. Glycemic index.
  (1) The glycemic index compares the rise in blood sugar after the ingestion of simple sugars and complex carbohydrates with the rise that occurs after the absorption of glucose.
  (2) Equal amounts of starches do not give the same rise in plasma glucose (pasta equal in calories to a baked potato causes a smaller rise than the potato); thus, it is helpful to know the glycemic index of a particular food product.
2. Exercise.
  a. Exercise increases the cellular glucose uptake by increasing the number of cell receptors.
  b. The following points must be considered:
    (1) The exercise program must be individualized and built up slowly.
    (2) Insulin is more rapidly absorbed when injected into a limb that is then exercised, and this can result in hypoglycemia.
3. Weight loss.
  a. Weight loss to ideal body weight if the patient is overweight.
  b. This is the single most important goal of the nonpharmacologic arm of management.

Pharmacologic Therapy

1. When nonpharmacologic measures fail to normalize the serum glucose, pharmacologic therapy must be instituted.
  a. Oral hypoglycemic agents (e.g., metformin, glitazones, or a sulfonylurea) should be added to the regimen in type 2 DM.
  b. Table 5-9 describes commonly used oral hypoglycemic agents.
  c. The sulfonamides and the biguanide metformin are the oldest and most commonly used classes of hypoglycemic drugs.
  d. Insulin is used in patients whose hyperglycemia cannot be controlled otherwise.
  e. The goal of treatment is to achieve a stable HbA_{1c} under 6.5%.
2. Oral hypoglycemic agents.
  a. Metformin.
    (1) The primary mechanism is to decrease hepatic glucose output.
    (2) Because metformin does not cause hypoglycemia when used as a monotherapy, it is preferred for most patients.
    (3) It is contraindicated in patients with renal insufficiency (i.e., creatinine >1.5 mg/dL).
    (4) It is used with caution in patients with chronic liver disease or congestive heart failure (CHF).

b. Glitazones.
   (1) Pioglitazone and rosiglitazone increase insulin sensitivity and are useful as single agents or in addition to other agents in type 2 diabetics whose hyperglycemia is inadequately controlled.
   (2) Serum transaminase levels should be obtained before starting therapy and monitored periodically.
   (3) Edema is a common complication.
c. Sulfonylureas and meglitinides.
   (1) Sulfonylureas and meglitinides are insulin secretagogues.
   (2) Meglitinides work best when given before meals because they increase the postprandial output of insulin from the pancreas.
   (3) All sulfonylureas are relatively contraindicated in patients allergic to sulfa.
d. Acarbose and miglitol.
   (1) Acarbose and miglitol work by competitively inhibiting pancreatic amylase and small intestinal glucosidases to delay gastrointestinal absorption of carbohydrates, thereby reducing alimentary hyperglycemia.
   (2) The major side effects are flatulence, diarrhea, and abdominal cramps.
e. Incretin hormones (e.g., sitagliptin) are becoming available, but their place in the management of elderly diabetic patients remains to be defined.
3. Insulin.
a. Insulin is indicated for the treatment of all T1DM and T2DM patients whose diabetes cannot be adequately controlled with diet and oral agents.
b. Table 5-10 describes commonly used types of insulin.
c. Risks of insulin therapy.
   (1) Weight gain.
   (2) Hypoglycemia.
   (3) Allergic or cutaneous reactions (rare).
d. Replacement insulin therapy should mimic normal release patterns.
   (1) Long-acting insulin.
      (a) Approximately 50% to 60% of daily insulin should be a basal type.
      (b) Intermediate-acting insulin (neutral protamine Hagedorn [NPH]), is injected once or twice daily.
      (c) Among long-acting insulins, once-daily bedtime insulin glargine is as effective as once- or twice-daily NPH but has a lower risk of nocturnal hypoglycemia and less weight gain.
   (2) Short-acting or rapid-acting insulin.
      (a) The remaining 40% to 50% of daily insulin should be short-acting or rapid-acting insulin (regular, aspart, lispro) to cover mealtime carbohydrates and correct elevated current glucose levels.
      (b) When using short-acting insulins, insulin aspart and insulin lispro are more effective in lowering postprandial glucose levels than regular insulin.
   (3) Continuous subcutaneous insulin infusion (CSII, or insulin pump).

Table 5-9 **Oral Antidiabetic Agents as Monotherapy**

Drug Type	Generic Name	Mode of Action	Preferred Patient Type	Therapeutic			
				↓ Hb A$_{1c}$* (%)	↓ FPG* (mg /dL)	↓ PPG* (mg /dL)	Insu Leve
Sulfonylureas	Glimepiride, glyburide, glipizide, chlorpropamide, tolbutamide	↑ ↑ Pancreatic insulin secretion chronically	Diagnosis age >30 yr, lean, diabetes <5 yr, insulinopenic	1-2	50-70	~90	↑
Biguanides	Metformin	↓ ↓ HGP; ↓ peripheral IR; ↓ intestinal glucose absorption	Overweight, IR, fasting hyperglycemia, dyslipidemia	1-2	50-80	80	—
α-Glucosidase inhibitors	Acarbose, miglitol	Delays PP digestion of carbohydrates and absorption of glucose	PP hyperglycemia, insulinopenic	0.5-1	15-30	40-50	—
Thiazolidinediones	Rosiglitazone, pioglitazone	↓↓ Peripheral IR; ↑↑ glucose disposal; ↓ HGP	Overweight, IR, dyslipidemia, renal dysfunction	0.8-1	25-50	—	—
Meglitinides	Repaglinide, nateglinide	↑↑ Pancreatic insulin secretion acutely	PP hyperglycemia, insulinopenic	1-2	40-80	30	↑

↑ Increased; ↓, decreased; —, unchanged; bw, body weight; FPG, fasting plasma gluco HDL, high-density lipoprotein; HGP, hepatic glucose production; IR, insulin resistan LDL, low-density lipoprotein; PP, postprandial; PPG, postprandial plasma gluco TG, triglyceride.
*Values combined from numerous studies; values are also dose dependent.
Modified from Andreoli TE (ed): *Cecil Essentials of Medicine*, ed 5. Philadelphia, WB Saunde 2001.

fects							
eight	Lipids	Side Effects	Dose(s) /Day	Max Daily Dose (mg)	Range/ Dose (mg)	Optimal Administration Time	Main Site of Metabolism and Excretion
	—	Hypo-glycemia	1-3	Depends on agent	Depends on agent	~30 min premeal (some with food, others on empty stomach)	Hepatic/ renal fecal
↓		Diarrhea, lactic acidosis	2-3	25-50	500-1000	With meal	Not metab-olized/ renal
		Abdominal pain, flatulence, diarrhea	1-3	150 (<60-kg bw) 300 (>60-kg bw)	25-50 (<60-kg bw) 25-100 (>60-kg bw)	With first bite of meal	Only 2% absorbed /fecal
↑	↑ Large "fluffy" LDL ↑ HDL	Idiosyncratic hepato-toxicity with trogli-tazone; edema	1	Depends on agent	Depends on agent	With meal (break-fast)	Hepatic /fecal
	—	Hypo-glycemia (low risk)	1-4+	16 (repaglin-ide), 360 (nateglin ide)	0.5-4, (repaglin-ide), 60-120 (nateglin-ide)	Prefer-ably <15 (0-30 min) premeals (omit if no meal)	Hepatic/ fecal

Table 5-10 **Types of Insulin**

Insulin Type	Generic Name	Preprandial Injection Timing (h)	Onset (h)	Peak (h)	Duration (h)	Blood Glucose Nadir (h)
Rapid acting	Lispro*	0-0.2	0.2-0.5	0.5-2	<5	2-4
Short acting	Regular	0.5-(1)	0.3-1	2-6	(≤16)	(Pre-next meal)
	Lente		1-2	4-12		
Intermediate acting	NPH	0.5-(1)	1-3	6-15	16-26	6-13
Long acting†	Clargine	0.5-(1)	2-3	NA	24	NA
Mixed short and intermediate acting	70/30 50/50	0.5(1)	0.5-1	3-12	16-24	3-12

Note: Times depend on several factors including dose, anatomic site of injection, method (SQ, IM, IV), duration of diabetes, degree of insulin resistance, level of activity, and body temperature. Some time ranges are wide to include data from several separate studies. Preprandial injection depends on pre-meal BG values as well as insulin type. If BG is low, the patient might need to inject insulin and eat immediately (carbohydrate portion of meal first). If BG is high, the patient may delay the meal after insulin injection and eat the carbohydrate portion last.
*Insulin analogue with reversal of lysine and proline at positions 28 and 29 on the β chain.
†Insulin glargine (rDNA origin) is a newer, once-daily insulin analogs (Lantus) that provides 24-hour basal glucose-lowering with once-a-day bedtime dosing. Onset of action is 2-3 h, duration of action is 24+ h.
70/30, 70% NPH, 30% regular; 50/50, 50% NPH, 50% regular; BG, blood glucose; NPH, neutral protamine Hagedorn.
Data from Andreoli TE (ed): Cecil Essentials of Medicine, ed 5. Philadelphia, WB Saunders, 2001.

(a) CSII provides better glycemic control than does conventional therapy.

(b) CSII provides comparable or slightly better control than multiple daily injections.

(c) It should be considered for patients presenting with diabetes in childhood or adolescence and during pregnancy, but it has little use in geriatrics.

4. Combination therapy of various hypoglycemic agents is commonly used when monotherapy does not produce adequate glycemic control.

5. Low-dose aminosalicylic acid to decrease the risk of cerebrovascular disease is beneficial for diabetics older than 30 years who have other risk factors (hypertension, dyslipidemia, smoking, obesity).

Monitoring

1. Blood glucose: The United Kingdom Prospective Diabetes Study (UKPDS) confirmed the benefit of tight glycemic control.

2. Lipids.
   a. A fasting serum lipid panel should be obtained yearly on all adult diabetic patients.
   b. Tight lipid control (LDL <70 mg/dL) is indicated in all diabetics.
   c. Statins are often necessary to achieve therapeutic goals.

3. BP.
   a. The UKPDS also demonstrated that BP control in patients with DM is as important as glycemic control.
   b. Target BP control in patients with DM is 130/80 or lower.
   c. Angiotensin-converting enzyme (ACE) inhibitors (or angiotensin-receptor blockers [ARBs] if ACE inhibitors are not tolerated) are the antihypertensive agents of choice in patients with DM.
   d. Verapamil is a good second-line choice if needed as combined or monotherapy.

Complications

1. Kidneys.
   a. Nephropathy occurs in 35% to 45% of patients with T1DM and in 20% with T2DM.
   b. The first sign of renal involvement in patients with DM is most often microalbuminuria, which is classified as incipient nephropathy.
   c. ACE inhibitors are effective in slowing the progression of renal disease in both T1DM and T2DM, independently of the reduction in BP.
   d. ARBs and nondihydropyridine CCBs are also effective in protecting against the progression of nephropathy in diabetics, especially in T2DM.

2. Eyes.
   a. Retinopathy occurs in approximately 15% of diabetic patients after 15 years and increases 1%/year after diagnosis.
   b. Diabetic patients should be advised to have annual ophthalmologic examination.
   c. In T1DM, ophthalmologic visits should begin within 3 to 5 years of disease onset.
   d. T2DM patients should be seen from disease onset.

3. Feet.
   a. Podiatric care can reduce the rate of foot infections and amputations in patients with DM.

    b. Noninfected neuropathic foot ulcers require debridement and reduction of pressure.
4. Infections are generally more common in diabetics because of multiple factors, such as impaired leukocyte function, decreased tissue perfusion secondary to vascular disease, repeated trauma because of loss of sensation, and urinary retention secondary to neuropathy.
5. Nervous system.
    a. The frequency of neuropathy in type 2 diabetics approaches 70% to 80%.
    b. Gabapentin (900-3600 mg/day) is effective for the symptomatic treatment of peripheral neuropathic pain.
    c. Amitriptyline, duloxetine, and carbamazepine can also be effective.

SUGGESTED READINGS

American Diabetes Association: Position statement: Standards of medical care for patients with diabetes mellitus. *Diabetes Care* 25:S33-S49, 2002.

Barr RG, Nathan DM, Meigs JB, Singer DE: Tests of glycemia for the diagnosis of type 2 diabetes mellitus. *Ann Intern Med* 137:263-272, 2002.

Beckman JA, Creager MA, Libby P: Diabetes and atherosclerosis: Epidemiology, pathophysiology, and management. *JAMA* 287:2570-2581, 2002.

Boulton AJ, Kirsner RS, Vilekyte L: Clinical practice. Neuropathic diabetic foot ulcers. *N Engl J Med* 351:48-55, 2004.

DeWitt DE, Hirsch IB: Outpatient insulin therapy in type 1 and type 2 diabetes mellitus: Scientific review. *JAMA* 289:2254-2264, 2003.

Holmboe ES: Oral antihyperglycemic therapy for type 2 diabetes: Clinical applications. *JAMA* 287:373-376, 2002.

Mayfield J, White R: Insulin therapy for type 2 diabetes: Rescue, augmentation, and replacement of beta-cell function. *Am Fam Phys* 70:489-500, 2004.

Nathan DM: Clinical practice. Initial management of glycemia in type 2 diabetes mellitus. *N Engl J Med* 347:1342-1349, 2002.

Remuzzi G, Schieppati A, Ruggementi P: Clinical practice. Nephropathy in patients with type 2 diabetes. *N Engl J Med* 346:1145-1151, 2002.

Stern MP, Williams K, Haffner SM: Identification of persons at high risk for type 2 diabetes mellitus: Do we need the oral glucose tolerance test? *Ann Intern Med* 136:575-581, 2002.

US Preventive Services Task Force: Screening for type 2 diabetes mellitus in adults: Recommendations and rationale. *Ann Intern Med* 138:212-214, 2003.

Zandbergen AA, Baggen MG, Lamberts SW, et al: Effect of losartan on microalbuminuria in normotensive patients with type 2 diabetes mellitus. *Ann Intern Med* 139:90-96, 2003.

HYPERCHOLESTEROLEMIA

Tom J. Wachtel and Beth J. Wutz

Definitions

Hypercholesterolemia refers to a blood cholesterol measurement higher than 200 mg/dL.
1. A cholesterol level of 200 to 239 mg/dL is considered borderline high.
2. A level of 240 mg/dL or higher is considered to be a high cholesterol measurement.

Epidemiology

1. Incidence and prevalence.
    a. More than 100 million Americans have a total serum cholesterol higher than 200 mg/dL.

 b. Elevated cholesterol requires drug therapy in about 60 million Americans.

 c. Prevalence of hypercholesterolemia increases with increasing age.

 d. The majority of cardiovascular events occur in people older than 65 years. According to the Framingham Heart Study:

  (1) The lifetime cumulative incidence of coronary artery disease (CAD) is 34% in men and 20% in women older than 60 years when the total cholesterol level is less than 200 mg/dL.

  (2) The lifetime cumulative incidence of CAD is 51% in men and 36% in women older than 60 years when the total cholesterol level is greater than 240 mg/dL.

2. Risk factors.

 a. Diet.

 b. Genetic predisposition.

 c. Sedentary lifestyle.

 d. Associated secondary causes.

Clinical Findings

1. Most patients have no physical findings.

2. Possible findings, particularly in the familial forms, include:

 a. Tendon xanthomas.

 b. Xanthelasma.

 c. Arcus corneae.

 d. Arterial bruits in young adults.

 e. History of coronary heart disease, cerebrovascular disease, or peripheral arterial disease.

Etiology

1. Primary.

 a. Genetics.

 b. Obesity.

 c. Diet.

2. Secondary.

 a. Diabetes.

 b. Alcohol consumption.

 c. Oral contraceptive use.

 d. Hypothyroidism.

 e. Glucocorticoid use.

 f. Most diuretics.

 g. Nephrotic syndrome.

 h. Hepatoma.

 i. Extrahepatic biliary obstruction.

 j. Primary biliary cirrhosis.

Diagnosis

See Tables 5-11 through Table 5-13.

Treatment

Treatment is based on the National Cholesterol Education Program Adult Treatment Panel (ATP) III recommendations.

1. Prevention.

 a. Primary prevention: Monitor patients without atherosclerosis or DM.

Table 5-11 LDL Cholesterol Goals and Cutpoints for Therapeutic Lifestyle Changes and Drug Therapy in Different Risk Categories

Risk Category	Goal (mg/dL)	Low-Density Lipoprotein	
		Level at which to Initiate TLCs (mg/dL)	Level at which to Consider Drug Therapy (mg/dL)
CHD or CHD risk equivalents (10-y risk >20%)	<100	≥100	≥130 (100-129: drug optional)*
2+ Risk factors (10-y risk 20%)	<130	≥130	10-y risk 10%-20% ≥130 10-y risk <10%: ≥160
0-1 Risk factor†	<160	≥160	≥190 (160-189: LDL-lowering drug optional)

*Some authorities recommend use of LDL-lowering drugs in this category if an LDL cholesterol level of <100 mg/dL cannot be achieved by TLCs. Others prefer to use drugs that primarily modify triglycerides and HDL (e.g., nicotinic acid or fibrate). Clinical judgment also might call for deferring drug therapy in this subcategory.
†Almost all people with 0-1 risk factor have a 10-year risk <10%; thus, 10-year risk assessment in people with 0-1 risk factor is not necessary.
CHD, coronary heart disease; LDL, low-density lipoprotein, TLC, therapeutic lifestyle changes.
Data from Expert Panel on Detection, Evaluation, and Treatment of High Blood Cholesterol in Adults: Executive Summary of the Third Report of the National Cholesterol Education Program (NCEP) Expert Panel on Detection, Evaluation, and Treatment of High Blood Cholesterol in Adults (Adult Treatment Panel III). *JAMA* 285:2486-2497, 2001.

Table 5-12 Comparison of LDL Cholesterol and Non-HDL Cholesterol Goals for Three Risk Categories

Risk Category	LDL Goal (mg/dL)	Non-HDL Goal (mg/dL)
CHD and CHD risk equivalent (10-y risk for CHD >20%)	<70	<130
Multiple (2+) risk factors and 10-y risk 20%	<130	<160
0-1 Risk factor	<160	<190

CHD, coronary heart disease; HDL, high-density lipoprotein; LDL, low-density lipoprotein.
Data from Expert Panel on Detection, Evaluation, and Treatment of High Blood Cholesterol in Adults: Executive Summary of the Third Report of the National Cholesterol Education Program (NCEP) Expert Panel on Detection, Evaluation, and Treatment of High Blood Cholesterol in Adults (Adult Treatment Panel III). *JAMA* 285:2486-2497, 2001.

Table 5-13 **ATPIII Classification of LDL, Total, and HDL Cholesterol (mg/dL)**

Measurement (mg/dL)	Analysis
LDL Cholesterol	
<100	Optimal
100-129	Near or above optimal
130-159	Borderline high
160-189	High
≥190	Very high
Total Cholesterol	
<200	Desirable
200-239	Borderline high
≥240	High
HDL Cholesterol	
<40	Low
≥60	High

ATP, Adult treatment panel; HDL, high-density lipoprotein, LDL, low-density lipoprotein.
Data from Expert Panel on Detection, Evaluation, and Treatment of High Blood Cholesterol in Adults: Executive Summary of the Third Report of the National Cholesterol Education Program (NCEP) Expert Panel on Detection, Evaluation, and Treatment of High Blood Cholesterol in Adults (Adult Treatment Panel III). *JAMA* 285:2486-2497, 2001.

(1) Total cholesterol lower than 200 mg/dL and the HDL higher than 40: Repeat the test in 5 years.
(2) Total cholesterol 200 to 239 mg/dL and the HDL higher than 40.
   (a) Discuss diet modification.
   (b) Repeat the test in 1 to 2 years.
(3) Total cholesterol higher than 240 mg/dL or the HDL lower than 40 mg/dL.
   (a) Perform a fasting lipid profile (cholesterol, HDL, triglycerides).
   (b) Calculate LDL from the fasting lipid profile:

   $$LDL = (total\ cholesterol - HDL - triglycerides)/5$$

(4) Fasting lipid profile with LDL lower than 130 mg/dL and one or no risk factors for CAD.
   (a) Dietary guidance.
   (b) Repeat the profile in 5 years.
(5) Fasting lipid profile with LDL 130 to 159 mg/dL (borderline high risk) and one or no risk factors for CAD.
   (a) Diet modification and exercise.
   (b) Repeat the profile in 12 weeks.
(6) Fasting LDL 130 to 159 mg/dL and two or more CAD risk factors, or LDL 160 to 189 with one or no risk factors.
   (a) Diet modification and exercise.
   (b) Consider drug option.
   (c) Repeat the profile in 12 weeks.

(7) Fasting lipid profile with LDL 160 to 189 mg/dL and two or more risk factors for CAD or LDL 190 mg/dL or higher.
  (a) Diet modification and exercise.
  (b) Drug therapy.
  (c) Monitor lipid profile every 3 months until goal is achieved, then monitor yearly.
  b. Secondary prevention in patients with atherosclerosis or DM:
    (1) All patients: Fasting lipid profile
    (2) LDL lower than 100 mg/dL.
      (a) Instruct patient on diet and exercise.
      (b) Repeat the profile annually.
    (3) LDL higher than 100 mg/dL: Drug therapy is required.
    (4) Some authorities/guidelines suggest drug therapy when LDL is greater than 70 mg/dL.
3. Intervention.
  a. Nonpharmacologic therapy.
    (1) First line of treatment is dietary therapy (Table 5-14).
      (a) Low-cholesterol, low-fat diet (limit fat intake to 30% or less of the total calorie intake).
      (b) Saturated fats less than 7% of total calories.
      (c) No more than 200 mg/day of cholesterol.
    (2) Increased activity with aerobic exercise: Encourage at least 20 to 30 min of aerobic exercise three to four times a week.

Table 5-14 Nutrient Composition of the TLC Diet

Nutrient	Recommended Intake
Saturated fat*	<7% of total calories
Polyunsaturated fat	Up to 10% of total calories
Monounsaturated fat	Up to 20% of total calories
Total fat	25%-35% of total calories
Carbohydrate†	50%-60% of total calories
Fiber	20-30 g/day
Protein	Approximately 15% of total calories
Cholesterol	<200 mg/day
Total calories‡	Balance energy intake and expenditure to maintain desirable body weight and to prevent weight gain

*Trans fatty acids are another LDL-raising fat that should be kept at a low intake.
†Carbohydrates should be derived predominantly from foods rich in complex carbohydrates, including grains, especially whole grains, fruits, and vegetables.
‡Daily energy expenditure should include at least moderate physical activity (contributing approximately 200 kcal/day).
TLC, therapeutic lifestyle changes.
Data from Expert Panel on Detection, Evaluation, and Treatment of High Blood Cholesterol in Adults: Executive Summary of the Third Report of the National Cholesterol Education Program (NCEP) Expert Panel on Detection, Evaluation, and Treatment of High Blood Cholesterol in Adults (Adult Treatment Panel III). *JAMA* 285:2486-2497, 2001.

    (3) Smoking cessation is strongly encouraged.

    (4) Counsel the patient on CAD risk factors.

  b. Pharmacologic therapy.

    (1) Specific indications.

      (a) Bile acid sequestrants to lower LDL.

      (b) Niacin to lower LDL and triglycerides and raise HDL.

      (c) HMG-CoA reductase inhibitors to lower LDL.

      (d) Fibric acids work to lower triglycerides more than LDL.

      (e) Check the transaminase level at baseline, after 3 months of treatment, then yearly.

    (2) Medication in primary prevention.

      (a) Needed for patients on dietary therapy who have:

        i. LDL higher than 190 mg/dL but no risk factors.

        ii. LDL higher than 160 mg/dL and two or more risk factors.

        iii. HDL lower than 30 mg/dL.

      (b) Considered for patients who have:

        i. LDL higher than 160 mg/dL.

        ii. LDL 130 to 159 mg/dL and two or more risk factors for CAD.

    (3) Medication in secondary prevention is needed for patients who have LDL higher than 70 mg/dL plus:

      (a) Known CAD.

      (b) Vascular disease.

      (c) Diabetes.

    (4) The Prospective Study of Pravastatin in the Elderly at Risk (PROSPER) suggests a treatment benefit in patients aged 70 to 82 years only if the HDL cholesterol is lower than 45 mg/L and when, in that subgroup of patients, a significant reduction in the ratio of LDL to HDL is achieved. Treatment is more efficacious in men than in women. Such new evidence can help to prioritize treatment choices, particularly in patients with polypharmacy issues.

    (5) Medications and their effects (Table 5-15).

      (a) Bile acid sequestrants (poorly tolerated) reduce LDL by 15% to 30%.

      (b) Niacin (poorly tolerated) reduces LDL by 5% to 25%.

      (c) HMG-CoA reductase inhibitors (statins) reduce LDL by 20% to 55%.

      (d) Fibric acids reduce LDL by 5% to 20%.

      (e) Cholesterol absorption inhibitors (ezetimibe) reduce LDL by 20%.

4. Follow-up.

  a. After initiating therapy, repeat laboratory tests in 12 weeks and titrate medication as necessary.

  b. Once goal is achieved, lifelong medication and blood lipid monitoring once or twice a year, are needed although patients who are successful at modifying their lifestyle and able to lose weight can occasionally ease off their pharmacologic therapy.

  c. Diet modification should continue with drug therapy.

  d. Repeat review for additional cardiovascular risk factors.

Table 5-15   Drugs Affecting Lipoprotein Metabolism

Agent and Daily Doses	Expected Lipoprotein Effects	Side Effects	Contraindications
HMG-CoA Reductase Inhibitors (Statins)			
Atorvastatin (10–80 mg)	LDL ↓18%–55%	Myopathy	*Absolute*
Fluvastatin (20–80 mg)	HDL ↑5%–15%	Increased liver enzymes	Active or chronic liver disease
Lovastatin (20–80 mg)	TG ↓7%–30%		
Pravastatin (20–80 mg)			*Relative*
Rosuvastatin (5–40 mg)			Concomitant use of certain drugs*
Simvastatin (20–80 mg)			
Bile Acid Sequestrants			
Cholestyramine (4–16 g)	LDL ↓15%–30%	Gastrointestinal distress	*Absolute*
Colesevelam (2.6–3.8 g)	HDL ↑3%–5%	Constipation	Dysbetalipoproteinemia
Colestipol (5–20 g)	TG No change or increase	Decreased absorption of other drugs	TG >400 mg/dL
			Relative
			TG >200 mg/dL
Nicotinic Acid (Niacin)			
Immediate-release (crystalline) nicotinic acid (1.5–3 g)	LDL ↓5–25%	Flushing	*Absolute*
	HDL ↑15%–35%	Hyperglycemia	Chronic liver disease
	TG ↓20%–50%	Hyperuricemia (or gout)	Severe gout

		Side effects	Contraindications
Extended-release nicotinic acid (Niaspan) 1-2 g		Upper GI distress	*Relative*
Sustained-release nicotinic acid (1-2 g)		Hepatotoxicity	Diabetes
			Hyperuricemia
			Peptic ulcer disease
Fibric Acids			*Absolute*
Gemfibrozil (600 mg bid)	LDL[†] ↓5%-20%	Dyspepsia	Severe renal disease
Fenofibrate (160 mg qd)	HDL ↑10%-20%	Gallstones	Severe hepatic disease
Clofibrate (1000 mg bid)	TG ↓20%-50%	Myopathy	
Cholesterol Absorption Inhibitors			
Ezetimibe (10 mg qd)	LDL ↓18%	Abdominal pain	Severe hepatic disease
	HDL ↑1%	Myalgias	
	TG ↓7%-8%		

*Cyclosporine, macrolide antibiotics, various antifungal agents, and cytochrome P450 inhibitors (fibrates and niacin should be used with appropriate caution).

[†]May be increased in patients with high TG.

CoA, coenzyme A; GI, gastrointestinal; HDL, high-density lipoprotein; HMG, 3-hydroxy-3 methylglutaryl; LDL, low-density lipoprotein; TG, triglyceride.

Data from Expert Panel on Detection, Evaluation, and Treatment of High Blood Cholesterol in Adults: Executive Summary of the Third Report of the National Cholesterol Education Program (NCEP) Expert Panel on Detection, Evaluation, and Treatment of High Blood Cholesterol in Adults (Adult Treatment Panel III). *JAMA* 285:2486-2497, 2001.

SUGGESTED READINGS

Allen Maycock CA, Muhlestein JB, Horne BD, et al: Intermountain Heart Collaborative Study. Statin therapy is associated with reduced mortality across all age groups of individuals with significant coronary disease, including very elderly patients. *J Am Coll Cardiol* 40(10):1777-1785, 2002.

Expert Panel on Detection, Evaluation, and Treatment of High Blood Cholesterol in Adults: Executive Summary of the Third Report of the National Cholesterol Education Program (NCEP) Expert Panel on Detection, Evaluation, and Treatment of High Blood Cholesterol in Adults (Adult Treatment Panel III). *JAMA* 285:2486-2497, 2001.

Hunt D, Young P, Simes J, et al: Benefits of pravastatin on cardiovascular events and mortality in older patients with coronary heart disease are equal to or exceed those seen in younger patients: Results from the LIPID trial. *Ann Intern Med* 134:931-940, 2001.

Roberts CGP, Rodriguez A: Lipid-lowering medications in the elderly. *Clinical Geriatrics* 10:36-44, 2005.

Safeer R, Ugalat P: Cholesterol treatment guidelines update. *Am Fam Physician* 65:871-880, 2002.

Shepherd J, Blauw GJ, Murphy MB, et al: PROSPER study group. Prospective Study of Pravastatin in the Elderly at Risk; Pravastatin in elderly individuals at risk of vascular disease (PROSPER): A randomized controlled trial. *Lancet* 360:1623-1630, 2002.

HYPERTHYROIDISM

Fred F. Ferri and Tom J. Wachtel

Definition

Hyperthyroidism (or thyrotoxicosis) is a hypermetabolic state resulting from excess thyroid hormone.

Epidemiology

1. Hyperthyroidism affects 2% of women and 0.2% of men in their lifetime.
2. Toxic multinodular goiter usually occurs in women older than 55 years and is more common than Graves' disease in the elderly.

Clinical Findings

1. Patients with hyperthyroidism generally present with the following clinical manifestations:
   a. Tachycardia.
   b. Tremor.
   c. Hyperreflexia.
   d. Anxiety.
   e. Irritability.
   f. Emotional liability.
   g. Panic attacks.
   h. Heat intolerance.
   i. Sweating.
   j. Increased appetite.
   k. Diarrhea.
   l. Weight loss.
2. The presentation may be different in elderly patients (see later).
3. Patients with Graves' disease can present with:
   a. Exophthalmos.

    b. Lid retraction.

    c. Lid lag (Graves' ophthalmopathy). The following signs and symptoms of ophthalmopathy may be present.

        (1) Blurring of vision.

        (2) Photophobia.

        (3) Increased lacrimation.

        (4) Double vision.

        (5) Deep orbital pressure.

    d. Clubbing of fingers associated with periosteal new bone formation in other skeletal areas (Graves' acropachy) and pretibial myxedema may also be noted.

3. Elderly hyperthyroid patients may have only subtle signs (weight loss, tachycardia, fine skin, brittle nails).

    a. This form is known as apathetic hyperthyroidism and manifests with lethargy rather than hyperkinetic activity.

    b. An enlarged thyroid gland may be absent.

    c. Coexisting medical disorders (most commonly, cardiac disease) can also mask the symptoms.

    d. These patients often have unexplained CHF, worsening of angina, new-onset atrial fibrillation resistant to treatment, or systolic hypertension.

4. Subclinical hyperthyroidism.

    a. Subclinical hyperthyroidism is defined as a normal serum free T_4 and free T_3 levels with a TSH level suppressed below the normal range.

    b. These patients usually do not present with signs or symptoms of overt hyperthyroidism.

    c. Treatment options include observation or a therapeutic trial of low-dose antithyroid agents for 6 months in attempt to induce remission.

Etiology

1. Graves' disease (diffuse toxic goiter).
2. Toxic multinodular goiter (Plummer's disease).
3. Toxic adenoma (hot nodule).
4. Iatrogenic and factitious.
5. Transient hyperthyroidism (subacute thyroiditis, Hashimoto's thyroiditis).
6. Rare causes.

    a. Hypersecretion of TSH (e.g., pituitary neoplasms).

    b. Struma ovarii.

    c. Ingestion of a large amount of iodine by a patient with preexisting thyroid hyperplasia or adenoma (jodbasedow phenomenon).

    d. Carcinoma of thyroid.

    e. Amiodarone therapy.

Differential Diagnosis

1. Anxiety disorders and depression.
2. Dementia.
3. Pheochromocytoma.

4. All causes of weight loss including:
   a. Cancer.
   b. Tuberculosis.
   c. Diabetes.
5. Perimenopausal state (hot flushes).

Work-up

Suspected hyperthyroidism requires laboratory confirmation and identification of its etiology because treatment varies with its cause.
1. Laboratory tests.
   a. Elevated TT_4 with elevated T_3 resin uptake (T_3RU).
   b. Elevated free T_4.
   c. Elevated free T_3.
   d. Low TSH (unless hyperthyroidism is a result of the exceptionally rare hypersecretion of TSH from a pituitary adenoma).
   e. Thyroid autoantibodies can be useful in selected cases to differentiate Graves' disease from toxic multinodular goiter (absent thyroid antibodies).
2. Imaging studies.
   a. A 24-hour radioactive iodine uptake and thyroid scan are useful to distinguish hyperthyroidism from iatrogenic thyroid hormone synthesis (thyrotoxicosis factitia) and from thyroiditis.
   b. An overactive thyroid usually shows increased uptake.
   c. Iatrogenic thyroid ingestion and thyroiditis may reveal normal or decreased uptake.
   d. The scan results reveal the etiology of the hyperthyroidism.
      (1) Graves' disease: increased homogeneous uptake.
      (2) Multinodular goiter: increased heterogeneous uptake.
      (3) Hot nodule: single focus of increased uptake.
   e. The 24-hour radioactive iodine uptake is also generally performed before the therapeutic administration of radioactive iodine to determine the appropriate dose.

Treatment

1. Antithyroid drugs (thionamides).
   a. Propylthiouracil (PTU) and methimazole (Tapazole).
      (1) PTU and methimazole inhibit thyroid hormone synthesis by blocking production of thyroid peroxidase.
      (2) PTU inhibits peripheral conversion of T_4 to T_3.
      (3) Dosage.
         (a) PTU 50 to 100 mg PO tid.
         (b) Methimazole 10 to 20 mg PO tid or 30 to 60 mg/day given as a single dose.
   b. Antithyroid drugs can be used as the primary form of treatment or as adjunctive therapy before radioactive therapy or surgery or later if the hyperthyroidism recurs.
   c. Common side effects.
      (1) Skin rash (3% to 5% of patients).
      (2) Arthralgias.
      (3) Myalgias.
      (4) Granulocytopenia (0.5%).

    d. Rare side effects.

      (1) Aplastic anemia.

      (2) Hepatic necrosis from PTU.

      (3) Cholestatic jaundice from methimazole.

    e. When antithyroid drugs are used as primary therapy, they are usually given for 6 to 24 months; prolonged therapy can cause hypothyroidism.

    f. The use of antithyroid drugs before radioactive iodine therapy is best reserved for patients in whom exacerbation of hyperthyroidism after radioactive iodine therapy is hazardous (e.g., elderly patients with CAD or significant coexisting morbidity). In these patients the antithyroid drug can be stopped 2 days before radioactive iodine therapy, resumed 2 days later, and continued for 4 to 6 weeks.

    g. Follow-up.

      (1) Patients undergoing treatment with antithyroid drugs should be seen every 1 to 3 months until euthyroidism is achieved and every 3 to 4 months while they remain on antithyroid therapy.

      (2) After treatment is stopped, periodic monitoring or thyroid function tests with TSH every 3 months for 1 year, then every 6 months for 1 year, then annually is recommended.

2. Radioactive iodine (RAI).

    a. RAI (^{131}I) is the treatment of choice for patients older than 21 years.

    b. Radioiodine is also used in hyperthyroidism caused by toxic adenoma or toxic multinodular goiter.

    c. A single dose of RAI is effective in inducing euthyroid state in nearly 80% of patients.

    d. There is a high incidence of post-RAI hypothyroidism (>5% within first year and 2%/year thereafter). Therefore, these patients should be screened annually or when symptomatic for the onset of hypothyroidism.

3. Surgical therapy (subtotal thyroidectomy).

    a. Indications.

      (1) Obstructing goiters.

      (2) Any patient who refuses RAI and cannot be adequately managed with antithyroid medications (e.g., patients with toxic adenoma or toxic multinodular goiter).

    b. Patients should be rendered euthyroid with antithyroid drugs before surgery.

    c. Complications of surgery include hypothyroidism (28% to 43% after 10 years), hypoparathyroidism, and vocal cord paralysis (1%).

    d. Hyperthyroidism recurs after surgery in 10% to 15% of patients.

4. Adjunctive therapy.

    a. Propranolol alleviates the β-adrenergic symptoms of hyperthyroidism.

    b. Initial dose is 20 to 40 mg PO bid to qid.

    c. Dosage is gradually increased until symptoms are controlled.

    d. Major contraindications to propranolol are CHF and bronchospasm.

SUGGESTED READINGS

Kearns AE, Thompson GB: Medical and surgical management of hyperthyroidism. *Mayo Clin Proc* 77:87-91, 2002.

Shrier DK, Burman KD: Subclinical hyperthyroidism: Controversies in management. *Am Fam Physician* 65:431-438, 2002.

Toft AD: Clinical practice. Subclinical hyperthyroidism. *N Engl J Med* 345:512-516, 2001.

HYPOTHYROIDISM

Fred F. Ferri and Tom J. Wachtel

Definition

Hypothyroidism is a disorder caused by the inadequate secretion of thyroid hormone.

Epidemiology

1. Incidence is 1.5% to 2% of women and 0.2% of men
2. Predominant age.
   a. Incidence of hypothyroidism increases with age.
   b. Among persons older than 60 years, 6% of women and 2.5% of men have laboratory evidence of hypothyroidism (TSH more than twice normal).

Clinical Findings

1. Hypothyroid patients generally present with the following signs and symptoms:
   a. Fatigue.
   b. Lethargy.
   c. Weakness.
   d. Constipation.
   e. Weight gain.
   f. Cold intolerance.
   g. Muscle weakness.
   h. Slow speech.
   i. Cognitive impairment.
2. Skin.
   a. Dry, coarse, thick, cool, and sallow (yellow color caused by carotenemia).
   b. Nonpitting edema in skin of eyelids and hands (myxedema) secondary to infiltration of subcutaneous tissues by a hydrophilic mucopolysaccharide substance.
3. Hair.
   a. Brittle and coarse.
   b. Loss of outer one third of eyebrows
   c. Facies.
   d. Dulled expression.
   e. Thickened tongue.
   f. Thick, slow-moving lips.
4. Thyroid gland might or might not be palpable (depending on the cause of the hypothyroidism).
5. Heart sounds are distant, with possible pericardial effusion.
6. Bradycardia.
7. Neurologic.
   a. Delayed relaxation phase of the deep tendon reflexes.
   b. Cerebellar ataxia.
   c. Hearing impairment.

    d. Poor memory.

    e. Peripheral neuropathies with paresthesia.

8. Musculoskeletal.

    a. Carpal tunnel syndrome.

    b. Muscle stiffness.

    c. Weakness.

Etiology

1. Primary hypothyroidism (thyroid gland dysfunction) accounts for more than 90% of the cases of hypothyroidism.

    a. Hashimoto's thyroiditis is the most common cause of hypothyroidism after 8 years of age.

    b. Idiopathic myxedema (nongoiter form of Hashimoto's thyroiditis).

    c. Previous treatment of hyperthyroidism (radioiodine therapy, subtotal thyroidectomy).

    d. Subacute thyroiditis.

    e. Radiation therapy to the neck (usually for malignant disease).

    f. Iodine deficiency or excess.

    g. Drugs.

        (1) Lithium.

        (2) Periodic acid–Schiff.

        (3) Sulfonamides.

        (4) Phenylbutazone.

        (5) Amiodarone.

        (6) Thiourea.

    h. Congenital (approximately 1 case per 4000 live births).

    i. Prolonged treatment with iodides.

2. Secondary hypothyroidism.

    a. Pituitary dysfunction.

    b. Postpartum necrosis.

    c. Neoplasm.

    d. Infiltrative disease causing deficiency of TSH.

3. Tertiary hypothyroidism: Hypothalamic disease causing deficiency of TRH.

    a. Granuloma.

    b. Neoplasm.

    c. Irradiation.

4. Tissue resistance to thyroid hormone is rare.

Differential Diagnosis

1. Depression.

2. Dementia from other causes.

3. Systemic disorders (e.g., nephrotic syndrome, CHF, amyloidosis).

Laboratory Tests

1. Increased TSH: TSH may be normal or low if the patient has secondary or tertiary hypothyroidism, is receiving dopamine or corticosteroids, or the level is obtained following severe illness.

2. Decreased free T_4.

3. Other common laboratory abnormalities.

    a. Hyperlipidemia.

b. Hyponatremia.

c. Anemia.

4. Increased antimicrosomal and antithyroglobulin antibody titers are useful when autoimmune thyroiditis is suspected as the cause of the hypothyroidism.

Treatment

1. Replacement therapy with levothyroxine (Synthroid, Levothroid).

   a. Therapy should begin with 25 µg/day, depending on the patient's age and the severity of the disease.

   b. The dose may be increased by 25-µg/day increments every 6 to 8 weeks, depending on the clinical response and serum TSH level.

   c. Elderly patients with CAD should be started with 12.5 µg/day (higher doses can precipitate angina).

2. Monitoring.

   a. TSH levels.

      (1) Periodic monitoring of TSH level is an essential part of treatment.

      (2) Patients should be evaluated initially with an office visit and TSH levels every 6 to 8 weeks until the patient is clinically euthyroid and the TSH level is normalized.

      (3) The frequency of subsequent visits and TSH measurement can then be decreased to every 6 to 12 months.

   b. Therapy.

      (1) For monitoring therapy in patients with secondary or tertiary hypothyroidism, measurement of serum free T_4 level is appropriate.

      (2) Free T_4 should be maintained in the upper half of the normal range.

3. Patients should be educated regarding hypothyroidism and its possible complications. Patients should also be instructed about the need for lifelong treatment and monitoring for signs of thyroid dysfunction.

4. Admission to the hospital is recommended in all patients with myxedema coma.

5. Subclinical hypothyroidism.

   a. Subclinical hypothyroidism occurs in as many as 15% of elderly patients.

   b. It is characterized by an elevated serum TSH and a normal free T_4 level.

   c. Treatment is individualized.

   d. Generally, replacement therapy is recommended for all patients with serum TSH greater than 10 mU/L and with the presence of goiter or thyroid autoantibodies, and in patients with cognitive impairment (dementia).

   e. Occasionally, patients who were thought to be asymptomatic before treatment report feeling more energetic when euthyroidism is restored.

SUGGESTED READINGS

Cooper DS: Clinical practice. Subclinical hypothyroidism. *N Engl J Med* 345:
260-265, 2001.

Hueston WJ: Treatment of hypothyroidism. *Am Fam Physicians* 64:1717-1724, 2001.

OSTEOPOROSIS

Tom J. Wachtel

Definitions

1. Osteoporosis is a systemic skeletal disease characterized by low bone mass and microarchitectural deterioration of bone tissue resulting in reduced bone strength and increased risk of fracture.
2. Other definitions.
   a. Bone strength is defined as bone density plus bone quality (bone mineral density accounts for 70% of bone strength).
   b. Bone density is grams of mineral per volume.
   c. Bone mineral density is grams of mineral per area.
   d. Bone quality is factors that influence bone strength, including microarchitecture, turnover, damage accumulation, and mineralization.
   e. Microarchitecture describes number of trabeculae, trabecular thickness, trabecular spacing, etc.
   f. Macroarchitecture also affects bone strength but is not related to osteoporosis.

Epidemiology

1. About 44 million adults in the United States have abnormally low bone mass (osteopenia or osteoporosis).
2. About 40% of all women and 25% of all men will experience a fragility (or low-impact) fracture in their lifetime.
3. About 80% of all osteoporotic persons are women.
4. Osteoporosis (and osteopenia) accounts for 800,000 vertebral compression fractures, 300,000 hip fractures, and 250,000 wrist fractures annually.
5. The consequences of those fractures are significant for the patients.
   a. Hip fracture.
      (1) The mortality for hip fracture is 24% in the first 12 months.
      (2) Of those who survive, 50% fail to regain full ambulatory capability and 25% need long-term institutional care.
   b. Vertebral fracture.
      (1) Vertebral fractures can be asymptomatic but they can also be associated with back pain (2-fold increased risk of back pain associated with vertebral fractures).
      (2) Vertebral fractures may require reduced activity or bed rest.
      (3) Vertebral fractures are responsible for 70,000 annual U.S. hospital admissions and increased mortality.
6. Impact.
   a. Osteoporotic fractures are responsible for 4.1 million hospital days, 44.6 million nursing home days, and 3.4 million outpatient visits.
   b. Their economic impact is $20 billion annually.

Risk Factors for Primary Osteoporosis and Fragility Fractures

1. Personal history of a prior fragility fracture is the strongest predictor of a subsequent fracture regardless of bone density.
2. Family history of fracture.
3. Cigarette smoking.

4. Low body mass index and poor nutrition.
5. Female gender.
6. Early menopause (natural or surgical).
7. Age.
8. Alcoholism.
9. Low calcium intake.
10. Sedentary lifestyle.
11. General fragility.
12. Race/ethnicity (whites and Asians at higher risk than African Americans and Latin Americans).
13. Excessive caffeine intake.
14. History of falls.
15. Unsteady gait.
16. Risk factors for falls and unsteady gait such as impaired vision, vertigo, orthostatic hypotension, arthritis, neurologic disorders, dementia medications.

Etiology

1. Primary osteoporosis.
   a. Multifactorial resulting from a combination of factors including:
      (1) Nutrition.
      (2) Peak bone mass.
      (3) Genetics.
      (4) Level of physical activity.
      (5) Age of menopause (spontaneous vs. surgical).
      (6) Estrogen status.
   b. Postmenopausal osteoporosis is by far the most common form of primary osteoporosis. Increased bone resorption results in net bone loss, most rapidly during the first 5 years following menopause.
   c. In men, osteoporosis is also related to decreasing levels of sex hormones.
2. Secondary osteoporosis.
   a. Endocrine/metabolic.
      (1) Vitamin D deficiency.
      (2) Primary hyperparathyroidism.
      (3) Thyrotoxicosis.
      (4) Hypercortisolism (Cushing's syndrome).
      (5) (Male) hypogonadism.
      (6) T1DM.
      (7) Anorexia nervosa.
      (8) Hyperprolactinemia.
      (9) Porphyria.
      (10) Hypophosphatasia.
   b. Gastrointestinal.
      (1) Malabsorption syndromes.
      (2) Chronic liver disease.
      (3) Inflammatory bowel disease.
   c. Malignancies.
      (1) Multiple myeloma.
      (2) Lymphoma.

     (3) Paraneoplastic syndromes.

     (4) Other malignancies.

  d. Rheumatoid arthritis and variants.

  e. Chronic obstructive pulmonary disease (COPD).

  f. Renal failure.

  g. Marfan's syndrome.

  h. Homocystinuria.

  i. Mastocytosis.

  j. Osteogenesis imperfecta.

  k. Drugs.

     (1) Glucocorticoids.

     (2) Thyroid hormones.

     (3) Anti-epileptic drug (e.g., phenytoin and phenobarbital).

     (4) Loop diuretics.

     (5) Gonadotropin-releasing hormone (GnRH) antagonists.

Physical Findings

1. Osteoporosis is often silent, with no signs or symptoms. The prevalence of osteoporosis is 22% in white women aged 60 to 69 years, 38% in those aged 70 to 79 years, and 70% in those 80 years and older. This means that osteoporosis should be presumed to exist in all very elderly women until proven otherwise.
2. Height loss.
   a. The most common sign of osteoporosis is height loss.
   b. All elderly women (and probably men also) should be measured yearly.
   c. Most people know their adult height (or what it used to be).
3. Other signs.
   a. Thoracic kyphosis (dowager's hump).
   b. Back pain associated with vertebral compression fractures (osteoporosis without resulting fractures does not cause back pain).
   c. Symptoms and signs associated with the causes of secondary osteoporosis.
4. The consequence of osteoporosis is an increased risk (incidence) of fractures.

Types of Fractures

1. Traumatic fracture resulting from a force that exceeds the strength of normal bone.
2. Pathologic fractures involving a bone whose strength is weakened by a disease other than osteoporosis including:
   a. Primary bone cancer.
   b. Metastatic bone cancer.
   c. Benign bone tumor.
   d. Paget's disease.
   e. Osteomalacia.
   f. Osteopetrosis and other acquired causes of brittle bone.
3. Osteoporotic (or fragility or low-impact) fractures.

Work-up

1. Diagnosis of osteoporosis is made by densitometry. It is indicated in:
   a. All women 65 years and older.

   b. Postmenopausal women younger than 65 years with osteoporosis risk factors.

   c. All adults with fragility fractures.

   d. Anyone expected to be treated with glucocorticoids for longer than 3 months (cumulative).

   e. Selectively in adults with known diseases associated with secondary osteoporosis.

   f. Men 70 years and older (controversial).

2. Technologies for measuring bone mineral density (BMD).

   a. Quantitative ultrasound.

     (1) Advantages.

       (a) Low cost.

       (b) Safe (no radiation).

     (2) Disadvantages.

       (a) Only peripheral sites (finger, wrist, heel).

       (b) Imprecise.

   b. Dual-energy x-ray absorptiometry (DEXA).

     (1) Advantages.

       (a) The gold standard.

       (b) Epidemiologic studies have correlated and standardized BMD data obtained by DEXA with fracture risk.

       (c) Can measure peripheral and central sites (hip and spine).

       (d) Precise.

     (2) Disadvantages.

       (a) More costly than quantitative ultrasound.

       (b) Radiation exposure.

       (c) Variable results among different machines.

       (d) Any dense structure between the radiation source and film (e.g., osteophytes or vascular calcifications) will give a false high reading, because density is measured from a two-dimensional image.

   c. Quantitative CT.

     (1) Advantages.

       (a) Central or peripheral site.

       (b) Precise.

       (c) Measures the intended targeted bone only as a three-dimensional structure.

     (2) Disadvantages.

       (a) Most expensive technology.

       (b) Radiation exposure.

       (c) Not yet fully standardized.

3. Interpretation.

   a. All BMD measurement results are expressed in t scores (standard deviations or percentage above or below values for young normal persons) and z scores (standard deviations or percentage above or below age-matched values) regardless of what technology is used.

   b. World Health Organization Criteria for the Diagnosis of Osteoporosis are shown in Table 5-16.

   c. DEXA values are reported by comparison to age and gender reference groups with t scores and z scores (Fig. 5-3).

Table 5-16 **World Health Organization Criteria for Diagnosis of Osteoporosis**

Diagnosis	*t* Score
Normal	>–1
Osteopenia	–1 to –2.5
Osteoporosis	≤–2.5
Severe osteoporosis	<–2.5 plus fragility fracture(s)

(1) A *t* score more than 2 standard deviations below young normal persons indicates an increased risk for fracture and should lead to consideration of active therapy to prevent further bone loss.

(2) A *z* score more than 1 to 2 standard deviations below the age-matched mean value signifies a BMD that is much lower than expected for the patient's age and should prompt a thorough evaluation for secondary causes of bone loss.

d. The work-up for secondary causes of osteoporosis is presented in Table 5-17 (low *z* score work-up).

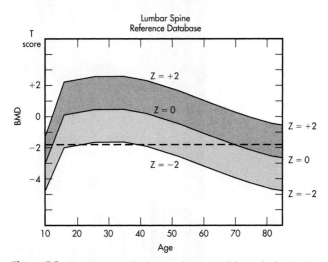

Figure 5-3   Natural history of lumbar spine bone mineral density, lumbar spine in girls and women age 10 through 85. The band is a mean ±2–standard deviation representation of bone density. The X axis represents age, the Y axis represents bone density in *t* scores. The middle of the ribbon represents a *z* score of 0 (i.e., the statistical average woman's bone density as she ages). (From Wachtel TJ: *Geriatrics Clinical Advisor*, Philadelphia, Mosby, 2006.)

Table 5-17 Work-up for the Secondary Cause of Osteoporosis (Low z Score)

Differential Diagnosis	Screening	Positive Screen	Confirmatory Test
Endocrine/Metabolism			
Hypercortisolism	FBS, K^+	$\uparrow$ FBS, $\downarrow K^+$	Overnight dexamethasone suppression test
Hyperparathyroidism	Ca^{2+}, P	$\uparrow Ca^{2+}$ and/or $\downarrow$ Phos	PTH level
Hyperthyroidism	TSH	$\downarrow$ TSH	TT_4, TT_3, T_3 RU
Hypogonadism in men	T, FSH, LH	$\downarrow$ T, $\uparrow$ FSH, $\uparrow$LH	
Hypogonadism in premenopausal women	FSH, LH	$\uparrow$ FSH, $\uparrow$LH	
Low vitamin D state*	Ca^{2+}, P	Lowish Ca^{2+} and $\downarrow$ P	25-OH-D level
Neoplasia			
Leukemia	CBC	$\uparrow$WBC	Bone marrow aspirate
Lymphoma	CBC, ? Imaging	Anemia, lymphadenopathy	More imaging
Metastatic cancer	N/A		
Multiple myeloma	CBC, ESR, Ca^{2+}, Creat	Anemia, $\uparrow$ ESR, $\uparrow Ca^{2+}$ or $\uparrow$ Creat	SPEP, UEP

Chronic Illness		
Hepatic failure	ALT, Alk phos, PT	Abn LFTs	Variable
Renal failure	Creat	↑ Creat	Variable
Rheumatoid arthritis	Steroid use (for longer than 3 months)		
Gastrointestinal		
Malabsorption	CBC, PT, carotene	Anemia, ↑ PT, ↓ carotene	D-xylose absorption
			Anemia evaluation
Drugs		
Dilantin	Medication history		
Glucocorticoids			
Loop diuretics			
Thyroid hormone			

*In high-risk populations (e.g., nursing home, northern latitude residence), a screening 25-OH-D level is recommended.
Abn LFTs, abnormal liver function tests; Alk phos, alkaline phosphatase; ALT, alanine transaminase; CBC, complete blood cell count; Creat, creatinine; ESR, erythrocyte sedimentation rate; FBS, fetal bovine serum; LH, luteinizing hormone; 25-OH-D, 25-hydroxyvitamin D; P, phosphorus; PT, prothrombin time; PTH, parathyroid hormone; RU, resin sponge uptake; SPEP, serum protein electrophoresis; T, testosterone; T_3, triiodothyronine; TSH, thyroid-stimulating hormone; TT_3, total triiodothyronine; TT_4, total thyroxine; UEP, urine electrophoresis.
Data from Wachtel TJ: *Geriatric clinical advisor.* Philadelphia, Mosby, 2006.

Treatment

The goal of treatment is fracture prevention. The strongest predictors of fracture are previous fracture, falls and fall risk, low BMD, and advancing age.

1. Nonpharmacologic management.
   a. Resistive exercises.
      (1) Walking.
      (2) Rowing machine.
      (3) Weight lifting.
      (4) Evidence suggests that the strongest predictor of compliance with exercise is enjoyability, which therefore should always be considered in providing recommendations.
   b. Fall prevention.
      (1) Assess gait and fall risk.
      (2) Consider referral for gait training, lower extremity muscle strengthening, and balance training.
      (3) Home safety evaluation.
      (4) Assistive devices as appropriate.
   c. Hip protectors.
   d. Supplements.
      (1) Calcium.
          (a) Provide 1500 mg/day from diet and/or supplements.
          (b) Examples of dietary sources include:
              i.   Milk: 300 mg per cup.
              ii. Yogurt: 350 mg per cup.
              iii. Cheese: 200 mg per oz.
              iv. Broccoli: 100 mg per cup.
          (c) Calcium preparations.
              i.   Calcium carbonate.
              ii. Calcium citrate.
              iii. Calcium gluconate.
      (2) Vitamin D.
          (a) Patient should obtain 800 1U/day from diet, sun exposure, and/or supplements.
          (b) Many calcium supplements also contain Vitamin D.
2. Pharmacologic treatment.
   a. Indication for treatment (according to the National Osteoporosis Foundation).
      (1) t Score less than −2.0 by central DEXA.
      (2) t Score less than −1.5 by central DEXA plus at least one additional fracture risk factor.
      (3) Patients with any prior history of fragility, or vertebral or hip fracture should be treated, even if a DEXA is not available.
      (4) Preventive treatment for osteoporosis and treatment of osteopenia are controversial, even though some drugs have Food and Drug Administration (FDA) approval for prevention.
   b. Antiresorptive (antiosteoclastic) treatments.
      (1) Estrogen.
          (a) Estrogen is effective in preventing hip and vertebral fractures.
          (b) The dose of conjugated estrogens is 0.625 mg daily; however, the overall risk outweighs the benefit.

    (c) This treatment is no longer recommended for osteoporosis either as single therapy or combined with progesterone.

(2) Selective estrogen receptor modulators (SERMs).

    (a) Raloxifene.

        i. Dose is 60 mg daily.

        ii. Approved for treatment (and prevention) of osteoporosis.

        iii. Evidence exists that raloxifene is effective in reducing the risk of vertebral fractures.

        iv. It is not known if it can reduce the risk of hip fracture.

        v. Reduces the risk of breast cancer.

    (b) Tamoxifen.

        i. Dose is 20 mg daily.

        ii. Not approved for treatment (and prevention) of osteoporosis.

        iii. Reduces the risk of breast cancer.

    (c) Side effects.

        i. Hot flushes.

        ii. Leg cramps.

        iii. Increased risk of deep vein thrombosis.

        iv. Increased risk of endometrial cancer.

(3) Calcitonin nasal spray.

    (a) A dose of 200 IU per day reduces the risk of vertebral fractures.

    (b) It is not known if it can reduce the risk of hip fracture.

    (c) The drug is well tolerated but is probably less effective than other agents.

(4) Bisphosphonates.

    (a) Several bisphosphonates are available, but only three are widely used for treatment or prevention of osteoporosis.

        i. Alendronate 70 mg PO weekly or 10 mg PO daily.

        ii. Risedronate 35 mg PO weekly or 5 mg PO daily.

        iii. Ibandronate 150 mg PO once monthly or 2.5 mg PO daily.

    (b) All three drugs are efficacious in reducing the risk of vertebral and extravertebral fractures.

    (c) The principal side effects for these drugs are potential esophageal ulceration and diarrhea.

    (d) Alendronate may be marginally more potent at increasing bone density and risedronate may have better gastrointestinal tolerability, but all three drugs are probably interchangeable.

    (e) They are considered the first line of pharmacologic treatment for osteoporosis.

c. Bone-building treatments (osteoblastic stimulant).

  (1) Recombinant human parathyroid hormone (rh-PTH or teriparatide) is a potent stimulant of osteoblastic cells when administered as pulse therapy.

  (2) Continuous exposure to parathormone stimulates osteoclasts more than osteoblasts and results in a net bone loss.

  (3) Teriparatide is administered at the dose of 20 µg SC daily.

  (4) The drug reduces vertebral and nonvertebral fractures (not specifically hip fractures, as is the case for alendronate and risedronate).

(5) Teriparatide can cause osteosarcoma at high doses in rats.

(6) It is very expensive.

3. Monitoring treatment.

a. No evidence currently exists to demonstrate effectiveness of a monitoring strategy.

b. Most clinicians recommend a central DEXA at baseline and at 2 years and 4 years into treatment (the technology is not precise enough to recommend shorter intervals).

c. Treatment success can be defined by an improvement or no change in BMD over time and no fracture.

(1) A decline in BMD over time does not necessarily indicate failure.

(2) Treatment trials show efficacy in fracture reduction compared with placebo even in subjects with declining BMD.

(3) Many clinicians consider declining BMD and/or fracture to indicate treatment failure and need to change treatment.

d. Evidence to support combined treatment is not yet convincing.

e. Markers of bone turnover are used by some clinicians to monitor response to treatment.

(1) The most common markers of bone resorption include acid phosphatase, hydroxyproline, and N-telopeptide (a metabolite of collagen cross-links).

(2) The most common markers of bone formation are alkaline phosphatase and osteocalcin.

(3) Change in those markers only takes 3 months to observe, but such changes correlate only poorly with fracture risk.

4. Osteoporosis in men.

a. Twenty percent of all osteoporotic persons in the United States are men.

b. Secondary causes (e.g., hypogonadism or vitamin D deficiency) are more likely in men (women typically have primary osteoporosis).

c. Bisphosphonates, calcitonin, and teriparatide are used to treat osteoporotic men.

d. Only alendronate and teriparatide are approved by the FDA for this indication.

5. Duration of treatment.

a. Most treatment trials were not conducted for periods longer than 5 years, but alendronate has 10-year data from trial extension open-label studies.

b. Some clinicians hesitate to treat for longer than 5 years for lack of any evidence base.

c. Some clinicians treat indefinitely because BMD declines after treatment withdrawal.

SUGGESTED READINGS

Bone HG, Hosking D, Devogetaer JP, et al: Ten years' experience with alendronate for osteoporosis in postmenopausal women. *N Eng J Med* 350:1189-1199, 2004.

Cauley JA, Robbins J, Chen Z, et al: Effects of estrogen plus progestin on risk of fracture and bone mineral density: The Women's Health Initiative randomized trial. *JAMA* 290:1729-1738, 2003.

Elliott ME, Binkley NC, Carnes M, et al: Fracture risks of women in long-term care: High prevalence of calcaneal osteoporosis and hypovitaminosis D. *Pharmacotherapy* 23:702-710, 2003.

Greenspan SL, Schneier DL, McClung MR, et al: Alendronate improves bone mineral density in elderly women with osteoporosis residing in long-term care facilities: A randomized, double-blind, placebo-controlled trial. *Ann Intern Med* 136:742-746, 2002.

Jolly EE, Bjamason NH, Neven P, et al: Prevention of osteoporosis and uterine effects in postmenopausal women taking raloxifene for 5 years. *Menopause* 10:337-344, 2003.

Keller MI: Treating osteoporosis in post-menopausal women: A case approach. *Cleveland J of Med* 71:829-837, 2004.

Kiebzak GM, Miller PD: Determinants of bone strength. *J Bone Miner Res* 18:383-384, 2003.

Lindsay R, Silverman SL, Cooper C, et al: Risk of new vertebral fracture in the year following a fracture. *JAMA* 285:320-323, 2001.

Marshall D, Johnell O, Wedel H: Meta-analysis of how well measures of bone mineral density predict occurrence of osteoporotic fractures. *BMJ* 312:1254-1259, 1996.

National Osteoporosis Foundation: *Physician's Guide to Prevention and Treatment of Osteoporosis.* Washington, DC, National Osteoporosis Foundation, 2003.

Neer RM, Arnaud CD, Zanchetta JR, et al: Effect of parathyroid hormone (1-34) on fractures and bone mineral density in postmenopausal women with osteoporosis. *N Eng J Med* 344:1434-1441, 2001.

Raisz LG: Screening for osteoporosis. *N Engl J Med* 353:164-171, 2005.

Rosen CJ: Postmenopausal osteoporosis. *N Engl J Med* 353:595-603, 2005.

Roux C, Seeman E, Eastell R, et al: Efficacy of risedronate on clinical vertebral fractures within six months. *Curr Med Res Opin* 20:433-439, 2004.

Siris ES, Miller PD, Barrett-Connor E, et al: Identification and fracture outcomes of undiagnosed low bone mineral density in postmenopausal women: Results from the National Osteoporosis Risk Assessment. *JAMA* 286:2815-2822, 2001.

Sorensen OH, Crawford GM, Mulder H, et al: Long-term efficacy of risedronate: A 5-year placebo-controlled clinical experience. *Bone* 32:120-126, 2003.

Zimmerman SI, Girman CJ, Buie VC, et al: The prevalence of osteoporosis in nursing home residents. *Osteoporos Int* 9:151-157, 1999.

5.3 Otorhinolaryngology

ALLERGIC RHINITIS
Michael P. Gerardo

Definitions

1. Allergic rhinitis is an inflammatory disorder involving the upper respiratory tract. It is characterized by itching of the eyes, nose, and palate and by nasal congestion.
   a. It is *seasonal* if this complex of symptoms occurs at a particular time of the year. Common seasonal allergens include trees, grass, weeds, pollen, fungi, and molds.
   b. It is *perennial* if the symptoms occur year round. Perennial rhinitis is often caused by dust mites, cockroaches, animal proteins, and fungi.

Epidemiology

Studies estimate the prevalence in the United States at between 9% and 40% of the population.

Clinical Findings

1. Patients can present with any combination of the following:
   a. Rhinorrhea.
   b. Nasal congestion.

   c. Postnasal drip.
   d. Maxillary and frontal sinus pressure.
   e. Pharyngitis.
   f. Cough.
   g. Watery eyes.
   h. Itchy eyes.
   i. Ear blockage or popping.
   j. Vertigo.
   k. Sneezing.
2. In patients with active rhinitis, the nasal mucosa must be visualized to evaluate nasal anatomy for discharge, polyps, and tumors.
3. Nasal inflammation can lead to obstruction of the osteomeatal complex. This obstruction predisposes patients to as many as 30% of acute and 80% of chronic bacterial infections of the sinuses.
4. Epistaxis.
   a. Epistaxis is usually benign.
   b. It can be associated with rhinitis and lead to significant blood loss.
   c. It can also rarely signal a nasopharyngeal malignancy.

Differential Diagnosis

1. In general, history can differentiate allergic rhinitis from the following:
   a. Infectious rhinitis (Table 5-18).
   b. Vasomotor rhinitis (idiopathic).
   c. Occupational rhinitis.
   d. Rhinitis medicamentosa.

Table 5-18 Allergic Rhinitis: Differentiation of Symptoms

Symptom	Upper Respiratory Infection	Allergic Rhinitis
Cough	Common	Sometimes
Aches	Occasional	Never
General fatigue, weakness	Sometimes	Sometimes
Itchy eyes	Rare	Common
Sneezing	Usual	Usual
Pharyngitis	Common	Sometimes
Rhinorrhea	Common	Common
Nasal congestion	Common	Common
Fever	Common	Rare
Duration of symptoms	3-14 days	Weeks; note seasonal recurrences
Treatment	Decongestants, acetaminophen, rest, fluids	Antihistamines (Rx or OTC), nasal steroids, decongestants
Possible complications	Sinusitis, otitis media	Sinusitis, asthma, otitis media

OTC, over the counter; Rx, prescription.

2. Patients who have a history of upper respiratory tract symptoms at the same time every year probably have allergic rhinitis rather than infection.

Treatment

1. Nonpharmacologic therapy consists of preventive measures.
    a. Allergen avoidance: Identifying allergens may be difficult but in many cases can be done by history alone.
    b. Environmental measures.
        (1) Measures that have been successful in previous research include:
            (a) Maintaining the humidity at no greater than 50%.
            (b) Hot water washing of bedding once per week.
        (2) Use of bed covers impermeable to dust mite allergens has not been shown to alleviate rhinitis.
        (3) High-efficiency particulate air (HEPA) filters might reduce animal and dust allergens, but they do not control symptoms.
2. Pharmacologic therapy (Table 5-19).
    a. Intranasal medications.
        (1) Corticosteroids: Intranasal corticosteroid therapy is considered first-line therapy for allergic rhinitis because of its limited side-effect profile and significantly greater relief of nasal symptoms, sneezing, itch, and postnasal drip than oral antihistamines.
        (2) Antihistamines.
            (a) Azelastine (Astelin), a topical intranasal second-generation antihistamine, also relieves the total allergic symptom profile including rhinorrhea, sneezing, postnasal drip, itchy eyes/ears/throat, and nasal congestion.
            (b) It is probably less effective than intranasal corticosteroids.
            (c) In several randomized trials, monotherapy with azelastine was as effective as dual therapy of azelastine plus loratadine or fexofenadine.
        (3) α-Adrenergic agonists.
            (a) Intranasal decongestant therapy prepared with a topical α-adrenergic agonist (e.g., oxymetazoline) reduces nasal congestion.
            (b) It is appropriate for relieving severe symptoms (e.g., vertigo).
            (c) α-Adrenergic agonists should not be used routinely due to risk of nasal hyperreactivity and rebound swelling.
            (d) Any use should be limited to 3 days.
        (4) Intranasal anticholinergic medication with ipratropium (Atrovent nasal) is particularly useful for managing rhinorrhea.
    b. Systemic medications.
        (1) In the elderly, systemic treatments should be reserved for patients who fail intranasal therapy.
        (2) Antihistamines.
            (a) First-generation oral antihistamines.
                i. First-generation antihistamines should be avoided due to their anticholinergic and sedating effects.
                ii. They also have a negative effect on cognitive function.

Table 5-19 **Pharmacological Treatments for Specific Allergic Rhinitis Symptoms**

Drug Class	Sneezing and Itching	Rhinorrhea	Congestion	Eye Symptoms
Oral antihistamines	Yes	Yes	Yes ±	Yes
Intranasal antihistamines	Yes	Yes	Yes ±	No
Oral decongestants	No	No	Yes	No
Intranasal decongestants	No	No	Yes	No
Intranasal corticosteroids	Yes	Yes	Yes	Yes
Intranasal anticholinergics	No	Yes	No	No
Antileukotrienes	Yes	Yes	Yes ±	Yes ±

±, limited effectiveness.

(b) Second-generation oral antihistamines (loratadine, deslora-tadine, fexofenadine).
  i. These are less sedating than the first-generation medications and are effective in relieving sneezing, rhinorrhea, and itch.
  ii. Cetirizine may be more effective in relieving the symptoms of sneezing, rhinorrhea, and itch but is associated with more sedation than other second-generation oral antihistamines.
  iii. In general, the second-generation medications are minimally effective against nasal congestion.
  iv. Montelukast, a leukotriene antagonist, is indicated as medical therapy for allergic rhinitis.
(3) Pseudoephedrine.
  (a) Some over-the-counter decongestants contain pseudo-ephedrine, which increases pulse pressure and systolic BP and should be avoided in persons with CAD and hypertension.
  (b) Pseudoephedrine also tightens the urinary bladder outlet and can worsen lower urinary tract symptoms in men with benign prostatic hyperplasia (BPH).
  (c) An additive adverse effect on the lower urinary tract is seen with the oral combination of decongestant and antihistamine especially in men with BPH.
3. Referral.
  a. Patients with symptoms not amenable to medical treatment should be evaluated by allergist or immunologist for allergen identification and possibly immunotherapy.
  b. An otorhinolaryngologist should evaluate patients with suspected or visualized structural abnormality when rhinoscopy is required for possible biopsy or surgery.

SUGGESTED READINGS

Berger WE: Weighing the pros and cons of a wide array of therapies: How to get your patient's allergic rhinitis under control. *J Resp Dis* 26:150-161, 2005.

Dykewicz MS: Rhinitis and sinusitis. *J Allerg Clin Immunol* 111:S520-S529, 2003.

Kaszuba SM, Baroody FM, DeTineo M: Superiority of intranasal corticosteroids compared with an oral antihistamine in the as-needed treatment of seasonal allergic rhinitis. *Arch Intern Med* 161:2581-2592, 2001.

HEARING LOSS

Fred F. Ferri

Incidence

1. Hearing loss is the most common sensory impairment in the elderly.
2. It affects 28% of elderly persons and is more prevalent in men.

Classification

Hearing loss can be classified according to the component of the auditory system being disrupted.

1. Conductive hearing loss is disruption of sound transmission from external ear to inner ear (e.g., otitis media, Paget's disease, damage to the tympanic membrane).

2. Sensorineural hearing loss is caused by dysfunction of hair cells or the cochlear nerve (e.g., Meniere's disease, drugs, acoustic neuroma).
3. Central hearing loss is secondary to lesions of the auditory centers of the brain (e.g., cerebrovascular accident, neoplasms).

Etiology

1. Frequent causes of hearing loss in the elderly.
   a. Cerumen impaction in the external canal represents a significant reversible factor in 30% of the elderly.
   b. Drugs.
      (1) Aminoglycosides.
      (2) Vancomycin.
      (3) Furosemide.
      (4) Ethacrinic acid.
      (5) Cisplatin.
      (6) Nitrogen mustard.
      (7) NSAIDs.
      (8) Antimalarials.
   c. Paget's disease of bone.
   d. Meniere's disease.
   e. Acoustic neuroma, meningioma.
   f. Otosclerosis, otitis media, trauma.
2. Most common diagnosis of hearing loss is presbycusis.
   a. Characterized by slowly progressive bilateral and symmetric high-frequency hearing loss.
      (1) The patient experiences significant difficulty understanding high-pitched voices (e.g., young children).
      (2) Background noise (e.g., in restaurants) also significantly impairs speech understanding.
   b. Four types of presbycusis, based on the selective atrophy of different morphologic structures in the cochlea, are shown in Table 5-20.

Table 5-20 **Types of Presbycusis**

| Type | Location in Cochlea | Audiometric Profile | |
		Pure Tones	Discrimination
Sensory	Basal end	High-tone abrupt slope	Related to frequency range
Neural	All turns	All frequencies	Severe loss
Strial	Apical region	All frequencies	Minimal loss
Cochlear conductive	All turns basal > apical	High-tone gradual slope	Related to steepness of slope

Data from Goldstein J, Kashima H, Koopmann C (eds): *Geriatric Otorhinolaryngology.* Philadelphia, BC Decker, 1989.

Evaluation

1. Initial screening in the office setting can be performed with a tuning fork and a portable audioscope (sensitivity 90%, specificity 80%).
2. Audiologic evaluation with pure-tone threshold audiometry will further define extent of loss and potential for rehabilitation.
   a. Figure 5-4 illustrates audiograms of patients with sensory presbycusis (note *abrupt* sloping high-tone hearing loss).
   b. Figure 5-5 shows an audiometric profile of patients with cochlear conductive presbycusis (*gradual* sloping high-tone hearing loss).
3. Hearing Handicap In Elderly Screening (HHIE-S).
   a. This is a communication-specific self-assessment scale on social and emotional consequences of hearing loss (Fig. 5-6).
   b. It is an accurate screening method to detect hearing loss (specificity is 96% for a score greater than 24).

Implications of Hearing Loss in the Elderly

1. Hearing loss results in interference with activities of daily living, reduced socialization, and decreased ability to live independently.
2. Misinterpretation of hearing loss as a cognitive, affective, or personality disorder is common.
3. Several studies suggest an increased prevalence of hearing impairment among patients with dementia.
   a. Seriously hearing-impaired persons have a greater chance of being demented.
   b. Current evidence is inconclusive that poor hearing is associated with cognitive decline in normal elderly persons.

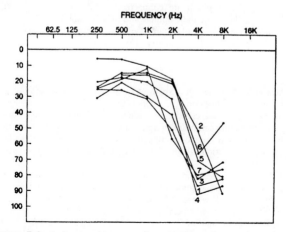

Figure 5-4 Audiogram of seven ears from six subjects showing abrupt sloping high-tone hearing losses. (From Goldstein J, Kashima H, Koopmann C (eds): *Geriatric Otorhinolaryngology.* Philadelphia, BC Decker, 1989.)

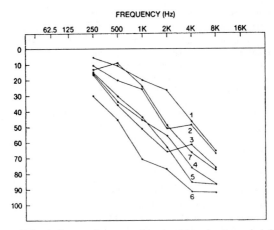

Figure 5-5 Audiogram of seven ears from six subjects showing gradual sloping high-tone hearing losses. (From Goldstein J, Kashima H, Koopmann C (eds): *Geriatric Otorhinolaryngology*. Philadelphia, BC Decker, 1989.)

Hearing Aids

1. Twenty percent of patients older than 80 use hearing aids.
2. Five major types of hearing aids.
   a. In-the-ear aids are the most popular type.
   b. Behind-the-ear aids are connected to the ear canal by flexible tubing. These are more durable and easier to adjust.
   c. In-the-canal aids are contained entirely within the ear canal.
   d. Eyeglass units (the popularity of these models has declined significantly).
   e. Aids worn on the body are usually reserved for more severe hearing loss.
3. Hearing aids can be very expensive (average price is over $500). Their purchase should be conditional on a 30-day trial.
   a. Hearing aids dispensed by an audiologist and purchased in a not-for-profit facility can result in significant cost savings to the consumer.
   b. Diagnostic testing for hearing aids is covered by Medicare, but hearing aid selection, fitting, dispensing, and follow-up are not covered services.
4. Patients should be informed of the limitations of hearing aids.
   a. Significant hearing improvement can be achieved if hearing loss is 55 to 80 dB, whereas if loss is greater than 80 dB, only limited improvement can be expected.
   b. Poor discrimination also limits usefulness of a hearing aid.
   c. Successful use of a hearing aid also depends on:
      (1) Hearing aid orientation by relistening and auditory-visual communication training.

	Yes (4)	Sometimes (2)	No (0)
1. Does a hearing problem cause you to feel embarrassed when meeting new people?	___	___	___
2. Does a hearing problem cause you to feel frustrated when talking to members of your family?	___	___	___
3. Do you have difficulty hearing when someone speaks in a whisper?	___	___	___
4. Do you feel handicapped by a hearing problem?	___	___	___
5. Does a hearing problem cause you difficulty when visiting friends, relatives, or neighbors?	___	___	___
6. Does a hearing problem cause you to attend religious services less often than you would like?	___	___	___
7. Does a hearing problem cause you to have arguments with family members?	___	___	___
8. Does a hearing problem cause you difficulty when listening to TV or radio?	___	___	___
9. Do you feel that any difficulty with your hearing limits or hampers your personal or social life?	___	___	___
10. Does a hearing problem cause you difficulty when in a restaurant with relatives or friends?	___	___	___

Figure 5-6 Hearing-handicap inventory for the elderly—screening version (HHIE-S). Range of total points: 0 to 40; 0 to 8: no self-perceived handicap; 10 to 22: mild to moderate handicap; 24 to 40: significant handicap. (From Ventry IM, Weinstein BE: ASHA 25:37-42, 1983. Reprinted with permission from American Speech-Language-Hearing Association. All rights reserved.)

(2) Counseling of the hearing-impaired and significant others.
5. Telephone, television, radio, and stereo amplifiers are useful to increase loudness of the signal.
   a. Telephone amplifiers.
      (1) These are usually available from the telephone company.
      (2) They can be built into the handset of the telephone, or they can be portable.
      (3) Telephone devices for the deaf and telephone caption units are also commonly available.
   b. Television, radio, or stereo amplifiers.
      (1) These may be connected directly to the audio input.
      (2) The listener may use standard headphones or pillow speakers.

VERTIGO

Fred F. Ferri, with revisions by Tom J. Wachtel

Definitions

1. Dizziness is a vague term used by patients to describe various sensations (e.g., vertigo, lightheadedness, unsteadiness, near syncope, malaise).
2. Lightheadedness is the sensation of faintness or giddiness. The patient does not have true vertigo but has a perception of difficulty maintaining balance.
3. Vertigo is the sensation of motion of either the patient with respect to the environment or vice versa. It is usually accompanied by symptoms of nausea, vomiting, nystagmus, and staggering.

Diagnostic Approach

1. Vertigo may be multifactorial. Examples include:
   a. Drug toxicity.
   b. Infection.
   c. Metabolic abnormalities.
   d. Nerve conduction abnormalities.
   e. Hypoxia.
   f. Mass effect.
2. The history should include the following:
   a. Drug and alcohol use.
   b. Past and current illnesses, including:
      (1) Diabetes.
      (2) CHF.
      (3) COPD.
      (4) Cerebrovascular accident.
   c. Duration and lateralization of symptoms, including provoking factors.
   d. History of trauma, hearing difficulty, head pain.
   e. Intermittent versus continuous symptoms.
3. Physical exam should focus on:
   a. Presence or absence of orthostatic changes in BP and pulse.
   b. Romberg and cerebellar evaluation.
   c. Examination for nystagmus. Provocative head movement tests (e.g., the Nylen–Bárány test or Dix–Hallpike maneuver) can be helpful for diagnosis.
      (1) The fast component of nystagmus is to the "good" ear.
      (2) The slow component is to the affected ear.
   d. Hearing testing and tuning fork (including Weber's and Rinne's tests).
4. Peripheral vertigo can be distinguished from central vertigo by observing nystagmus and which direction the patient tends to fall.
   a. Peripheral vertigo.
      (1) Nystagmus is accentuated by looking toward the unaffected ear and is improved by visual fixation.
      (2) The patient tends to fall away from the fast component of the nystagmus.
   b. Central vertigo.
      (1) Nystagmus is accentuated by looking toward the side of the lesion and is not improved by visual fixation.
      (2) The patient falls toward the fast component of the nystagmus.

5. Electronystagmography can measure nystagmus and distinguish peripheral from central vestibular lesions.

Diagnosis

1. Peripheral vertigo.
   a. Acute labyrinthitis.
      (1) Often follows a viral syndrome.
      (2) Symptoms.
         (a) Vertigo, nausea, and vomiting, with onset over several hours.
         (b) Symptoms usually peak within 24 hours, then resolve gradually over several weeks.
         (c) Tinnitus may be present.
         (d) During the first day, the patient usually has difficulty focusing the eyes because of spontaneous nystagmus.
         (e) Symptoms are exacerbated by head movement or position changes.
      (3) Physical exam.
         (a) Nystagmus, usually more prominent on looking toward the good ear.
         (b) Vertigo worsening with head movement.
         (c) Abnormal caloric tests.
         (d) Possible hearing loss in the affected ear.
         (e) Normal otoscopic examination typically.
         (f) Otherwise normal neurologic examination.
      (4) Prognosis.
         (a) Usually has a benign course, with complete recovery within 1 to 3 months.
         (b) Some older patients have chronic dizziness that persists for many months.
   b. Benign positional vertigo.
      (1) Brief (few seconds) episodes of vertigo occur on assumption of a particular head position.
      (2) No hearing loss is found, caloric testing is normal.
      (3) Disorder is usually self-limited but can last several months.
   c. Meniere's disease.
      (1) Classic triad of vertigo, tinnitus, and deafness is seen.
      (2) Hearing loss is initially fluctuating.
      (3) Vertigo usually lasts 1 or 2 hours.
   d. Vestibular neuronitis.
      (1) Duration of vertigo may be prolonged (several days).
      (2) Deafness or tinnitus is generally not present.
      (3) Symptoms are exacerbated by position changes and head movement.
      (4) Caloric testing reveals hypofunction of affected side.
      (5) May be a symptom of multiple sclerosis.
   e. Drug toxicity.
2. Central vertigo.
   a. Vertebrobasilar insufficiency.
   b. Acoustic neuroma.
      (1) Symptoms.
         (a) Unilateral hearing loss.

         (b) Tinnitus.
         (c) Dizziness.
      (2) Diagnosis.
         (a) Brainstem evoked response.
         (b) CT or MRI directed to cerebellopontine angle and internal auditory canals.
   c. Neoplasms of cerebellopontine angle (primary or metastatic).
   d. Cerebellar-brainstem hemorrhage/infarction.
   e. Basilar migraine: Vertigo associated with occipital headache, tinnitus, and visual disturbances.
   f. Other common causes of central vertigo in the elderly are alcohol and other drug toxicity, electrolyte abnormalities, and hyperventilation.

Treatment

1. Peripheral vertigo.
   a. Phenergan or other antiemetics are effective.
   b. Vestibular suppressant.
      (1) Meclizine 12.5 to 25 mg qid is often used.
      (2) Scopolamine patch is also effective.
      (3) Wean off vestibular suppressant therapy as soon as possible.
      (4) Caution should be used in the elderly because the risk of potential side effects (urinary retention, delirium, lethargy, falls) is higher in the geriatric population.
   c. Methylprednisolone 100 mg/day for 3 days, with slow taper over 3 weeks.
   d. Valacyclovir has not been shown to be helpful.
2. Benign positional vertigo: Treatment is symptomatic with meclizine prn.
3. Meniere's disease.
   a. Treatment includes sedatives, antiemetics, antihistamines, diuretics, and sodium restriction.
   b. Surgical intervention is controversial.
4. Vestibular neuronitis: Treatment is symptomatic.
5. Drug toxicity: Eliminate any suspected drugs.
6. Central vertigo.
   a. Acoustic neuroma: Surgical excision or palliative subtotal resection depending on the size of the tumor, severity of symptoms. and overall medical status of patient.
   b. Drug toxicity: Eliminate any suspected drugs.

SUGGESTED READINGS

Labriguen RH: Initial evaluation of vertigo. *Am Fam Physician* 73:244-251, 2006.
Strupp M, Zingler VC, Arbusow V, et al: Methylprednisolone, valacyclovir, or the combination for vestibular neuritis, *N Engl J Med* 351(4):354-361, 2004.

5.4 Ophthalmology

CATARACTS

Fred F. Ferri

Definition

1. Cataracts are an opacity in the lens of the eye, usually from denaturation of lens protein caused by aging.

2. The opacity can occur in the cortex, the nucleus of the lens, or the posterior subcapsular region, but usually it is in a combination of areas.

3. The major age-related changes in the eye are illustrated in Figure 5-7.

Prevalence

1. Some stage of cataract development is present in more than 50% of persons aged 65 to 74 years and in 65% to 70% of those older than 75 years.

2. Cataract removal is the most common surgical procedure in patients 65 years or older (1.3 million operations per year with an annual cost of approximately $3 billion).

Contributing Factors

1. Diabetes mellitus.
2. Ultraviolet B light (cortical cataract).
3. Systemic corticosteroids (posterior subcapsular cataract).
4. Familial incidence.
5. Prolonged glaucoma therapy with topical medications.
6. Ocular trauma.
7. Intraocular surgery.

Symptoms and Signs

1. The visual abnormalities caused by cataracts vary with the location and stage of the cataract (e.g., distance visual acuity is most significantly impaired by nuclear cataracts).

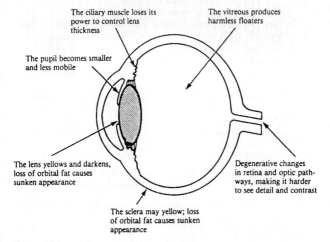

The ciliary muscle loses its power to control lens thickness

The vitreous produces harmless floaters

The pupil becomes smaller and less mobile

The lens yellows and darkens, loss of orbital fat causes sunken appearance

Degenerative changes in retina and optic pathways, making it harder to see detail and contrast

The sclera may yellow; loss of orbital fat causes sunken appearance

Figure 5-7   Aging changes of the eye. (From Bosker G, Schwartz GR, Jones JS, et al (eds): *Geriatric emergency medicine*. St Louis, Mosby, 1990.)

2. The sclerotic lens results in myopia, which temporarily corrects presbyopia, causing a misconception that eyesight is improving (e.g., patient may be able to read newspaper without glasses). This phenomenon is called "second sight."

Surgical Correction

1. Indications.
   a. Corrected visual acuity in the affected eye is greater than 20/50 in absence of other ocular disease.
   b. Surgery may be justified when visual acuity is 20/40 or better in specific situations (e.g., disabling glare, monocular diplopia).
2. In 90% of patients vision improves by two lines or more on a Snellen chart; mental status and timed performance of manual tasks also improve.
3. Cataract surgery is generally performed with the patient under local anesthesia on an outpatient basis. It can be accomplished by two methods.
   a. Extracapsular extraction (>95% of cataract operations).
      (1) Standard procedure.
          (a) The central portion of the anterior capsule is removed.
          (b) The contents of the lens are aspirated.
          (c) The posterior capsule of the lens is left behind and an intraocular lens (IOL) is implanted on or within the capsular bag.
      (2) Small-incision phacoemulsification is a newer technique that involves fragmenting the lens nucleus with ultrasonic vibrations and then aspirating the lens material.
      (3) Complications.
          (a) The most common complication of extracapsular extraction is late opacification of the posterior capsule, which occurs in 35% to 50% of patients over a 3-year postoperative period.
          (b) It manifests by gradual decline in visual acuity, usually 3 to 18 months after surgery.
          (c) Treatment consists of opening the posterior capsule using a Nd:YAG (neodymium:yttrium-aluminum-garnet) laser in the outpatient setting.
   b. Intracapsular extraction.
      (1) The entire cataract and surrounding capsule are removed in a single piece.
      (2) Because there is no posterior lens capsule to secure an implant, most surgeons use an anterior chamber implant.
      (3) Intracapsular extraction is rarely done in the United States and is usually reserved for cases of phacoanaphylaxis and subluxation of the lens.

SUGGESTED READINGS

Congdon N, Vingerling JR, Klein BE, et al: Prevalence of cataract and pseudophakia/aphakia among adults in the United States. Arch Ophthalmol 122(4):487-494, 2004.

Consultation section: Cataract surgical problem. J Cataract Refract Surg 28:577-588, 2002.

Solomon R, Donnenfeld ED: Recent advances and future frontiers in treating age-related cataracts, JAMA 290:248-251, 2003.

Wong TY, Klein BE, Klein R, Tomany SC: Relation of ocular trauma to cortical, nuclear and posterior subcapsular cataracts, Br J Ophthalmol 86:152-155, 2002.

GLAUCOMA

Fred F. Ferri

Definitions

1. Glaucoma is a group of disorders characterized by increased intraocular pressure that can lead to cupping and atrophy of the optic nerve head with visual field loss.
2. Glaucoma can be primary or secondary.
   a. Primary glaucoma can be subdivided into open-angle (90%) and angle-closure (10%) types.
   b. Secondary glaucoma is due to processes that anatomically or functionally block the outflow channels (e.g., trauma, diabetes, occlusion of the central retinal vein, uveitis, ocular tumors, cataract extraction).

Prevalence

1. Glaucoma increases with age and is more common in men than women.
2. Can be found in 2% of the population older than 40 years and in 5% to 10% of elderly persons in the eighth decade of life.
3. Ten percent of all blindness in the United States is due to glaucoma.
4. It is the second leading cause of blindness in the United States and the leading cause of blindness in African Americans.

Open-Angle Glaucoma

1. Etiology and diagnosis.
   a. Examination of the affected eyes reveals:
      (1) An increase in intraocular pressure.
      (2) Anatomically normal anterior chamber angle (as determined by gonioscopy).
      (3) Cupping of the optic nerve.
      (4) Visual field defects.
   b. The block to the outflow of the aqueous humor in the drainage channels (trabecular meshwork) is poorly understood.
   c. The visual loss is of insidious onset, slowly progressive, and asymptomatic until very late. Most people are not aware that there is a problem until the disease is far advanced, hence the importance of regular eye care for the elderly.
   d. The visual loss involves the peripheral field initially, followed by loss of central visual acuity in late stages.
2. Medical therapy.
   a. Ophthalmic β-blockers (e.g., timolol, levobunolol, betaxolol).
      (1) Mechanism of action: Suppression of production of aqueous humor in the eye.
      (2) Systemic side effects.
         (a) Bronchospasm.
         (b) Bradycardia.
         (c) CHF.
   b. Systemic inhibitors of carbonic anhydrase (e.g., acetazolamide).
      (1) Mechanism of action: Decreased production of aqueous humor.
      (2) Systemic side effects.
         (a) Paresthesias.
         (b) Anorexia.

        (c) Nausea and fatigue.
        (d) Metabolic acidosis.
        (e) Renal calculi.
        (f) Bone marrow suppression.
        (g) Cutaneous reactions.
  c. Ophthalmic miotics (e.g., pilocarpine, carbachol).
    (1) Mechanism of action.
        (a) Pupillary constriction.
        (b) Stimulation of muscle fibers of the ciliary body.
        (c) Improvement of flow through the trabecular meshwork.
    (2) Systemic side effects.
        (a) Headache.
        (b) Nausea.
        (c) Bronchospasm.
        (d) Increased salivation.
        (e) Increased perspiration.
  d. Ophthalmic adrenergics (e.g., epinephrine).
    (1) Mechanism of action.
        (a) Decreased production of aqueous humor.
        (b) Increased flow through trabecular meshwork.
    (2) Systemic side effects.
        (a) Hypertension.
        (b) Tachycardia.
        (c) Dysrhythmias.
        (d) Anxiety.
        (e) Headaches.
3. Surgical therapy.
  a. Argon laser trabeculoplasty.
    (1) This is the therapeutic step most commonly used after failure of medical therapy.
    (2) It improves drainage of aqueous humor from the eye by using laser burns to create openings on or next to the trabecular meshwork.
  b. Conventional surgery.
    (a) A fistula is created between the anterior chamber and the subconjunctival space, allowing passage of the aqueous humor.
    (b) The fistula is sometimes augmented by silicone implants.

Angle-Closure Glaucoma

1. Etiology and diagnosis.
  a. Results from forward displacement of the iris against the cornea, closing the chamber angle and blocking flow of aqueous humor out of the eye.
  b. Clinical presentation can be dramatic, with redness and pain in or about the eye associated with abrupt onset of blurred vision.
  c. Patient may see rainbow-colored haloes around lights, followed by a dramatic loss of vision in the involved eye.
  d. Systemic symptoms of nausea, vomiting, and abdominal pain can accompany acute angle-closure glaucoma.
  e. Examination of the eye reveals tenderness and firmness of the affected globe, increased intraocular pressure, and fixed, semidilated pupil.

2. Therapy.
   a. Medication.
      (1) Immediate and frequent instillation of miotics.
      (2) Parenteral or oral administration of acetazolamide or hyperosmotics (glycerol, mannitol).
   b. Definitive treatment is laser iridotomy, allowing free flow of aqueous humor.

SUGGESTED READINGS

Foster PJ, Aung T, Nolan WP, et al: Defining "occludable" angles in population surveys: Drainage angle width, peripheral anterior synechiae, and glaucomatous optic neuropathy in East Asian people. *Br J Ophthalmol* 88(4):486-490, 2004.

Fraser S, Bunce C, Wormald R, Brunner E: Deprivation and late presentation of glaucoma: Case control study. *BMJ* 322:639-643, 2001.

Gazzard G, Foster PJ, Devereux JG, et al: Intraocular pressure and visual field loss in primary angle closure and primary open angle glaucomas. *Br J Ophthalmol* 87(6):720-725, 2003.

Gordon MO et al: The Ocular Hypertension Treatment Study: Baseline factors that predict the onset of primary open-angle glaucoma. *Arch Ophthalmol* 120:714-720, 2002.

Heijl A, Leske MC, Bengtsson B, et al: Reduction of intraocular pressure and glaucoma progression: Results from the Early Manifest Glaucoma Trial. *Arch Ophthalmol* 120:1268-1279, 2002.

Higginbotham EJ et al: The Ocular Hypertension Treatment Study: Topical medication delays or prevents primary open-angle glaucoma in African American individuals. *Arch Ophthalmol* 122(6):813-820, 2004.

Kapur SB: The lens and angle-closure glaucoma. *J Cataract Refract Surg* 27(2): 176-177, 2001.

Lam DS, Tham CC, Chiu T, et al: Angle-closure glaucoma. *Ophthalmology* 109:1-2, 2002.

Rezaie T, Child A, Hitchings R, et al: Adult-onset primary open-angle glaucoma caused by mutations in optineurin, *Science* 295:1077-1079, 2002.

LOSS OF VISION

Michael D. Stein

Overview

1. Acute loss of vision is a medical emergency.
2. Gradual loss is more commonly encountered in the primary care setting.

History

Ask about:
1. Onset.
2. Eye pain.
3. Unilateral or bilateral symptoms.
4. Scotomas (blurred or partially blind areas).
5. Other medical conditions (diabetes mellitus, multiple sclerosis).
6. Trauma.
7. Headache, jaw claudication, temporal or scalp pain (temporal arteritis).

Examination

1. Inspect eyes, including conjunctiva, cornea, and sclera.
2. Check pupillary reflex to determine if there is an afferent defect (no response to direct light), which suggests optic neuritis or acute angle-closure glaucoma.

3. Check confrontation visual field for defects.
4. Perform funduscopic examination.

Differential Diagnosis

1. Sudden loss.
   a. Vitreous hemorrhage (often caused by diabetes mellitus).
   b. Vascular occlusion of retina.
   c. Acute angle-closure glaucoma.
   d. Optic neuritis (inflammatory, multiple sclerosis).
   e. Amaurosis fugax (carotid ischemia).
   f. Hysteria.
   g. Occipital infarct (can cause bilateral blindness, homonymous hemianopia).
2. Gradual loss.
   a. Presbyopia (corrects with refraction).
   b. Chronic or open-angle glaucoma.
   c. Cataract.
   d. Macular degeneration.
   e. Diabetic retinopathy.
   f. Corneal degeneration.
   g. Corneal opacity.

Treatment

1. Depends on the diagnosis.
2. Referral to an ophthalmologist is often recommended.

MACULAR DEGENERATION

Fred F. Ferri

Prevalence

1. Affects nearly 30% of the geriatric population (women > men).
2. Most common cause of legal blindness (visual acuity 20/200 or less).

Etiology

1. Exact etiology is unknown.
2. Vascular.
   a. The macular area of the retina depends on the choroidal capillaries for nutrition.
   b. It is believed that a disruption of the vascular supply to the macula results in changes in the retinal pigmented epithelium (RPE).
      (1) Separation of the RPE–sensory retina interface.
      (2) Subsequent death of cone photoreceptor cells in the macula and loss of central vision.
3. Hyaline deposits (drusen) can accumulate beneath the RPE and are visible as yellow-white pinhead-sized lesions on ophthalmologic exam.
4. Leakage or bleeding from retinal neovascularization (choroidal neovascular membranes) can result in further damage to the RPE–sensory retina interface.
5. Possible factors may be ultraviolet light and retinal adsorption.

Signs and Symptoms

1. Painless progressive loss of central vision with complaint of difficulty reading.

2. Peripheral vision is unaffected.
3. Therefore, total blindness does not occur.

Clinical Classification and Therapy

1. Nonexudative (dry type).
   a. Much more common (90% of cases) than exudative type.
   b. Generally less severe (usual visual acuity reduction to 20/50 to 20/100) than exudative type.
   c. Ophthalmoscopic exam might reveal drusen and areas of depigmentation alternating with zones of hyperpigmentation.
   d. No specific therapy is available for this type of macular degeneration. Ocuvite with zinc antioxidants may be useful.
2. Exudative (wet type).
   a. Responsible for 10% of cases of age-related macular degeneration.
   b. Results in much more severe loss of visual acuity than the dry type. It causes 90% of cases of legal blindness from macular degeneration.
   c. Ophthalmoscopic exam might reveal a detachment of the sensory retina in the macular area.
   d. Fluorescein angiography can identify hemorrhagic areas.
   e. Therapy with laser photocoagulation may be useful in some patients with focal areas of neovascularization.
   f. Patients with exudative macular degeneration are monitored on a regular basis with self-testing using an Amster grid to detect early distortion in central vision (curvy appearance of the lines or missing squares), which indicates hemorrhage and/or retinal detachment (Fig. 5-8).

SUGGESTED READINGS

Friedman DS, O'Colmain BJ, Munoz B, et al: Prevalence of age-related macular degeneration in the United States. *Arch Ophthalmol* 122(4):564-572, 2004.

Gottlieb JL: Age-related macular degeneration. *JAMA* 288:2233-2236, 2002.

Jonas JB: Verteporfin therapy of subfoveal choroidal neovascularization in age-related macular degeneration. *Am J Ophthalmol* 133(6):857-859, 2002.

Liu M, Regillo CD: A review of treatments for macular degeneration: A synopsis of currently approved treatments and ongoing clinical trials. *Curr Opin Ophthalmol* 15(3):221-226, 2004.

Mackenzie PJ, Chang TS, Scott IU, et al: Assessment of vision-related function in patients with age-related macular degeneration. *Ophthalmology* 109(4):720-729, 2002.

Ting TD, Oh M, Cox TA, et al: Decreased visual acuity associated with cystoid macular edema in neovascular or age-related macular degeneration. *Arch Ophthalmol* 120(6):731-737, 2002.

5.5 Rheumatology

ARTHRITIS

Tom J. Wachtel

Definition

Arthritis specifically refers to an inflammatory or a degenerative process in a joint.

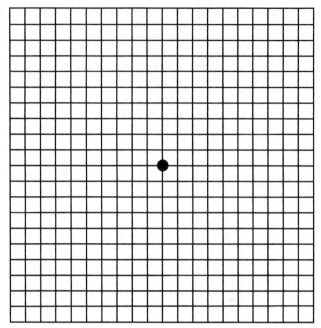

Figure 5-8   Amsler grid. The patient examines the Amsler grid with each eye (patients who wear glasses keep their glasses on for this test). The grid is placed on wall or desk at comfortable distance normally used for reading. (From Yoshikawa TT, Cobbs EL, Brummel-Smith K [eds]: *Ambulatory geriatric care.* St Louis, Mosby, 1993.)

Overview

1. Musculoskeletal complaints are among the most common reasons for patients to seek medical attention.
2. Laypersons often use the term *arthritis* to describe a wide variety of painful experiences involving the musculoskeletal system.
3. Differential diagnosis.
   a. Arthritis may be mimicked by:
      (1) Bursitis.
      (2) Tendinitis.
      (3) Bone pathologic conditions.
      (4) Cellulitis.
      (5) Phlebitis.
      (6) Myalgia.
      (7) Neuralgia.
      (8) Ischemia.
   b. History and physical exam should always include a complete assessment of any painful limb to ascertain the integrity of the vascular

system, nervous system, bones, muscles, and other soft tissue structures of the relevant limb.

c. Once the physician is convinced that the complaint is generated by arthritis, the next step is to differentiate between inflammatory and noninflammatory arthritis. This can be done by looking for the classic signs of inflammation (rubor, calor, tumor, dolor) and asking the patient about the pattern of pain.

(1) Inflammatory arthritis.
  (a) Made worse by rest and improved by exercise.
  (b) Morning stiffness has a 1- to 2-hour loosening-up period.
  (c) Tends to be acute or subacute.
(2) Degenerative arthritis.
  (a) Worsened by exercise.
  (b) Morning stiffness lasts only 10 to 15 minutes.
  (c) Tends to be chronic.

Monoarticular Arthritis

Diagnosis

1. Acute inflammatory arthritis.
   a. The first step in evaluating monoarticular arthritis is to determine whether signs of acute inflammation (pain, swelling, erythema, heat, and loss of function) are present.
   b. The key test is arthrocentesis with joint fluid examination for cell count and differential, Gram stain, culture and sensitivity, and a search for crystals (under polarized light).
2. Noninflammatory arthritis.
   a. Noninflammatory monoarticular arthritis can occur as a result of recent trauma; usually the patient gives a history of the traumatic event.
   b. Monoarticular osteoarthritis can affect a joint that is subject to repeated microtrauma (occupation or sport), a congenitally abnormal joint, or a joint previously damaged by trauma or infection.
   c. Neoplastic disorders (e.g., synovial sarcoma or pigmented villonodular synovitis) can mimic monoarticular arthritis with or without signs of inflammation. A biopsy is required for diagnosis.

Differential Diagnosis

1. Infectious arthritis.
   a. Bacterial.
      (1) Nongonococcal.
         (a) *Staphylococcus aureus* (60%).
         (b) Non–group A β-hemolytic streptococci (15%).
         (c) Gram-negative pathogens (18%).
      (2) Gonococcal.
   b. Lyme disease.
      (1) Large joints.
      (2) Intermittent swelling more than pain.
   c. Viral.
      (1) HIV.
      (2) Hepatitis B.
   d. Mycobacterial: Evidence of pulmonary tuberculosis is present in only 50% of patients with mycobacterial infection.

2. Crystal-induced arthritis.
   a. Gout (urate).
   b. Pseudogout (calcium pyrophosphate).
   c. Hydroxyapatite arthropathy.
   d. Calcium oxalate arthropathy.
3. Trauma.
   a. Fracture.
   b. Hemarthrosis (acquired or congenital clotting disorders).
4. Osteoarthritis.
   a. Chronic.
   b. Made worse after overuse or minor trauma.
5. Systemic diseases.
   a. Rheumatoid arthritis.
   b. SLE.
   c. Inflammatory bowel disease.
   d. Reiter's syndrome.
   e. Psoriasis.

Work-up

1. Lab tests.
   a. CBC and cultures of blood, skin lesions, cervix, urethra, and urine are important if infectious arthritis is suspected.
   b. Serum uric acid levels can be misleading and may be consistently normal even with gout.
   c. Arthrocentesis should be performed in nearly every patient, particularly if infection is suspected. Synovial fluid should be examined for:
      (1) Total leukocyte count and differential.
      (2) Gram stain and culture.
      (3) Crystal examination.
      (4) Interpretation.
         (a) Normal synovial fluid contains <180 cells/mL.
         (b) Most patients with osteoarthritis have <500 cells/mL.
         (c) As the leukocyte count increases, so does the possibility of infection, especially with more than 50,000 cells/mL.
         (d) More than 90% polymorphonuclear neutrophil leukocytes (PMNs) suggests infection or crystals.
         (e) Cultures are positive in only 25% of patients with gonococcal arthritis.
2. Radiology.
   a. X-ray studies are usually not helpful.
      (1) Fractures, tumors and chronic osteoarthritis can be discerned.
      (2) Chondrocalcinosis may be seen with pseudogout.
   b. MRI can help with sacroiliac involvement, meniscal tears, and ligament damage.

Treatment

1. Acute monoarticular inflammatory arthritis is a medical emergency because septic arthritis must be treated immediately if present.
2. Septic and crystalline arthritides are very painful, and treatment should begin as soon as possible.

Septic Arthritis

Diagnosis

1. Septic arthritis.
   a. Septic arthritis is characterized by a cell count greater than 50,000 with more than 90% PMNs.
   b. Previously injured joints are more susceptible to infection; therefore, a patient with underlying rheumatoid arthritis who presents with fever, chills, and flare-up in a single joint should be evaluated in the same manner.
   c. The most common organism is *Staphylococcus aureus*, but any pathogenic bacterium may be encountered.
2. Gonococcal arthritis.
   a. Disseminated gonococcemia, rare in the elderly, can affect joints and/or the skin.
   b. When arthralgia is present, examination of the joint can simply reveal tenosynovitis or an effusion. Effusion, if present, should be tapped.
   c. Both the Gram stain and culture may be falsely negative in gonococcal arthritis; therefore, empirical treatment is indicated if the index of suspicion is high (unusual in geriatrics).

Treatment

1. Empirical antibiotic therapy is required until cultures are completed if the synovial fluid Gram stain is negative.
2. Normal hosts should be treated for gram-positive organisms (e.g., *Staphylococcus aureus*).
3. Daily closed drainage is mandatory for patients with septic arthritis.
4. The joint should be immobilized as long as joint fluid reaccumulates.
5. Arthroscopic or open drainage should be considered if the response to antibiotics is slow.

Crystalline Arthritis

Diagnosis

1. Differential.
   a. Crystalline arthritis is characterized by fewer cells per milliliter (5000 to 20,000) with a predominance of PMNs.
   b. The shape and polarizing characteristics of the crystals make the diagnosis of gout or pseudogout.
   c. Tapping the first metatarsophalangeal joint in podagra may be difficult or refused by the patient.
   d. If the diagnosis of gout versus pseudogout is uncertain, the patient should be treated with indomethacin, an adequate treatment for either condition.
2. Acute gout (see later section "Gout").
3. Joint diseases caused by other chemical species of crystals.
   a. Calcium pyrophosphate deposition disease (pseudogout).
      (1) Joints involved.
         (a) Knees.
         (b) Wrists.
      (2) Crystal characteristics.
         (a) Rhomboid or polymorphic-shaped.

(b) Weakly positive.
(c) Birefringent.
(3) Treatment.
(a) NSAIDs.
(b) Joint immobilization.
(c) Intraarticular steroids.
b. Hydroxyapatite arthropathy.
(1) Joints involved.
(a) Knees.
(b) Hips.
(c) Shoulders.
(2) Crystal characteristics.
(a) Crystals form nonbirefringent clumps with synovial fluid when placed on slide.
(b) Diagnosis often requires electron microscopy because the crystals are small.
(3) Treatment.
(a) NSAIDs.
(b) Joint immobilization.
(c) Intraarticular steroids.
c. Calcium oxalate–induced arthritis.
(1) Joints involved.
(a) Distal interphalangeal (DIP) joints of hands.
(b) Proximal interphalangeal (PIP) joints of hands.
(2) Crystal characteristics.
(a) Bipyramidal shaped.
(b) Positive.
(c) Birefringent.
(3) Treatment.
(a) NSAIDs.
(b) Joint immobilization.
(c) Intraarticular steroids.
d. Steroids can crystallize following an intraarticular injection and provoke an inflammatory response.

Polyarticular Arthritis
Inflammatory Polyarticular Arthritides
1. Evaluation.
   a. The evaluation of inflammatory arthritis varies with the acuteness of the disease. The history can provide some clues, but the help of the laboratory may be needed when the symptoms do not resolve rapidly or blossom into a readily recognized clinical entity.
   b. Rheumatoid arthritis is the prototype of chronic inflammatory arthritides.
      (1) The prevalence is 3% in female patients and 1% in male patients.
      (2) The course and prognosis vary in severity; spontaneous long-term remissions can occur, but the disease should be considered incurable.
2. Differential diagnosis.
   a. Acute arthritis.

(1) Rheumatic fever (rare in adults, exceptional in geriatric patients).
  (a) Recent strep throat.
  (b) Antistreptolysin titer greater than 200 Todd units.
  (c) Involvement of lower extremity joints.
(2) Serum sickness.
  (a) Recent administration of a drug.
  (b) Rash.
(3) Prodrome of hepatitis: Liver function tests and hepatitis serology.
(4) Lyme arthritis.
  (a) Recent tick bite.
  (b) Characteristic rash may be absent.
(5) Onset of rheumatoid arthritis.
(6) Infectious enterocolitis.
b. Chronic arthritis.
(1) Rheumatoid arthritis (see "Rheumatoid arthritis" later).
(2) Rheumatoid variants.
  (a) Still's disease.
  (b) Sjögren's syndrome.
  (c) Inflammatory bowel disease.
  (d) Psoriatic arthritis.
  (e) Reiter's disease.
(3) Connective tissue disease (e.g., lupus, scleroderma).
(4) Sarcoidosis.
(5) Amyloidosis.
(6) Behçet's syndrome.
(7) Whipple's disease.

Osteoarthritis

1. Definition.
   a. Osteoarthritis is a noninflammatory disorder of movable joints.
   b. It is characterized by deterioration and abrasion of articular cartilage and by formation of new bone on the surfaces of the joints.
2. Diagnosis.
   a. The diagnosis of degenerative joint disease is generally easy.
   b. The disease affects mostly the weight-bearing joints (knees, hips, lumbosacral and cervical spine), DIP joints, and carpometacarpal joints.
   c. Symptoms are mostly pain and limitation of function, confirmed on examination by decreased range of motion.
   d. Unfortunately, symptoms (occurring in 20% of the U.S. adult population) correlate poorly with radiographic evidence of osteoarthritis (present in 80% of patients aged 80 years or older).
3. Clinical manifestations and management: See "Osteoarthritis" later.

BURSITIS, TENDINITIS, AND SELECTED SOFT TISSUE SYNDROMES

Tom J. Wachtel

Definitions

1. A *bursa* is a sac lined with synovial membrane that secretes synovial fluid, which acts as lubricant between moving structures (e.g., tendons ligaments, bones).

2. *Bursitis* is inflammation of a bursa.
3. *Tendon* is the noncontractile portion of a muscle; it usually inserts on bone.
4. *Tendinitis* is inflammation of a tendon.
5. *Capsule* is the fibrous tissue that holds a joint together.
6. *Ligament* is a reinforced component of a capsule.

Bursitis and Tendinitis

1. Sometimes specific involvement of a bursa or tendon produces a classic bursitis or tendinitis syndrome (see examples later). More commonly, the distinction between tendinitis and bursitis is tentative at best.
2. The etiology of both conditions is the same, for example, repetitive microtrauma or mechanical stresses to the structure associated with the patient's occupation or leisure activities.
3. Osteoarthritis and other chronic arthritic conditions predispose patients to the periarticular syndromes that can account for symptoms misinterpreted as a flare-up of the underlying arthritic disease.
   a. Rarely, bursitis or tendinitis is associated with rheumatologic conditions such as rheumatoid arthritis and variants, crystalline arthritis, or infection.

Differential Diagnosis

The presence of known degenerative joint disease does not make the diagnosis of tendinitis or bursitis less likely. Common examples of tendinitis, bursitis, and related syndromes are listed in Table 5-21.

1. Degenerative joint disease.
2. Cellulitis (if bursitis is septic).
3. Infectious arthritis.

Treatment

1. Discontinue the causing activity; rest.
2. Cold compresses early to provide analgesia and reduce swelling; heat application may be helpful during the recovery phase.
3. NSAIDs for 2 weeks.
4. Failure to respond to this treatment is best approached with needle aspiration (in bursitis) and injection of corticosteroid/local anesthetic solutions (e.g., 20 to 40 mg prednisolone or triamcinolone with 2 or 3 mL of 1% to 2% xylocaine) inside the bursa in bursitis or in the tendon sheath at the tendon insertion (trigger point) in tendinitis.
5. Exercise.
   a. Mobilization should begin as soon as the inflammation (i.e., pain) has subsided, beginning with passive range of motion and stretching and progressing to active movements.
   b. Heat application should be recommended especially before exercises.
   c. Exercise performed alone or in physical therapy is excessive if any induced pain persists for longer than 30 minutes following completion.
6. Occasionally, refractory bursitis needs aspiration if excessive fluid volume is present, followed by application of a compression dressing to

Table 5-21 Common Examples of Tendinitis, Bursitis, and Related Syndromes

Bursitis or Tendinitis	Area of Tenderness	Reproducing Syndromes
Shoulder		
Supraspinatus tendinitis	Posterolateral humeral head below acromion	Abduction External rotation
Bicipital tendinitis	Upper medial humerus	Forceful supination with elbow held in flexion
Adhesive capsulitis (frozen shoulder)	Variable	Progressive limitation of all shoulder movements
Elbow		
Tennis elbow	Lateral epicondyle wrist extensor tendon	Forceful extension of wrist and fingers
Olecranon bursitis	Posterior point of elbow	Full elbow flexion
Hip		
Weavers' bursitis	Ischial tuberosities	Sitting on hard surfaces
Trochanteric bursitis	Greater trochanter	External rotation
Knee		
Anserine bursitis	Medial proximal tibia	Ascending and descending stairs
Iliotibial band syndrome	Lateral distal femur	Repetitive knee flexion and extension (running)
Prepatellar bursitis	Anterior knee	Flexion of knee
Foot		
Heel spur or plantar fasciitis	Achilles tendon	Walking or running

prevent fluid reaccumulation (repeat aspiration may be required). Most bursal sacs dry up eventually.
7. Treatment of septic bursitis.
   a. Appropriate antibiotic coverage and drainage.
   b. Aspiration of purulent fluid with a large-bore needle. If there is no rapid clinical response, incision and drainage are indicated.

Other Soft Tissue Syndromes

1. Stenosing tenosynovitis.
   a. Restriction of tendon movement by a fibrotic nodule on the tendon and/or stenosis of a tendon sheath.
   b. Examples.
      (1) Trigger finger.
      (2) De Quervain's disease of the thumb abductor longis and extensor brevis.
   c. Treatment is the same as for tendinitis.
2. Nerve entrapment syndromes.
   a. Mononeuropathy caused by fibrous tissue compression and resulting nerve degeneration.
   b. Example is carpal tunnel syndrome.
   c. Treatment.
      (1) Wrist splint.
      (2) NSAIDs.
      (3) Local steroid injections.
      (4) Surgical decompression.
3. Reflex sympathetic dystrophy (causalgia or regional pain syndrome).
   a. Unexplained pain and swelling of an extremity sometimes associated with trauma, myocardial infarction, or stroke. Focal osteoporosis, muscular atrophy, and rarely contractures of the involved extremity can occur.
   b. Work-up.
      (1) X-ray might show patchy osteoporosis only in the affected limb.
      (2) Bone scan might light up in a periarticular distribution.
   c. Treatment.
      (1) Analgesics, β-blockers, CCBs, gabapentin.
      (2) Oral corticosteroids.
      (3) Nerve or stellate ganglion block.
      (4) Gradual physical therapy.
4. Thoracic outlet syndrome.
   a. Subclavian artery and/or nerve compression by a cervical rib or by scalene muscles causing symptoms of arterial insufficiency and/or neuropathy.
   b. Treatment is surgical decompression when symptoms are severe.
5. Raynaud's syndrome.
   a. Upper extremity vasomotor phenomenon often triggered by cold exposure and resulting in the following clinical temporal sequence:
      (1) Hand pallor.
      (2) Hand cyanosis.
      (3) Erythema and pain caused by hyperemia.
   b. Most cases are idiopathic, but the syndrome may be associated with a collagen vascular disease (scleroderma).

   c. Treatment.
      (1) Avoid precipitating factors (e.g., cold).
      (2) CCBs, except in scleroderma.
6. Dupuytren's contracture.
   a. Idiopathic hypertrophic fibrosis of the palmar fascia progressing over several years and resulting in a painless flexion contracture of the involved hand.
   b. It is often bilateral, may be hereditary, and is more common in alcoholics.
   c. Treatment is surgery.

SUGGESTED READINGS

Barr KP: Rotator cuff disease. *Phys Med Rehabil Clin N Am* 15:475-491, 2004.

Cole CC, Seto C, Gazewood J: Plantar fasciitis: Evidence-based review of diagnosis and therapy. *Am Fam Physician* 72:2237-2242, 2005.

Dawson DM: Entrapment neuropathies of the upper extremities. *N Engl J Med* 329:2013-2018, 1993.

Fireman HH: Don't forget anserine bursitis. *CMAJ* 165:1300, 2001.

Gnanadesigan N, Smith RL: Knee pain: Osteoarthritis or anserine bursitis? *J Am Med Dir Assoc* 4:164-166, 2003.

Mehta S, Gimbel JA, Soslowsky LJ: Etiologic and pathogenetic factors for rotator cuff tendinopathy. *Clin Sports Med* 22:791-812, 2003.

Raja SN, Grabow TS: Complex region pain syndrome 1 (reflex sympathetic dystrophy). *Anesthesiology* 96:1254-1260, 2002.

Schwartzman RJ: New treatments for reflex sympathetic dystrophy. *N Engl J Med* 343:654-656, 2000.

Stevens JC, Beard CM, O'Fallon WM, Kurland LT: Conditions associated with carpal tunnel syndrome. *Mayo Clin Proc* 67:541-548, 1992.

Tortolani PJ, Carbone JJ, Quartararo LG: Greater trochanteric pain syndrome in patients referred to orthopedic spine specialists. *Spine* 2:251-254, 2002.

Van Mieghem IM, Boets A, Sciot R, Van Brueseghem I: Ischiogluteal bursitis: An uncommon type of bursitis. *Skeletal Radiol* 33:413-436, 2004.

Veldman PH, Reynen HM, Arntz IE, Goris RJ: Signs and symptoms of reflex sympathetic dystrophy: Prospective study of 829 patients, *Lancet* 342:1012-1016, 1993.

Webner D, Drezner JA: Lesser trochanteric bursitis: A rare cause of anterior hip pain. *Clin J Sport Med* 14:242-244, 2004.

Wilson JJ, Best TM: Common overuse tendon problem: A review and recommendations for treatment. *Am Fam Physician* 72:811-818, 2005.

GOUT

Lonnie R. Mercier

Definitions

1. Gout is a clinical disorder in which crystals of monosodium urate become deposited in tissue as a result of hyperuricemia.
2. Gout and hyperuricemia can be classified as either primary or secondary if they result from another disorder.

Epidemiology

1. Prevalence: 3 cases/1000 persons.
2. Predominant sex: 95% male; gout is rare in women before menopause.

Clinical Findings

1. Usually, the initial attack is in a single joint or an area of tenosynovium.
2. Gout is mainly a disease of the lower extremities.

a. The first site of involvement, classically, is the metacarpophalangeal joint of the great toe (podagra).

b. Another common site of acute attack is the extensor tenosynovium on the dorsum of the midfoot.

3. Severe pain and inflammation may be precipitated by exercise, dietary indiscretions, and physical or emotional stress.

4. Attacks can occur following illness or surgery.

5. Signs and symptoms.

a. Swelling, heat, redness, and other signs of inflammation (the physical findings simulating cellulitis).

b. Exquisite soft tissue tenderness.

c. Fever, tachycardia, and other constitutional symptoms.

d. Eventually, deposits of urate crystals (tophi) in the subcutaneous tissue.

Etiology

1. Hyperuricemia and gout develop from excessive uric acid production, a decrease in the renal excretion of uric acid, or (rarely) both.

2. Primary gout results from an inborn error of metabolism and may be attributed to several biochemical defects.

3. Secondary hyperuricemia can develop as a complication of acquired disorders (e.g., leukemia) or as a result of the use of certain drugs (e.g., diuretics).

Differential Diagnosis

1. Pseudogout.

2. Rheumatoid arthritis and other monoarticular flare-up of inflammatory polyarticular diseases (e.g., SLE, psoriatic arthritis).

3. Osteoarthritis.

4. Cellulitis.

5. Infectious arthritis including Lyme arthritis.

6. Hemarthrosis.

Work-up

1. Mild leukocytosis.

2. Elevated ESR.

3. Hyperuricemia is the rule but may be absent.

4. Synovial aspirate.

a. Usually cloudy and markedly inflammatory.

b. Urate crystals in fluid are needle-shaped and birefringent under polarized light.

5. X-rays are not typically helpful in early gouty arthritis but can reveal characteristic punched-out lesions and joint destruction in late disease.

Treatment

Treatments for gout are shown in Box 5-3.

1. Acute treatment.

a. NSAIDs such as ibuprofen are the preferred treatment in the absence of contraindications.

b. Colchicine given PO or IV.

c. Corticosteroids or adrenocorticotropic hormone (ACTH) for those who are intolerant of NSAIDs or colchicine.

BOX 5-3   Treatment of Gout

Acute Gout

THERAPEUTIC GOAL
Terminate acute inflammatory attack.

PHARMACOLOGIC THERAPY
NSAIDs (preferred): Indomethacin, 50 mg qid, or ibuprofen, 800 mg tid (or other NSAIDs in full doses) (lower dose in renal insufficiency; contraindicated with PUD).

or

Colchicine, oral (used infrequently): 0.6-1.2 mg (1-2 tablets), then 0.6 mg (1 tablet) q1-2h until attack subsides or until nausea, diarrhea, or GI cramping develops. Maximum total dose, 4-6 mg. If ineffective in 48 h, do not repeat.

Colchicine, IV (only if oral medication is precluded): 1-2 mg in 20 mL 0.9% saline infused slowly (extravasation causes tissue necrosis); dose may be repeated once in 6 h. Few GI symptoms with IV use. Maximum total dose, 4 mg per attack. Monitor blood counts.

Steroids (if NSAIDs or colchicines are contraindicated or if oral medication is precluded, e.g., postoperatively): Triamcinolone acetonide, 60 mg IM, or ACTH, 40 U IM or 25 U by slow IV infusion, or prednisone, 20-40 mg daily. Intra-articular steroids may be used to treat a single inflamed joint: triamcinolone hexacetonide, 5-20 mg, or dexamethasone phosphate, 1-6 mg.

Hypouricemic agents: Of no benefit for inflammatory attack and can initiate recurrent attack. Should not be started until attack has resolved, but ongoing use should not be interrupted during an attack.

Long-Term Treatment

THERAPEUTIC GOAL
Prevent attacks, resolve tophi, maintain serum urate at ≤6 mg/dL.

PHARMACOLOGIC THERAPY
Colchicine, oral: 0.6-1.2 mg daily for 1-2 wk before initiating hypouricemic therapy and for several months afterward to prevent recurrent attacks during the initial period of hypouricemic therapy.

Allopurinol: Dose is variable; usually 300 mg qd, but up to 900 mg may be needed in occasional patient. Dose should be reduced to 100 mg daily or every other day in patients with renal insufficiency.

or

Uricosuric agent (reduced efficacy if creatinine clearance <80 mL; ineffective if <30 mL): Probenecid 0.5-1 g bid, or sulfinpyrazone 100 mg tid or qid. Usually well tolerated, but can cause headache, GI upset, rash.

Continued

BOX 5-3   Treatment of Gout—cont'd

OTHER THERAPY

Diet: moderate protein, low fat, avoid excessive alcohol.

Treat hypertension if present.

For uric acid overexcretors or when initiating uricosuric agent: high fluid intake, particularly at night, to promote uric acid excretion in a dilute urine.

Acetazolamide, 250 mg at bedtime, may be used to keep urine pH >6.

Interval Gout

THERAPEUTIC GOAL

Prevent recurrent attacks.

PHARMACOLOGIC THERAPY

Colchicine, oral: 0.6-1.2 mg daily as prophylaxis against recurrent attacks.

Hypouricemic agent: Start only if indicated by frequent attacks, severe hyperuricemia, presence of tophi, urolithiasis, or urate overexcretion.

OTHER THERAPY

Diet: Moderate protein, low fat, avoid excessive alcohol.

Treat hypertension if present.

High fluid intake to promote uric acid excretion in a dilute urine (for uric acid overexcretors).

ACTH, adrenocorticotropic hormone; GI, gastrointestinal; NSAIDs, nonsteroidal antiinflammatory drugs.

From Goldman L, Ausiello D (eds): *Cecil textbook of medicine*, ed 22. Philadelphia, WB Saunders, 2004.

    d. Intraarticular cortisone when oral medication cannot be given.
    e. General measures, such as rest, elevation, and analgesics as needed until acute pain subsides.
2. Chronic treatment.
    a. Nonpharmacologic therapy.
      (1) Modification of diet by avoiding foods high in purines, such as:
        (a) Anchovies.
        (b) Organ meat.
        (c) Liver.
        (d) Spinach.
        (e) Mushrooms.
        (f) Asparagus.
        (g) Oatmeal.
        (h) Cocoa.
        (i) Sweetbreads.
      (2) Lifestyle modification.
        (a) Treatment for obesity.
        (b) Moderation in alcohol intake, no more than two drinks per day.

(3) Hypertension and its management, requiring careful assessment and possibly nondiuretic drugs.
  b. Pharmacologic therapy.
    (1) Prevention is achieved through normalization of serum urate concentration.
    (2) The main indication for prophylaxis is recurrent attacks or gouty joint inflammation, three or more per year.
    (3) Uricosuric agents (e.g., probenecid) or xanthine oxidase inhibitors (allopurinol) are used in patients with recurrent attacks despite adequate dietary restrictions.
    (4) Colchicine.
      (a) Colchicine is indicated for acute gout prophylaxis before starting hyperuricemic therapy.
        i. Dosing for acute prophylaxis is 0.6 mg bid.
        ii. It is generally discontinued 6 to 8 weeks after normalization of serum urate levels.
      (b) Long-term colchicine therapy (0.6 mg qd or bid) may be necessary in patients with frequent gout attacks despite the use of uricosuric agents.
    (5) A 24-hour urine collection is useful in deciding which antihyperuricemic agent is indicated.
      (a) Allopurinol is generally used if the uric acid output is greater than 900 mg/day on a regular diet.
      (b) Hyperuricemic therapy should not be started for at least 2 weeks after the acute attack has resolved, because it can prolong the acute attack and it can also precipitate new attacks by rapidly lowering the serum uric acid level.
    (6) Urinary uric acid hypoexcretors (<700 mg/day) can be given probenecid to block absorption of uric acid.
      (a) Start with 250 mg bid for 1 week, then increase to 500 mg bid.
      (b) Start probenecid only after the acute attack of gout has completely subsided.
    (7) Surgery is usually limited to excision of large tophi and, occasionally, arthroplasty.
    (8) Renal disease is the most common complication of gout after arthritis. Most gouty patients develop renal disease as a result of parenchymal urate deposition, but the involvement is only slowly progressive and often has no effect on life expectancy.
    (9) Incidence of urolithiasis is increased, with 80% of calculi being uric acid stones.

SUGGESTED READINGS

Agudelo CA, Wise CM: Gout: Diagnosis, pathogenesis, and clinical manifestations. *Curr Opin Rheumatol* 13:234-239, 2001.

Terkeltaub RA: Clinical practice. Gout. *N Engl J Med* 349:1647-1655, 2003.

Velilla-Moliner J, Martinez-Burgui JA, Cobeta-Garca JC, Fatahi-Bandpey ML: Podagra, is it always gout? *Am J Emerg Med* 22(4):320-321,2004.

Wallace KL, Riedel AA, Joseph-Ridge N, Wortmann R: Increasing prevalence of gout and hyperuricemia over 10 years among older adults in a managed care population, *J Rheumatol* 31(8):1582-1587, 2004.

HIP FRACTURE
Lonnie R. Mercier and Tom J. Wachtel

Definition
A femoral neck fracture occurs within the capsule of the hip joint between the base of the head and the intertrochanteric line.

Epidemiology
1. Prevalence: Lifetime risk in women is approximately 16%.
2. Prevalent sex: Female-to-male ratio is 3:1.
3. Prevalent age: About 90% of hip fractures occur in persons older than 60 years.

Clinical Findings
1. Hip or groin pain.
2. In displaced fractures, the affected limb is usually shortened and externally rotated.
3. In impacted fractures, there is possibly no deformity and only mild pain with hip motion.
4. Mild external bruising.

Etiology
1. Trauma.
2. Age-related bone weakness, usually caused by osteoporosis.
3. Increased risk of fractures in elderly (decline in muscle function, use of psychotropic medication, etc.).
4. About 5% of hip fractures occur spontaneously and cause the fall. About 95% of hip fractures are caused when the patient falls and hits the hip.
5. Previous falls and previous fractures are strong risk factors for future falls and fractures.

Differential Diagnosis
1. Osteoarthritis of the hip.
2. Pathologic fracture.
3. Lumbar disc syndrome with radicular pain.
4. Insufficiency fracture of the pelvis.

Work-up
1. Diagnosis is usually obvious based on clinical and radiographic findings.
2. Imaging studies.
   a. Standard x-rays consisting of an anteroposterior film of the pelvis and a cross-table lateral film of the hip to confirm the diagnosis.
   b. If the initial x-rays are negative and an occult femoral neck fracture is suspected, hospital admission and further radiographic assessment with either bone scanning or MRI.
   c. Bone scanning is most sensitive after 48 to 72 hours.

Treatment
1. Surgery is indicated in most cases, usually within 24 hours, unless the patient was not ambulatory before the fracture. The usual procedure is open reduction internal fixation or total or partial hip arthroplasty.
2. Complications are nonunion and avascular necrosis.

3. Give deep venous thrombosis prophylaxis.
4. Intracapsular fractures occasionally occur in nonambulatory patients.
   a. Usually treated nonsurgically, especially in the patient with dementia and limited pain perception.
   b. Early bed-to-chair mobilization and vigilant nursing care to avoid skin breakdown.
   c. Fracture is usually pain free in a short time, even if solid bony healing does not occur.

Prevention

1. Elimination of environmental hazards (poor lighting, loose rugs).
2. Regular exercise for balance and strength.
3. Patient education about fall prevention, including medication review.
4. Prevention and treatment of osteoporosis.
   a. A low-impact fracture is an osteoporosis-defining event.
   b. Dual energy x-ray absorptiometry (DEXA) is not necessary to diagnose osteoporosis in this setting, but it can be useful to monitor response to treatment.

Prognosis

1. Mortality rate within 1 year in elderly patients is 25% to 30%.
2. Dementia is a particularly poor prognostic sign, in part because cooperation with rehabilitation is difficult and the patient might forget how to walk during the time of non–weight-bearing status (which should be minimized).

SUGGESTED READINGS

Bettelli G, Bianchi G, Marinelli A, et al: Relationship between mortality and proximal femur fractures in the elderly. *Orthopedics* 26:1045-1049, 2003.

Feldstein AC, Nichols GA, Elmer PJ, et al: Older women with fractures: Patients falling through the cracks of guideline-recommended osteoporosis screening and treatment. *J Bone Joint Surg Am* 85:2294-2302, 2003.

Kaufman JD, Bolander ME, Bunta AD, et al: Barriers and solutions to osteoporosis care in patients with hip fracture. *J Bone Joint Surg Am* 85:1837-1843, 2003.

Lawrence VA, Hilsenbeck SG, Noveck H, et al: Medical complications and outcomes after hip fracture repair. *Arch Intern Med* 162:2053-2057, 2002.

McClung MR, Geusens P, Miller PD, et al: Effect of risedronate on the risk of hip fracture in elderly women. Hip Intervention Program Study Group. *N Engl J Med* 344(5):333-340, 2001.

McKinley JC, Robinson CM: Treatment of displaced intracapsular fractures with total hip arthroplasty. *J Bone Joint Surg Am* 84:2010-2015, 2002.

Rao SS, Cherukuri M: Management of hip fracture: The family physician's role. *Am Fam Physician* 73:2195-2200, 2006.

Stevens JA, Olson S: Reducing falls and resulting hip fractures among older women. *Home Care Provid* 5(4):134-139, 2000.

LOW BACK PAIN

Tom J. Wachtel

Epidemiology

1. Low back pain is very common.
   a. About 75% of all people experience low back pain sometime during their lives.

b. It is the third most frequent office complaint among patients older than 75 years.

c. About 40% of nursing home patients who report pain complain of their backs.

2. There are 20 million new cases per year in the United States, and 6.5 million patients are bedridden with low back pain every day.

Etiology

1. Musculoskeletal causes (Table 5-22).
   a. Acute (lasting up to 6 weeks).
   b. Subacute (lasting 6 to 12 weeks).
   c. Chronic (lasting more than 3 months).
   d. Most common etiologies are age dependent.
2. Visceral causes (Table 5-23): Any intraabdominal painful process can radiate to the low back or cause pain primarily in the low back.

Clinical Findings

Acute Low Back Pain

1. Consider visceral causes first.
   a. Rule out an infectious process by checking for fever and chills, and if they are present, obtain a CBC.

Table 5-22 Musculoskeletal Causes of Low Back Pain

Cause	Duration	Typical Age of Onset
Ankylosing spondylitis and variants	Chronic	Young adult
Compression fracture (secondary to malignancy or osteoporosis)	Acute to chronic	Elderly
Disk herniation	Acute to chronic	Young adult
Diskitis	Acute	Any age
Epidural abscess	Acute	Any age
Facet joint disease	Acute or chronic	Young adult
Fibromyalgia	Chronic	Any age
Malingering	Chronic	Any age
Muscle strain	Acute	Young adult
Osteomyelitis (bacterial or tuberculous)	Acute	Any age
Osteoarthritis/spinal stenosis	Chronic	Elderly
Paget's disease	Chronic	Elderly
Poor posture	Chronic	Any age
Sickle cell crisis	Acute	Young adult
Spinal tumor	Subacute	Any age
Spinal tumor with cord compression	Acute	Any age
Spine deformities (e.g., scoliosis)	Chronic	Any age
Spondylolisthesis	Acute to chronic	Young adult
Trauma	Acute	Young adult

Table 5-23 Visceral Causes of Low Back Pain

Cause	Duration	Age
Abdominal Aortic Aneurysm		
Expanding	Subacute to chronic	Elderly
Ruptured	Acute	Elderly
Aortic Dissection	Acute	Elderly
Renal Pathology		
Pyelonephritis	Acute	Any age
Renal colic	Acute	Any age
Renal cancer	Subacute	Middle age to elderly
Pancreatic Pathology		
Pancreatitis	Acute	Any age
Pancreatic cancer	Subacute	Middle age to elderly
Retroperitoneal Mass		
Lymphoma	Subacute to chronic	Any age
Soft tissue sarcomas	Subacute to chronic	Middle age to elderly
Metastatic cancer (uterine, prostate, testicular)	Subacute to chronic	Middle age to elderly
Gynecologic and Obstetric		
Cervical pathology	Subacute to chronic	Young adult to middle age
Endometrial pathology	Subacute to chronic	Postmenopausal
Ovarian tumor	Subacute to chronic	Middle age to elderly
Pelvic inflammatory disease	Acute	Young adult
Uterine leiomyoma	Chronic	Middle age

    b. Rule out renal pathology by asking about urinary symptoms and obtaining a urinalysis and renal function test.
    c. Inquire about female genital symptoms and perform a pelvic exam if there is any question of pelvic pathologic conditions.
    d. Consider intraabdominal pathology such as pancreatic disease.
    e. Consider abdominal aortic aneurysm.
2. History.
    a. Is onset sudden or insidious?
    b. Relation to exercise.
    c. Recent trauma (even minor).
    d. History of fractures.
    e. Lower extremity symptoms.
    f. History of symptoms of malignancy.
3. Examine spine and lumbar plexus.
    a. Inspect spine for deformities.
    b. Note patient's posture.

    c. Palpate and percuss lumbar spine.

    d. Inquire about symptoms of sciatica (pain, numbness, or weakness in buttocks and lower extremities).

    e. Perform straight leg raising test.

    f. Perform sensory, motor, and reflex examination of lower extremities; new objective neurologic abnormalities require urgent attention and/or neurosurgical referral.

4. Ancillary tests.

    a. Unlike young adults, low threshold for CBC, calcium, ESR, and liver function tests.

    b. Lumbosacral spine x-ray may be useful to rule out osteoporosis, compression fractures, Paget's disease, osteoarthritis, vertebral cancer.

    c. Additional tests may be indicated.

       (1) Parathormone level.

       (2) Serum and urine protein electrophoresis.

       (3) Bone scan.

       (4) MRI of spine.

5. Management.

    a. Most patients have a negative or nonspecific exam. They should be treated empirically for acute low back syndrome if screening tests are negative (even if sciatica is present).

    b. Bed rest for 2 days if pain is severe.

    c. Analgesics.

       (1) Aspirin.

       (2) Acetaminophen.

       (3) NSAIDSs.

       (4) Opioids.

    d. Muscle relaxants (avoid benzodiazepines).

       (1) Chlorzoxazone (Parafon Forte).

       (2) Cyclobenzaprine (Flexeril).

       (3) Carisoprodol (Soma).

    e. Physical therapy is *not* proven effective in management of acute low back syndrome. Examples:

       (1) Exercise programs.

       (2) Traction.

       (3) Diathermy.

       (4) Heat or cold application.

       (5) Ultrasound.

       (6) Transcutaneous electrical nerve stimulation.

    f. Chiropractic or osteopathic manipulative therapy is popular and may be as effective as traditional allopathic management.

    g. Prevention of recurrent episodes.

       (1) Exercises to strengthen abdominal and paraspinal musculature.

       (2) Pelvic tilt exercises.

       (3) Flexion exercises if spinal stenosis is likely.

       (4) Improve posture.

          (a) Weight loss if indicated.

          (b) Avoid high heels.

     (c) Avoid standing still. If that is not possible, use a footstool for one foot when standing (or for both feet when sitting).

  (5) Teach proper lifting techniques (i.e., use thighs, not back).

Subacute Low Back Pain

1. Some cases of acute low back pain become subacute.
   a. About 10% of patients with acute low back syndrome continue to be symptomatic after 6 weeks of conservative treatment. They now have subacute low back pain.
   b. At this point, efforts to establish a definitive diagnosis must be made. Often this is done with imaging using CT or MRI technology that can provide information about the spine, spinal cord, paraspinal soft tissue, retroperitoneal space, and abdominal and pelvic viscera.
2. Disk disease (onset usually before age 40 years).
   a. Pathogenesis.
      (1) When a person lifts a heavy object using a lumbar extension effort, the anterior aspect of the vertebral bodies and intravertebral disks become the fulcrum of a lever where considerable force tends to squeeze and express the disk backward.
      (2) If structural disk injury occurs, the process of disk herniation (posterior bulging) will begin.
   b. Clinical course.
      (1) Stage 1.
         (a) Stretching the sensory receptors in the posterior ligament causes an acute low back syndrome, which should be managed as described earlier.
         (b) The pain is aggravated by flexion.
      (2) Stage 2.
         (a) Further herniation irritates and then compresses lumbar plexus nerve roots and causes a dermatomal (radicular) neuropathy called *sciatica*.
         (b) Lumbar disks most likely to herniate are L4-L5 (L5 root) and L5-S1 (S1 root) (98% of all cases).
      (3) Rule out cauda equina syndrome by inquiring about urine and fecal continence and by checking rectal sphincter tone.
      (4) Any objective neurologic deficit requires urgent diagnostic evaluation and treatment, albeit not necessarily surgical.
      (5) Stage 3.
         (a) Scarring occurs.
         (b) Back pain can decrease or become chronic.
         (c) Neurologic deficits become fixed.
   c. Signs of sciatica.
      (1) Subjective pain and sensory abnormalities. Subjective symptoms are most likely to be proximal, and objective findings are more likely to be distal (test with light touch or pinprick).
         (a) L5 root: Buttock, posterior thigh, lateral leg, dorsum of foot, and great toe.
         (b) S1 root: Buttock, posterior thigh, lateral aspect of ankle and foot, and lateral toes.

       (2) Deep tendon reflexes.
          (a) L5 root: None.
          (b) S1 root: Ankle jerk.
       (3) Motor function: Toe walking and heel walking are adequate tests.
       (4) Straight leg raising test.
          (a) The dura is stretched around the sciatic nerves at angles of 30 to 70 degrees.
          (b) A positive test is obtained when raising the contralateral leg reproduces sciatic pain on the affected side (better than 95% probability of disk disease).
          (c) Detecting malingering.
             i. Distracting the patient produces inconsistent results.
             ii. When the leg is lowered to an angle where the sciatic pain disappears, a patient with organic disease should complain on foot dorsiflexion performed at this point.
   d. Management.
       (1) Stage 1: Managed as a nonspecific acute low back syndrome.
       (2) Stage 2.
          (a) Patient may be a candidate for neurosurgery.
          (b) Surgery is very successful at relieving the radiculopathy if performed within 12 weeks of onset of the neurologic deficit.
          (c) Surgery is no more than 50% effective at resolving the back pain.
       (3) Stage 3: Treatment is mainly aimed at pain control, rehabilitative therapy (i.e., exercises), and resolving psychosocial comorbidities.
3. Osteoarthritis.
   a. Many elderly patients with low back pain are found to have radiologic evidence of osteoarthritis.
   b. However, poor correlation between symptoms and radiologic findings is the rule rather than the exception in osteoarthritis.
4. Spinal stenosis.
   a. Special considerations should be given to the possibility of spinal stenosis, a potentially reversible complication of spinal osteoarthritis.
   b. These patients have back pain and bilateral leg pain on standing or walking.
   c. Pain is resolved by spine flexion.
       (1) Sitting (pseudoclaudication).
       (2) Bending (shopping cart sign).
   d. Lumbosacral spine x-rays are suggestive, and CT scan or MRI is diagnostic.
   e. Surgical treatment may be required.
5. Osteoporosis.
   a. Osteoporosis per se does not produce symptoms.
   b. Osteoporosis predisposes patients to acute vertebral compression fractures that can occur spontaneously or during trauma.
6. Compression fractures.
   a. Sudden onset of low back pain in older women might result from a compression fracture.
   b. Compression fracture can often be confirmed by a simple x-ray of the spine.

   c. A radiologic diagnosis of a new compression fracture may be difficult in a patient with previous vertebral fracture or severe degenerative changes.

     (1) Pain is variable in severity but may be very severe.

     (2) Treatment is symptomatic as in any low back syndrome; however, the first few days following fracture may be complicated by an intestinal ileus often exacerbated by use of narcotic analgesics. Prophylactic stool softeners should be prescribed.

     (3) There is no evidence that back braces or corsets are effective, but many patients report some comfort from their use.

7. Malignant spine lesions.

   a. Plain x-ray might reveal malignant disease involving spine.

   b. Primary osteosarcoma is unusual in this location, but multiple myeloma should always be considered as a potential cause of osteoporosis or lytic lesions.

   c. Diagnosis can be made by ordering an ESR for screening, followed by serum protein electrophoresis, immunoelectrophoresis, and a urine protein electrophoresis.

   d. Metastatic lesions of the spine usually originate from lung (lytic lesions), prostate (blastic lesions), kidney (lytic lesions), breast (blastic or lytic lesions), or thyroid (blastic or lytic lesions).

   e. Malignant lesions of the spine can cause pain without a compression fracture. This should be suspected when back pain occurs at rest.

   f. They also can cause extrinsic cord or root compression, a neurosurgical oncologic emergency.

8. Ankylosing spondyloarthropathies (onset exceptional after age 40 years).

   a. Presentation.

     (1) Young men more commonly and severely affected than women.

     (2) They present with back pain, occasionally with hip, knee, or ankle pain with stiffness, worse in the morning as in any inflammatory arthritis.

     (3) A positive family history may be elicited.

   b. Clinical findings.

     (1) Reduced chest expansion.

     (2) Increased finger-to-toe distance.

     (3) Inability to perform the occiput to wall test.

     (4) Sacroiliac joint tenderness.

   c. Extraarticular manifestations.

     (1) Cardiac complications (arteriovenous block, aortic regurgitation).

     (2) Iritis.

     (3) Pulmonary fibrosis.

     (4) Amyloidosis.

     (5) Psoriasis or inflammatory bowel disease can coexist.

   d. Diagnosis of ankylosing spondylitis confirmed by:

     (1) Elevated sedimentation rate.

     (2) Evidence of sacroiliitis on pelvic x-ray.

     (3) Evidence of syndesmophytes or common ligament calcification (bamboo spine) on a spine x-ray.

     (4) Presence of an HLA-B27 antigen.

e. Treatment.
   (1) Symptomatic relief can be achieved with aspirin and NSAIDs.
   (2) Physical therapy should be performed to preserve mobility or permit ankylosing in the most functional position.
f. By the time the patient is elderly, the disease usually will have stabilized and the patient will often experience the same problems as those seen in degenerative disease of the spine.

9. Osteomyelitis, diskitis, and epidural abscess.
   a. Bacterial infections or, more rarely, tuberculosis can involve the spine and adjacent structures through the hematogenous route or from spread of a continuous focus of infection. Infection may be acute (e.g., staphylococcal diskitis) or chronic (e.g., tuberculous osteomyelitis, known as *Pott's disease*).
   b. Pain is characteristically worse at night.
   c. The patient might have particular risk factors (e.g., IV drug abuse) and might have obvious or subtle signs of infection.
   d. Imaging studies are needed to establish a definitive diagnosis.

10. Posterior facet joint syndrome.
    a. Because posterior articular facets meet each other at an angle, those joints are subjected to a constant shearing force in the erect position.
    b. Pain is typically of sudden onset (acute lumbago) and rarely lasts more than 1 week.
    c. Posterior facet joint syndrome should be suspected when pain is aggravated by spinal extension.
    d. It is diagnosed more frequently by chiropractors than by allopathic physicians and may be improved by manipulative therapy.

11. Fibromyalgia.
    a. Although not restricted to the low back, this controversial condition manifests itself by soft tissue aching and chronic stiffness aggravated by stress.
    b. Young and middle-aged women are most commonly affected, but it can persist into older age groups.
    c. It is characterized by the presence of trigger points that, according to some authorities, must be quite specific.
    d. Many patients complain of insomnia and waking up unrefreshed in the morning; a substantial fraction of patients also display other depressive symptoms.
    e. Some patients respond to antidepressant drugs, psychotherapy, NSAIDs, or physical therapy. However, as might be expected in a condition where somatization plays an important part, many patients do not improve and pursue an erratic health care–seeking course.
    f. An association with vitamin D deficiency has been described and should be ruled out with a 25-hydroxyvitamin D level.

Chronic Low Back Pain

1. Some cases of acute back pain become chronic.
   a. Overall, 5% of all cases of acute back pain become chronic.
   b. The percentage is far greater in the elderly because of the high prevalence of osteoarthritis and vertebral collapse fractures.
   c. Patients often make frequent doctor visits and can cause great bidirectional frustration in the physician-patient relationship.

   d. Ideally, workup will have been completed during the subacute phase; if not, it should be done at once.
2. Whether an incurable organic cause is diagnosed (e.g., osteoarthritis, osteoporosis with compression fractures) or patient has unexplained chronic refractory back pain, management should be supportive.
   a. Nonaddictive analgesic agents.
   b. Exercises.
   c. Attention to psychosocial ills, perhaps a trial of antidepressants.
   d. Protection from excessive diagnostic procedures, surgery, and doctor shopping.
3. Therapeutic success is enhanced by setting realistic expectations for symptom and functional improvement with the patient.

SUGGESTED READINGS

Biyani A, Andersson GB: Low back pain: Pathophysiology and management. *J Am Acad Orthop Surg* 12:106-115, 2004.
Brodke DS, Ritter SM: Nonsurgical management of low back pain and lumbar disk degeneration. *Instr Course Lec* 54:279-286, 2005.

OSTEOARTHRITIS

Lonnie R. Mercier and Tom J. Wachtel

Definition

1. Osteoarthritis (OA) or degenerative joint disease (known in Europe as osteoarthrosis) is a joint condition in which degeneration and loss of articular cartilage occur, leading to pain and deformity.
2. Two forms are usually recognized: primary (idiopathic) and secondary.
   a. The primary form may be localized or generalized.
   b. The secondary forms are generally localized.

Epidemiology

1. Prevalence is 2% to 6% of general population. Radiologic evidence of OA can exist without symptoms.
2. Predominant sex: None (female = male).
3. Predominant age is older than 50 years.

Clinical Findings

1. Symptoms.
   a. Similar symptoms in most forms: stiffness, pain, and crepitus.
   b. Joint tenderness and swelling.
   c. Decreased range of motion.
2. Physical examination.
   a. Crepitus with motion.
   b. Bony hypertrophy.
   c. Pain with range of motion.
   d. DIP joint involvement possibly leading to development of nodular swellings called *Heberden's nodes*.
   e. PIP joint involvement possibly leading to development of nodular swellings called *Bouchard's nodes*.

Etiology

1. Primary OA is of unknown cause.
2. Secondary OA can result from a number of disorders including trauma, metabolic conditions, and other forms of arthritis.

Differential Diagnosis

1. Bursitis, tendinitis.
2. Back pain (see earlier).
3. Inflammatory arthritis.
4. Crystalline arthropathy.
5. Infectious arthritis.
6. Radiculopathy and peripheral neuropathy with pain.
7. Peripheral arterial disease.
8. Peripheral venous disease.
9. Myopathies.
10. Bone pain (malignancy, Paget's disease, fractures).
11. Soft tissue sarcomas (chondrosarcoma, liposarcoma, fibrosarcoma, rhabdomyosarcoma).

Work-up

1. No diagnostic test exists for degenerative joint disease.
2. Laboratory evaluation is normal.
3. Rheumatoid factor, ESR, CBC, and antinuclear antibody tests may be required if an inflammatory component is present.
4. Synovial fluid examination is generally normal.
5. Radiologic evaluation reveals:
   a. Joint space narrowing.
   b. Subchondral sclerosis.
   c. New bone formation in the form of osteophytes.

Treatment

1. Nonpharmacologic therapy.
   a. Rest, restricted use or weightbearing, heat.
   b. Walking aids such as a cane (often helpful for weight-bearing joints).
   c. Suitable footwear.
   d. Gentle range-of-motion and strengthening exercise.
   e. Local creams and liniments to provide a counterirritant effect.
   f. Education, reassurance.
2. Pharmacologic therapy.
   a. Mild analgesics for joint pain (e.g., acetaminophen).
   b. NSAIDs if inflammation is present.
   c. Occasional local corticosteroid injections (usually limited to three times per year).
   d. Viscosupplementation (injection of hyaluronic acid products into the degenerative joint) is of uncertain benefit.
   e. Nutritional supplements (glucosamine and chondroitin) may be helpful.
3. Surgery.
   a. Surgical intervention is generally helpful in degenerative joint disease.
   b. Arthroplasty, arthrodesis, and realignment osteotomy are the most common procedures performed.
   c. Arthroscopic debridement (of the knee) appears to be of only limited value.

Prognosis

1. Rate of progression is variable.

2. Symptoms and x-ray are only poorly correlated.
3. The decision to perform surgery depends on the functional and quality-of-life impact of OA on an individual patient.

SUGGESTED READINGS

Callaghan JJ, Templeton JE, Liu SS, et al: Results of Charnley total hip arthroplasty at a minimum of thirty years. A concise follow-up of a previous report. *J Bone Joint Surg Am* 86:690-695, 2004.

Hartofilakidis G, Karachalios T: Idiopathic osteoarthritis of the hip: Incidence, classification and natural history of 272 cases. *Orthopedics* 26:161-166, 2003.

Hinton R, Moody RL, Davis AW, Thomas SF: Osteoarthritis: Diagnosis and therapeutic considerations. *Am Fam Physician* 65:841-848, 2002.

Olsen NJ: Tailoring arthritis therapy in the wake of the NSAID crisis. *N Engl J Med* 352:2578-2580, 2005.

Wang C, Lin J, Chang CJ, et al: Therapeutic effects of hyaluronic acid in osteoarthritis of the knee. A meta-analysis of randomized controlled trials. *J Bone Joint Surg Am* 86:538-545, 2004.

Wegman A, van der Windt D, van Tulder M, et al: Nonsteroidal antiinflammatory drugs or acetaminophen for osteoarthritis of the hip or knee? A systematic review of evidence and guidelines. *J Rheumatol* 31:344-354, 2004.

PAGET'S DISEASE OF BONE

Lonnie R. Mercier and Tom J. Wachtel

Definition

1. Paget's disease (a.k.a. osteitis deformans) of the bone is a nonmetabolic disease of bone characterized by repeated episodes of osteolysis and excessive attempts at repair that results in a weakened bone of increased mass.
2. Monostotic (solitary lesion) and polyostotic (numerous lesions) disease are both described.
3. It is viewed by some as a benign neoplasm or a preneoplastic disease.

Epidemiology

1. Prevalence: Localized lesions in 3% of patients older than 50 years.
2. Prevalent age: Rare before 40 years.
3. Prevalent sex: Male-to-female ratio of 2:1.

Clinical Findings

1. Symptoms.
   a. May be asymptomatic.
   b. Onset is variable.
   c. Skeletal pain, especially hip and pelvis.
2. Signs and physical findings result mainly from the effects of complications:
   a. Bowing of long bones, sometimes leading to pathologic fracture.
   b. Increased heat of the extremity (resulting from increased vascularity).
   c. Skull enlargement and spinal involvement caused by characteristic bone enlargement, which can produce neurologic complications (vision problems, hearing loss, radicular pain, and cord compression).
   d. Thoracic kyphoscoliosis.
   e. Secondary osteoarthritis, especially of the hip.
   f. Heart failure as a result of chest and spine deformity and blood shunting.

Etiology

Unknown.

Differential Diagnosis

1. Skeletal neoplasm (primary or metastatic).
2. OA.
3. Hyperparathyroidism.
4. Vertebral hemangioma.

Work-up

1. Laboratory tests.
   a. Elevated serum alkaline phosphatase.
   b. Normal serum calcium and phosphorus levels.
   c. Increased urinary excretion of pyridinoline cross-links, although the test is expensive and not usually required in routine cases.
2. Imaging studies.
   a. Targeted radiographs reflect the characteristic radiolucency and opacity.
   b. Bone scanning usually reflects the activity and extent of the disease.
3. Bone biopsy is useful in uncertain cases or if sarcomatous degeneration is suspected.

Treatment

1. Nonpharmacologic therapy.
   a. Counseling regarding home environment to prevent falls.
   b. Cane for balance and weight-bearing pain.
   c. Referrals.
      (1) For dental evaluation if there is involvement of the mandible or maxilla.
      (2) For ear, nose, and throat (ENT) evaluation if there is hearing loss.
      (3) For ophthalmologic evaluation if there is impaired vision.
      (4) For orthopedic consultation for assessment of pain in bone or joint.
2. Pharmacologic therapy.
   a. Calcitonin.
   b. Bisphosphonates.
   c. NSAIDs for pain relief.
   d. General indications for treatment.
      (1) All symptomatic patients.
      (2) Asymptomatic patients with high level of metabolic activity or those at risk for deformity.
      (3) Preoperative, if surgery involves pagetic site.

Prognosis

1. Many monostotic lesions remain asymptomatic.
2. Progression of the disease is common.
3. Malignant degeneration occurs in less than 1% of patients and should be considered when there is a sudden increase in pain. It carries a poor prognosis.

SUGGESTED READINGS

Kotocvicz MA: Paget disease of bone: Diagnosis and indications for treatment. *Aust Fam Physician* 33(3):127-131, 2004.

Langston AL, Ralston SH: Management of Paget's disease of bone. *Rheumatology* (Oxford) 43(8):955-959, 2004.

Lin JT, Lane JM: Bisphosphonates. *J Am Acad Orthop Surg* 11:1-4, 2003.

Schneider D, Hofmann MT, Peterson JA: Diagnosis and treatment of Paget's disease of bone. *Am Fam Physician* 65:2069-2072, 2002.

POLYMYALGIA RHEUMATICA

Fred F. Ferri and Tom J. Wachtel

Definition

Polymyalgia rheumatica is a clinical syndrome predominantly involving persons older than 50 years and characterized by pain and stiffness involving mainly the shoulders, pelvic girdle, musculature, and torso.

Epidemiology

1. Prevalence: 600 cases per 100,000 persons.
2. Incidence after age 50: 52.5 new cases per 100,000 persons.

Clinical Manifestations

1. Symmetric polymyalgias, arthralgias, and stiffness involving back, shoulder, neck, and pelvic girdle muscles.
2. Duration is generally longer than 1 month.
3. Constitutional symptoms (fever, malaise, weight loss).
4. Headache in patients with coexisting temporal arteritis.
5. Symptoms are worse in the morning (difficulty getting out of bed) and at night.
6. Muscle strength usually is within normal limits, but pain can impair testing.
7. Crescendo of symptoms over several weeks or months.

Laboratory Findings

Laboratory findings are the same as for temporal arteritis.

Diagnostic Criteria

1. Age older than 50 years.
2. ESR greater than 50 mm.
3. At least 1 month of aching and morning stiffness in at least two of the following areas:
   a. Neck and torso.
   b. Hips and thighs.
   c. Shoulders and upper arms.
4. Other diseases have been excluded.

Treatment

1. Abolish symptoms.
   a. Low-dose corticosteroids (e.g., prednisone 10 to 20 mg/day) generally produce dramatic relief of symptoms within 48 hours and confirm the diagnosis.
      (1) Failure to improve within 1 week suggests other diagnoses (e.g., fibromyalgia, polymyositis, viral myalgias, hypothyroidism, depression rheumatoid arthritis, occult neoplasm, or infection).
      (2) Rarely, the dose of prednisone must be as high as 40 mg/day.

b. Corticosteroid dosage is then gradually tapered over several months based on repeated clinical observation and monitoring of ESR.
   c. In patients with mild symptoms, NSAIDs may be used instead of corticosteroids.
2. Monitor closely for possible development of temporal arteritis.
   a. Instruct patient to immediately report any visual or neurologic symptoms.
   b. As many as one third of patients can develop temporal arteritis within 1 year of onset of polymyalgia rheumatica.

SUGGESTED READINGS

Mandell BF: Polymyalgia rheumatica: Clinical presentation is key to diagnosis and treatment. *Cleve Clin J Med* 71:489-495, 2004.
Salvarani C, Cantini F, Boiardi L, Hunder GG: Polymyalgia rheumatica and giant-cell arteritis. *N Engl J Med* 347:261-271, 2002.

RHEUMATOID ARTHRITIS

Lonnie R. Mercier, with adaptations by Tom J. Wachtel

Definition

Rheumatoid arthritis (RA) is a systemic disorder characterized by chronic joint inflammation that most commonly affects peripheral joints. This process results in the development of pannus, a destructive tissue that damages cartilage.

Epidemiology

1. Prevalence: 5 cases/1000 adults.
2. After age 50 years, the sex difference is less marked than the female-to-male ratio of 3:1 noted in younger adults.

Clinical Findings

1. Arthropathy.
   a. Usually gradual onset; common prodromal symptoms of weakness, fatigue, and anorexia.
   b. Initial presentation is multiple symmetric joint involvement, most often in the hands and feet, usually metacarpophalangeal, metatarsophalangeal, and PIP joints.
   c. Joint effusions, tenderness, and restricted motion usually present early in the disease.
   d. Eventual characteristic deformities:
      (1) Subluxations.
      (2) Dislocations.
      (3) Joint contractures.
2. Extraarticular manifestations.
   a. Tendon sheaths and bursae are commonly affected by chronic inflammation.
   b. Findings of carpal tunnel syndrome resulting from flexor tenosynovitis (possible tendon rupture).
   c. Rheumatoid nodules over bony prominences such as the elbow and shaft of the ulna.
   d. Splenomegaly, lymphadenopathy, pericarditis, pleuritis, pulmonary fibrosis, lung nodules, vasculitis, episcleritis, Sjögren's syndrome.
   e. Weight loss, fever, sweats, fatigue, anemia.

3. According to the American College of Rheumatology, RA exists when four of seven criteria are present; the first four criteria must be present for at least 6 weeks.
   a. Morning stiffness longer than 1 hour.
   b. Arthritis in three or more joints with swelling.
   c. Arthritis of hand joints with swelling.
   d. Symmetric arthritis.
   e. Rheumatoid nodules.
   f. Roentgenographic changes typical of RA.
   g. Positive serum rheumatoid factor.

Etiology

1. Etiology is unknown.
2. There is increasing evidence that the inflammation and destruction of bone and cartilage that occurs in many rheumatic diseases are the result of the activation by some unknown mechanism of proinflammatory cells that infiltrate the synovium. These cells, in turn, release various substances, such as cytokines and tumor necrosis factor α (TNFα) which subsequently cause the pathologic changes typical of this group of diseases. Many of the newer therapeutic agents are directed at suppressing these final mediators of inflammation.

Differential Diagnosis

1. SLE.
2. Lyme arthritis.
3. Hepatitis B.
4. Seronegative spondyloarthropathies (i.e., ankylosing spondylitis).
5. Psoriatic arthritis.
6. Palindromic rheumatism.
7. Polymyalgia rheumatica.
8. Relapsing polychondritis.
9. Behçet's disease.
10. Acute rheumatic fever.
11. Reiter's disease.
12. Sarcoidosis.
13. Scleroderma.
14. Reactive arthritis.
15. Enteropathic arthropathy.
16. Fibromyalgia.
17. Crystal deposition disease (occasionally polyarticular involvement).

Work-up

1. Laboratory tests.
   a. Positive rheumatoid factor in 80% of cases; rheumatoid factor can also be present in the normal population (i.e., false-positive test).
   b. Possible mild anemia and mild leukocytosis.
   c. Usually, elevated acute phase reactants (ESR, C-reactive protein).
   d. Joint fluid is usually turbid and forms a poor mucin clot.
   e. Elevated cell count with an increase in polymorphonuclear leukocytes.
2. Imaging studies.
   a. Plain x-rays can reveal soft-tissue swelling and osteoporosis early.

    b. Eventually, joint space narrowing, erosion, and deformity are visible on x-ray as a result of continued inflammation and cartilage destruction.

Treatment

1. Patient education is important.
   a. Remissions and exacerbations are common, but the condition is chronically progressive in many cases.
   b. Joint degeneration and deformity can lead to disability.
   c. Early diagnosis and treatment are important and can improve quality of life.
   d. Rest with proper exercise and splinting can prevent or correct joint deformities.
   e. Diet to control obesity.
   f. Close cooperation among primary physician, therapist, rheumatologist, and orthopedist.
2. Pharmacologic therapy.
   a. NSAIDs.
      (1) NSAIDs are used as the initial treatment to relieve inflammation.
      (2) Aspirin is the drug of choice for most patients, but other NSAIDs are also effective.
3. Disease-modifying antirheumatic drugs (DMARDs).
   a. DMARDs are traditionally begun when NSAIDs are not effective.
   b. Current recommendations favor early aggressive treatment with DMARDs, seeking to minimize long-term joint damage.
   c. Commonly used agents are methotrexate, cyclosporine, hydroxychloroquine, sulfasalazine, leflunomide, and infliximab.
   d. Most of these are associated with potential toxicity and require close monitoring.
   e. They are also slow-acting drugs that require more than 8 weeks to become effective (Table 5-24).
4. Oral prednisone.
5. Intrasynovial steroid injections.
6. Etanercept (Enbrel).
   a. Etanercept, a TNFα-blocker, is indicated in moderately to severely active RA in patients who respond inadequately to DMARDs.
   b. The combination of etanercept and methotrexate has been reported to be effective and promising in the treatment of RA.

SUGGESTED READINGS

Edwards JC, Szczepanski L, Szechinski J, et al: Efficacy of B-cell-targeted therapy with rituximab in patients with rheumatoid arthritis. *N Engl J Med* 350:2572-2581, 2004.

Gardner GC, Kadel NJ: Ordering and interpreting rheumatologic laboratory tests. *J Am Acad Orthop Surg* 11:60-67, 2003.

Genovese MC, Bathon JM, Martin RW, et al: Etanercept versus methotrexate in patients with early rheumatoid arthritis: Two-year radiographic and clinical outcomes. *Arthritis Rheum* 46:1443-1450, 2002.

Kremer JM: Rational use of new and existing disease-modifying agents in rheumatoid arthritis. *Ann Intern Med* 134:695-706, 2001.

Maini SR: Infliximab treatment of rheumatoid arthritis, *Rheum Dis Clin North Am* 30:329-347, 2004.

Olsen NJ, Stein CM: New drugs for rheumatoid arthritis. *N Engl J Med* 350:2167-2179, 2004.

Table 5-24 Selected Disease-Modifying Antirheumatic Drugs

Generic (Trade) Name	Route	Recommended Dosages	Toxic Effects	Recommended Monitoring
Gold Compounds				
Aurothiomalate (Myochrysine)	IM	10 mg followed by 25 mg 1 wk later, then 25-50 mg weekly to toxicity, major clinical improvement, or cumulative dose = 1 g. If effective, interval between doses is increased	Pruritis, dermatitis (frequent: ⅓ of pts), stomatitis, nephrotoxicity, blood dyscrasias, "nitritoid" reaction (flushing), weakness, nausea, dizziness 30 min after injection	CBC, platelet count before every other injection. U/A before each dose
Aurothioglucose (Solganal)	IM	Initial dose, 10 mg; 2nd and 3rd doses, 25 mg; 4th and subsequent doses, 50 mg. Interval between doses, 1 wk. If improvement and no toxicity, decrease dose to 25 mg or increase interval between doses	Dermatitis, stomatitis, nephrotoxicity, blood dyscrasias	CBC, platelet count every 2 wk. Urinalysis before each dose
Auranofin (Ridaura)	PO	3 mg bid or 6 mg qd May increase to 3 mg tid after 6 months	Loose stools, diarrhea (up to 50%), dermatitis	Baseline CBC, platelet count, U/A, renal, liver function, at onset Then CBC with platelet count, U/A at 9 mo

Continued

Table 5-24 Selected Disease-Modifying Antirheumatic Drugs—cont'd

Generic (Trade) Name	Route	Recommended Dosages	Toxic Effects	Recommended Monitoring
Antimalarial				
Hydroxychloroquine (Plaquenil)	PO	400-600 mg qd with meals, then 200-400 mg qd	Retinopathy, dermatitis, muscle weakness, hypoactive DTRs, CNS	Ophthalmologic examination every 3 mo (visual acuity, slit lamp, funduscopic, visual field tests), neuromuscular examination
Alkylating Agents				
Cyclophosphamide (Cytoxan)	PO	50-100 mg daily up to 2.5 mg/kg/d	Leukopenia, thrombocytopenia, hematuria, GI, alopecia, rash, bladder cancer, non-Hodgkin's lymphoma, infection	CBC with platelet count, regularly hCG as needed
Chlorambucil (Leukeran)	PO	0.1-0.2 mg/kg/d	Bone marrow suppression, GI, CNS, infection	CBC with platelet count every wk. WBCs 3-4 days after each CBC during 1st 3-6 wk of therapy, hCG as needed
Cyclosporine (Sandimmune)	PO	2.5-5 mg/kg/d	Nephrotoxicity, tremor, hirsutism, hypertension, gum hyperplasia	Renal function, liver function
Pyrimidine Synthesis Inhibitors				
Leflunomide (Arava)	PO	Loading dose: 100 mg/d for 3 days	Hepatotoxicity, carcinogenesis	LFTs every month, drug levels after

Drug	Route	Dose	Adverse effects	Monitoring
		Maintenance therapy: 20 mg/d; if not tolerated, 10 mg/d	Immunosuppression, long half-life	discontinuation (after 1 mo therapy, remains in blood for 2 y without use of cholestyramine)
Other Drugs				
Azathioprine (Imuran)	PO	50-100 mg qd, increase at 4-wk intervals by 0.5 mg/kg/d up to 2.5 mg/kg/d	Leukopenia, thrombocytopenia, GI, neoplastic if previous Rx with alkylating agents	CBC with platelet count, wkly × 1 mo, 2×/mo × 2 mo, then monthly hCG as needed
Methotrexate (Rheumatrex)	PO	7.5-15 mg weekly	Pulmonary toxicity, ulcerative stomatitis, leukopenia, thrombocytopenia, GI distress, malaise, fatigue, chills, fever, CNS, elevated LFTs/liver disease, lymphoma, infection	CBC with platelet count, LFTs weekly × 6 wk, then monthly LFTs, U/A periodically, hCG as needed
Penicillamine (Cuprimine, Depen)	PO	125-250 mg qd, then increasing at monthly intervals by 125-250 mg doses to max 750-1000 mg	Pruritus, rash/mouth ulcers, bone marrow depression, proteinuria, hematuria, hypogeusia, myasthenia, myositis, GI distress, pulmonary toxicity, teratogenic	CBC every 2 wk until dose stable, then every mo. U/A weekly until dose is stable, then every mo. hCG as needed
Sulfasalazine (Azulfidine)	PO	500 mg daily, then increase up to 3 g daily	GI, skin rash, pruritus, blood dyscrasias, oligospermia	CBC, U/A q 2 wk × 3 mo, then monthly × 9 mo, then every 6 mo

CBC, complete blood count; CNS, central nervous system; DTR, deep tendon reflex; GI, gastrointestinal; hCG, human chorionic gonadotropin; LFT, liver function test; pts, patients; U/A, urinalysis; WBC, white blood cell count.
From Rakel RE (ed): *Principles of family practice*, ed 6, Philadelphia, 2002, WB Saunders.

Smith JB, Haynes MK: Rheumatoid arthritis—a molecular understanding. *Ann Intern Med* 136:908-922, 2002.

Van Everdingen AA, Jacobs JW, Siewertsz Van Reesema DR, Bijlsma JW: Low-dose prednisone therapy for patients with early active rheumatoid arthritis: Clinical efficacy, disease-modifying properties, and side effects: A randomized, double-blind, placebo-controlled clinical trial. *Ann Intern Med* 136:1-12, 2002.

TEMPORAL ARTERITIS

Fred F. Ferri and Tom J. Wachtel

Definition

Temporal (giant cell) arteritis is a systemic segmental granulomatous inflammation predominantly involving the arteries of the carotid system in patients older than 50 years. However, it can involve any large- or medium-sized arteries.

Epidemiology

1. Prevalence: 200 cases per 100,000 persons.
2. Incidence after age 50 years: Ranges from 17 to 23.3 new cases per 100,000 persons per year.

Clinical Manifestations

1. Headache, often associated with marked scalp tenderness.
2. Tenderness, decreased pulsation, and nodulation of temporal arteries.
3. Constitutional symptoms (fever, weight loss, anorexia, fatigue).
4. Polymyalgia syndrome (aching and stiffness of the trunk and proximal muscle groups).
5. Visual disturbances (visual loss, blurred vision, diplopia, amaurosis fugax).
6. Intermittent claudication of jaw and tongue on mastication.
7. Cough.

Laboratory Findings

1. Elevated ESR.
   a. ESR is usually higher than 50 mm/hour by the Westergren method.
   b. A normal ESR does not exclude the diagnosis.
2. Mild to moderate normochromic normocytic anemia, elevated platelets.
3. Liver function test abnormalities (elevation of alkaline phosphatase most common).

Diagnosis

The presence of any three of the following five items allows the diagnosis of temporal arteritis with a sensitivity of 94% and a specificity of 91%.

1. Age of onset 50 years or older.
2. New onset or new type of headache.
3. Temporal artery tenderness or decreased pulsation on physical exam.
4. Westergren ESR ≥50 mm/hour.
5. Artery biopsy with vasculitis and mononuclear cell infiltrate or granulomatous changes.
   a. Because of potential skip lesions in the artery, the biopsy segment of the temporal artery should be at least 2 cm long.
   b. A negative biopsy in a patient with classic features of temporal arteritis presents a difficult clinical dilemma that requires individualized management judgment.

Treatment

1. Prednisone.
   a. In stable patients without ocular involvement, prednisone is prescribed at 40 to 60 mg/day continued for a few weeks until symptoms resolve and ESR returns to normal.
   b. If the ESR remains normal, prednisone can be reduced by 5 mg every other week until a dose of 20 mg/day is reached.
   c. Subsequent dose reductions should be by 2.5 mg/day every 2 to 4 weeks.
   d. When the total dose reaches 5 mg/day, reduction should be by 1 mg every 2 to 4 weeks as tolerated.
   e. Usual length of prednisone treatment is 6 months to 2 years. Do not delay treatment while the temporal artery biopsy is pending.
2. Methylprednisolone: In very ill patients and patients with significant ocular involvement (e.g., visual loss in one eye), rapid aggressive treatment with large doses of IV methylprednisolone is indicated to provide optimum protection to the uninvolved eye and offer some chance of visual recovery in the involved eye.
3. Follow-up.
   a. Temporal arteritis is associated with risk of aortic aneurysm, which is often a late complication and can cause death.
   b. Patients with a history of temporal arteritis should have an annual exam, including palpation of the abdominal aorta, perhaps an abdominal ultrasound, and an annual radiograph of the chest including a lateral view.

SUGGESTED READINGS

Salvarani C, Cantini F, Boiardi L, Hunder GG: Polymyalgia rheumatica and giant-cell arteritis. N Engl J Med 347:261-271, 2002.
Smetana GW, Shmerling RH: Does this patient have temporal arteritis? JAMA 287:92-101, 2002.

5.6 Cardiovascular Disorders

ACUTE CORONARY SYNDROMES
Michael P. Gerardo

Overview

The full spectrum of coronary artery disease (CAD) includes asymptomatic disease, chronic stable angina, and the acute coronary syndromes (ACS). The ACS are unstable angina and myocardial infarction (MI). The ACS are caused by a number of mechanisms including plaque disruption, thrombosis, and vasospasm. Age is the single strongest predictor of morbidity and mortality among MI patients with ST elevation.

Diagnosis of ACS is often delayed in older persons compared to younger patients; this delay in MI presentation is strongly associated with poorer outcomes. Older persons might have difficulty in recognizing symptoms consistent with ACS; providers should discuss the varied presentation of ACS in older adults and the importance of seeking medical attention for any acute chest pain. For institutionalized older adults, stat ECG and cardiac enzymes may be a reasonable alternative to evaluation by emergency department physicians.

Definitions

The ACS are unstable angina and myocardial infarction.
1. Unstable angina.
   a. Unstable angina is any recent chest pain that is a change from previous episodes.
   b. The pain can occur at rest (rest angina) or can be of increasing intensity, frequency, or duration (crescendo angina).
2. MI is defined by the following criteria:
   a. Biochemical markers (troponin or CK-MB) consistent with myocardial necrosis plus one of the following:
      (1) Ischemic symptoms.
      (2) New Q waves on ECG.
      (3) ST segment elevation or depression.
      (4) Coronary angioplasty.
   b. Pathologic evidence of acute myocardial infarction.
3. ST elevation MI (STEMI) indicates full thickness myocardial necrosis. STEMI should immediately be considered for reperfusion therapy (see later).
4. Non–ST elevation MI occurs as a result of myocardial necrosis from plaque rupture with subsequent embolization. Non–ST elevation MI can evolve into a STEMI.

Epidemiology

1. More than 500,000 MIs occur per year in the United States.
2. Eighty-five percent of MI deaths occur in those older than 65 years.
3. At least one third of all MIs are clinically unrecognized.
4. The risk of silent MI is greatest for women, diabetics, and older adults.

Differential Diagnosis

The differential diagnosis of chest pain is discussed later under "Coronary Artery Disease and Angina Pectoris."

Initial Evaluation

1. History and physical exam.
   a. Chest pain lasting longer than 30 minutes suggests an ACS or a noncardiac source for the pain.
   b. Markers of more severe disease include signs and symptoms consistent with heart failure.
   c. The pain from ACS is most likely to occur at rest.
   d. Pain from ACS is often associated with lightheadedness, syncope, nausea, vomiting, diaphoresis, and apprehension.
2. Laboratory exam.
   a. Causes of demand ischemia.
      (1) Older persons are at increased risk for demand ischemia, a condition where myocardial damage can occur during periods of high oxygen requirements such as gastrointestinal bleeding, infection, or other pathophysiologic stressors.
      (2) An investigation for these causes should be done when appropriate in a person presenting with acute chest pain.

   b. Cardiac markers.
     (1) CK-MB and cardiac troponin (troponin I and troponin T) are not clinically evident within the first 6 hours of an ischemic event.
     (2) They should therefore be checked every 8 hours three times to rule out a myocardial infarction.
     (3) Cardiac troponin levels are very specific for myocardial injury.
   c. ECG.
     (1) In STEMI, the progression begins with inverted T waves (ischemia), followed by elevated ST segments (injury), and finally Q waves (infarction).
     (2) In unstable angina/non–ST elevation MI, T wave inversion occurs, the Q waves are absent, and the ST segment can show evolving changes.
3. Imaging studies.
   a. Chest x-ray is useful in verifying the presence or absence of pulmonary congestion.
   b. Bedside echocardiography provides information related to left ventricular (LV) function and valvular morphology.
   c. Doppler echocardiography is useful in identifying postinfarction mitral regurgitation or ventricular septal defect.

Acute Care Management

1. Reperfusion therapy.
   a. STEMI.
     (1) Primary angioplasty.
       (a) Primary angioplasty is the treatment of choice for any older patient who presents within 12 hours of chest pain with a STEMI at a skilled center that can provide rapid (door to balloon <90 minutes) primary percutaneous transluminal coronary angioplasty (PTCA).
       (b) Stenting in concert with glycoprotein IIb/IIIa antagonists is the most commonly used primary percutaneous coronary intervention.
       (c) The threat of vessel occlusion has been reduced by the use of glycoprotein IIb/IIIa inhibitors (abciximab), drug-eluting (sacrolimus, paclitaxel) stents, and antithrombotic therapy (chronic acetylsalicylic acid [ASA] and clopidogrel for up to 1 year).
     (2) Thrombolytic therapy.
       (a) Thrombolytic therapy (alteplase, reteplase, tenecteplase) should be considered in persons who present within 12 hours of chest pain and in centers without onsite PTCA.
       (b) The greatest benefit is seen if thrombolytic therapy is initiated within the first 3 hours of chest pain.
       (c) Patients without STEMI do not benefit from thrombolytic therapy.
       (d) Contraindications.
         i. Previous hemorrhagic stroke.
         ii. Any stroke within the past year.
         iii. Intracranial neoplasm.
         iv. Active internal bleeding.

  (e) Relative contraindications.
        i. Systolic BP (SBP) greater than 180 mm Hg.
        ii. Major surgery within the past 3 weeks.
        iii. Diabetic retinopathy.
        iv. Use of anticoagulation.
        v. Noncompressible venipuncture.
        vi. History of hypertensive urgency.
        vii. Prior exposure or allergic reaction to streptokinase or anistreplase within the past 2 years. Streptokinase is a non–fibrin-specific thrombolytic and is not commonly used the acute management of STEMI.
  b. Unstable angina and non–ST elevation MI.
      (1) Patients with an unstable angina or non–ST elevation MI are traditionally offered either the early invasive or noninvasive approach for assessing the patient's post-MI risk.
      (2) A growing body of evidence suggests that the early invasive approach with catheterization and revascularization is superior to the noninvasive approach.
      (3) The benefits gained from the early invasive approach are most dramatic for those at highest risk of death, indicated by positive cardiac enzymes, symptoms consistent with heart failure, and ventricular arrhythmias.
      (4) The Thrombolysis in Myocardial Infarction (TIMI) risk score and Global Registry of Acute Coronary Events (GRACE) risk score identify patients who would benefit from the early invasive strategy (www.timi.org, www.umassmed.edu/outcomes/grace).
2. Pharmacologic therapy.
  a. Aspirin and clopidogrel.
      (1) Aspirin at a dose of 162 mg to 325 mg should be administered to all patients with ST elevation MI, even patients who take a daily aspirin.
      (2) Patients who have a contraindication to ASA should receive clopidogrel 300 mg as the first dose.
      (3) Patients on clopidogrel who undergo angiography need to delay surgical revascularization by 5 days.
  b. Heparin.
      (1) Heparin or low molecular weight (LMW) heparin should be started when a patient presents with ACS.
      (2) Unfractionated heparin and LMW heparin have equivalent rates of coronary deaths and coronary events in sites that can offer early intervention.
      (3) Most centers use enoxaprin 1 mg/kg subcutaneous administration q12h.
  c. Oxygen should be administered if the oxygen saturation is low (i.e., less than 92%).
  d. Morphine.
      (1) Morphine is often used in conjunction with nitrates to medically manage the chest pain of an acute MI.
      (2) Physicians should first try to control the pain with nitrates and use narcotics (morphine or meperidine) as adjunctive therapy.

   e. β-Blocker therapy.
- (1) β-Blocker therapy is beneficial in reducing short-term morbidity and mortality.
- (2) β-Blockade should be avoided in persons with:
  - (a) Decompensated heart failure.
  - (b) Severe asthma.
  - (c) Second-degree or third-degree heart block.

   f. Angiotensin converting enzyme inhibitors.
- (1) ACE inhibitors have both short-term and long-term mortality benefits.
- (2) The greatest benefit is seen in patients with:
  - (a) Low ejection fraction (EF).
  - (b) Large or anterior infarctions.
  - (c) Decompensated heart failure.

   g. Nitrates.
- (1) Nitrates reduce chest pain related to ischemia and reduce pulmonary congestion.
- (2) Nitrates do not provide a mortality benefit and should not be administered to people without chest pain.
- (3) It is important to ask male patients if they have taken phosphodiesterase inhibitors (sildenafil, vardenafil, and tadalafil) within the past 24 hours because the combination of the two can result in severe hypotension or death.

   h. CCBs.
- (1) CCBs should not be used as first-line therapy for hypertension or ischemia.
- (2) CCBs can result in increased coronary related mortality.
- (3) If CCBs are going to be administered, long-acting CCBs can be used in persons who are intolerant to β-blockers or nitrates.

   i. Statins.
- (1) Hydroxymethylglutaryl coenzyme A (HMG-CoA) reductase inhibitors (statins) should be started within the first days of an acute coronary syndrome.
- (2) More intensive therapy with atorvastatin 80 mg was shown to be effective in reducing both the short-term and long-term mortality for persons with ACS regardless of low-density lipoprotein (LDL) level.

3. Discharge therapy.
   a. Before discharge, all patients with ACS should undergo risk stratification, thereby identifying which patients might benefit from coronary angiography.
- (1) Coronary angiogram is indicated in the following circumstances:
  - (a) Recurrent ischemia.
  - (b) Hemodynamic instability.
  - (c) Ventricular arrhythmias.
  - (d) LV dysfunction.
- (2) A submaximal stress test administered prior to the discharge of patients who received thrombolytic therapy identifies which patients require a coronary angiogram.

(3) All other patients should undergo a submaximal stress test prior to discharge or a maximal stress test within 3 to 6 months after discharge.

b. Pharmacologic therapy.

(1) Pharmacologic therapy should focus on secondary prevention of coronary-related morbidity and mortality.

(2) LDL goal should be maintained below 100 mg/dL with a target goal of 70 mg/dL.

(3) Chronic β-blocker therapy improves long-term survival and should be administered to patients who do not have a contraindication to therapy.

(4) Antiplatelet therapy should include aspirin (81 mg to 325 mg daily) and clopidogrel (75 mg daily for up to 1 year).

(5) ACE inhibitors should be administered to all patients who do not have a contraindication to therapy, because trials have shown reductions in coronary events, stroke, and death.

(6) The benefit of ACE-inhibitor therapy was greatest for patients with LV dysfunction.

(7) CCBs have not been shown to improve long-term survival and should not be used in secondary prevention.

c. All patients should discontinue smoking.

d. Trials of cardiac rehabilitation programs have shown favorable effects on the long-term prognosis and should be offered to all post-MI patients.

SUGGESTED READINGS

Andersen HR, Nielsen TT, Rasmussen K, et al: A comparison of coronary angioplasty with fibrinolytic therapy in acute myocardial infarction. N Engl J Med 349:733-742, 2003.

Antman EM, Anbe DT, Armstrong PW, et al: ACC/AHA guidelines for the management of patients with ST-elevation myocardial infarction—executive summary. A report of the American College of Cardiology/American Heart Association Task Force on Practice Guidelines (Writing Committee to revise the 1999 guidelines for the Management of Patients with Acute Myocardial Infarction). J Am Coll Cardiol 44:671-719, 2004.

Becker R: Antithrombotic therapy after myocardial infarction. N Engl J Med 347:1019-1022, 2002.

Braunwald E, Antman EM, Beasley JW, et al: ACC/AHA 2002 guideline update for the management of patients with unstable angina and non-ST-segment elevation myocardial infarction—summary article: A report of the American College of Cardiology/American Heart Association Task Force on Practice Guidelines (Committee on the Management of Patients with Unstable Angina). J Am Coll Cardiol 40:1366-1374, 2002.

Cannon CP, Braunwald E, McCabe CH, et al: Intensive versus moderate lipid lowering with statins after acute coronary syndromes. N Engl J Med 350:1495-1504, 2004.

Dickstein K, Kjekshus J; OPTIMAAL Steering Committee of the OPTIMAAL Study Group: Effects of losartan and captopril on mortality and morbidity in high-risk patients after acute myocardial infarction: The OPTIMAAL randomized trial. Optimal Trial in Myocardial Infarction with Angiotensin II Antagonist Losartan. Lancet 360:752-760, 2002.

Meier MA, Al-Badr WH, Cooper JV, et al: The new definition of myocardial infarction. Arch Intern Med 162:1585-1589, 2002.

Newby LK, Kristinsson A, Bhapkar MV, et al: Early statin initiation and outcomes in patients with acute coronary syndromes. JAMA 287:3087-3095, 2002.

Rapaport E; ACC/AHA American College of Cardiology/American Hearth Association: Guidelines for the acute coronary syndromes. *Curr Cardiol Rep* 3:289-298, 2001.

Sabatine MS et al: CLARITY-TIMI 28 Investigators: Addition of Clopidogrel to Aspirin and Fibrinolyic Therapy for Myocardial Infarction with ST-segment Elevation. *N Engl J Med* 346:957-966, 2005.

Stone GW, Grines CL, Cox DA, et al: Comparison of angioplasty with stenting, with or without abciximab, in acute myocardial infarction. *N Engl J Med* 346:957, 2002.

Wiviott SD, Braunwald E: Unstable angina and non–ST-segment elevation myocardial infarction. *Am Fam Physician* 70:535-538, 2004.

ANEURYSM AND ABDOMINAL AORTA

Pranav M. Patel, Wen-Chih Wu, and Tom J. Wachtel

Definition

An abdominal aortic aneurysm (AAA) is a permanent localized dilation of the abdominal aortic artery to at least 50% when compared with the normal diameter. The normal diameter in men is 2.3 cm, and in women it is 1.9 cm.

Epidemiology

1. The incidence of AAAs has been rising from 12.2 cases/100,000 persons in 1951 to 36.2 cases/100,000 persons in 1980.
2. The prevalence ranges from 2% to 5% in men older than 60 years.
3. AAA is predominantly a disease of the elderly, affecting men more than women (4:1).
4. Rupture of an AAA is the tenth leading cause of death in men older than 55 years (15,000 deaths/year in the United States).

Clinical Findings

1. Symptoms.
   a. Abdominal pain radiating to the back, flank, and groin.
      (1) The pain is thought to be caused by rapid expansion of the aneurysm as it stretches the overlying peritoneum.
      (2) AAA must be considered in the differential of anyone presenting with abdominal pain or back pain.
   b. Early satiety, nausea, and vomiting due to compression of adjacent bowel.
   c. Rarely, flank and groin pain from ureteral obstruction and hydronephrosis.
2. Physical exam.
   a. The exam is not very sensitive for AAA smaller than 5 cm, but it has a sensitivity of 82% for detecting AAA larger than 5 cm.
   b. Pulsatile epigastric mass that may or may not be tender.
   c. Venous thrombosis from iliocaval venous compression.
   d. Discoloration and pain of the feet with distal embolization of the thrombus within the aneurysm.
   e. Shock, hypoperfusion, and abdominal distention if rupture occurs.
   f. Rare presentations include hematemesis or melena with abdominal and back pain in patients with aortoenteric fistulas. Aortocaval fistula produces loud abdominal bruits.

Etiology

1. Atherosclerosis (degenerative or nonspecific).
2. Genetic syndromes.
   a. Ehlers-Danlos syndrome.
   b. Cystic medial necrosis (Marfan's syndrome).
3. Trauma.
4. Inflammatory arteritis.
5. Mycotic, infected (septic) artery.
6. Syphilis.

Differential Diagnosis

Almost 75% of abdominal aneurysms are asymptomatic and are discovered on routine examination or serendipitously when ordering studies for other complaints. AAA should be considered in patients complaining of abdominal pain or back pain.

Work-up

1. Abdominal ultrasound.
   a. Abdominal ultrasound is nearly 100% accurate in identifying an aneurysm and estimating the size to within 0.3 to 0.4 cm.
   b. It is not very good in estimating the proximal extension to the renal arteries or involvement of the iliac arteries.
2. CT.
   a. CT scan is recommended for preoperative aneurysm imaging and estimating the size to within 0.3 mm.
   b. There are no false negatives.
   c. The CT scan can localize the proximal extent, detect the integrity of the wall, and rule out rupture.
3. Angiography.
   a. Angiography gives detailed arterial anatomy, localizing the aneurysm relative to the renal and visceral arteries.
   b. This is the definitive preoperative study for surgeons.
4. MRI can also be used, but it is more expensive and not as readily available.

Treatment

Treatment focuses on risk-factor modification (diet and exercise for BP, cholesterol, and diabetes, and abstinence from tobacco) and surgery.

1. Surveillance.
   a. Serial studies have shown that expansion rates are faster in current smokers than ex-smokers.
   b. After AAA is diagnosed, surveillance ultrasound for sizing is safe, with very low rates of AAA rupture (<1%).
   c. The most commonly used predictor of rupture is the maximum diameter of the AAA. Recommended screening intervals are shown in Table 5-25.
   d. The β-blocker propranolol has demonstrated a trend toward fewer surgeries in patients with asymptomatic small AAAs (3.0 to 5.0 cm).
2. Surgery.
   a. Abdominal aortic rupture is an emergency. Surgery is the only chance for survival.

Table 5-25 Recommended Screening Intervals for Abdominal Aortic Aneurysm

Baseline Diameter	Screening Interval (months)
<3.5 cm	36
4.0 cm	24
4.5 cm	12
5 cm	3

b. Vascular surgical referral should be made in asymptomatic patients with aneurysms 4 cm or greater or in rapidly expanding aneurysms (expansion rate of 0.7 to 1 cm/year), especially if symptoms are present.

c. Recent randomized trials found no reduction in mortality from repairing AAAs smaller than 5.5 cm in patients at low operative risk.

d. Prophylactic surgery is recommended for AAA larger than 5.5 cm.

e. For aneurysms 5.5 cm or greater, prosthetic graft replacement is recommended, providing there is no contraindication (e.g., MI within 6 months, refractory CHF, life expectancy <2 years, severe sequelae from cerebrovascular accident, severe dementia).

f. For the high-risk patient deemed unsuitable for prosthetic graft, endovascular stent-anchored grafts under local anesthesia have provided an alternative approach.

g. Infrarenal AAAs.
   (1) Most AAAs are infrarenal.
   (2) Surgical risk is increased in patients with:
      (a) Coexisting CAD.
      (b) Pulmonary disease (PaO_2 <50 mm Hg, forced expiratory volume in one second [FEV_1] <11).
      (c) Liver cirrhosis.
      (d) Chronic renal failure (creatinine >3 mg/dL).

h. Cardiac preoperative evaluation with radionuclide perfusion studies for ischemia and aggressive perioperative hemodynamic monitoring help identify high-risk patients and decrease postoperative complications.

i. In patients with dementia, postoperative delirium should be anticipated and managed.

Prognosis

1. It is estimated that AAAs smaller than 5 cm expand at a rate of 0.4 cm/year.
2. Risk of rupture.
   a. The risk of rupture is 0% per year in aneurysms smaller than 4 cm.
   b. Risk is 0.6% to 1%/year in aneurysms 4.0 to 5.5 cm.
   c. Risk is 4.4%/year in aneurysms 5.5 to 5.9 cm.
   d. Risk is 10.2%/year in aneurysms 6.0 to 6.9 cm.
   e. Risk is 32.5%/year in aneurysms larger than 7 cm in diameter.

3. Mortality.
    a. Mortality after rupture is greater than 90%.
    b. Of those patients who reach the hospital, it is estimated 50% will survive.
    c. Elective repair of the nonruptured aorta has a 4% mortality rate.

SUGGESTED READINGS

Lederle FA, Wilson SE, Johnson GR, et al: Immediate repair compared with surveillance of small abdominal aortic aneurysms, *N Engl J Med* 346:1437-1444, 2002.

Lederle FA, Johnson GR, Wilson SE, et al: Rupture rate of large abdominal aortic aneurysms in patients refusing or unfit for elective repair, *JAMA* 287:2968-2972, 2002.

Lederle FA: Ultrasonographic screening for abdominal aortic aneurysm. *Ann Intern Med* 139:516-522, 2003.

Powell J, Brady A: Detection, management and prospects for medical treatment of small abdominal aortic aneurysms. *Arterioscler Thromb Vasc Biol* 24:241-245, 2004.

Powell J, Greenhalgh R: Clinical practice. Small abdominal aortic aneurysms. *N Engl J Med* 348:1895-1901, 2003.

The Propranolol Aneurysm Trial Investigators: Propranolol for small abdominal aortic aneurysms: Results of a randomized trial. *J Vasc Surg* 35:72-79, 2002.

Sparks AR, Johnson PL, Meyer MC: Imaging of abdominal aortic aneurysms. *Am Fam Physician* 65:1565-1570, 2002.

The United Kingdom Small Aneurysm Trial Participants: Long-term outcomes of immediate repair compared with surveillance of small abdominal aortic aneurysms. *N Engl J Med* 346:1445-1452, 2002.

AORTIC DISSECTION
Lynn Bowlby and Tom J. Wachtel

Definition
Aortic dissection occurs when an intimal tear allows blood to dissect between medial layers of the aorta. The term "dissecting aneurysm" should not be used because a dissection is not an aneurysm.

Classification
Because the majority of aortic dissections originate in the ascending or descending aorta, there are two major classifications.
1. DeBakey (Fig. 5-9).
    a. Type I ascending and descending aorta.
    b. Type II ascending aorta.
    c. Type III descending aorta.
2. Stanford.
    a. Type A ascending aorta (proximal).
    b. Type B descending aorta (distal).

Epidemiology
1. Predominant sex: Male more than female.
2. Peak incidence: Ages 60 to 80 years.
3. Risk factors.
    a. Hypertension, atherosclerosis, and family history of aortic aneurysms.
    b. Inflammatory diseases that cause a vasculitis.
    c. Disorders of collagen (Marfan's syndrome, Ehlers-Danlos syndrome).
    d. Bicuspid aortic valve.

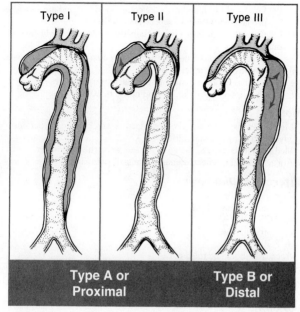

Figure 5-9 Classification systems for aortic dissection. (From Isselbacher EM, Eagle KA, DeSanctis RW: Disease of the aorta. In Braunwald E [ed]: *Heart disease: a textbook of cardiovascular medicine*, ed 5. Philadelphia, WB Saunders, 1997.)

    e. Aortic coarctation.
    f. Turner's syndrome.
    g. Crack cocaine.
    h. Trauma.

Clinical Findings

1. History.
    a. Sudden onset of very severe chest pain. Pain is at its peak at onset, differentiating it from angina, which is usually crescendo-decrescendo.
    b. Little radiation to neck, shoulder, or arm.
    c. Sharp, tearing, or ripping pain.
    d. Ascending aortic dissection with anterior chest pain.
    e. Descending aortic dissection with back pain.
    f. Syncope, abdominal pain, CHF, and malperfusion may occur.
2. Physical exam.
    a. BP.
        (1) Most patients have severe hypertension.
        (2) About 25% have hypotension (SBP <100), which can indicate bleeding, cardiac tamponade, or severe aortic regurgitation.

(3) Pulse and BP differentials are common (38%) and are caused by partial compression of subclavian arteries.

b. Cardiac and neurologic systems are the most commonly involved organ systems.

c. Aortic regurgitation occurs in 18% to 50% of cases of proximal dissection.

d. Pericarditis occurs in less than 5%.

e. Myocardial ischemia caused by coronary artery compression.

f. Cerebral ischemia/stroke is found in 5% to 10% of patients.

Etiology

1. Mechanism is unknown, but risk factors are known. Hypertension affects arterial wall composition.
2. Medial degeneration of the aorta appears to be the culprit.
3. Aortic dissection reflects systemic illness of vasculature.

Differential Diagnosis

1. Aortic dissection is known as a great imitator.
   a. Pulmonary embolism.
   b. ACS.
   c. Aortic stenosis.
   d. Pericarditis.
2. Acute MI should be ruled out.
3. Other causes of chest pain (e.g., esophageal spasm, costochondritis, anxiety disorders).
4. Aortic aneurysm.

Work-up

1. ECG is helpful to rule out MI, but findings are generally nonspecific.
2. Laboratory tests.
   a. CBC, cardiac enzymes, oxygen saturation.
   b. Serum biochemical marker: Smooth muscle myosin heavy chain is high in the first 6 hours after onset.
3. Imaging studies.
   a. Chest x-ray might show nonspecific widened mediastinum (62%) and displacement of aortic intimal calcium.
   b. Transesophageal echocardiography.
      (1) Transesophageal echocardiography has a sensitivity 97% to 100%.
      (2) It can detect aortic insufficiency and pericardial effusion.
      (3) It is the study of choice in unstable patients, but it is operator dependent.
   c. MRI.
      (1) Sensitivity is 90% to 100%.
      (2) MRI is the gold standard.
      (3) The length of the test and difficult access are not suitable for unstable patients.
      (4) MRI gives best information for surgeons.
   d. CT.
      (1) Sensitivity 83% to 100%.
      (2) Involves IV contrast.
   e. Aortography is rarely done anymore.
   f. Transthoracic echocardiography has poor sensitivity.

Treatment

1. Medical.
   a. Admit the patient to the intensive care unit for hemodynamic monitoring.
   b. Distal dissections are treated only medically unless distal organ ischemia or impending rupture occurs (type III or B).
   c. Chronic aortic dissection (>2 weeks) is followed with aggressive BP control.
2. Pharmacologic.
   a. Propanolol 1 mg every 3 to 5 minutes or metoprolol 5 mg IV every 5 minutes, followed by nitroprusside 0.3 to 10 mg/kg/min, with target SBP 100 to 120 mm Hg.
   b. Decrease contractility and BP with IV β-blocker; β-blocker is the cornerstone of treatment.
   c. IV labetalol can be used instead, 20 mg IV, then 40 to 80 mg every 10 minutes.
   d. IV CCBs or ACE inhibitors may be used.
3. Surgical.
   a. Proximal dissections (DeBakey type I, II or Stanford type A) require emergent surgery to prevent rupture or pericardial effusion.
   b. Endovascular stent placement is a new treatment, especially for older high-risk surgical patients.

Prognosis

1. Natural history of untreated aortic dissection is 85% mortality within 2 weeks.
2. Proximal aortic dissection is a surgical emergency. Time is critical; mortality is 1% to 3% per hour.
3. Patients who have had surgical repair or have a chronic aneurysm should be followed with imaging at 1, 3, 6, 9, and 12 months.
4. Overall, in-hospital mortality is 30% in patients with proximal dissections and 10% in patients with distal dissections.

SUGGESTED READINGS

Hagan PG, Nienaber CA, Isselbacher EM, et al: The International Registry of Acute Aortic Dissection: New insights into an old disease. *JAMA* 283:897-903, 2000.

Khan IA, Nair CK: Clinical, diagnostic, and management perspectives of aortic dissection. *Chest* 122(1):311-328, 2002.

Moore AG, et al: Choice of computed tomography, transesophageal echocardiography, magnetic resonance imaging, and aortography in acute aortic dissection: International Registry of Acute Aortic Dissection (IRAD). *Am J Cardiol* 89:1235-1238, 2002.

Nienaber CA, Eagle KA: Aortic dissection: New frontiers in diagnosis and management. Part I: From etiology to diagnostic strategies. *Circulation*, 108(6):628-635, 2003.

Nienaber CA, Eagle KA: Aortic dissection: New frontiers in diagnosis and management. Part II: Therapeutic management and follow-up. *Circulation* 108(6): 772-778, 2003.

AORTIC REGURGITATION

Fred F. Ferri

Definition

Aortic regurgitation is retrograde blood flow into the left ventricle from the aorta secondary to an incompetent aortic valve.

Epidemiology

1. The most common cause of isolated severe aortic regurgitation is aortic root dilation. Other causes include a congenital bicuspid valve, rheumatic fever, connective tissue diseases, and aortitis including syphilis.
2. Infectious endocarditis is also a common cause of acute aortic regurgitation.

Clinical Findings

The clinical presentation varies depending on whether aortic insufficiency is acute or chronic.

1. Chronic aortic insufficiency.
   a. Chronic aortic insufficiency is well tolerated except when it is secondary to infective endocarditis, and these patients remain asymptomatic for years.
   b. Common manifestations after significant deterioration of LV function are:
      (1) Dyspnea on exertion.
      (2) Syncope.
      (3) Chest pain.
      (4) CHF.
   c. Physical findings.
      (1) Widened pulse pressure.
         (a) Markedly increased SBP.
         (b) Decreased diastolic BP (DBP).
      (2) Bounding pulses, head bobbing with each systole (de Musset's sign).
      (3) Water hammer or collapsing pulse (Corrigan's pulse) can be palpated at the wrist or on the femoral arteries (pistol shot femoral pulse) and is caused by rapid rise and sudden collapse of the arterial pressure during late systole.
      (4) Capillary pulsations (Quincke's pulse) can occur at the base of the nail beds.
      (5) A to-and-fro double Duroziez's murmur may be heard over femoral arteries with slight compression.
      (6) Popliteal systolic pressure is increased over brachial systolic pressure by least 40 mm Hg (Hill's sign).
      (7) Cardiac auscultation reveals:
         (a) Displacement of cardiac impulse downward and to the patient's left.
         (b) S_3 heard over the apex.
         (c) Decrescendo, blowing diastolic murmur heard along left sternal border.
         (d) Low-pitched apical diastolic rumble (Austin Flint murmur) caused by contrast of the aortic regurgitant jet with the LV wall.
         (e) Early systolic apical ejection murmur.
2. Acute aortic insufficiency.
   a. In patients with acute aortic insufficiency, both the wide pulse pressure and the large stroke volume are absent.

b. A short blowing diastolic murmur may be the only finding on physical examination.

c. Acute aortic insufficiency manifests primarily with hypotension caused by a sudden fall in cardiac output.

d. A rapid rise in LV diastolic pressure results in a further decrease in coronary blood flow.

Etiology

1. Infective endocarditis.
2. Rheumatic fibrosis.
3. Trauma with valvular rupture.
4. Congenital bicuspid aortic valve.
5. Myxomatous degeneration.
6. Syphilitic aortitis.
7. Rheumatic spondylitis.
8. SLE.
9. Aortic dissection.
10. Takayasu's arteritis, granulomatous arteritis.

Differential Diagnosis

1. Patent ductus arteriosus.
2. Pulmonary regurgitation.
3. Other valvular abnormalities.

Work-up

1. Medical history and physical examination focus on the following clinical manifestations:
   a. Dyspnea on exertion.
   b. Syncope.
   c. Chest pain.
   d. CHF.
2. Chest x-ray.
   a. LV hypertrophy (chronic aortic regurgitation).
   b. Aortic dilation.
   c. Normal cardiac silhouette with pulmonary edema is possible in patients with acute aortic regurgitation.
3. ECG: LV hypertrophy.
4. Echocardiography.
   a. Coarse diastolic fluttering of the anterior mitral leaflet.
   b. LV hypertrophy in patients with chronic aortic regurgitation
5. Cardiac catheterization.
   a. Assesses degree of LV dysfunction.
   b. Confirms the presence of a wide pulse pressure.
   c. Assesses surgical risk.
   d. Determines if there is coexistent CAD.

Treatment

1. Medical therapy.
   a. Digitalis, diuretics, ACE inhibitors, and sodium restriction for CHF.
   b. Nitroprusside in patients with acute aortic regurgitation.
   c. Long-term vasodilator therapy with ACE inhibitors or nifedipine for reducing or delaying the need for aortic valve replacement in

   asymptomatic patients with severe aortic regurgitation and normal
   LV function.
   d. Bacterial endocarditis prophylaxis for surgical and dental procedures.
2. Surgery is reserved for:
   a. Symptomatic patients with chronic aortic regurgitation despite
      optimal medical therapy.
   b. Patients with acute aortic regurgitation (infective endocarditis)
      producing LV failure.
   c. Evidence of LV systolic failure.
      (1) Echocardiographic fractional shortening greater than 25%.
      (2) Echocardiographic diastolic dimension greater than 55 mm.
      (3) Angiographic ejection fraction less than 50% or end-systolic
          volume index greater than 60 mL/m².
   d. Evidence of diastolic failure.
      (1) Pulmonary pressure greater than 45 mm Hg systolic.
      (2) LV end-diastolic pressure greater than 15 mm Hg at catheter-
          ization.
      (3) Pulmonary hypertension detected on examination.
   e. In general, the "55 rule" has been used to determine the timing
      of surgery: Surgery should be performed before ejection fraction
      falls to less than 55% or end-systolic dimension increases to greater
      than 55 mm.
   f. The operative mortality rate for aortic regurgitation is 3% to 5%.

AORTIC STENOSIS

Fred F. Ferri and Tom J. Wachtel

Definitions

1. Aortic stenosis (AS) is obstruction to systolic LV outflow across the
   aortic valve.
2. Symptoms appear when the valve orifice decreases to less than 1 cm²
   (normal orifice is 3 cm²).
3. The stenosis is considered severe when the orifice is less than 0.5 cm²
   or the pressure gradient is 50 mm Hg or higher.

Epidemiology

1. AS is the most common valve lesion in adults in Western countries.
2. Calcific stenosis (most common cause in patients older than 60 years)
   occurs in 75% of patients.

Clinical Findings

1. A rough, loud systolic diamond-shaped murmur.
   a. Best heard at the base of the heart and transmitted into the neck
      vessels.
   b. Often associated with a thrill or ejection click.
   c. Might also be heard well at the apex.
2. Absence or diminished intensity of sound of aortic valve closure
   (in severe AS).
3. Late, slow-rising carotid upstroke with decreased amplitude.
4. Strong apical pulse.
5. Narrowing of pulse pressure in later stages of AS.

6. Some patients with AS experience bleeding into the gastrointestinal tract or skin. This is caused by an acquired defect in von Willebrand's factor. Aortic valve replacement restores normal hemostasis.

Etiology

1. Rheumatic inflammation of aortic valve.
2. Progressive stenosis of congenital bicuspid valve (found in 1% to 2% of population).
3. Idiopathic calcification of the aortic valve.
4. Congenital.

Differential Diagnosis

1. Hypertrophic cardiomyopathy.
2. Mitral regurgitation.
3. Ventricular septal defect.
4. Aortic sclerosis.
   a. AS is distinguished from aortic sclerosis by the degree of valve impairment.
   b. In aortic sclerosis, the valve leaflets are abnormally thickened, but obstruction to outflow is minimal.

Work-up

1. Medical history focusing on symptoms and potential complications:
   a. Angina.
   b. Syncope (particularly with exertion).
   c. CHF.
   d. Gastrointestinal bleeding in patients with associated hemorrhagic telangiectasia (arteriovenous [AV] malformation).
2. Chest x-ray examination.
   a. Poststenotic dilation of the ascending aorta.
   b. Calcification of aortic cusps.
   c. Pulmonary congestion (in advanced stages of aortic stenosis).
3. ECG.
   a. LV hypertrophy is found in more than 80% of patients.
   b. ST-T wave changes.
   c. Atrial fibrillation is common.
4. Doppler echocardiography.
   a. Thickening of the LV wall.
   b. If the patient has valvular calcifications, multiple echoes may be seen from within the aortic root and there is poor separation of the aortic cusps during systole.
   c. Gradient across the valve can be estimated but is less precise than with cardiac catheterization.
5. Cardiac catheterization.
   a. Indicated in symptomatic patients.
   b. It confirms the diagnosis and estimates the severity of the disease by measuring the gradient across the valve, allowing calculation of the valve area.
   c. It also detects coexisting coronary artery stenosis that might need bypass at the same time as aortic valve replacement.

Treatment

1. Medical.
   a. Diuretics and sodium restriction are needed if CHF is present; digoxin is used only to control rate of atrial fibrillation.
   b. ACE inhibitors are relatively contraindicated.
   c. CCB verapamil may be useful only to control rate of atrial fibrillation.
   d. Antibiotic prophylaxis is necessary for surgical and dental procedures.
2. Surgical.
   a. Valve replacement.
      (1) Valve replacement is the treatment of choice in symptomatic patients because the 5-year mortality rate after onset of symptoms is extremely high, even with optimal medical therapy.
      (2) Valve replacement is indicated if cardiac catheterization establishes a pressure gradient greater than 50 mm Hg and valve area less than 1 cm^2.
      (3) The surgical mortality rate for valve replacement is 3% to 5%; however, it varies with the patient's age (>8% in patients older than 75 years).
   b. Balloon aortic valvotomy for adult acquired aortic stenosis is useful only for short-term reduction in severity of aortic stenosis when surgery is contraindicated, because restenosis occurs rapidly.

Prognosis

1. The 5-year survival rate in adults is 40%.
2. The average duration of symptoms before death is as follows:
   a. Angina, 60 months.
   b. Syncope, 36 months.
   c. CHF, 24 months.
3. About 75% of patients with symptomatic aortic stenosis will be dead 3 years after onset of symptoms unless the aortic valve is replaced.

SUGGESTED READINGS

Alpert JS: Aortic stenosis: A new face for an old disease. *Arch Intern Med* 163: 1769-1770, 2003.
Carabello BA: Clinical practice: Aortic stenosis. *N Engl J Med* 346:677-682, 2002.

ATRIAL FIBRILLATION

Fred F. Ferri and Tom J. Wachtel

Definition

Atrial fibrillation is chaotic atrial activity caused by simultaneous discharge of multiple atrial foci.

Epidemiology

The prevalence of atrial fibrillation increases with age. It is 2% in the general population, 5% in patients older than 60 years, and 9% of those 80 years or older.

Clinical Findings

1. Patients are commonly asymptomatic.

2. Most common complaint is palpitations.
3. Fatigue, dizziness, and lightheadedness occur in some patients.
4. CHF (often diastolic).
5. Cardiac auscultation reveals irregularly irregular rhythm.

Etiology

1. Idiopathic ("lone" atrial fibrillation).
2. CAD.
3. Mitral and/or aortic valve disease.
4. Thyrotoxicosis.
5. Pneumonia.
6. Pulmonary embolism.
7. COPD.
8. Pericarditis.
9. Myocarditis, cardiomyopathy.
10. Tachycardia-bradycardia syndrome.
11. Alcohol abuse ("holiday heart").
12. MI.
13. Wolff-Parkinson-White syndrome.
14. Other causes.
   a. Left atrial myxoma.
   b. Atrial septal defect.
   c. Carbon monoxide poisoning.
   d. Pheochromocytoma.
   e. Hypoxia.
   f. Hypokalemia.
   g. Sepsis.

Work-up

1. Thyroid stimulating hormone, CBC, glucose, creatinine, sodium, potassium, ALT, alkaline phosphatase, calcium.
2. ECG.
   a. Irregular, nonperiodic wave forms (best seen in V_1) reflecting continuous atrial reentry.
   b. Absence of P waves.
   c. Conducted QRS complexes showing no periodicity.
3. Echocardiography to evaluate left atrial size and detect valvular disorders in all patients.
4. Holter monitoring is useful only in selected patients to evaluate paroxysmal atrial fibrillation.

Treatment
General Principles[1]

The American Academy of Family Physicians and the American College of Physicians provide the following recommendations for the management of newly detected atrial fibrillation.

1. Rate control with chronic anticoagulation is the recommended strategy for the majority of patients with atrial fibrillation.
   a. Rhythm control has not been shown to be superior to rate control (with chronic anticoagulation) in reducing morbidity and mortality and may be inferior in some patient subgroups to rate control.

    b. Rhythm control is appropriate when based on other special considerations, such as patient symptoms and exercise tolerance.

2. Patients with atrial fibrillation should receive chronic anticoagulation with adjusted-dose warfarin unless they are at low risk for stroke or have a specific contraindication to the use of warfarin, including:
   a. Thrombocytopenia.
   b. Recent trauma or surgery.
   c. Alcoholism.
   d. Very old age with frailty and fall risk.
3. Rate-control medication.
   a. The following drugs are recommended for their demonstrated efficacy in rate control during exercise and while at rest (drugs listed alphabetically within class):
      (1) Atenolol.
      (2) Metoprolol.
      (3) Diltiazem.
      (4) Verapamil.
   b. Digoxin is only effective for rate control at rest and therefore should only be used as a second-line agent for rate control in atrial fibrillation.
4. For patients who elect to undergo acute cardioversion to achieve sinus rhythm in atrial fibrillation, both direct-current cardioversion and pharmacologic conversion are appropriate options.
5. Either of the following management strategies is appropriate for patients who elect to undergo cardioversion.
   a. Transesophageal echocardiography with short-term prior anticoagulation followed by early acute cardioversion (in the absence of intracardiac thrombus) with postcardioversion anticoagulation.
   b. Delayed cardioversion with pre- and postcardioversion anticoagulation.
6. Maintenance therapy.
   a. Most patients converted to sinus rhythm from atrial fibrillation should not be placed on rhythm maintenance therapy because the risks outweigh the benefits.
   b. In a selected group of patients whose quality of life is compromised by atrial fibrillation, the recommended pharmacologic agents for rhythm maintenance are amiodarone, disopyramide, propafenone, and sotalol (drugs listed in alphabetical order).
   c. The choice of agent depends on the specific risk of side effects based on patient characteristics.

Nonpharmacologic Therapy

1. Avoidance of alcohol in patients with suspected excessive alcohol use.
2. Avoidance of caffeine and nicotine.

Pharmacologic Therapy

1. New-onset atrial fibrillation.
   a. Cardioversion in the hemodynamically unstable patient.
      (1) Emergency synchronized cardioversion may be required following immediate conscious sedation with a rapid, short-acting sedative (e.g., midazolam).
      (2) Cardioversion is indicated if the ventricular rate is higher than 140 bpm and the patient is symptomatic (particularly in acute

MI or with chest pain, dyspnea, CHF) or when there is no conversion to normal sinus rhythm after 3 days of pharmacologic therapy.

(3) Clinical thromboembolism following cardioversion.

   (a) The likelihood of cardioversion-related clinical thromboembolism is low in patients with atrial fibrillation lasting less than 48 hours.

   (b) Patients with atrial fibrillation lasting longer than 2 days have a 5% to 7% risk of clinical thromboembolism if cardioversion is not preceded by several weeks of warfarin therapy.

   (c) If transesophageal echocardiography reveals no atrial thrombus, cardioversion may be performed safely after only a short period of anticoagulant therapy.

   (d) Anticoagulant therapy should be continued for at least 1 month after cardioversion to minimize the incidence of adverse thromboembolic events following conversion from atrial fibrillation to sinus rhythm.

b. If the patient is hemodynamically stable, treatment options include the following in a hospital setting:

(1) Diltiazem.

   (a) IV diltiazem 0.25 mg/kg given over 2 minutes, followed by a second dose of 0.35 mg/kg 15 minutes later if the rate is not slowed.

   (b) May then follow with IV infusion 10 mg/h (range, 5-15 mg/hour).

   (c) Onset of action following IV administration is usually within 3 minutes, with peak effect most often occurring within 10 minutes.

   (d) After the ventricular rate is slowed, the patient can be changed to oral diltiazem 60 to 90 mg q6h.

(2) Verapamil.

   (a) IV verapamil 2.5 to 5 mg initially, then 5 to 10 mg IV 10 minutes later if the rate is still not slowed.

   (b) After the ventricular rate is slowed, the patient can be changed to oral verapamil 80 to 120 mg q6-8h.

(3) Esmolol, metoprolol, and atenolol are β-blockers that are available in IV preparations that can be used in atrial fibrillation.

(4) Other medications useful for converting atrial fibrillation to sinus rhythm are ibutilide, flecainide, propafenone, disopyramide, amiodarone, and quinidine.

(5) Digoxin.

   (a) Digoxin is not a very potent AV-nodal blocking agent and cannot be relied upon for acute control of the ventricular response.

   (b) Give 0.5 mg IV loading dose (slow), then 0.25 mg IV 6 hours later.

   (c) A third dose may be needed after 6 to 8 hours.

   (d) The daily dose varies from 0.125 to 0.25 mg (decrease dosage in patients with renal insufficiency and in elderly patients).

   (e) Digoxin should be avoided in Wolff-Parkinson-White patients with atrial fibrillation. Procainamide is the preferred pharmacologic agent in these patients.

  (6) Loop diuretics and oxygen are used for CHF.

  (7) If the patient is asymptomatic or if the only symptom is palpitation or mild CHF, treatment may be initiated on an outpatient basis with any of the above medications given orally.

2. IV heparin or SC LMW heparin.
 a. For hospitalized patients.
 b. Sometimes omitted for outpatients.

3. Anticoagulate with warfarin (unless the patient has specific contraindications).

4. Long-term anticoagulation.
 a. Long-term anticoagulation with warfarin (adjusted to maintain an international normalized ratio of 2 to 3) is indicated in all patients with atrial fibrillation.
 b. The safety of long-term anticoagulation with warfarin in the long-term care setting and in very old patients is not established and should therefore be individualized.
 c. The risk of hemorrhage (particularly intracranial) is increased by the propensity to fall and by cerebral atrophy, which stretches subdural veins.

5. Aspirin 325 mg/day may be a suitable alternative to warfarin in patients older than 70 years of age with increased risk of bleeding.

6. The efficacy of clopidogrel (Plavix) is not known.

7. Medical cardioversion.
 a. Attempts at medical (pharmacologic) intervention should be considered only after proper anticoagulation because cardioversion can lead to systemic emboli. Following successful cardioversion, anticoagulation with warfarin should be continued for 4 weeks. However, spontaneous cardioversion can occur any time.
 b. Useful agents for medical cardioversion are quinidine, flecainide, propafenone, amiodarone, ibutilide, sotalol, dofetilide, and procainamide.
 c. Amiodarone.
  (1) Amiodarone appears to be the most effective agent for converting to sinus rhythm in patients who do not respond to other agents.
  (2) Amiodarone therapy should be considered for patients with recent atrial fibrillation and structural heart disease, particularly those with LV dysfunction.
  (3) Amiodarone should also be considered for patients with refractory conditions who do not have heart disease, before therapies with irreversible effects such as AV nodal ablation are attempted.
 d. Factors associated with maintenance of sinus rhythm following cardioversion.
  (1) Left atrium diameter less than 60 mm.
  (2) Absence of mitral valve disease.
  (3) Short duration of atrial fibrillation.

8. Catheter-based radiofrequency ablation procedures designed to eliminate atrial fibrillation represent newer approaches to atrial fibrillation.

9. Implantable pacemakers and defibrillators.
   a. These devices combine pacing and cardioversion therapies to prevent and treat atrial fibrillation.
   b. They are likely to have an increasing role in the management of atrial fibrillation.

REFERENCE

1. Adapted from Snow V, Weiss KB, Lefevre M, et al: Management of newly detected atrial fibrillation: A clinical practice guideline from the American Academy of Family Physicians and the American College of Physicians. *Ann Intern Med* 139(12):1009-1017, 2003.

SUGGESTED READINGS

Cooper JM, Katcher MS, Orlov MV: Implantable devices for the treatment of atrial fibrillation, *N Engl J Med* 346:2062-2068, 2002.

Ezekowitz M, Falk RH: The increasing need for anticoagulation therapy to prevent stroke in patients with atrial fibrillation. *Mayo Clin Proc* 79(7):904-913, 2004.

Falk RH: Atrial fibrillation. *N Engl J Med* 344:1067-1078, 2001.

Hart RG: Atrial fibrillation and stroke prevention. *N Engl J Med* 349:1015-1016, 2003.

Hylek EM, Go AS, Chang Y, et al: Effect of intensity of oral anticoagulation on stroke severity and mortality in atrial fibrillation. *N Engl J Med* 349:1019-1026, 2003.

Klein AL, Grimm RA, Murray RD, et al: Use of transesophageal echocardiography to guide cardioversions in patients with atrial fibrillation. *N Engl J Med* 344:1411-1420, 2001.

Snow V, Weiss KB, Lefevre M, et al: Management of newly detected atrial fibrillation: A clinical practice guideline from the American Academy of Family Physicians and the American College of Physicians. *Ann Intern Med* 139(12):1009-1017, 2003.

CONGESTIVE HEART FAILURE

Fred F. Ferri and Tom J. Wachtel

Definitions

1. Congestive heart failure (CHF) is a pathophysiologic state characterized by congestion in the pulmonary or systemic circulation. It is caused by the heart's inability to pump sufficient oxygenated blood to meet the metabolic needs of the tissues.
2. The American College of Cardiology and the American Heart Association describe the following four stages of heart failure:
   a. At high risk for heart failure, but without structural heart disease or symptoms of heart failure (e.g., CAD, hypertension).
   b. Structural heart disease but without symptoms of heart failure.
   c. Structural heart disease with prior or current symptoms of heart failure.
   d. Refractory heart failure requiring specialized interventions.
3. The New York Heart Association (NYHA) defines the following functional classes:
   a. Asymptomatic.
   b. Symptomatic with moderate exertion.
   c. Symptomatic with minimal exertion.
   d. Symptomatic at rest.

Epidemiology

1. Annual mortality ranges from 10% in stable patients with mild symptoms to more than 50% in symptomatic patients with advanced disease.

2. CHF is the most common admission diagnosis (20%) in elderly patients.
3. Heart failure occurs in 4.7 million persons in the United States and is the discharge diagnosis in 3.5 million hospitalizations annually.
4. One in three patients with CHF has diastolic heart failure.
   a. The ratio increases with age. The highest incidence is in patients older than 75 years.
   b. The mortality rate is about half that of systolic heart failure.
   c. Morbidity (e.g., hospitalization) is the same for diastolic and systolic heart failure.

Clinical Findings

1. Symptoms.
   a. Dyspnea on exertion initially, then with progressively less strenuous activity, and eventually manifesting when the patient is at rest. Dyspnea is caused by increasing pulmonary congestion.
   b. Orthopnea caused by increased venous return in the recumbent position.
   c. Paroxysmal nocturnal dyspnea (PND) resulting from multiple factors.
      (1) Increased venous return in the recumbent position.
      (2) Decreased PaO_2.
      (3) Decreased adrenergic stimulation of myocardial function.
   d. Fatigue, reduced exercise tolerance, lethargy resulting from low cardiac output, deterioration in activities of daily living.
   e. Cognitive impairment, new, or worsening of underlying dementia (delirium).
2. Physical exam.
   a. Patients with left heart failure might have the following abnormalities on physical examination:
      (1) Pulmonary rales.
      (2) Tachypnea.
      (3) S_3 gallop.
      (4) Cardiac murmurs.
         (a) Aortic stenosis.
         (b) Aortic regurgitation.
         (c) Mitral regurgitation (MR).
      (5) Paradoxical splitting of S_2.
   b. Patients with right heart failure present with:
      (1) Jugular venous distention.
      (2) Peripheral edema.
      (3) Perioral and peripheral cyanosis.
      (4) Congestive hepatomegaly.
      (5) Ascites.
      (6) Hepatojugular reflux.
   c. In patients with heart failure, elevated jugular venous pressure and a third heart sound each are independently associated with adverse outcomes.
   d. Acute precipitants of CHF exacerbations include:
      (1) Noncompliance with salt restriction.
      (2) Pulmonary infections.
      (3) Arrhythmias.

(4) Medications (e.g., CCBs, antiarrhythmic agents).
(5) Failed attempts at reductions in CHF therapy.

Etiology

1. LV failure.
   a. Systemic hypertension.
   b. Valvular heart disease (AS, aortic regurgitation, MR).
   c. Cardiomyopathy, myocarditis.
   d. Bacterial endocarditis.
   e. Myocardial infarction.
   f. Idiopathic hypertrophic subaortic stenosis (IHSS).
   g. LV failure is further differentiated according to systolic dysfunction (low ejection fraction) and diastolic dysfunction (normal or high ejection fraction), or "stiff ventricle."
      (1) It is important to make this distinction because treatment is different (see "Treatment").
      (2) Patients with heart failure and a normal ejection fraction have abnormalities in active relaxation and passive stiffness.
      (3) Normal ejection fraction is usually defined as greater than 50%.
      (4) An ejection fraction lower than 40% suggests systolic heart failure.
      (5) Both mechanisms of LV failure can coexist.
   h. Patients with diastolic heart failure have low stroke volume despite normal ejection fraction.
   i. Passive stiffness caused by:
      (1) Increased myocardial mass (hypertensive patient).
      (2) Alteration in collagen (CAD patient).
   j. Impaired active relaxation: When chamber compliance is reduced, a small increase in blood volume causes a large increase in left atrial pressure.
   k. Tachycardia.
      (1) Tachycardia may be somewhat helpful to patients with systolic dysfunction, but it is deleterious when the cause of heart failure is diastolic dysfunction.
      (2) A stiff ventricle needs more time to fill during diastole.
      (3) Thus, tachycardia is similar in effect to a pump that loses its prime.
   l. Common causes of systolic dysfunction.
      (1) Myocardial infarction.
      (2) Cardiomyopathy.
      (3) Myocarditis.
   m. Causes of diastolic dysfunction.
      (1) Hypertensive cardiovascular disease.
      (2) Restrictive cardiomyopathy.
      (3) Ischemic heart disease.
2. Right ventricular (RV) failure.
   a. Valvular heart disease (mitral stenosis).
   b. Pulmonary hypertension.
   c. Bacterial endocarditis (right-sided).
   d. RV infarction.
3. Biventricular failure.
   a. LV failure.

   b. Cardiomyopathy.
   c. Myocarditis.
   d. Arrhythmias.
   e. Anemia.
   f. Thyrotoxicosis.
   g. AV fistula.
   h. Paget's disease of bone.

Precipitants of Heart Failure

1. Uncontrolled hypertension.
2. Atrial fibrillation and other causes of tachycardia (particularly important in diastolic heart failure).
3. Myocardial ischemia.
4. Medication noncompliance.
5. Dietary noncompliance (salt).
6. Anemia.
7. Renal failure.
8. Hypoxia.
9. NSAIDs including cyclooxygenase-2 (COX-2) inhibitors.
10. Thioglitazones.

Work-up

1. Laboratory.
   a. CBC.
   b. BUN, creatinine, sodium, and potassium.
   c. ALT and alkaline phosphatase.
   d. TSH.
   e. Cardiac enzymes (for acute decompensation).
   f. B-type natriuretic peptide (BNP).
      (1) BNP is a cardiac neurohormone specifically secreted from the ventricles in response to volume expansion and pressure overload.
      (2) Elevated levels indicate CHF.
      (3) Bedside measurement of BNP is useful in establishing or excluding the diagnosis of CHF in patients with acute dyspnea.
2. Standard 12-lead ECG is useful to diagnose ischemic heart disease and obtain information about rhythm abnormalities.
3. Chest x-ray examination can reveal:
   a. Pulmonary venous congestion.
   b. Cardiomegaly with dilation of the involved heart chamber.
   c. Pleural effusions.
4. Echocardiography.
   a. Two-dimensional echocardiography is critical to assess global and regional LV function and estimate ejection fraction.
   b. The current standard of care requires echocardiography as part of the management of CHF.
5. Exercise stress testing may be useful for evaluating concomitant coronary disease and assessing degree of disability in selected patients.
6. Cardiac catheterization.
   a. Cardiac catheterization is an excellent way to evaluate ventricular diastolic properties, significant CAD, or valvular heart disease.
   b. However, it is invasive.

   c. The decision to perform cardiac catheterization should be individualized.

7. Uncommon causes of heart failure (e.g., amyloidosis, myocarditis) can require additional testing to establish an etiologic diagnosis.

Treatment

Nonpharmacologic Therapy

1. Identify and correct precipitating factors.
   a. Anemia.
   b. Thyrotoxicosis.
   c. Infections.
   d. Increased sodium load.
   e. β-Blockers.
   f. Medical noncompliance.
2. Decrease cardiac workload (restrict patients' activity) only during periods of acute decompensation.
   a. The risk of thromboembolism during this period can be minimized by using heparin 5000 U SC q12h in hospitalized patients.
   b. In patients with mild to moderate symptoms, aerobic training can improve symptoms and exercise capacity.
3. Restrict sodium intake to no more than 3 g/day.
4. Restricting fluid intake to 2 L or less may be useful in patients with hyponatremia.

Pharmacologic Therapy

1. Treatment of CHF secondary to systolic dysfunction.
   a. Diuretics.
      (1) Diuretics are indicated in patients with systolic dysfunction and volume overload.
      (2) The most useful approach to selecting the dose of, and monitoring the response to, diuretic therapy is by measuring body weight, preferably on a daily basis.
      (3) Selected medications.
         (a) Furosemide.
            i. Treatment with 20 to 80 mg/day produces prompt venodilation and diuresis.
            ii. In decompensated patients, IV therapy can produce diuresis when oral therapy has failed.
            iii. After successful diuresis, when changing from IV to oral furosemide, doubling the dose is usually necessary to achieve an equal effect.
            iv. Monitor serum potassium every 6 months (every 3 months if digitalis is also used).
         (b) Thiazides.
            i. Thiazides are not as powerful as furosemide but are useful in mild to moderate CHF.
            ii. Monitor serum potassium every 12 months (every 6 months if digitalis is also used).
            iii. Thiazides are not effective when creatinine clearance is less than 20 mL/min.

(c) Metolazone.
   i. The addition of metolazone to furosemide enhances diuresis.
   ii. Monitor potassium frequently.
(d) Spironolactone and ACE inhibitors.
   i. Blockade of aldosterone receptors by spironolactone used in conjunction with ACE inhibitors reduces mortality and morbidity in patients with severe CHF.
   ii. Treat with spironolactone 12.5 to 25 mg qd.
   iii. Spironolactone is generally not associated with hyperkalemia when used in low doses.
   iv. Serum electrolytes and renal function should be monitored after initiation of therapy and when titrating doses.
   v. Spironolactone use should be considered in patients with recent or recurrent NYHA class IV symptoms.
(e) Fluid intake.
   i. Elderly patients have a blunted thirst sensation. They also may have restricted access to water because of mobility impairment or cognitive deficits. As a result, IV volume depletion and prerenal failure is a common complication of diuretic therapy.
   ii. Patients with mild baseline renal failure (e.g., diabetic nephropathy) and patients dependent on others for fluid intake (e.g., nursing home patients) are particularly at risk.
   iii. Monitor these patients closely for clinical signs of dehydration and laboratory evidence of prerenal failure (high BUN/creatinine ratio).
   iv. Monitoring fluid intake and output (I&O) is important and appropriate in the hospital. If a urinary catheter is used for this purpose, its duration should be minimized.
   v. In the nursing home setting, I&O is often unreliable and in outpatients it is impractical. Daily to weekly weight should be monitored in such situations instead of I&O. For reliable patients, a weight-based diuretic sliding scale can be recommended.
b. Angiotensin converting enzyme (ACE) inhibitors.
   (1) ACE inhibitors cause dilation of the arteriolar resistance vessels and venous capacity vessels, thereby reducing both preload and afterload.
   (2) They are associated with decreased mortality and improved clinical status.
   (3) They can be used as first-line therapy or they can be added to diuretics.
   (4) Therapy with ACE inhibitors.
      (a) Initiate therapy at a low dose (e.g., captopril 6.25 mg tid or enalapril 2.5 mg bid) to prevent hypotension.
      (b) Titrated up to higher doses if tolerated.
   (5) Contraindications.
      (a) Renal insufficiency (creatinine > 3.0 or creatinine clearance < 30 mL/min).
      (b) Renal artery stenosis.

(c) Persistent hyperkalemia ($K^+ > 5.5$ mEq/L).

(d) Symptomatic hypotension.

(e) History of adverse reactions (e.g., angioedema).

(6) ACE inhibitors and β-blockers may be used together.

c. Angiotensin receptor blockers (ARBs).

(1) ARBs block the angiotensin II type 1 receptor, which is responsible for many of the deleterious effects of angiotensin II.

(2) These receptors are potent vasoconstrictors that can contribute to the impairment of LV function.

(3) ARBs are useful in patients unable to tolerate ACE inhibitors because of angioedema or intractable cough.

(4) They can also be used in combination with a β-blocker.

d. β-Blockers.

(1) All patients with stable NYHA class II or III heart failure caused by LV systolic dysfunction should receive a β-blocker unless they have a contraindication to its use or are intolerant to it.

(2) β-Blockers are especially useful in patients who remain symptomatic despite therapy with ACE inhibitors and diuretics.

(3) Effective agents are started at the following doses and titrated upward as tolerated.

(a) Carvedilol (Coreg) 3.125 mg bid.

(b) Bisoprolol 1.25 mg qd.

(c) Metoprolol 12.5 mg bid.

e. Digitalis.

(1) Digitalis is useful because of its positive inotropic and vagotonic effects in patients with CHF secondary to systolic dysfunction.

(2) It is of limited value in patients with mild CHF and normal sinus rhythm.

(3) It is more beneficial in patients with rapid atrial fibrillation, severe CHF, or ejection fraction of 30% or less.

(4) It can be added to diuretics and ACE inhibitors in patients with severe CHF.

(5) In patients with chronic heart failure and normal sinus rhythm, digoxin does not reduce mortality, but it does reduce the rate of hospitalization both overall and for worsening heart failure.

(6) Its beneficial effects are found with a low dose that results in a serum concentration of approximately 0.7 ng/mL.

(7) Higher doses may be detrimental.

f. Direct vasodilating drugs (hydralazine, isosorbide) are useful in the therapy of systolic dysfunction with CHF because they can reduce the systemic vascular resistance and pulmonary venous pressure, especially when used in combination.

g. Anticoagulants.

(1) Anticoagulation is not recommended for patients in sinus rhythm and no prior history of stroke, LV thrombi, or arteriolar emboli.

(2) Anticoagulation therapy is appropriate for patients with heart failure and atrial fibrillation or a history of embolism.

(3) Aspirin is appropriate for all patients with ischemic heart disease.

h. Surgical revascularization should be considered in patients with both heart failure and severe limiting angina.

    i. Atriobiventricular pacing significantly improves exercise tolerance and quality of life in patients with chronic heart failure and intraventricular conduction delay.

    j. Obstructive sleep apnea has an adverse effect on heart failure. Recognition and treatment of coexisting obstructive sleep apnea by continuous positive airway pressure reduces SBP and improves LV systolic function.

    k. Additional points.

       (1) Sudden death secondary to ventricular arrhythmias occurs in more than 40% of patients with heart failure.

       (2) An implantable cardiac defibrillator device should be considered in selected patients.

       (3) In patients with advanced heart failure and a prolonged QRS interval, cardiac-resynchronization therapy decreases the combined risk of death from any cause or first hospitalization and, when combined with an implantable defibrillator, significantly reduces mortality.

       (4) Intensive home care by nurses with expertise in managing heart failure can improve symptoms control and reduce hospitalization.

       (5) Cardiac transplantation has a 5-year survival rate of more than 70% in many centers and represents a viable option in selected patients.

2. Treatment of CHF secondary to diastolic dysfunction.

    a. There is no evidence-based treatment of diastolic heart failure.

    b. Pulmonary edema associated with diastolic heart failure.

       (1) Diuretics.

       (2) Oxygen.

       (3) Morphine.

       (4) Nitrates.

       (5) Treat ischemia if present.

       (6) Treat severe hypertension (hypertensive crisis) if present.

       (7) Treat tachycardia (may require urgent cardioversion of atrial fibrillation).

    c. Chronic management for patients with diastolic heart failure.

       (1) Reduce the congestive state.

         (a) Salt restriction.

         (b) Diuretics.

         (c) ACE inhibitors.

         (d) ARBs.

       (2) Maintain atrial contraction and prevent tachycardia.

         (a) β-Blockers.

         (b) CCBs.

         (c) Cardioversion of atrial fibrillation.

         (d) Sequential atrioventricular pacing.

         (e) Radiofrequency ablation modification of atrioventricular node and pacing.

       (3) Treat and prevent myocardial ischemia.

         (a) Nitrates.

         (b) β-Blockers.

         (c) CCBs.

  (d) Coronary artery bypass surgery, percutaneous coronary intervention.

 (4) Control hypertension with antihypertensive agents.

 d. Treatment of CHF secondary to structural cardiac abnormalities.

  (1) AS.

   (a) Diuretics.

   (b) Contraindicated medications.

    i. ACE inhibitors.

    ii. ARBs.

    iii. Nitrates.

    iv. Digitalis (except to control rate of atrial fibrillation).

   (c) Aortic valve replacement in patients with critical stenosis.

  (2) Aortic insufficiency and MR.

   (a) ACE inhibitors increase cardiac output and decrease pulmonary wedge pressure. They are agents of choice along with diuretics.

   (b) Hydralazine combined with nitrates can be used if ACE inhibitors are not tolerated.

   (c) Surgery.

  (3) IHSS.

   (a) β-Blockers or verapamil.

   (b) Medications that are contraindicated because they increase outlet obstruction by decreasing the size of the left ventricle in end systole.

    i. Diuretics.

    ii. Digitalis.

    iii. ACE inhibitors.

    iv. ARBs.

    v. Hydralazine.

   (c) Restoration of intravascular volume with IV saline solution if necessary in acute pulmonary edema.

   (d) Septal myotomy and DDD pacing are useful in selected patients.

  (4) Treatment of CHF secondary to mitral stenosis.

   (a) Diuretics.

   (b) Control of the heart rate and atrial fibrillation with digitalis, verapamil, and/or β-blockers is critical to allow emptying of the left atrium and relief of pulmonary congestion.

   (c) Repairing or replacing the mitral valve is indicated if CHF is not readily controlled by these measures.

   (d) Balloon valvuloplasty is useful in selected patients.

SUGGESTED READINGS

Aurigemma GP, Gaasch WH: Diastolic heart failure. *N Engl J Med* 351:1097-1105, 2004.

Bristow MR, Saxon LA, Boehmer J, et al: Cardiac-resynchronization therapy with or without an implantable defibrillator in advanced chronic heart failure. *N Engl J Med* 350:2140-2150, 2004.

Goldstein S: Benefits of beta-blocker therapy in heart failure: Weighing the evidence. *Arch Intern Med* 162:641-648, 2002.

Gutierrez C, Blanchard DG: Diastolic heart failure: Challenges of diagnosis and treatment. *Am Fam Physician* 69:2609-2616, 2004.

Jessup M, Brozena S: Heart failure. *N Engl J Med* 348:2007-2018, 2003.

King DE et al: Acute management of atrial fibrillation: Part I. Rate and rhythm control. *Am Fam Physician* 66:249-256, 2002.

Kukin ML: Beta blockers in chronic heart failure: Considerations for selecting an agent. *Mayo Clin Proc* 77:1199-1206, 2002.

Maisel AS, Krishnaswamy P, Nowak RM, et al: Rapid measurement of B-type natriuretic peptide in the emergency diagnosis of heart failure. *N Engl J Med* 347:161-167, 2002.

Mueller C, Scholer A, Laule-Kilian K, et al: Use of B-type natriuretic peptide in the evaluation and management of acute dyspnea. *N Engl J Med* 350:647-654, 2004.

Nohria A, Lewis E, Stevenson LW: Medical management of advanced heart failure. *JAMA* 287:628-640, 2002.

Redfield MM: Understanding "diastolic" heart failure. *N Eng J Med* 350:1930-1931, 2004.

Vasan RS: Diastolic heart failure. *BMJ* 4:80-84, 2004.

Zile MR, Baicu CF, Gaasch WH: Diastolic heart failure—abnormalities in active relaxation and passive stiffness of the left ventricle. *N Engl J Med* 350:1953-1959, 2004.

CORONARY ARTERY DISEASE AND ANGINA PECTORIS

Michael P. Gerardo

Overview

Atherosclerotic coronary artery disease (CAD) results in ischemia when the oxygen demand of myocardial muscle exceeds the coronary artery supply.

1. Three features characterize ischemia.
   a. The location of the pain is either substernal or precordial.
   b. The pain is precipitated by exertion.
   c. Relief of the pain occurs with rest or after the administration of sublingual nitroglycerin.
2. If the three criteria are met, the patient has typical (classic) angina.
3. Atypical angina is defined as meeting two of the three criteria.
4. If none or one of the criteria is met, the patient has nonanginal chest pain.
5. This characterization of ischemic symptoms is the same for older adults, but the fraction of atypical and nonanginal presentations of ischemia increases with age.

Definitions

Angina may be classified into one of the following categories:

1. Chronic stable angina.
   a. Chronic stable angina occurs in a predictable fashion.
   b. The pain is brought on by an identified precipitant like climbing a certain number of stairs or walking a known distance.
   c. The severity of the pain is the same as on previous episodes.
   d. The relief of the pain is with an expected dose of sublingual nitroglycerin or a recognized time of rest.
2. Unstable angina.
   a. Unstable angina is any recent chest pain that has changed in character from previous episodes.
   b. The pain can occur at rest (rest angina).
   c. The pain can be of increasing intensity, frequency, or duration (crescendo angina).

    d. Unstable angina and acute MI are described in greater detail in "Acute Coronary Syndromes."

3. Prinzmetal's variant angina.
    a. Prinzmetal's variant angina is caused by coronary artery vasospasm.
    b. It most often affects women younger than 50 years.
    c. It occurs at rest either in the presence or absence of CAD.

4. Microvascular angina.
    a. Microvascular angina (syndrome X) is any chest pain that is associated with a positive exercise stress test, but the coronary angiogram is normal.
    b. The symptoms are related to an inadequate flow in the coronary microvascularization.
    c. These patients have an excellent prognosis.

5. Refractory angina.
    a. Refractory angina occurs in a subset of patients in whom medical therapy and revascularization do not relieve anginal symptoms or progression of ischemia.
    b. Physicians should consider referral.
      (1) Noninvasive interventions.
        (a) Enhanced extracorporeal counterpulsation.
        (b) Transcutaneous electrical nerve stimulation.
        (c) Spinal cord stimulation.
      (2) Invasive interventions.
        (a) Transmyocardial revascularization.
        (b) Percutaneous myocardial revascularization.
      (3) These interventions can reduce the anginal burden, but they have not been shown to improve either the quantity or quality of life.

6. Nonobstructive causes of angina include:
    a. Severe myocardial hypertrophy.
    b. Severe AS or aortic regurgitation.
    c. Mitral valve prolapse.
    d. Any increase in metabolic demand as is seen with cocaine use (also causes coronary vasospasm), marked anemia, hypoxia, and hyperthyroidism.

Epidemiology

1. CAD affects more than 13 million Americans and is responsible for one in five deaths.
2. Increasing age is an independent risk factor for ischemic-related morbidity and mortality.
3. Approximately 27% of men and 17% of women older than 80 years have CAD.
4. Men are more likely to be affected during the middle and older ages.
5. Postmenopausal women are affected more than premenopausal women.

Differential Diagnosis

A thorough history can localize a noncardiac source of the pain.

1. Pulmonary diseases can mimic ischemic pain.
    a. Pulmonary hypertension.
    b. Pulmonary embolism.
    c. Pneumothorax.
    d. Pneumonia.

2. Gastrointestinal disorders account for a significant number of emergency department presentations of acute chest pain.
   a. Reflux disease.
   b. Peptic ulcer disease (PUD).
   c. Esophageal spasm.
   d. Pancreatitis.
   e. Cholelithiasis.
   f. Cholecystitis.
3. Symptoms of musculoskeletal syndromes are usually replicated with movement of the arm or shoulder.
   a. Arthritis.
   b. Costochondritis.
   c. Trauma.
   d. Muscle strain.
4. Aortic dissection classically presents with abrupt and severe retrosternal chest pain and reaches maximum intensity immediately after onset, most often radiating to the back.
5. Pericarditis can cause chest pain that is related to position.
6. Anxiety/panic disorders and primary hyperventilation.

Initial Evaluation

1. History.
   a. CAD risk factors.
      (1) Modifiable risk factors.
   b. Hypertension.
   c. Current tobacco use.
   d. Dyslipidemia.
   e. Diabetes mellitus.
   f. Obesity.
   g. Lack of exercise.
      (1) Nonmodifiable risk factors.
   h. Increasing age.
   i. Male sex.
   j. Family history of CAD (the risk of CAD is greater the younger the onset of CAD in a first-degree relative).
   k. Characterization of the pain and associated symptoms.
      (1) The pain should be characterized as typical, atypical, or nonanginal chest pain (see earlier).
      (2) Patients most often describe the substernal chest pain as dull, aching, burning, tight, heavy, pressure-like, or squeezing.
      (3) The pain can last anywhere from 30 seconds to 30 minutes and is often accompanied by nausea, diaphoresis, dyspnea, and radiation of pain to the jaw, left shoulder, or arm.
      (4) Ischemic chest pain is uncommonly associated with pleurisy or pulmonary disease. Pleuritic chest pain should direct the physician to pulmonary causes of the chest pain.
   l. Functional status and quality of life.
      (1) The NYHA's Functional Classification of Angina is often used to assess the impact of angina on the patient's functional status.
         (a) Class I: Anginal symptoms occur with strenuous activity.

(b) Class II: Anginal symptoms occur with prolonged or slightly more than usual activity.

(c) Class III: Anginal symptoms occur with usual activity of daily living.

(d) Class IV: Anginal symptom occur at rest.

(2) Providers should discuss the influence of these symptoms on the patient's quality of life because both of these issues can alter the preference for further testing and/or surgical intervention.

d. Any previous evaluation with ECG, stress test, or coronary angiogram is extremely helpful in verifying the diagnosis, determining a change from baseline, and identifying new ischemic insults when compared to repeated studies.

2. Physical examination.

The physical exam is of minimal use in diagnosing CAD.

a. The cardiac exam is often normal in CAD.

b. The physician should examine and comment on heart sounds that suggest valvular disease or cardiac disease related to diastolic or systolic dysfunction. These findings can be confirmed and their severity can be evaluated with echocardiography.

c. Reproducible chest pain and tenderness associated with repositioning suggest a musculoskeletal etiology for the chest pain.

3. Laboratory testing.

a. Patients should have appropriate screening for diabetes mellitus and dyslipidemia.

b. High sensitivity C-reactive protein testing is available for clinical use and can be helpful in determining which patients at intermediate risk (based on Framingham 10-year risk of heart disease) would benefit from more aggressive LDL management.

c. Homocysteine level and lipoprotein(a) are also markers of CAD; however, their role in CAD management and risk stratification has yet to be determined.

4. Pretest probability.

a. The probability of CAD is determined by assessing the patient's age, sex, and characterization of chest pain.

b. Patients with intermediate pretest probability should undergo risk stratification with further testing (e.g., exercise ECG, stress echocardiogram, or nuclear perfusion testing) to determine who might benefit from cardiac catheterization.

c. Patients with a high pretest probability for CAD should be considered for direct catheterization when appropriate.

5. Imaging studies.

a. Exercise ECG.

(1) Exercise ECG remains the test of choice per current guidelines.

(2) Comorbid illness common in the older population (e.g., COPD, arthritis, deconditioning) can preclude the use of exercise stress testing.

(3) For patients who cannot perform an exercise protocol, pharmacologic-based stress testing is achieved with dobutamine, adenosine, or dipyridamole.

   b. Myocardial scintigraphy.
- (1) Stress (exercise or pharmacological based) echocardiography and myocardial nuclear perfusion testing (scintigraphy) are both more costly than exercise ECG, but they provide additional information related to the location of lesion and LV dysfunction.
- (2) Myocardial scintigraphy distinguishes between ischemic and infarcted myocardium.
- (3) Physicians should use these modalities when the baseline ECG is abnormal (i.e., resting ST depression, left bundle branch block, LV hypertrophy with strain, paced rhythms).
- (4) Either test is appropriate, with equivalent sensitivity and specificity, for diagnosing significant CAD.

   c. Coronary angiogram is discussed later.

Management

1. Overview.
   - a. When treating an older person with known CAD, care should focus on developing a patient-centered plan because individual differences in drug pharmacokinetics, complex disease management due to comorbid illness, and preferences for care affect the decision to undergo revascularization.
   - b. In patients with asymptomatic CAD, the goal of care should be to reduce risk factors such as smoking, treatment of dyslipidemia, exercise, and hypertension. These measures have been shown to delay the progression of disease, and in some cases the treatment of dyslipidemia can produce regression of atherosclerotic lesions.
2. Nonpharmacologic therapy.
   - a. All patients should discontinue smoking.
   - b. Diet and exercise have favorable effects on BP, glucose, and cholesterol levels.
   - c. Patients can be provided with dietary guidelines published by the U.S. Department of Health and Human Services and the U.S. Department of Agriculture in January 2005.
2. Pharmacologic therapy.
   - a. Aspirin.
     - (1) Aspirin at a dose of 81 to 325 mg per day reduces the risk of subsequent MI.
     - (2) A dose of 81 mg daily can minimize the risk of bleeding associated with antiplatelet therapy.
     - (3) Patients on warfarin should not receive more than 81 mg/day.
     - (4) Current guidelines recommend all persons older than 45 years who have one or more CAD risk factors be treated with daily aspirin therapy, if there are no contraindications to ASA.
     - (5) For patients intolerant to aspirin, clopidogrel may be used as antiplatelet therapy.
   - b. β-Blockers.
     - (1) β-Blocker therapy should be instituted as treatment in patients without a contraindication to β-blockade (severe reactive airway disease, bradycardia, high-degree heart block).

(2) As tertiary prevention, β-blockers reduce all-cause mortality and reinfarction in persons with a previous MI or ischemic left systolic dysfunction.

(3) Side effects of β-blocker therapy include:

    (a) Heart block, bradycardia, and exacerbation of acute heart failure.

    (b) Depression.

    (c) Impotence.

    (d) Constipation.

    (e) Exacerbation of bronchospasm.

c. ACE inhibitors.

(1) ACE inhibitors reduce mortality, coronary events, and stroke in persons with a prior MI or ischemic systolic dysfunction.

(2) A reduction in cardiovascular deaths, stroke, and nonfatal stroke was also seen in high-risk patients, including those with diabetes, peripheral artery disease, and previous stroke.

(3) Current recommendations are that providers consider ACE inhibitors in patients with systolic dysfunction, diabetes, prior MI, or hypertension.

(4) Serum electrolytes and renal function should be monitored when the drug is started, during period of illness, and when the dose is changed, because the elderly may be more susceptible to kidney dysfunction associated with the use of ACE inhibitors.

(5) ARBs should be considered for those persons who are intolerant to ACE inhibitors (cough or angioedema).

d. Nitrates.

(1) Nitrates are very effective antianginal agents.

(2) Caution must be taken when prescribing nitrates, because older persons may be more susceptible to the orthostatic hypotension related to nitrate use.

(3) Patients should be advised to not take phosphodiesterase inhibitors with nitrates because of the risk of severe hypotension and death from a combination of the two therapies.

(4) The main limitation to chronic nitrate therapy is the development of tolerance, which can be avoided by including an 8- to 10-hour period of the day without nitrates.

(5) Other side effects include headache, hypotension, nausea, and lightheadedness.

e. Calcium-channel blockers.

(1) CCBs are not first-line therapy for management of symptoms related to ischemia.

(2) CCBs have not been shown to reduce mortality after infarction.

(3) Only amlodipine has been shown to be safe in patients with heart failure.

(4) Short-acting dihydropyridines (nifedipine) should never be used in persons with CAD.

(5) Other CCBs may be used as antianginal or rate-controlling agents in those intolerant to β-blockers.

(6) Diltiazem and verapamil are preferable because they produce less reflex tachycardia.

   f. Lipid-lowering agents.

     (1) Lipid-lowering agents, such as the HMG-CoA reductase inhibitors (statins), reduce the number of coronary events, stroke, and coronary deaths in persons with known CAD, persons with diabetes and peripheral artery disease, and those with elevated LDL.

     (2) Routine monitoring of liver function with enzyme studies is recommended.

   g. Narcotics for pain control should also be considered in older adults in whom coronary revascularization is not an option and standard medical therapy does not relieve the angina.

3. Invasive procedures.

   a. Coronary angiography.

     (1) Coronary angiography should be considered in patients who are candidates for coronary revascularization.

     (2) The decision to undergo cardiac catheterization is often based on medical comorbidity, cognitive decline, and individual preference for care.

     (3) The physician should meet with the family or medical proxy to discuss the risks associated with coronary revascularization prior to recommending coronary angiography in persons with dementia.

       (a) Perioperative and postoperative mortality.

       (b) Worsening cognitive status.

       (c) Slower recovery times.

     (4) Persons with dementia may be unable to tolerate the time required to perform a percutaneous angioplasty.

   b. Revascularization.

     (1) Coronary artery bypass grafting (CABG).

       (a) CABG is reserved for persons with left main disease, three-vessel disease, and LV dysfunction.

       (b) Previous studies have shown an advantage of CABG over PTCA in diabetics, but these trials preceded the common use of drug-eluting stents.

       (c) CABG has a very low mortality rate (1% to 3%) in patients with normal ejection fraction. The mortality rate in older persons is 4% to 8%.

       (d) Surgical intervention should result in elimination of symptoms, reduction in the use antianginal medications, and improved LV function.

       (e) Careful consideration of the benefit of CABG in the very old is warranted, because higher morbidity and mortality rates have been demonstrated for persons older than 70 years.

       (f) The increase in morbidity and mortality is compounded for persons with poor health (chronic kidney disease and diabetes) and in patients undergoing repeat procedures.

       (g) Minimally invasive surgical techniques, including sternotomy, lateral thoracotomy, or thoracoscopy, offer the benefit of quicker discharge and shorter recovery time, but there are limited data describing the efficacy of these techniques.

(2) Percutaneous coronary intervention.
  (a) PTCA is the procedure of choice for the revascularization of single-vessel disease.
  (b) Optimal lesions for PTCA are proximal, noneccentric, nonbranching, and uncalcified.
  (c) The threat of vessel occlusion has been reduced by the use of glycoprotein IIb/IIIa inhibitors (abciximab, eptifibatide, tirofiban), drug eluting stents (sacrolimus, paclitaxel) and antithrombotic therapy (chronic ASA and clopidogrel for up to 1 year).
  (d) Restenosis can occur within the first 6 months after intervention and is treated with repeat PTCA.
  (e) In-stent restenosis is treated with brachytherapy or restenting with drug-eluting stents.

SUGGESTED READINGS

Eagle KA, Guyton RA, Davidoff R, et al: AC/AHA 2004 Guideline update for coronary artery bypass graft surgery: Summary article: A report of the American College of Cardiology/American Heart Association Task Force on Practice Guidelines Committee to Update the 1999 Guidelines on Coronary Artery Bypass Graft Surgery. Circulation 110;e340-e347, 2004.

Gibbons RJ, Abrams J, Chatterjee K, et al: ACC/AHA 2002 guideline update for the management of patients with chronic stable angina—summary article: A report of the American College of Cardiology/American Heart Association Task Force on Practice Guidelines (Committee on the Management of Patients with Chronic Stable Angina). J Am Coll Cardiol 41:159-168, 2003.

Hu FB, Willett WC: Optimal diets for prevention of coronary heart disease. JAMA 288:2569-2578, 2002.

Levinson SS, Elin RJ: What is C-reactive protein telling us about coronary artery disease? Arch Intern Med 162:389-392, 2002.

Ridker PM, Rifai N, Rose L, et al: Comparison of C-reactive protein and low-density lipoprotein cholesterol levels in the prediction of first cardiovascular events. N Engl J Med 347:1557-1565, 2002.

Smith SJ Jr, Blair SN, Bonow RO, et al: AHA/ACC Scientific Statement: AHA/ACC guidelines for preventing heart attack and death in patients with atherosclerotic cardiovascular disease: 2001 update: A statement for healthcare professionals from the American Heart Association and the American College of Cardiology. Circulation 104:1577-1579, 2001.

Snow V, Barry P, Fihn SD, et al: Evaluation of primary care patients with chronic stable angina: guidelines from the American College of Physicians. Ann Intern Med 141:57-64, 2004.

TIME Investigators. Trial of invasive versus medical therapy in elderly patients with chronic symptomatic coronary-artery disease (TIME): A randomized trial. Lancet 358:951-957, 2001.

Yang E, Barsness GW, Gersh BJ, et al: Current and future treatment strategies for refractory angina. Mayo Clinic Proc 79(10):1284-1292, 2004.

HYPERTENSION

Fred F. Ferri and Tom J. Wachtel

Definitions

1. The Joint National Committee on Prevention, Detection, Evaluation, and Treatment of High Blood Pressure (JNC 7) classifies normal BP in adults as less than 120 mm Hg systolic and less than 80 mm Hg diastolic.

2. Prehypertension is defined as SBP 120 to 139 mm Hg or DBP 80 to 89 mm Hg.
3. Stage 1 hypertension is SBP 140 to 159 mm Hg or DBP 90 to 99 mm Hg.
4. Stage 2 hypertension is SBP 160 mm Hg or higher or DBP 100 mm Hg or higher.

Epidemiology

1. Prevalence of hypertension in persons older than 60 years is 65%.
2. Two thirds have isolated systolic hypertension, which is no longer considered a separate clinical entity.
3. About 90% of persons age 55 years will develop hypertension in their lifetime.
4. About 50 million persons in the United States and approximately 1 billion persons worldwide meet the criteria for diagnosis of hypertension.

Clinical Findings

1. History.
   a. Age of onset of hypertension, previous antihypertensive therapy.
   b. Family history of hypertension, stroke, cardiovascular disease.
   c. Diet, salt intake, alcohol, drugs (e.g., NSAIDs, decongestants, steroids).
   d. Occupation, lifestyle, socioeconomic status, psychological factors.
   e. Other cardiovascular risk factors.
      (1) Hyperlipidemia.
      (2) Obesity.
      (3) Diabetes mellitus.
      (4) Carbohydrate intolerance.
   f. Symptoms of secondary hypertension.
      (1) Headache, palpitations, excessive perspiration (possible pheochromocytoma).
      (2) Weakness, polyuria (consider hyperaldosteronism).
      (3) Claudication of lower extremities (seen with coarctation of aorta).
2. Physical examination.
   a. Physical examination may be entirely within normal limits except for the presence of hypertension.
   b. The initial physical examination on a hypertensive patient should include the following:
      (1) Measure height and weight.
      (2) Evaluate skin for the presence of striae (Cushing's syndrome).
      (3) Perform funduscopic examination: Check for papilledema, retinal exudates, hemorrhages, arterial narrowing, AV compression.
      (4) Examine the neck for carotid bruits, distended neck veins, or enlarged thyroid gland.
      (5) Perform cardiopulmonary examination: Check for loud aortic component of S_2, S_4, ventricular lift, murmurs, arrhythmias.
      (6) Check abdomen for masses (pheochromocytoma, polycystic kidneys), presence of bruits over the renal artery (renal artery stenosis), dilation of the aorta.
      (7) Obtain two or more BP measurements separated by 2 minutes with the patient either supine or seated and after standing for at least 2 minutes. (The latter is to check for orthostatic hypotension.) Measure BP in both upper extremities (if values are discrepant,

use the higher value). BP should be measured at least twice (on separate visits) in the sitting position before making a diagnosis of hypertension.

(8) Examine arterial pulses (dilated or absent femoral pulses and BP greater in upper extremities than lower extremities suggest aortic coarctation).

(9) Note the presence of truncal obesity (Cushing's syndrome) and pedal edema (CHF, nephrosis).

(10) Perform neurologic assessment.

(11) The clinical evaluation should help determine if the patient has primary or secondary (possibly reversible) hypertension, if there is target organ disease present, and if there are cardiovascular risk factors in addition to hypertension.

Etiology

1. Essential (primary) hypertension (90%).
2. Drug-induced or drug-related (5%).
3. Renal parenchymal disease (3%).
4. Renovascular hypertension (<2%).
5. Primary aldosteronism (0.5%).
6. Pheochromocytoma (0.2%).
7. Cushing's syndrome and chronic steroid therapy (0.2%).
8. Hyperparathyroidism or thyroid disease (0.2%).
9. Coarctation of the aorta (0.2%).

Work-up

1. Urinalysis for evidence of renal disease.
2. BUN and creatinine to rule out renal disease. High serum creatinine is a predictor of cardiovascular risk in essential hypertension.
3. Serum electrolyte levels: Low potassium suggests primary aldosteronism, diuretic use, or Cushing's syndrome.
4. Fasting serum glucose to screen for Cushing's syndrome.
5. Screening for coexisting diseases that may adversely affect prognosis.
   a. Serum lipid panel, uric acid, calcium.
   b. If pheochromocytoma is suspected: 24-hour urine for vanillylmandelic acid and metanephrines.
6. ECG to check for presence of LV hypertrophy with strain pattern.
7. Echocardiogram in selected cases.
8. Magnetic resonance angiography (MRA) of the renal arteries in suspected renovascular hypertension (renal artery stenosis).

Management

Nonpharmacologic Therapy: Lifestyle Modifications

1. Lose weight if overweight.
2. Limit alcohol intake to 1 oz of ethanol per day in men or 0.5 oz in women.
3. Exercise (aerobic) regularly (30 min/day, most days).
4. Reduce sodium intake.
5. Maintain adequate dietary intake potassium (>3500 mg/day).
6. Stop smoking and reduce dietary saturated fat and cholesterol intake for overall cardiovascular health.
7. Consume diet rich in fruits and vegetables.

Pharmacologic Therapy

1. Approach.
   a. The choice of antihypertensive treatment should take comorbidities into account, particularly in older patents who are at risk for polypharmacy.
   b. Home BP monitoring (e.g., once weekly) with a digital measuring device is gaining in popularity. The device should be checked against the physician's equipment from time to time. A BP log should be maintained by the patient. This strategy eliminates white coat hypertension and provides a better sampling of BP measurements. However, no one knows what are optimal home BPs.
   c. According to the Seventh Report of the Joint National Committee on Detection, Evaluation, and Treatment of High Blood Pressure:
      (1) Antihypertensive drug therapy should be initiated in patients with stage 1 hypertension. Diuretics or β-blockers are preferred for initial therapy because a reduction in morbidity and mortality has been demonstrated and because of their lower cost.
      (2) ACE inhibitors, ARBs, CCBs, and α/β-blockers are also effective.
      (3) Two-drug combination is necessary for most patients with stage 2 hypertension. Fixed dose combinations may improve compliance and cut cost.
2. Medications.
The major advantages and limitations of each class of drugs are described as follows:
   a. Diuretics.
      (1) Advantages: Inexpensive, once per day dosing. Useful in edema states, CHF, chronic renal disease (decreased incidence of hip fractures in patients taking thiazide diuretics, opposite effect for loop diuretics).
      (2) Disadvantages: Significant adverse metabolic effects, increased risk of cardiac arrhythmias, sexual dysfunction, possible adverse effects on lipids and glucose levels. Avoid in patients with urinary incontinence. Thiazides are not effective when creatinine clearance is less than 20 mL/min. (Note: Low creatinine clearance can coexist with normal creatinine levels in very old patients.)
   b. β-Blockers.
      (1) Advantages: Ideal in hypertensive patients with ischemic heart disease or after MI. Favored in hyperkinetic, young patients (resting tachycardia, wide pulse pressure, hyperdynamic heart) and stable (class II-III) CHF patients.
      (2) Disadvantages: Adverse effect on quality of life (increased incidence of fatigue, depression, impotence, bronchospasm, hypoglycemia, peripheral vascular disease; adverse effects on lipids; masking of signs and symptoms of hypoglycemia in diabetics).
   c. CCBs.
      (1) Advantages.
         (a) Helpful in hypertensive patients with ischemic heart disease.
         (b) Generally favorable effect on quality of life; can be used in patients with bronchospastic disorders, renal disease, peripheral vascular disease, metabolic disorders, and salt sensitivity.

(c) Nondihydropyridine CCBs (verapamil, diltiazem) are useful in reducing proteinuria.

(2) Disadvantages.

    (a) Diltiazem and verapamil should be avoided in patients with CHF because of their negative chronotropic and inotropic effects.

    (b) Pedal edema can occur with nifedipine and amlodipine.

    (c) Constipation can be a problem in patients receiving verapamil.

d. ACE inhibitors.

(1) Advantages.

    (a) Well tolerated, favorable impact on quality of life.

    (b) Useful in hypertension complicated by CHF.

    (c) Helpful in prevention of diabetic renal disease.

    (d) Effective in decreasing LV hypertrophy.

(2) Disadvantages.

    (a) Cough is a common side effect (5% to 20% of patients).

    (b) Hyperkalemia can occur in patients with diabetes or severe renal insufficiency.

    (c) Hypotension can occur in volume-depleted patients.

(3) In patients with hypertension and chronic renal insufficiency, it is not uncommon to see a small rise in serum creatinine as the BP is lowered. Some physicians respond by decreasing the dose of the medication or by discontinuing it. This approach is not optimal for the long-term preservation of renal function because a small, nonprogressive increase in serum creatinine in the context of improved BP control indicates successful reduction of the intraglomerular pressure. The same applies to ARBs.

e. ARBs.

(1) Advantages.

    (a) Well tolerated, favorable impact on quality of life.

    (b) Useful in patients unable to tolerate ACE inhibitors because of persistent cough and in CHF and diabetic patients.

    (c) Single daily dose.

(2) Disadvantages.

    (a) Cost.

    (b) Hypotension can occur in volume-depleted patients.

f. α_1-Adrenergic blockers.

(1) Advantages.

    (a) No adverse effect on blood lipids or insulin sensitivity.

    (b) Helpful in BPH.

    (c) May be less effective than other agents.

(2) Disadvantages.

    (a) Postural hypotension.

    (b) Syncope can be avoided by giving an initial low dose at bedtime.

g. Other agents (e.g., hydralazine, reserpine, guanfacine, methyldopa, minoxidil, clonidine) are infrequently used.

h. Start with a low dose and titrate upward slowly, monitoring for orthostatic hypotension. Consider titrating down if BP is consistently below 120/80 mm Hg.

3. Treatment of renovascular hypertension (RVH): The therapeutic approach varies with the cause of the RVH.
   a. Medical therapy is advisable in elderly patients with atheromatous RVH. Useful agents are:
      (1) β-Blockers: Very effective in patients with elevated plasma renin.
      (2) ACE inhibitors: Very effective; however, they should be avoided in patients with bilateral renal artery stenosis and in patients with solitary kidney and renal stenosis.
      (3) Diuretics are often used in combination with ACE inhibitors.
   b. Surgical revascularization is generally reserved for atheromatous RVH in patients responding poorly to medical therapy (uncontrolled hypertension, deteriorating renal function).
4. Malignant hypertension, hypertensive emergencies, and hypertensive urgencies.
   a. Malignant hypertension is a potentially life-threatening situation.
      (1) The rate of BP rise is a critical factor.
      (2) The clinical manifestations are grade IV hypertensive retinopathy (exudates, hemorrhages, and papilledema), cardiovascular and/or renal compromise, and encephalopathy.
      (3) It requires rapid BP reduction (not necessarily into normal ranges) to prevent or limit target organ disease.
   b. Hypertensive emergencies are situations that require immediate (within 1 h) lowering of BP to prevent end-organ damage. The choice of therapeutic agents in malignant hypertension varies with the cause.
      (1) Nitroprusside is the drug of choice in hypertensive encephalopathy, hypertension and intracranial bleeding, malignant hypertension, hypertension and heart failure, dissecting aortic aneurysm (used in combination with the propranolol). Its onset of action is immediate.
      (2) Fenoldopam is a newer vasodilator agent useful for the short-term (up to 48 h) management of severe hypertension when rapid but quickly reversible reduction of BP is required.
      (3) The following are important points to remember when treating hypertensive emergencies:
         (a) Introduce a plan for long-term therapy at the time of the initial emergency treatment.
         (b) Agents that reduce arterial pressure can cause the kidney to retain sodium and water; therefore, the judicious administration of diuretics should accompany their use.
         (c) The initial goal of antihypertensive therapy is not to achieve a normal BP but rather to gradually reduce the BP. Cerebral hypoperfusion can occur if the mean BP is lowered by more than 40% in the initial 24 hours.
         (d) Hypertensive emergencies can be treated with oral clonidine 0.1 mg q 20 min (to a maximum of 0.8 mg) or IV medication.

SUGGESTED READINGS

ALLHAT Officers and Coordinators for the ALLHAT Collaborative Research Group: Major outcomes in high-risk hypertensive patients randomized to angiotensin-converting enzyme inhibitor of calcium channel blocker vs diuretic: The Antihypertensive and Lipid-Lowering Treatment to Prevent Heart Attack Trail (ALLHAT) (published erratum appears in JAMA 2003;289:178). JAMA 288:2981-2997, 2002.

Aronow WS: Treatment of older persons with hypertension. *Clin Geriatrics* 13:12-16, 2005.

Chobanian AV, Bakris GL, Black HR, et al: The Seventh Report of the Joint National Committee on Prevention, Detection, Evaluation, and Treatment of High Blood Pressure: The JNC 7 report. JAMA 289:2560-2572, 2003.

Dickerson LM, Gibson MV: Management of hypertension in older persons. *Am Fam Physician* 71:469-476, 2005.

Francos GC, Schairer HL Jr: Hypertension. Contemporary challenges in geriatric care. *Geriatrics* 58:44-49, 2003.

Franklin SS, Jacobs MJ, Wong ND, et al: Predominance of isolated systolic hypertension among middle-aged and elderly US hypertensives: Analysis based on National Health and Nutrition Examination Survey (NHANES) III. *Hypertension* 37:869-874, 2001.

Gueyffier F, Bulpitt C, Boissel JP, et al: Antihypertensive drugs in very old people: A subgroup meta-analysis of randomised controlled trials. *Lancet* 353:793-796, 1999.

Magill MK, Gunning K, Saffel-Shrier S, Gay C: New developments in the management of hypertension. *Am Fam Physician* 68:853-858, 2003.

Malacco E, Mancia G, Rappelli A, et al: Treatment of isolated systolic hypertension: The SHELL study results. *Blood Press* 12:160-167, 2003.

Oparil S, Zaman MA, Calhoun DA: Pathogenesis of hypertension. *Ann Intern Med* 139:761-776, 2003.

Staessen JA, Gasowski J, Wang JG, et al: Risks of untreated and treated isolated systolic hypertension in the elderly: Meta-analysis of outcome trials. *Lancet* 355:865-872, 2000.

Wing LM, Reid CM, Ryan P, et al: A comparison of outcomes with angiotensin-converting-enzyme inhibitors and diuretics for hypertension in the elderly. *N Engl J Med* 348:583-592, 2003.

Wright JT Jr, Dunn JK, Cutler JA, et al: Outcomes in hypertensive black and nonblack patients treated with chlorthalidone, amlodipine, and lisinopril. JAMA 293:1595-1608, 2005.

MITRAL REGURGITATION

Fred F. Ferri

Definition

Mitral regurgitation (MR) is retrograde blood flow through the left atrium secondary to an incompetent mitral valve. Eventually, there is an increase in left atrial and pulmonary pressures, which can result in RV failure.

Epidemiology

The prevalence of MR has increased since the 1970s; however, this may be because of increasing availability of echocardiography rather than any real increases in this condition.

Clinical Findings

1. Patients with MR generally present with the following symptoms:
   a. Fatigue, dyspnea, orthopnea, frank CHF.
   b. Hemoptysis (caused by pulmonary hypertension).
   c. Possible systemic emboli in patients with left atrial mural thrombi associated with atrial fibrillation.
2. Hyperdynamic apex, often with palpable left ventricular lift and apical thrill.

3. Holosystolic murmur at the apex with radiation to the base or to the left axilla; poor correlation between the intensity of the systolic murmur and the degree of regurgitation.
4. Apical early- to mid-diastolic rumble (rare).

Etiology

1. Papillary muscle dysfunction (as a result of ischemic heart disease).
2. Ruptured chordae tendineae.
3. Infective endocarditis.
4. Calcified mitral valve annulus.
5. LV dilation.
6. Rheumatic valvulitis.
7. Primary or secondary mitral valve prolapse.
8. Hypertrophic cardiomyopathy.
9. Idiopathic myxomatous degeneration of the mitral valve.

Differential Diagnosis

1. Hypertrophic cardiomyopathy.
2. Pulmonary regurgitation.
3. Tricuspid regurgitation.
4. Ventricular septal defect.

Work-up

1. Echocardiography: Enlarged left atrium, hyperdynamic left ventricle (erratic motion of the leaflet is seen in patients with ruptured chordae tendineae); Doppler electrocardiography shows evidence of MR. The most important aspect of the echocardiographic examination is the quantification of the LV systolic performance.
2. Chest x-ray study.
   a. Left atrial enlargement (usually more pronounced in mitral stenosis).
   b. LV enlargement.
   c. Possible pulmonary congestion.
3. ECG.
   a. Left atrial enlargement.
   b. LV hypertrophy.
   c. Atrial fibrillation.

Treatment

1. Medical therapy.
   a. Medical therapy is primarily directed toward treatment of complications (e.g., atrial fibrillation) and prevention of bacterial endocarditis.
   b. Consider digitalis for inotropic effect and to control ventricular response if atrial fibrillation with fast ventricular response is present.
   c. Afterload reduction (to decrease the regurgitant fraction and to increase cardiac output) may be accomplished with nifedipine, hydralazine plus nitrates or ACE inhibitors.
   d. Anticoagulants if atrial fibrillation occurs.
   e. Antibiotic prophylaxis before dental and surgical procedures.
2. Surgery.
   a. Surgery is the only definitive treatment for MR.
   b. Transesophageal echocardiography allows accurate assessment of the feasibility of valve repair and is indicated before surgical intervention.

c. The timing of surgical repair is controversial; generally, surgery should be considered early in symptomatic patients despite optimal medical therapy and in patients with moderate to severe MR and minimal symptoms if there is echocardiographic evidence of rapidly progressive increase in left ventricular end-systolic dimension (echocardiographic evidence of systolic failure includes end-systolic dimension >55 mm and fractional shortening <31%).

d. Surgery is also indicated in asymptomatic patients with preserved ventricular function if there is a high likelihood of valve repair or if there is evidence of pulmonary hypertension or recent atrial fibrillation.

Prognosis

Prognosis is generally good unless there is significant impairment of the left ventricle or significantly elevated pulmonary artery pressures. Most patients remain asymptomatic for many years (average interval from diagnosis to onset of symptoms is 16 years).

SUGGESTED READING

Otto CM: Clinical practice. Evaluation and management of chronic mitral regurgitation, N Engl J Med 345:740-746, 2001.

MITRAL STENOSIS

Fred F. Ferri

Definitions

1. Mitral stenosis is a narrowing of the mitral valve orifice.
2. The cross section of a normal orifice measures 4 to 6 cm^2.
3. A murmur becomes audible when the valve orifice becomes smaller than 2 cm^2.
4. When the orifice approaches 1 cm^2, the condition becomes critical and symptoms become more evident.

Epidemiology

1. The occurrence of mitral valve stenosis has decreased worldwide since the 1970s (particularly in developed countries) as a result of declining incidence of rheumatic fever.
2. The incidence of mitral stenosis is higher in women.

Clinical Findings

1. Exertional dyspnea initially, followed by orthopnea and PND.
2. Acute pulmonary edema can develop after exertion.
3. Systemic emboli.
   a. Caused by stagnation of blood in the left atrium.
   b. Can occur in patients with associated atrial fibrillation.
4. Hemoptysis may be present as a result of persistent pulmonary hypertension.
5. Prominent jugular A waves are present in patients with normal sinus rhythm.
6. Opening snap.
   a. Opening snap occurs in early diastole.
   b. A short (<0.07 sec) A_2-to–opening snap interval indicates severe mitral stenosis.

7. Apical mid-diastolic or presystolic rumble that does not radiate is present.
8. Accentuated S_1 (because of delayed and forceful closure of the valve) is present.
9. Pulmonary hypertension.
   a. There may be an accentuated P2 and/or a soft, early diastolic decrescendo murmur (Graham Steell murmur).
   b. The Graham Steell murmur is caused by pulmonary regurgitation.
   c. The murmur is best heard along the left sternal border and may be confused with aortic regurgitation.
10. A palpable RV heave may be present at the left sternal border.
11. Patients with mitral stenosis usually have symptoms of left-sided heart failure: dyspnea on exertion, PND, orthopnea.
12. RV dysfunction (in late stages) may be manifested by peripheral edema, enlarged and pulsatile liver, and ascites.

Etiology

1. Progressive fibrosis, scarring, and calcification of the valve.
2. Rheumatic fever.
   a. Rheumatic fever is still a common cause in less-developed countries.
   b. Heart valves most commonly affected in rheumatic heart disease (in descending order of occurrence):
      (1) Mitral.
      (2) Aortic.
      (3) Tricuspid.
      (4) Pulmonary.
3. Congenital defect (parachute valve).
4. Rare causes.
      (1) Endomyocardial fibroelastosis.
      (2) Malignant cardinoid syndrome.
      (3) SLE.

Differential Diagnosis

1. Left atrial myxoma.
2. Other valvular abnormalities (e.g., tricuspid stenosis, MR).
3. Atrial septal defect.

Work-up

1. Echocardiography.
   a. The characteristic finding on echocardiogram is a markedly diminished E to F slope of the anterior mitral valve leaflet during diastole.
   b. There is also fusion of the commissures, resulting in anterior movement of the posterior mitral valve leaflet during diastole.
   c. Calcification in the valve may also be noted.
   d. Two-dimensional echocardiogram can accurately establish the valve area.
2. Chest x-ray.
   a. Straightening of the left cardiac border caused by dilated left atrial appendage.
   b. Left atrial enlargement on lateral chest x-ray (appearing as double density of posteroanterior chest x-ray).

   c. Prominence of pulmonary device.

   d. Possible pulmonary congestion and edema (Kerley B lines).

3. ECG.

   a. RV hypertrophy.

   b. Right axis deviation caused by pulmonary hypertension.

   b. Left atrial enlargement (broad notched P waves).

   c. Atrial fibrillation.

4. Cardiac catheterization.

   a. Cardiac catheterization helps to establish the severity of mitral stenosis and diagnose associated valvular and coronary lesions.

   b. Findings on cardiac catheterization include:

     (1) Normal LV function.

     (2) Elevated left atrial and pulmonary pressures.

Treatment

1. Medical.

   a. If the patient is in atrial fibrillation, control and rate response with diltiazem, digitalis, or esmolol. Although digitalis is the drug of choice for chronic heart rate control, IV diltiazem or esmolol may be acutely preferable when a rapid decrease in heart rate is required.

   b. If the patient has persistent atrial fibrillation (because of large left atrium), permanent anticoagulation is indicated to decrease the risk of serious thromboembolism.

   c. Treat CHF with diuretics and sodium restriction.

   d. Give antibiotic prophylaxis with dental and surgical procedures.

2. Surgical.

   a. Valve replacement is indicated when the valve orifice is less than 0.7 to 0.8 cm^2 or if symptoms persist despite optimal medical therapy.

   b. Commissurotomy may be possible if the mitral valve is not calcified and if there is pure mitral stenosis without significant subvalvular disease.

   c. Operative mortality rates are 1% to 5%.

3. Percutaneous transvenous mitral valvotomy.

   a. This is becoming the therapy of choice for many patients with mitral stenosis who respond poorly to medical therapy, particularly those who are poor surgical candidates and whose valve is not heavily calcified.

   b. Balloon valvotomy gives excellent mechanical relief, usually resulting in prolonged benefit.

Prognosis

Prognosis is generally good except in patients with chronic pulmonary hypotension.

PERIPHERAL VASCULAR DISEASE

Tom J. Wachtel

Peripheral Arterial Occlusive Disease

Definition

Peripheral arterial occlusive disease (PAD) is an impairment of blood flow to one or more limbs, usually resulting from atherosclerosis, occasionally from thromboembolism, and rarely from arteritis.

Epidemiology

1. Rare in the third decade (0.5%).
2. Uncommon in those aged 30 to 60 years (3%).
3. Very common in persons older than 75 years (20%).
   a. Symptomatic PAD tends to peak 10 years after CAD onset.
   b. PAD is more common in men than women, whose prevalence rates mirror those of men 10 years later in life.
   c. PAD is associated with smoking, hypercholesterolemia, hypertension, diabetes, obesity, sedentary lifestyle, and family history.

Symptoms

1. Intermittent claudication.
   a. Cramping pain caused by ambulation and relieved by rest.
   b. Calf pain associated with superficial femoral or popliteal stenosis.
   c. Buttock, hip, and thigh pain associated with aortoiliac stenosis.
   d. Rest pain indicates more severe disease (narrower stenosis and more extensive stenosis, or fewer collateral arteries as occurs in more rapidly progressive disease).
2. Arterial leg ulcer.
   a. Painful.
   b. Often begins with trauma.
   c. Sites.
      (1) Toes.
      (2) Around first metatarsophalangeal joint.
      (3) Heel.
      (4) Lateral malleolus.
      (5) Distal pretibial region.
3. Examination.
   a. Abdominal or limb bruits.
   b. Diminished or absent pulses.
   c. Shiny, atrophic skin.
   d. Diminished hair growth.
   e. Brittle nails.
   f. Poor capillary filling when skin is blanched.

Diagnostic Tests

1. Noninvasive methods.
      (1) Segmental BP measurement using Doppler technology.
      (2) Ankle brachial index (ABI) used to stratify severity of PAD (ABI of 1 is normal, <0.4 is severe).
2. Invasive procedure: Arteriography is the gold standard test to diagnose PAD.

Treatment

1. Improve cardiovascular risk profile.
   a. Smoking cessation.
   b. Treat hypertension, hyperlipidemia, diabetes, and obesity.
2. Medication.
   a. Aspirin 88 mg to 650 mg daily.
   b. Cilostazol (Pletal) 50 to 100 mg PO bid.
   c. Pentoxifylline (Trental) 400 mg PO tid.

3. Surgery.
   a. Percutaneous angioplasty.
   b. Vascular reconstruction.
   c. Amputation.
4. Management of arterial ulcer.
   a. Do not elevate limb.
   b. Daily cleaning with saline solution.
   c. Debridement.
   d. Wet to wet dressings (apply wet, allow it to dry, but wet it again before removing) or wet to dry if continued debridement is desired.

Peripheral Venous Disorder

Varicose Veins

1. Definition and pathophysiology: Dilation of superficial veins that results from incompetent valves and reversal of blood flow.
2. Epidemiology prevalence: One third of women and one fifth of men in the United States.
3. Symptoms.
   a. Dilated, cosmetically displeasing veins.
   b. Calf aching or heaviness; similar symptoms in location of varicose veins.
   c. Acute symptom exacerbation with signs of inflammation and a palpable cord can signify superficial phlebitis.
4. Treatment.
   a. Avoid a stationary standing position whenever possible.
   b. Leg elevation.
   c. Support stockings.
   d. Weight loss if obese.
   e. Sclerosing therapy (cosmetic indication for small veins).
   f. Surgery (stripping).

Chronic Venous Insufficiency and Venous Ulcer

1. Definitions.
   a. Chronic venous insufficiency is a sequela of deep venous thrombosis during which deep vein valves are permanently disrupted.
   b. Other causes probably also lead to deep vein valve dysfunction because many patients with chronic venous insufficiency do not have a history of deep venous thrombosis.
   c. Stasis dermatitis results from chronic venous hypertension and capillary distention, allowing exudation of fibrinogen and red blood cells (RBCs), hence the fibrosis and local hemosiderosis that characterize stasis dermatitis.
2. Symptoms.
   a. Leg edema is often bilateral but asymmetrical.
   b. Erythema.
   c. Hyperpigmentation.
   d. Rarely, vesicles or bullae may be present.
   e. Dermal fibrosis and loss of skin elasticity (lower leg may look strangulated).
   f. Painless ulcer on the medial aspect of the leg.
3. Stasis is sometimes mistaken for cellulitis, but cellulitis is typically unilateral and stasis dermatitis is bilateral. However, secondary infection of

stasis dermatitis is possible (impetiginization) and should be managed as cellulitis.

4. Treatment.
   a. Stasis dermatitis.
      (1) Leg elevation as often and as high (above horizontal) as practical.
      (2) Weight loss if obese.
      (3) Support stockings.
      (4) Compression devices (e.g., Unna boot or pneumatic compression)
      (5) Moist compresses (Burow's solution) if skin weeps.
      (6) Corticosteroid cream such as hydrocortisone 1% cream.
   b. Venous ulcer.
      (1) Treat as for stasis dermatitis.
      (2) Clean ulcer daily with saline solution.
      (3) Wet to dry dressing if mild debridement is needed.
      (4) Wet to wet dressing if ulcer is free of any necrotic material.
      (5) Unna's boot dressing.
         (a) Apply once ulcer has begun to epithelialize (change weekly).
         (b) Contraindicated if there is any evidence of infection or arterial insufficiency.
      (6) Occlusive dressing such as foams, films, hydrocolloids, or hydrogels; dressing should be changed when fluid begins to leak.

SUGGESTED READINGS

Belch JJ, Topol EJ, Agnelli G, et al: Critical issues in peripheral arterial disease detection and management. *Arch Intern Med* 163:884-892, 2003.

Burns P, Gough S, Bradbury AW: Management of peripheral arterial disease in primary care. *BMJ* 326:584-588, 2003.

Gey DC, Lesho E, Manngold J: Management of peripheral arterial disease, *Am Fam Physician* 69:525-532, 2004.

Hiatt WR: Medical treatment if peripheral arterial disease and claudication. *N Engl J Med* 344:1608-1621, 2001.

Yuwono HS: Diagnosis and treatment of chronic venous insufficiency. *Clin Hemorheol Microcirc* 23:233-237, 2000.

SYNCOPE

Sean I. Savitz, Fred F. Ferri, and Tom J. Wachtel

Definition

Syncope is the temporary loss of consciousness resulting from an acute global reduction in cerebral blood flow.

Epidemiology

1. Syncope accounts for 3% to 5% of emergency department visits.
2. About 30% of the adult population will experience at least one syncopal episode during their lifetime.
3. The recurrence rate is 30%.

Clinical Findings

1. BP and heart rate should be recorded in the supine and standing positions.
   a. A drop of more than 20 mm Hg in systolic BP from supine to standing suggests orthostatic hypotension.
   b. Waiting a few minutes after the patient stands improves the sensitivity of the measurement.

   c. If there is a drop in BP and a rise in heart rate, the patient may be dehydrated or intravascular volume depleted. Dehydration is common and often subtle in the elderly.

   d. If there is a drop in BP but no change in heart rate, the patient may be on a β-blocker or might have an autonomic neuropathy.

   e. If BP is unequal in both arms (difference >20 mm Hg), consider subclavian steal or dissecting aneurysm.

   f. If back pain is present, consider a ruptured aortic aneurysm.

2. Unwitnessed loss of consciousness is consistent with syncope or seizure.

3. Dizziness characterized as lightheadedness (rather than vertigo) is often called *presyncope*. The differential diagnosis and work-up are the same as for syncope.

4. Heart.

   a. If murmurs are present and suggestive of AS or IHSS, consider syncope secondary to left ventricular outflow obstruction.

   b. If there are jugular venous distension and distant heart sounds, consider cardiac tamponade.

5. Pulse: If the patient has tachycardia, bradycardia, or irregular rhythm, consider arrhythmia.

6. Carotid sinus pressure can be diagnostic if it reproduces symptoms and other causes are excluded.

   a. A pause longer than 3 seconds is abnormal.

   b. A systolic BP drop greater than 50 mm Hg without symptoms or less than 30 mm Hg with symptoms when sinus pressure is applied separately on each side for less than 5 seconds is considered abnormal.

   c. This test should be avoided in patients with carotid bruits or cerebrovascular disease.

   d. ECG monitoring, IV access, and bedside atropine should be available when carotid sinus pressure is applied.

7. If the patient is diabetic, consider hypoglycemia.

8. If risk factors for venous thromboembolic disease exist (e.g., recent orthopedic surgery), consider pulmonary embolism.

9. Many medications can cause hypotension, lightheadedness, or syncope. Most notable on the list are all antihypertensive and all anticholinergic medications.

10. The history is crucial to diagnosing the cause of syncope and can suggest a diagnosis that can be evaluated with directed testing.

   a. Sudden loss of consciousness: Consider cardiac arrhythmias.

   b. Gradual loss of consciousness: Consider orthostatic hypotension, vasodepressor syncope, hypoglycemia.

   c. History of aura before loss of consciousness or prolonged confusion (>1 min), amnesia, or lethargy after loss of consciousness suggests seizure rather than syncope.

   d. Patient's activity at the time of syncope.

     (1) Micturition, coughing, postprandial, defecation: Consider syncope secondary to decreased venous return.

     (2) Turning head or while shaving: Consider carotid sinus syndrome.

     (3) Physical exertion in a patient with murmur: Consider aortic stenosis.

    (4) Arm exercise: Consider subclavian steal syndrome.
    (5) Assuming an upright position: Consider orthostatic hypotension.
  e. Associated events.
    (1) Chest pain: Consider MI or pulmonary embolism.
    (2) Palpitations: Consider arrhythmias.
    (3) Incontinence (urine or fecal) and tongue biting are associated with seizure or syncope.
    (4) Brief, transient shaking after loss of consciousness can represent myoclonus from global cerebral hypoperfusion and not seizures. However, sustained tonic-clonic muscle action is more suggestive of seizure.
    (5) Focal neurologic symptoms or signs point to a neurologic event such as a seizure with residual deficits (e.g., Todd's paralysis) or cerebral ischemic injury.
    (6) Psychological stress: Syncope may be vasovagal.

Etiology

1. The etiology of syncope is identified in >50% of cases during the initial evaluation.
2. A thorough history and physical examination are the most productive means of establishing a diagnosis in patients with syncope.
3. Neurally mediated syncope is usually associated with bradycardia.
  a. Psychophysiologic.
    (1) Emotional upset.
    (2) Panic disorders.
    (3) Hysteria.
  b. Visceral reflex.
    (1) Micturition.
    (2) Defecation.
    (3) Food ingestion.
    (4) Coughing.
    (5) Ventricular contraction.
    (6) Glossopharyngeal neuralgia.
  c. Carotid sinus pressure.
  d. Reduction of venous return caused by Valsalva maneuver.
4. Orthostatic hypotension.
  a. Hypovolemia (usually associated with tachycardia).
  b. Vasodilator medications.
  c. Autonomic neuropathy.
    (1) Diabetes.
    (2) Amyloid.
    (3) Parkinson's disease.
    (4) Multisystem atrophy.
  d. Pheochromocytoma.
  e. Carcinoid syndrome.
  f. Medication induced.
5. Cardiac.
  a. Reduced cardiac output.
    (1) Left ventricular outflow obstruction.
      (a) Aortic stenosis.
      (b) Hypertrophic cardiomyopathy.

      (2) Obstruction to pulmonary flow.
          (a) Pulmonary embolism.
          (b) Pulmonic stenosis.
          (c) Primary pulmonary hypertension.
      (3) MI with pump failure.
      (4) Cardiac tamponade.
      (5) Mitral stenosis.
      (6) Reduction of venous return.
          (a) Atrial myxoma.
          (b) Valve thrombus.
    b. Arrhythmias or asystole.
      (1) Extreme tachycardia (>160-180 bpm).
      (2) Severe bradycardia (<30-40 bpm).
      (3) Sick sinus syndrome.
      (4) Atrioventricular block (second- or third-degree block).
      (5) Ventricular tachycardia or fibrillation.
      (6) Long QT syndrome.
      (7) Pacemaker malfunction.
  6. Other causes.
    a. Hypoxia.
    b. Hypoglycemia.
    c. Anemia.
    d. Hyperventilation.
    e. Recreational drugs or alcohol.
  7. Cerebrovascular disease is a rare cause of syncope, unless a seizure is misinterpreted as syncope. When a seizure is misinterpreted as syncope, all the etiologies of seizures can be implicated.

Work-up

  1. Laboratory tests.
    a. CBC to rule out anemia.
    b. Electrolytes, BUN, creatinine, calcium.
    c. Serum glucose level.
    d. Cardiac isoenzymes should be obtained if the patient gives a history of chest pain before the syncopal episode.
    e. Arterial blood gas to rule out pulmonary embolus or hyperventilation when suspected.
    f. Evaluate drug and alcohol levels when suspected.
  2. Imaging studies.
    a. If the patient has head trauma or neurologic signs on examination, CT or MRI may be helpful.
    b. If seizure is suspected, CT scan or MRI of the head and electroencephalogram (EEG) may be useful.
    c. If pulmonary embolism is suspected, ventilation-perfusion scan or chest CT angiogram should be done.
    d. Noninvasive carotid studies are not usually necessary.
  3. Cardiology.
    a. ECG to rule out arrhythmias; may be diagnostic in 5% to 10% of patients.
    b. Echocardiography if structural or valvular heart disease (e.g., murmur) or heart failure is suspected.

   c. If arrhythmia or MI is suspected, a 24-hour hospital admission to a telemetry unit is appropriate.

   d. Holter monitoring.

     (1) Generally, Holter monitoring is rarely useful, revealing a cause for syncope in less than 3% of cases.

     (2) Fifteen-day or 30-day event recorders (activated after a syncopal episode to retrieve information about the cardiac rhythm during the preceding 4 minutes) can be helpful in patients with unexplained syncope.

   e. Electrophysiologic studies may be indicated in patients with structural heart disease and/or recurrent syncope.

4. Tilt-table testing is useful to support a diagnosis of neurally mediated syncope.

   a. Indications.

     (1) Patients with recurrent episodes of unexplained syncope.

     (2) The test is also useful for identifying patients with prominent bradycardic response who might benefit from implantation of a permanent pacemaker.

   b. Contraindications: Patients older than 50 years should have stress testing before tilt-table testing. Positive results preclude tilt-table testing.

   c. Testing.

     (1) Tilt-table testing is performed by keeping the patient in an upright posture on a tilt-table with footboard support.

     (2) The angle of the tilt table varies from 60 to 80 degrees.

     (3) The duration of upright posture during tilt-table testing varies from 25 to 45 minutes.

   d. Findings.

     (1) The hallmark of neurally mediated syncope is severe hypotension associated with a paradoxical bradycardia triggered by a specific stimulus.

     (2) The diagnosis of neurally mediated syncope is likely if upright tilt testing reproduces these hemodynamic changes in less than 15 minutes and causes presyncope or syncope.

Treatment

1. Dehydration.

   a. Ensure proper hydration.

   b. Consider thromboembolism-deterrent (TED) stockings and salt tablets.

2. Anemia should be corrected.

3. Eliminate medications that can induce hypotension.

4. Orthostatic hypotension.

   a. Teach the patient to rise slowly from lying to sitting to standing positions.

   b. Consider midodrine to promote venous return via adrenergic-mediated vasoconstriction.

   c. Treat intravascular volume depletion with volume replacement.

   d. Consider fludrocortisone (Florinef) for its mineralocorticoid effects to increase intravascular volume.

5. Panic disorder: Teach relaxation, and occasionally use a paper bag rebreathing technique if the diagnosis is panic disorder with primary hyperventilation.
6. Other underlying causes: Treat specific causes when identified (e.g., pacemaker in patients with syncope secondary to complete heart block).

SUGGESTED READINGS

Fenton AM, Hammill SC, Rea RF, et al: Vasovagal syncope. *Ann Intern Med* 133: 714-725, 2000.

Kapoor WN: Syncope. *N Engl J Med* 343:1856-1862, 2000.

Menozzi C, Brignole M, Garcia-Civera R, et al: Mechanism of syncope in patients with heart disease and negative electrophysiologic test. *Circulation* 105:2741-2745, 2002.

Soteriades ES, Evans JC, Larson MG, et al: Incidence and prognosis of syncope. *N Engl J Med* 347:878-885, 2002.

5.7 Dermatologic Disorders

ECZEMA

Tom J. Wachtel

Definitions

1. The term *eczema* means "bubbling over."
2. Eczema comprises several diseases.
   a. Contact dermatitis.
   b. Atopic dermatitis.
   c. Nummular dermatitis.
   d. Lichen simplex chronicus.
3. The term *dermatitis* is often used to describe an eczematous eruption.

Clinical Manifestations and Differential Diagnosis

1. The characteristic symptom in patients with eczema is pruritus.
2. Types of eczema.
   a. Contact dermatitis.
      (1) Contact dermatitis is an acute, subacute, or chronic inflammation of the epidermis and dermis caused by external agents, toxicity, or an allergic reaction.
      (2) Skin lesions.
          (a) Acute: Irregular, well-demarcated patches of erythema and edema with closely spaced vesicles, punctate erosions exuding serum, and crusts.
          (b) Subacute: Patches of mild erythema showing small dry scales or superficial desquamation.
          (c) Chronic: Patches of lichenification (thickening of the epidermis) with satellite small papules, excoriations, and hyperpigmented areas.
   b. Nummular (discoid) eczema.
      (1) Nummular eczema is a chronic, pruritic, inflammatory dermatitis occurring in the form of coin-shaped plaques composed of grouped small papules and vesicles on an erythematous base.

(2) Skin lesions.
   (a) Closely grouped small vesicles and papules that coalesce into round plaques, often more than 4 to 5 cm in diameter, with an erythematous base that has indistinct borders, crusts, and excoriations.
   (b) Dry scaly plaques that may be lichenified are often located on distal lower extremities.

c. Lichen simplex chronicus.
   (1) Lichen simplex is a circumscribed area of lichenification (skin thickening) resulting from repeated physical trauma (rubbing and scratching), occurring especially in women on the nuchal areas, arms, legs, and ankles and in the anogenital area.
   (2) Skin lesions.
      (a) A solid plaque of round or oval lichenification with minimal scaling.
      (b) The pruritus can be intense and scratching becomes pleasurable (mostly nocturnal).
      (c) The rubbing can become automatic and an unconscious habit.

d. Dyshidrotic eczema.
   (1) Dyshidrotic eczema is a vesicular type of hand and foot eczema.
   (2) It can be an acute, chronic, or recurrent dermatosis of the fingers, palms, and soles.
   (3) It is characterized by a sudden onset of deep-seated, pruritic, usually small (1.0 mm) clusters of clear vesicles.
   (4) Later, scaling, fissures, and lichenification can occur.

Treatment

1. General skin care.
   a. The rubbing and scratching must be stopped.
   b. The skin should be lubricated.
   c. Advise avoidance of irritants and other exacerbating factors such as detergents, perfumed skin care products and soaps, bubble baths, and woolen and nylon clothing.

2. Topical steroids.
   a. Description.
      (1) Topical steroids are the mainstay treatment for reducing inflammation and pruritus in all forms of eczema.
      (2) Ointments are more efficient at delivering the steroid, but creams are more acceptable to patients.
      (3) Topical steroids can be divided into low-, medium-, high-, and highest-potency products.
      (4) Prolonged use of topical steroids can result in skin atrophy, telangiectasia, striae, and bruising.
      (5) Box 5-4 lists commonly used topical steroids.
   b. Method.
      (1) Inflamed skin should be treated two or three times daily until the flares are controlled, then steroids should be tapered.
      (2) The face should be treated with low-potency products and for the shortest length of time possible.

BOX 5-4   Commonly Used Topical Glucocorticoids*

Low Strength

Desonide 0.05% (Desowen)
Hydrocortisone 1%

Medium Strength

Betamethasone dipropionate 0.05% (Diprosone)
Betamethasone valerate 0.1% (Valisone)
Fluocinolone acetonide 0.025% (Synalar)
Triamcinolone acetonide 0.1% (Aristocort or Kenalog)

High Strength

Fluocinonide 0.01% and 0.025% (Lidex)
Fluocinonide solution 0.05% (Lidex)
Halcinonide 0.1% (Halog)
Mometasone Furoate 0.1% (Elocon)

Highest Strength

Betamethasone dipropionate 0.05% in optimized vehicle (e.g., Diprolene)
Clobetasol propionate 0.5% (Clobex or Temovate)
Fluticasone propionate 0.05% (Cutivate)
Halobetasol propionate 0.05% (Ultravate)

---

*Ointments and creams unless otherwise specified.

(3) Other acute outbreaks can be treated with medium-potency topical steroids.
(4) High-potency products are reserved for resistant, chronic, or lichenified nonfacial lesions.
(5) Steroid lotions and shampoos can be used to treat scalp lesions.
3. Control of pruritus.
   a. The following topical medications can lessen pruritic symptoms and should be tried first:
      (1) Colloidal oatmeal (Aveeno Baths, Aveeno Anti-Itch cream or lotion).
      (2) Camphor and menthol (Sarna Anti-Itch) lotion.
   b. Antihistamines.
      (1) Hydroxyzine (Vistaril or Atarax).
         (a) Usual dose is 50 to 100 mg divided tid or qid.
         (b) Hydroxyzine is sedating and helps with nighttime itching.
         (c) It can impair cognition or cause delirium.
      (2) Diphenhydramine (Benadryl).
         (a) Usual dose is 25 mg p.r. tid.
         (b) Diphenhydramine is sedating and helps with nighttime itching.
         (c) It can impair cognition or cause delirium.

(3) Cetirizine (Zyrtec).
    (a) Usual dose is 5 to 10 mg once or twice a day.
    (b) It is nonsedating but may be less effective than diphenhydramine or hydroxyzine.
  c. Doxepin (Sinequan) 25 to 150 mg at bedtime can also be effective.
4. Treatment of infection.
  a. Superinfection (impetigo) is common.
  b. Mild or localized disease might respond to topical mupirocin 2% ointment (Bactroban).
  c. Systemic antibiotics such as cephalexin, diclooxocillin, or erythromycin are used for more severe or extensive secondary infections.
5. Treatment of refractory cases.
  a. Topical tacrolimus (Protopic).
    (1) Tacrolimus is a potent macrolide immunosuppressant.
    (2) It is a newer therapy shown to be effective for lesions refractory to topical steroid treatment.
    (3) Tacrolimus can be used on affected areas for short-term or extended intermittent therapy as a 0.1% or 0.03% ointment.
  b. Systemic corticosteroids are rarely indicated because of well-known side effects and rebound with discontinuation.

HERPES ZOSTER (SHINGLES)
Fred F. Ferri, with revisions by Tom J. Wachtel

Definition
Herpes zoster is a localized infection of peripheral nerves causes by reactivation of varicella-zoster virus that had been dormant in the dorsal root ganglia.

Epidemiology
1. Incidence increases with age (5 cases/1000 between ages 50 and 80 years, 10 cases/1000 after age 80 years), possibly secondary to age-related impairment of cell-mediated immunity.
2. Incidence also increased in immunocompromised hosts.
3. Persons with acute zoster are contagious to persons not immune to chickenpox (varicella).
4. Recurrence of zoster is possible but rare.

Clinical Findings
1. The first symptom is usually dysesthesia or paresthesia of the involved dermatome.
2. Rash.
  a. Sensory changes are usually followed by eruption of grouped vesicles involving one or several dermatomes.
  b. In unusual cases, prodromal symptoms are not followed by a rash (zoster sine herpete).
3. Constitutional symptoms (fever, malaise) usually accompany vesicular eruption.
4. Vesicles become pustular after 4 or 5 days. They subsequently dry up and crust in 7 to 10 days. Crusts fall off within 3 weeks.

Differential Diagnosis
1. Rash in herpes simplex and other viral infections.

2. Pain from herpes zoster may be confused with acute myocardial infarction, pulmonary embolism, pleuritis, pericarditis, or renal colic.

Complications

1. Postherpetic neuralgia occurs in more than 30% of patients older than 60 years.
2. Extensive dissemination occurs in 2% to 10%; these patients are generally immunocompromised because of immunosuppressive therapy, underlying malignancy, or acquired immunodeficiency syndrome (AIDS).
3. Eye involvement (keratoconjunctivitis, iritis) occurs in 40% to 50% of patients with ophthalmic zoster.
4. Ramsay Hunt syndrome.
   a. Caused by herpes zoster of the geniculate ganglion.
   b. It consists of facial palsy associated with vesicles in the pharynx and external auditory canal.
   c. Auditory nerve involvement occurs in 37% of patients, resulting in hearing deficits and vertigo.
5. Secondary infection.
   a. Secondary bacterial infections can occur, particularly in diabetic persons.
   b. Systemic antibiotics are indicated in suspected superinfection.

Treatment

1. Herpes zoster.
   a. Wet compresses (using Burow's solution or cool tap water) applied for 15 to 30 minutes 5 to 10 times a day are useful to break vesicles and remove serum and crust.
2. Oral antiviral agents can decrease acute pain, inflammation, and vesicle formation when treatment is begun within 48 hours of onset of rash. Treatment options are:
   a. Acyclovir (Zovirax) 800 mg 5 times daily for 7 to 10 days.
   b. Valacyclovir (Valtrex) 1000 mg tid for 7 days.
   c. Famciclovir (Famvir) 500 mg tid for 7 days.
2. Postherpetic neuralgia.
   a. Postherpetic neuralgia is defined as pain that persists more than 30 days after onset of rash.
   b. Incidence increases with age (30% by age 40 years, >70% by age 70 years).
   c. Treatment.
      (1) Antivirals, when used as early as possible, reduce the risk of postherpetic neuralgia.
      (2) Gabapentin 300 to 1800 mg qd (in one dose or divided) is effective for treating pain and sleep interference.
      (3) Pregabalin (Lyrica) 50 mg to 150 mg bid is also effective.
      (4) Lidocaine patch 5% (Lidoderm) can relieve postherpetic neuralgia. Patches are applied to intact skin to cover the most painful area for up to 12 hours within a 24-hour period.
      (5) Capsaicin 0.075% cream (Zostrix) can be useful. It is generally applied three times daily for several weeks after the crusts have fallen off.

3. A new vaccine is now available, but how effective it will prove to be in practice remains to be seen.

SUGGESTED READING

Gnann JW, Whitley RJ: Clinical practice. Herpes zoster. *N Engl J Med* 347:340-346, 2002.

PRURITUS

Fred F. Ferri

Pruritus is the most common dermatologic complaint in the elderly.

Etiology

1. Pruritus in the elderly is often due to dry skin (Box 5-5).
2. Other common causes.
   a. Drug reactions.
   b. Primary skin disorders.
   c. Psychogenic states.

Diagnostic Approach

1. Pruritus is generally associated with visible skin abnormalities (from the underlying cause or from scratching).
   a. Occasionally, pruritus precedes skin manifestations.
   b. When examining a patient complaining of pruritus, the skin exam should be complete and not limited to selected areas.
2. Medical history and laboratory evaluation should focus on potential drug reactions and metabolic disorders.
3. Underlying depression and anxiety can cause or exacerbate pruritus.
4. Scabies should be suspected when pruritus involves several members of an extended care facility.

Treatment

1. Eliminate underlying etiology. Pruritus caused by dry skin may be controlled with use of emollients to lubricate and hydrate the skin, modification of bathing procedures to limit excessive bathing time, and use of mild soaps.
2. Topical antipruritic lotions (e.g., pramoxine and hydrocortisone [Pramosone]) may be useful for localized pruritus.
3. Topical corticosteroids should be used only in the presence of prominent dermatitis.
4. Oral antihistamines (e.g., hydroxyzine) should be reserved for severe cases. Dosage should be decreased in half in geriatric patients to minimize excessive sedation.

PSORIASIS

Fred F. Ferri

Definition

1. Psoriasis is a chronic skin disorder of unknown origin.
2. It is characterized by excess proliferation of keratinocytes that results in the formation of thickened scaly plaques, itching, and inflammatory changes of the epidermis and dermis.
3. The various forms of psoriasis include guttate, pustular, and plaque.

BOX 5-5   Pruritus in the Elderly

Primary Skin Disorders

Acute dermatitis (any cause)
Bullous pemphigoid
Infection (varicella, candidiasis)
Infestations (scabies, lice)
Lichen planus
Lichen simplex chronicus (localized neurodermatitis)
Miliaria (prickly heat)
Papulosquamous disease (psoriasis)
Xerosis

Drug Reactions

Antidepressants
Aspirin
Opiates and derivatives

Circulatory

Stasis dermatitis

Metabolic

Diabetes mellitus
Hepatobiliary disease
Thyroid disease
Uremia

Hematopoietic

Hodgkin's disease
Iron deficiency anemia
Leukemia
Lymphomas
Polycythemia vera

Visceral Malignancies

Abdominal cancer
Central nervous system tumors

Other

Psychogenic states
Urticaria

Data from Bosker G, Schwartz GR, Jones JS, et al (eds): *Geriatric emergency medicine.*
St Louis, Mosby, 1990, p. 511.

Epidemiology

1. Psoriasis affects 1% to 3% of the world's population. Most patients have limited psoriasis involving less than 5% of their body surface.
2. There is a strong association between psoriasis and HLA B13, B17, and B27 (pustular psoriasis).
3. Peak age of onset is bimodal (adolescents and at 60 years of age).
4. Men and women are equally affected.

Clinical Findings

1. The primary psoriatic lesion is an erythematous papule topped by a loosely adherent scale. Scraping the scale results in several bleeding points (Auspitz's sign).
2. Chronic plaque psoriasis.
   a. Chronic plaque psoriasis generally manifests with symmetric, sharply demarcated, erythematous, silver-scaled patches affecting primarily the intergluteal folds, elbows, scalp, fingernails, toenails, and knees.
   b. This form accounts for 80% of psoriasis cases.
3. Nail involvement is common (pitting of the nail plate), resulting in hyperkeratosis, onychodystrophy with onycholysis.
4. Pruritus is variable but usually not severe.
5. Joint involvement can result in sacroiliitis and spondylitis or can mimic rheumatoid arthritis.

Differential Diagnosis

1. Contact dermatitis.
2. Atopic dermatitis.
3. Stasis dermatitis.
4. Tinea.
5. Nummular dermatitis.
6. Candidiasis.
7. Mycosis fungoides.
8. Cutaneous SLE.

Treatment

1. Sunbathing generally leads to improvement.
2. Patients with psoriasis benefit from a daily bath in warm water followed by application of a cream or ointment moisturizer. Regular use of an emollient moisturizer limits evaporation of water from the skin and allows the stratum corneum to rehydrate itself.
3. Patients with limited disease (<20% of the body) can be treated with the following:
   a. Topical steroids.
      (1) Disadvantages are brief remissions, expense, and decreased effect with continued use.
      (2) Salicylic acid can be compounded by pharmacist in concentrations of 2% to 10% and used in combination with a corticosteroid to decrease the amount of scale.
   b. Calcipotriene (Dovonex).
      (1) Calcipotriene is a vitamin D analogue.
      (2) It is effective for moderate plaque psoriasis.

    (3) Adults should comb the hair, apply solution to the lesions, and rub it in, avoiding uninvolved skin.

    (4) Disadvantages are its cost and potential burning and skin irritation.

    (5) It should not be used concurrently with salicylic acid because calcipotriene is inactivated by the acidic nature of salicylic acid.

  c. Tar products (Estar, LCD, Psorigel) can be used overnight and are most effective when combined with Ultraviolet B (UVB) light (Goeckerman regimen).

4. Therapeutic options for persons with generalized disease (affecting >20% of the body):

  a. UVB light exposure three times a week.

  b. Oral psoralen plus ultraviolet A (PUVA).

    (1) This treatment is effective for generalized disease.

    (2) It is administered two to three times weekly.

    (3) Many treatments are required, necessitating frequent office visits.

    (4) It may be associated with phototoxicity, such as erythema and blistering, and increased risk of skin cancer.

  c. Systemic treatments.

    (1) Methotrexate 25 mg every week for severe psoriasis.

    (2) Etretinate (Tegison).

      (a) Etretinate is a synthetic retinoid.

      (b) It is most effective for palmar–plantar pustular psoriasis.

      (c) Dose is 0.5 to 1 mg/kg per day.

      (d) It can cause liver enzyme and lipid abnormalities and is teratogenic.

5. Treatment with etanercept, a tumor necrosis factor (TNF) antagonist, for 24 weeks can lead to a reduction in severity of plaque psoriasis.

6. Efalizumab, a humanized monoclonal antibody that inhibits the activation of T cells, has also been reported to produce significant improvement in plaque psoriasis over a 24-week treatment period.

7. Eliminate triggering factors such as stress and certain medications (e.g., lithium, β-blockers, antimalarials).

SUGGESTED READINGS

Gordon KB, Papp KA, Hamilton TK, et al: Efalizumab for patients with moderate to severe plaque psoriasis. JAMA 290:3073-3080, 2003.

Lebwohl M, Tyring SK, Hamilton TK, et al: A novel targeted T-cell modulator, efalizumab, for plaque psoriasis. N Engl J Med 349:2004-2013, 2003.

Leonardi CL, Powers JL, Matheson RT, et al: Etanercept as monotherapy in patients with psoriasis. N Engl J Med 349:2014-2022, 2003.

SCABIES

Fred F. Ferri

Definition

Scabies is a contagious disease caused by the mite *Sarcoptes scabiei*.

Transmission

1. By direct skin contact with an infested patient.
2. Generally associated with poor living conditions.
3. It is very common in hospitals and nursing homes.

4. Isolation of infested nursing home patients and use of gowns and gloves when entering the infested patient's room are recommended.
5. Linens and recently worn clothing should be washed in hot water, although it is not known whether scabies can be acquired from infested clothing or bed linen.
6. Mites can survive out of human skin for approximately 36 hours.

Clinical Manifestations and Diagnosis

Signs and symptoms of scabies are shown in Box 5-6.
1. Primary lesions.
   a. Lesions are caused when the female mite burrows within the stratum corneum, laying eggs within the tract she leaves behind.
   b. The burrow (linear or serpiginous tract) ends with a minute papule or vesicle.
   c. Primary lesions are most commonly found in the web spaces of hands, wrists, buttocks, scrotum, penis, breasts, axillae, and knees (Fig. 5-10).
2. Secondary lesions result from scratching or infection.
3. Intense pruritus, especially nocturnal, is very common; caused by an acquired sensitivity to the mite or fecal pellets and is usually noted 1 to 4 weeks after the primary infestation.

Treatment

1. Following a warm bath or shower, lindane (Kwell, Scabene) lotion should be applied.
   a. Apply to all skin surfaces below the neck (can be applied to the face if the area is infested).
   b. Wash off 8 to 12 hours after application.
   c. A repeat application 1 week later is usually sufficient to eradicate infestation.
2. Pruritus.
   a. Pruritis generally abates 24 to 48 hours after treatment but can last up to 2 weeks.
   b. Oral antihistamines are effective in decreasing postscabeic pruritus.

BOX 5-6   Signs and Symptoms of Scabies

Diffuse eruption sparing the face
Generalized, severe itching
Nocturnal itching
Nodules on the penis and scrotum
Pinpoint erosions and crusts on the buttocks
Patient becomes better, then worse, after treatment with topical steroids
Patient develops more extensive rash despite treatment with antibiotics and topical medications
Rash is present in several members of the same family
Rash present for 4 to 8 weeks has suddenly become worse
Vesicles in the finger webs

Modified from Habif TP: *Clinical dermatology*, ed 3. St Louis, Mosby, 1996.

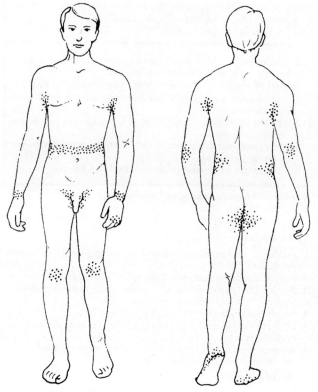

Figure 5-10 Distribution of scabies lesions. (From Habif TP: *Clinical dermatology*, ed 3. St Louis, Mosby, 1996.)

3. Topical corticosteroid creams can hasten resolution of secondary eczematous dermatitis.
4. Management of scabies epidemic in an extended care facility is described in Box 5-7.

SUGGESTED READING

Heukelbach J, Feldmeier H: Scabies. *Lancet* 367:1767-1774, 2006.

5.8 Infectious Diseases

BACTERIAL PNEUMONIA
Fred F. Ferri and Tom J. Wachtel

Definition

Bacterial pneumonia is an infection involving the lung parenchyma.

BOX 5-7   Management of Scabies Epidemic in an Extended Care Facility

1. Educate patients, staff, family, and frequent visitors about scabies and the need for cooperation in treatment.
2. Apply scabicide to all patients, staff, contact staff, and frequent visitors, symptomatic or not. Treat symptomatic family members of staff and visitors.
3. Launder all bedding and clothes worn in the last 48 hours in hot water (or dry clean).
4. Clean beds and floors with routine cleaning agents just before scabicide is removed.
5. Reexamine for treatment failures in 1 week and 4 weeks.

From Habif TP: *Clinical dermatology*, ed 3. St Louis, Mosby, 1996.

Epidemiology

1. Incidence of community-acquired pneumonia is 1/100 persons per year.
2. Incidence of nosocomial pneumonia is 0.8 cases/100 persons per year.
3. Primary care physicians see an average of 10 cases of pneumonia annually.
4. Hospitalization rate for pneumonia is 15% to 20%.
5. Most cases of community-acquired pneumonia occur in the winter and in elderly patients.
6. Aspiration pneumonia is perennial and the most common type of pneumonia in the nursing home population.

Clinical Findings

1. Usual symptoms are fever, tachypnea, chills, tachycardia, and cough.
2. Presentation varies with the cause of pneumonia, the patient's age, and the clinical situation.
   a. Patients with streptococcal pneumonia often present with:
      (1) High fever.
      (2) Chills.
      (3) Pleuritic chest pain.
      (4) Cough with production of purulent sputum.
   b. Very old, frail, or debilitated patients.
      (1) Sometimes present with only minimal symptoms (e.g., low-grade fever, confusion).
      (2) Respiratory symptoms are less commonly reported by older patients with pneumonia.
      (3) A drop in oxygen saturation by pulse oximetry compared with baseline should raise the possibility of pneumonia in a patient with cough and/or fever.
   c. Auscultation usually reveals crackles and diminished breath sounds in the involved lobe(s) of the lung.

d. Percussion dullness is present if the patient has pleural effusion. Dullness associated with lung consolidation is more difficult to detect.

Etiology

1. *Streptococcus pneumoniae.*
2. *Haemophilus influenzae.*
3. *Legionella pneumophila* (1% to 5% of adult pneumonias).
4. *Klebsiella, Pseudomonas, Escherichia coli.*
5. *Staphylococcus aureus.*
6. Pneumococcal infection is responsible for 50% to 75% of community-acquired pneumonias, whereas gram-negative organisms cause more than 80% of nosocomial pneumonias.
7. Gram-negative and anaerobic pathogens are often involved in aspiration pneumonitis.
8. Predisposing factors.
   a. COPD: *H. influenzae, S. pneumoniae, Legionella.*
   b. Seizures and neurodegenerative disorders (e.g., dementia, Parkinson's disease, multiple sclerosis, and cerebrovascular disease): Aspiration pneumonia.
   c. Compromised hosts: *Legionella,* gram-negative organisms.
   d. Alcoholism: *Klebsiella, S. pneumoniae, H. influenzae.*

Differential Diagnosis

1. Exacerbation of chronic bronchitis.
2. Pulmonary embolism/infarction.
3. Lung neoplasm.
4. Bronchiolitis.
5. Sarcoidosis.
6. Hypersensitivity pneumonitis.
7. Pulmonary edema.
8. Drug-induced lung injury.
9. Viral pneumonias.
10. Fungal pneumonias.
11. Parasitic pneumonias.
12. Atypical pneumonia.
13. Tuberculosis (TB).

Work-up

1. Laboratory tests.
   a. CBC: White blood cell (WBC) count is elevated, usually with left shift.
   b. Blood cultures are positive in approximately 20% of cases of pneumococcal pneumonia.
   c. Pulse oximetry or arterial blood gases: Hypoxemia with PO_2 less than 60 mm Hg while the patient is breathing room air is a standard criterion for hospital admission for the community-dwelling population.
   d. Direct immunofluorescent examination of sputum when suspecting *Legionella.* Direct fluorescent antibody stain is a specific and rapid test for detecting legionellae in sputum.

e. BUN, creatinine, and electrolytes to evaluate state of hydration.
f. Liver test abnormalities may be seen in *Legionella* pneumonia.
g. Brain natriuretic peptide may be useful to rule out CHF.
h. In hospitalized patients, attempt to obtain an adequate sputum specimen for Gram stain and cultures.
2. Imaging studies: Findings on chest x-ray vary with the stage and type of pneumonia and the hydration of the patient.
   a. Pneumococcal pneumonia typically manifests with a segmental lobe infiltrate.
   b. Diffuse infiltrates on chest x-ray can be seen with *L. pneumophila, M. pneumoniae,* viral pneumonias, *P. jiroveci,* miliary TB, aspiration, and aspergillosis.
   c. An initial chest x-ray is also useful to rule out the presence of any complication (pneumothorax, effusion/empyema, abscesses).
   d. Bibasillar or lower lobe infiltrates suggest aspiration pneumonia.
   e. Swallowing evaluation is appropriate when aspiration pneumonia is suspected.

Treatment

1. Nonpharmacologic therapy.
   a. Oxygen to maintain PaO_2 greater than 60 mm Hg or O_2 saturation at least 90% by pulse oximetry.
   b. IV hydration to correct dehydration.
   c. Assisted ventilation in patients with significant respiratory failure if not prohibited by an advance directive.
      (1) Noninvasive assisted ventilation with a face mask (e.g., continuous positive airway pressure [CPAP]) may be used.
      (2) Use of CPAP should be discussed with the patient or proxy when an advance directive says not to intubate (DNI).
2. Pharmacologic therapy.
   a. Initial antibiotic therapy should be based on clinical radiographic and laboratory evaluation.
   b. A macrolide (azithromycin or clarithromycin) or levofloxacin is recommended for empirical outpatient treatment of community-acquired pneumonia.
   c. Cefotaxime or a β-lactam/β-lactamase inhibitor can be added in patients with more severe presentation who insist on outpatient therapy.
   d. Duration of treatment ranges from 7 to 14 days.
3. Hospitalization.
   a. Indications for hospital admission of outpatients.
      (1) O_2 saturation less than 90% while the patient is breathing room air.
      (2) Hemodynamic instability.
      (3) Active coexisting condition requiring hospitalization.
   b. Indications for hospitalization for nursing home residents are unclear and depend on the condition of the patient as well as the ability of the facility to provide adequate care 24/7.
   c. In the hospital setting, a patient admitted to the general ward can be treated empirically with a second- or third-generation cephalosporin (ceftriaxone, cefotaxime, cefuroxime) plus a macrolide (azithromycin or clarithromycin) or doxycycline. An antipseudomonal

quinolone (levofloxacin, moxifloxacin, or gatifloxacin) may be substituted for the macrolide or doxycycline.

   d. In hospitalized patients at risk for *P. aeruginosa* infection, empirical treatment should consist of an antipseudomonal β-lactam (cefepime or piperacillin-tazobactam) plus an aminoglycoside plus an antipseudomonal quinolone or macrolide.

4. Causes of slowly resolving or nonresolving pneumonia.

   a. Difficult-to-treat bacterial and nonbacterial infections.

      (1) Viral pneumonia, *Legionella*, pneumonococci, or staphylococci with impaired host response.

      (2) TB.

      (3) Fungi.

   b. Underlying neoplasm.

      (1) Lung.

      (2) Lymphoma.

      (3) Metastases.

   c. CHF.

   d. Pulmonary embolism.

   e. Immunologic or idiopathic.

      (1) Wegener's granulomatosis.

      (2) Pulmonary eosinophilic syndrome.

      (3) SLE.

   f. Drug toxicity (e.g., amiodarone).

5. Follow-up: A follow-up chest x-ray 6 to 8 weeks after the acute event should be considered to rule out postobstructive pneumonia associated with an endobronchial lesion (e.g., lung cancer).

6. Prevention.

   a. Recommend influenza and pneumococcal vaccine.

   b. Feeding tubes (gastrostomy or jejunostomy) are not proven to prevent aspiration pneumonia.

SUGGESTED READINGS

Davidson R, Cavalcanti R, Brunton JL, et al: Resistance to levofloxacin and failure of treatment of pneumococcal pneumonia. *N Engl J Med* 346:747-750, 2002.

Dosa D: Should I hospitalize my resident with nursing home acquired pneumonia. *JAMDA* 6:327-333, 2005.

Halm EA, Teirstein AS: Management of community-acquired pneumonia. *N Engl J Med* 347:2039-2045, 2002.

Loeb M, Carusone SC, Goeree R, et al: Effect of a clinical pathway to reduce hospitalizations in nursing home residents with pneumonia: A randomized, controlled trial. *JAMA* 295:2503-2510, 2006.

Norman KM, Yoshikawa TT: Bacterial pneumonia acquired in nursing homes. *Ann Long-Term Care* 14:26-32, 2006.

CLOSTRIDIUM DIFFICILE COLITIS

Tom J. Wachtel

Definition

1. *Clostridium difficile* ("C diff") colitis, also known as *pseudomembranous colitis* or *antibiotic-associated colitis,* is an infection localized to the colon, caused by *C. difficile,* an anaerobic, gram-positive rod. It is usually associated with an antibiotic treatment within the preceding 6 weeks.

2. The typical symptom, diarrhea, is caused by production of a toxin.
3. Occasionally, the more serious form of the disease, pseudomembranous colitis, can be lethal.

Epidemiology

1. Community acquired.
2. Nosocomial outbreaks can be traced to transmission by hands.
3. Older patients are more susceptible.

Clinical Findings

1. The spectrum of disease ranges from asymptomatic to life threatening.
2. The typical patient experiences watery diarrhea with abdominal pain 4 to 9 days after starting to take an antimicrobial.
3. Diarrhea can begin after the antimicrobial has been discontinued.
4. Fever is often present.
5. Fever and abdominal pain can occur without diarrhea.
6. Hypovolemia or dehydration can be present.

Pathogenesis

1. Alteration in the intestinal flora secondary to antibiotic therapy, typically ampicillin, cephalosporins, or clindamycin.
2. Presence of C. difficile, usually from an exogenous source but sometimes in the patient's endogenous flora, which is capable of producing toxins A and B.

Work-up

1. Laboratory tests.
   a. CBC: leukocytosis (occasionally, leukemoid reaction, i.e., WBC >30,000).
   b. Low albumin.
   c. Positive stool occult blood.
   d. Positive fecal leukocytes.
   e. Positive stool for C diff toxin.
2. Sigmoidoscopy.
   a. Can show pseudomembranes but can miss colitis localized to the ascending colon.
   b. Abdominal CT scan can show colon thickening.

Treatment

1. Discontinue the causing antibiotic if possible, if it is still in use, or replace it with a quinolone if appropriate.
2. Fluid and electrolyte resuscitation if needed.
3. Antidiarrheal agents.
   a. Bismuth subsalicylate (Kaopectate).
   b. Loperamide (Imodium).
   c. Cholestyramine.
4. Oral metronidazole 500 mg tid for 10 days.
5. Vancomycin.
   a. Oral vancomycin 125 mg qid for 10 days.
   b. This should be used as a second course following metronidazole failure to cut down on vancomycin-resistant enterococcus occurrence; however, the reverse sequence is equally effective.

6. Restore the normal colon flora with administration of lactobacillus orally for 1 month (can use yogurt).
7. Relapse.
   a. About 20% of patients relapse within 4 weeks of completing therapy.
   b. Most relapses occur within 3 to 10 days after discontinuation of therapy.
   c. The frequency of relapse is the same whether vancomycin or metronidazole is used as initial therapy.
   d. Re-treatment of patients who relapse with oral vancomycin or metronidazole is usually effective.
   e. Treatment options for patients with multiple relapses.
      (1) Vancomycin plus rifampin for 10 to 14 days.
      (2) Vancomycin or metronidazole orally for 10 to 14 days followed by a 3-week course of cholestyramine, or cholestyramine plus lactobacilli, or vancomycin orally every other day.

SUGGESTED READINGS

Archibald LK, Banerjee SN, Jarvis WR: Secular trends in hospital-acquired *Clostridium difficile* disease in the United States, 1987-2001. *J Infect Dis* 189: 1585-1589, 2004.

Brown RB, Gantz NM: Antimicrobial-associated colitis. In Gantz NM, Brown RB, Berk SL, Myers JW (eds): *Manual of Clinical Problems in Infectious Disease.* Philadelphia, Lippincott Williams & Wilkins, 2006, pp. 454-458.

Do AN, Fridkin SK, Yechouron A, et al: Risk factors for early recurrent *Clostridium difficile*–associated diarrhea. *Clin Infect Dis* 26:954-959, 1998.

Fekety R: Guidelines for the diagnosis and management of *Clostridium difficile*–associated diarrhea and colitis. *Am J Gastroenterol* 92:739-750, 1997.

Fekety R, McFarland LV, Surawicz CM, et al: Recurrent *Clostridium difficile* diarrhea: characteristics and risk factors for patients enrolled in a prospective, randomized, double-blinded trial. *Clin Infect Dis* 24:324-333, 1997.

Johnson S, Gerding DN, Olson MM, et al: Prospective, controlled study of vinyl glove use to interrupt *Clostridium difficile* nosocomial transmission. *Am J Med* 88:137-140, 1990.

Manabe YC, Vinetz JM, Moore RD, et al: *Clostridium difficile* colitis: An efficient clinical approach to diagnosis. *Ann Intern Med* 123:835-840, 1995.

McFarland LV, Mulligan ME, Kwok RY, Stamm WE: Nosocomial acquisition of *Clostridium difficile* infection. *N Engl J Med* 320:204-210, 1989.

Simenshine RH, McDonald LC: *Clostridium difficile*–associated disease: New challenges from an established pathogen. *Cleve Clin J Med* 73:187-197, 2006.

INFLUENZA

Claudia L. Dade, with revisions by Tom J. Wachtel

Definition

Influenza (flu) is an acute febrile illness caused by infection with influenza type A or B virus.

Epidemiology

Annual incidence of influenza-related deaths is approximately 20,000 deaths/year in the United States, most occurring during winter outbreaks lasting 5 to 6 weeks.

Clinical Findings

1. Classic flu is characterized by abrupt onset of fever, headache, myalgias, anorexia, and malaise after a 1- to 2-day incubation period.

2. Clinical syndromes are similar to those produced by other respiratory viruses, including pharyngitis, common colds, tracheobronchitis, and bronchiolitis.
3. Respiratory symptoms such as cough, sore throat, and nasal discharge are usually present at the onset of the illness, but systemic symptoms tend to predominate.
4. Frail or debilitated elderly patients can experience fever, weakness, and confusion (delirium) without any respiratory complaints.
5. Influenza pneumonia should be considered when rapidly progressive cough, dyspnea, and cyanosis occur after typical flu onset.

Etiology

1. Variation in the surface antigens of the influenza virus, hemagglutinin, and neuraminidase leads to infection with variants to which resistance is inadequate in the population at risk.
2. The virus is transmitted by small-particle aerosols and is deposited on the respiratory tract epithelium.

Differential Diagnosis

1. Other viral infections, e.g., adenovirus, parainfluenza virus infection.
2. Secondary bacterial pneumonia or mixed bacterial-viral pneumonia.

Work-up

1. Laboratory tests.
   a. Virus isolation from nasal or throat swab or sputum specimens is the most rapid diagnostic method in the setting of acute illness.
   b. Specimens are placed into virus transport medium and processed by a reference laboratory.
   c. For serologic diagnosis:
      (1) Paired serum specimens, acute and convalescent, the latter obtained 10 to 20 days later.
      (2) Fourfold rises or falls in the titer of antibodies (various techniques) are considered diagnostic of recent infection.
      (3) In an institutional setting (e.g., nursing home), once three or four residents have been diagnosed serologically, all other symptomatic patients are presumed infected.
   d. If symptoms are severe, get CBC, pulse oximetry, and blood cultures.
2. Imaging studies.
   a. Chest x-ray examination may be indicated to demonstrate findings of viral pneumonia: peribronchial and patchy interstitial infiltrates in multiple lobes with atelectasis.
   b. Possible progression to diffuse interstitial pneumonitis or bacterial pneumonia complications.

Treatment

1. Bed rest.
2. Hydration.
3. Antipyretics.
4. Amantadine is no longer recommended because of resistance.
5. Neuraminidase inhibitors block release of virions from infected cells, resulting in shortened duration of symptoms and decrease in complications. They are effective against both influenza A and B.

    a. Zanamivir (Relenza) administered via inhaler, 10 mg bid.

    b. Oseltamivir (Tamiflu) administered orally 75 mg bid for 10 days; requires renal dosing adjustment. May cause delirium.

6. Rimantadine (Flumadine).

    a. Give 100 mg PO bid for adults younger than 65 years.

    b. Give once daily in patients older than 65 years.

    c. Further dose adjustments are needed with renal insufficiency.

7. Placebo-controlled studies have suggested that antiviral therapy with any of these agents must be initiated within 1 to 2 days of the onset of symptoms to reduce the duration of illness.

8. Antibiotics if bacterial pneumonia is present.

Prevention

1. Prevention of influenza in patients at high risk is an important goal of primary care.

2. Vaccines reduce the risk of infection and the severity of illness for about 6 months following inoculation.

    a. Antigenic composition of the vaccine is updated annually.

    b. Vaccination should be given at the start of flu season (October) for the following groups:

        (1) Adults at least 65 years of age.

        (2) Adults with chronic cardiac or pulmonary disease, including asthma.

        (3) Adults with diabetes mellitus.

        (4) Immunocompromised patients.

        (5) Household contacts of persons in the previous groups.

        (6) Health care workers.

    c. The only contraindication to vaccination is hypersensitivity to chicken eggs.

3. Chemoprophylaxis.

    a. Oseltamivir can be used in the prophylactic mode.

    b. Rimantadine is approved only for prophyaxis against influenza A; it is ineffective against influenza B.

    c. Consider chemoprophylaxis:

        (1) For high-risk patients in whom vaccination is contraindicated.

        (2) When the available vaccine is known not to include the circulating strain.

        (3) To provide added protection to immunosuppressed patients likely to have a diminished response to vaccination.

        (4) In the setting of an outbreak, when immediate protection of unvaccinated or recently vaccinated patients is desired (e.g., in a nursing home).

    d. Give for 2 weeks in the case of late vaccination and for the duration of the flu season in other patients.

SUGGESTED READINGS

Advisory Committee on Immunization Practices (AIP): Controlling influenza: Guidelines for using antiviral agents. *J Resp Dis* 27:43-46, 2006.

Colgan R et al: Antiviral drugs in the immunocompetent host: part II. Treatment of influenza and respiratory syncytial virus infections. *Am Fam Physician* 67(4): 763-766, 2003.

Montalto NJ: An office-based approach to influenza: Clinical diagnosis and laboratory testing, *Am Fam Physician* 67(1):111-118, 2003.

METHICILLIN-RESISTANT STAPHYLOCOCCUS AUREUS

Tom J. Wachtel

Definition

Staphylococcal resistance to methicillin and other semisynthetic penicillins is chromosomally linked and does not involve the inactivation of the antimicrobial. Instead, methicillin-resistant staphylococci produce a penicillin-binding protein that has reduced affinity for β-lactam antimicrobials, including the semisynthetic penicillins; this protein is called *penicillin-binding protein 2a*. Methicillin-resistant *Staphylococcus aureus* (MRSA) has the same virulence found in methicillin-susceptible staphylococci and can cause life-threatening disease in humans.

Epidemiology

1. Geographically variable prevalence.
2. There are now (since 2002) vancomycin-resistant strains of *S. aureus*.
3. More than 90% of all acute-care hospitals report having patients infected with this microbe.
4. Transmission.
   a. MRSA is usually introduced into a hospital by patients who are transferred from other institutions, especially nursing homes, in which the organisms are endemic. In fact, hospitals and nursing homes keep reinfecting each other.
   b. Physicians are also implicated as the source of interhospital spread.
   c. After introduction into a nursing home or a hospital, MRSA can disseminate rapidly and colonize patients and personnel, who then serve as sources of continued transmission.
   d. Diseases of the skin, including pressure ulcers, burns, surgical wounds, and chronic dermatitis, increase the probability of colonization.
   e. Colonization of the anterior nares of patients and hospital employees can also occur and facilitate the spread of MRSA.
   f. Colonization can progress to infection with MRSA among patients who are aged and debilitated.

Clinical Findings

1. Skin infection.
   a. Impetigo.
   b. Boils and carbuncles.
   c. Cellulitis.
   d. Infected surgical wounds or burns.
2. Endocarditis.
3. Upper and lower respiratory infection (e.g., bronchitis or pneumonia).
4. Osteomyelitis.
5. Septic arthritis.
6. Bacteremia.

Treatment

1. Vancomycin.
   a. Dosing.
      (1) Vancomycin is given at a dosage of 1 g every 12 hours.

(2) Because the drug is excreted by the kidneys, dosage adjustments are needed in patients with renal failure.

(3) Serum levels should be monitored, and peak concentrations of 30 to 40 μg/mL with trough levels of 5 to 10 μg/mL should be achieved.

b. Nephrotoxicity is rare unless another nephrotoxic drug is coadministered.

c. Creatinine levels should be monitored weekly during treatment.

d. Patients who fail to respond to therapy with vancomycin alone should be given a combination of vancomycin with rifampin to produce synergistic killing.

2. Some strains of MRSA are sensitive to trimethoprim–sulfamethoxazole, and the drug can be used to treat patients infected with MRSA.

3. Ciprofloxacin can be used in sensitive strains.

4. Linezolid, quinupristin-dalfopristin, and dapomycin are alternative agents for patients who fail or cannot tolerate vancomycin.

a. In one report, linezolid was more effective than vancomycin.

b. Linezolid (Zyvox) is given at a dose of 600 mg PO or IV q12h for 2 to 4 weeks.

c. Linezolid can cause myelosuppression, so weekly CBC is recommended during treatment..

d. *C. difficile* colitis can occasionally occur as a complication.

e. Linezolid is bacteriostatic, not bacteriocidal.

Infection Control

1. Emphasize hand hygiene using alcohol-based products.

2. Surveillance cultures (nares, axillae, groin, rectum) weekly.

3. Culture high-risk patients.

4. Patients colonized and/or infected with MRSA in a draining wound or in the sputum should be placed on contact isolation.

5. Patients who have MRSA in their sputum and are actively coughing require a mask on entering. Patients should be placed in private rooms or be cohorted with other patients who are MRSA positive.

6. Use gloves, gowns, and mask upon entering the room of a patient with MRSA.

7. MRSA patients must have a BP cuff, a stethoscope, vacuum collecting tube (Vacutainer) sleeve, and tourniquet in the room.

8. MRSA status should not restrict the patient's activity.

(1) Any wounds should be covered, with drainage contained before the patient leaves the room.

(2) Good personal hygiene should be stressed with the patient.

(3) If drainage and secretions cannot be contained, the patient should be restricted to his or her room.

9. When the patient is scheduled to go to another department (physical therapy, occupational therapy, radiology), the receiving department should be informed of the patient's MRSA status so appropriate precautions can be observed by the personnel in that department.

10. If standard infection control measures fail to arrest an outbreak of MRSA disease, surveillance cultures should be obtained to identify the colonized person who may be the source of continuous person-to-person transmission.

    a. Physicians, nursing personnel, and other persons in contact with patients who are infected or colonized with MRSA should be screened for carriage by culturing the anterior nares and cutaneous lesions.

    b. If the survey of personnel fails to detect MRSA carriage but the outbreak continues, additional cultures of health care workers' nares, throats, hands, axillae, rectums and inguinal regions should be considered.

    c. Occasionally, intensive care units must be closed to new admissions to control an outbreak of infection.

11. Antimicrobials should be used if an outbreak of MRSA disease is not terminated by alternate infection-control procedures because treatment of carriers is commonly associated with eradication of colonizing MRSA and control of epidemics.

    a. Topical 2% mupirocin (Bactroban) applied to the anterior nares two or three times daily for 5 to 7 days may be an effective means of eliminating the nasal carrier state.

    b. Minocycline (100 mg bid) together with mupirocin and rifampin also has been highly effective in eradicating the nasal carrier state.

    c. Follow-up cultures are necessary to ensure that MRSA has been eradicated from the colonized patients and health care workers.

SUGGESTED READINGS

Boyce JM, Havill NL, Kohan C, et al: Do infection control measures work for methicillin-resistant *Staphylococcus aureus*? *Infect Control Hosp Epidemiol* 25:395-401, 2004.

Cooper BS, Stone SP, Kibbler CC, et al: Isolation measures in the hospital management of methicillin resistant *Staphylococcus aureus* (MRSA): Systematic review of the literature. *BMJ* 329:1-8, 2004.

Crossley K: Long-term care facilities as sources of antibiotic-resistant nosocomial pathogens. *Curr Opin Infect Dis* 14:455-459, 2001.

Eady EA, Cove JH: Staphylococcal resistance revisited: Community-acquired methicillin resistant *Staphylococcus aureus*—an emerging problem for the management of skin and soft tissue infections. *Curr Opin Infect Dis* 16:103-124, 2003.

Eliopoulos GM: Quinupristin-dalfopristin and linezolid: Evidence and opinion. *Clin Infect Dis* 36:473-481, 2003.

Farr BM: Prevention and control of methicillin-resistant *Staphylococcus aureus* infections. *Curr Opin Infect Dis* 17:317-322, 2004.

Gantz NM: Methicillin-resistant *Staphylococcus aureus*. In Gantz NM, Brown BB, Berk SL, Myers JW (eds): *Manual of clinical problems in infectious disease*, ed 5. Philadelphia, Lippincott Williams & Wilkins, 2006, pp 263-268.

Henderson DK: Managing MRSA: A paradigm for preventing nosocomial transmission of resistant organism. *Am J Med* 119:545-552, 2006.

Howden BP, Ward PB, Charles PG, et al: Treatment outcomes for serious infections caused by methicillin-resistant *Staphylococcus aureus* with reduced vancomycin susceptibility. *Clin Infect Dis* 38:521-528, 2004.

Melzer M, Eykyn SL, Grandsden WR, Chinn S: Is methicillin-resistant *Staphylococcus aureus* more virulent than methicillin-susceptible *S. aureus*? A comparative cohort study of British patients with nosocomial infection and bacteremia. *Clin Infect Dis* 37:1453-1460, 2004.

Muto CA, Jernigan JA, Ostrowsky BE, et al: SHEA guideline for preventing nosocomial transmission of multidrug-resistant strains of *Staphylococcus aureus* and *Enterococcus*. *Infect Control Hosp Epidemiol* 24:362-386, 2003.

Palavecino E: Community-acquired methicillin-resistant *Staphylococcus aureus* infections. *Clin Lab Med* 24:403-418, 2004.

Rice LB: Antimicrobial resistance in gram-positive bacteria. Am J Med 119:S11-S19, 2006.

Richards LR: Preventing antimicrobial-resistant bacterial infection among older adults in long-term care facilities. J Am Dir Assoc 6:144-151, 2005.

TUBERCULOSIS

George O. Alonso and Tom J. Wachtel

Definition

Pulmonary tuberculosis (TB) is an infection of the lung caused by the bacterium *Mycobacterium tuberculosis*. Disseminated hematogenous disease caused by *M. tuberculosis* is called miliary TB. It can involve the lungs or be extrapulmonary and occur in virtually every organ site.

Epidemiology

1. Elderly patients account for approximately 30% of newly diagnosed TB cases yearly.
2. Persons older than 65 years have a TB case rate higher than any other population except HIV-positive persons.
3. More than 50% of new cases occur in persons older than 65 years.
4. Nursing home residents account for 20% of cases in the elderly.
5. Ninety percent of TB cases in the geriatric population are due to prior exposure or infection and reactivation.

Clinical Findings

1. Pulmonary TB.
   a. Primary pulmonary TB infection is generally asymptomatic.
   b. Reactivation pulmonary TB or progressive primary pulmonary TB.
      (1) Fever.
      (2) Night sweats.
      (3) Cough.
      (4) Hemoptysis.
      (5) Scanty nonpurulent sputum.
      (6) Weight loss.
   c. Pleurisy.
      (1) Pleuritic chest pain.
      (2) Fever.
      (3) Shortness of breath.
   d. Chest examination is nonspecific.
2. Miliary or disseminated TB.
   a. Systemic symptoms.
      (1) High intermittent fever (fever of unknown origin).
      (2) Night sweats.
      (3) Weight loss.
      (4) Malaise.
   b. Symptoms referable to individual organ systems might predominate.
      (1) Lungs.
         (a) Cough.
         (b) Shortness of breath.
      (2) TB meningitis.
         (a) Gradual-onset headache.
         (b) Minimal meningeal signs.

  (c) Change in mental status.
  (d) Cranial nerve VI palsy.
 (3) TB hepatitis.
  (a) Tender liver.
  (b) Obstructive enzymes (alkaline phosphatase) more elevated than hepatocellular enzymes (transaminase) and bilirubin.
 (4) TB pericarditis.
  (a) Chest pain.
  (b) Pericardial rub.
  (c) Cardiac tamponade.
  (d) Constrictive pericarditis.
 (5) Skeletal TB.
  (a) Large joint arthritis.
  (b) Bone lesions (especially ribs).
  (c) Pott's disease (spine).
 (6) Genitourinary TB.
  (a) Renal TB.
   i. Papillary necrosis and/or destruction of renal pelvis.
   ii. Strictures of upper third of ureters.
   iii. Hematuria.
   iv. Pyuria with negative or misleading bacterial cultures.
   v. Preserved renal function.
  (b) TB orchitis or epididymitis.
   i. Scrotal mass.
   ii. Draining abscess.
  (c) Prostatic TB.
 (7) Gastrointestinal TB is often difficult to distinguish from granulomatous bowel disease (Crohn's disease).
  (a) Bowel lesions.
   i. Circumferential ulcers.
   ii. Strictures.
   iii. Calcified granulomas.
   iv. TB mesenteric caseous adenitis.
   v. Abscess, but rare fistula formation.
  (b) Symptoms.
   i. Diarrhea.
   ii. Pain.
   iii. Obstruction.
   iv. Bleeding.
  (c) TB peritonitis is rare in geriatric patients.
 (8) Cutaneous TB.
  (a) Nodules or abscesses.
  (b) Tuberculids.
  (c) Erythema nodosum.
 (9) TB lymphadenitis (scrofula) can involve any node group.
 (10) Adrenal insufficiency is possible with M. *tuberculosis* infection of the adrenal gland.
 (11) Other rare presentations.
  (a) TB laryngitis.
  (b) TB otitis.
  (c) Ocular TB: choroidal tubercles, iritis, uveitis, episcleritis.

Etiology

1. M. *tuberculosis*, a slow-growing, aerobic, non–spore-forming bacillus.
2. Transmission is facilitated by close exposure to high-velocity cough (unprotected by proper mask or respirators) from patient with acid-fast bacillus (AFB)–positive sputum and cavitary lesions, producing aerosolized droplets containing AFB, which are inhaled directly into the alveoli. Humans are the only reservoir for M. *tuberculosis*.
3. Pathogenesis of pulmonary TB: AFB (M. *tuberculosis*) ingested by macrophages in alveoli, then transported to regional lymph nodes, where spread is usually contained.
4. Primary TB (asymptomatic, pneumonitis in lower or midlung fields, with hilar lymphadenopathy) essentially is an intracellular infection, resulting in multiplication of organisms for 2 to 12 weeks after exposure, until cell-mediated hypersensitivity matures and contains infection. AFB contained by T cell–mediated immune responses leads to pulmonary or extrapulmonary granulomas, wherein organisms can survive within macrophages but do not multiply and from which spread does not occur.
5. Progressive primary pulmonary disease types.
   a. May immediately follow the asymptomatic phase or take place later, depending largely on host condition (reactivation TB).
   b. Necrotizing pulmonary infiltrates.
   c. TB bronchopneumonia.
   d. Endobronchial TB.
   e. Interstitial TB.
   f. Widespread miliary lung lesions.
   g. TB pleurisy with pleural effusion.
6. Some AFB can reach the blood stream and disseminate widely (e.g., miliary TB).
7. Reactivation TB.
   a. Occurs months to years following primary TB.
   b. Preferentially involves the apical posterior segments of the upper lobes and superior segments of the lower lobes.
      (1) Associated with necrosis and cavitation of involved lung, hemoptysis, chronic fever, night sweats, weight loss.
      (2) Spread within lung occurs via cough and inhalation.

Differential Diagnosis

1. Pulmonary TB.
   a. Necrotizing pneumonia (anaerobic, gram negative).
   b. Histoplasmosis.
   c. Coccidioidomycosis.
   d. Interstitial lung diseases.
   e. Cancer.
   f. Sarcoidosis.
   g. Silicosis.
   h. Rare pneumonias (e.g., atypical mycobacteria).
2. Miliary/disseminated TB.
   a. Lymphoma.
   b. Typhoid fever.
   c. Brucellosis.
   d. Other tumors.

e. Collagen-vascular disease.
f. Widespread sites of possible dissemination result in multiple differential diagnostic possibilities.

Work-up

Pulmonary TB

1. Purified protein derivative (PPD).
   a. Recent conversion from negative to positive within 3 months of exposure is highly suggestive of recent infection.
   b. A single positive PPD is not diagnostic.
   c. Negative PPD never rules out acute TB.
   d. Positive PPD can reflect the booster phenomenon and can mimic a new skin test conversion. A prior positive PPD can become negative after several years and return to positive only after a second repeated PPD, usually done within 1 week.
   e. Induration is evaluated after 72 hours of intradermal injection of 0.1 mL of 5 TU-PPD. Positive PPD reaction is determined as follows:
      (1) A 5-mm induration in an HIV-positive close contact of a patient with active TB, fibrotic chest lesions.
      (2) A 10-mm induration if the patient is one of the following:
         (a) In a high-medical-risk group.
             i. Immunosuppressive disease or therapy.
             ii. Renal failure.
             iii. Gastrectomy.
             iv. Silicosis.
             v. Diabetes.
         (b) In a foreign-born high-risk group.
             i. Southeast Asia.
             ii. Latin America.
             iii. Africa.
             iv. India.
         (c) In a low socioeconomic group.
         (d) An IV drug addict.
         (e) A prisoner.
         (f) A health care worker.
      (3) A 15-mm induration if the patient is low risk.
   f. Anergy antigen testing (using mumps, *Candida*, or tetanus toxoid) can identify patients who are truly anergic to PPD and these antigens, but results are often confusing. Not recommended.
   g. Patients with TB may be selectively anergic only to PPD.
   h. Positive PPD indicates prior infection but does not diagnose active disease.
2. Laboratory tests.
   a. Sputum for AFB stains and culture (of induced sputum if the patient is not coughing productively).
   b. Sputum from bronchoscopy if there is high suspicion of TB with negative expectorated induced sputum for AFB.
      (1) Positive AFB smear is essential before or shortly after treatment to ensure subsequent growth for definitive diagnosis and sensitivity testing.

(2) Consider lung biopsy if sputum is negative, especially if infiltrates are predominantly interstitial.
  c. AFB stain-negative sputum might grow M. *tuberculosis* subsequently.
  d. Gastric aspirates in some cases.
  e. CBC has variable values and is rarely helpful.
    (1) WBCs: low, normal, or elevated (including leukemoid reaction: >50,000).
    (2) Normocytic anemia (of chronic disease).
    (3) Pancytopenia.
  f. ESR is usually elevated (not very useful).
  g. Thoracentesis.
    (1) Exudative effusion.
      (a) Elevated protein.
      (b) Decreased glucose.
      (c) Elevated WBCs (polymorphonuclear leukocytes early, replaced later by lymphocytes).
      (d) May be hemorrhagic.
    (2) Pleural fluid is usually AFB negative.
    (3) Pleural biopsy is often diagnostic.
    (4) Culture pleural biopsy tissue for AFB.
  h. Bone marrow biopsy may be helpful in difficult cases, especially miliary tuberculosis.
3. Imaging studies: Chest x-ray examination.
  a. Primary infection reflected by calcified peripheral lung nodule with calcified hilar lymph node.
  b. Reactivation pulmonary TB.
    (1) Necrosis.
    (2) Cavitation (especially on apical lordotic views).
    (3) Fibrosis and hilar retraction.
    (4) Bronchopneumonia.
    (5) Interstitial infiltrates.
    (6) Miliary pattern.
  c. TB pleurisy: Pleural effusion, often rapidly accumulating and massive.
  d. TB activity might not be established by a single chest x-ray examination.
  e. Serial chest x-ray examinations are excellent indicators of progression or regression.

Miliary/Disseminated/Extrapulmonary TB

1. CBC is often normal.
2. ESR is usually elevated.
3. PPD.
4. Fluid analysis and culture wherever available.
  a. Sputum.
  b. Urine.
  c. Cerebrospinal fluid.
  d. Pleural.
  e. Pericardial.
  f. Peritoneal.
  g. Gastric aspirates.

5. Chest x-ray examination (might or might not be positive).
6. CT scan or MRI of brain.
   a. Tuberculoma.
   b. Basilar arachnoiditis.
7. Barium studies of bowel.
8. Biopsy of any involved tissue is advisable to make immediate diagnosis.
   a. Transbronchial biopsy is preferred and easily accessible.
   b. Bone marrow.
   c. Lymph node.
   d. Scrotal mass if present.
   e. Any other involved site.
   f. Finding granulomas or AFB on biopsy specimen is diagnostic.

Treatment

General

1. Bedrest during acute phase of treatment.
2. High-calorie, high-protein diet to reverse malnutrition and enhance immune response to TB.
3. Isolation in negative-pressure rooms with high-volume air replacement and circulation (with health care providers wearing proper protective 0.5- to 1-μm filter respirators).
   a. Until three consecutive sputum AFB smears are negative, in pulmonary TB.
   b. Isolation is not required for closed-space (extrapulmonary) TB infections.
4. All contacts (especially close household contacts and infants) should be tested for PPD conversions more than 3 months following exposure.
5. Those with positive PPD should be evaluated for active TB and treated or given prophylaxis.

Antituberculous Antibiotics

1. Antituberculous antibiotics are listed in Table 5-26.
2. Compliance.
   a. Rigid adherence to the treatment regimen is the chief determinant of success.
   b. Required supervised directly observed therapy (DOT) is recommended for all patients and required for unreliable patients.
3. Preferred adult regimen.
   a. Thrice weekly for 6 months, all of the following:
      (1) Isoniazid (INH) 15 mg/kg (max 900 mg).
      (2) Rifampin 600 mg.
      (3) Ethambutol (EMB) 30 mg/kg (max 2500 mg).
      (4) Pyrazinamide (PZA).
         (a) Patients lighter than 50 kg: 2 g.
         (b) Patients 51 to 74 kg: 2.5 g.
         (c) Patients heavier than 75 kg: 3 g.
   b. Short-course daily therapy, 6 months total therapy.
      (1) For 2 months daily and until smear negative and sensitivity is confirmed.
         (a) INH 900 mg.
         (b) Rifampin 600 mg.

Table 5-26 Treatment Regimens for Patients with Pulmonary Tuberculosis Caused by Drug-Susceptible Organisms

| | Initiation Phase | | | Continuation Phase | |
Agents	Typical Dose	Schedule and Minimal Duration	Agents	Typical Dose	Schedule and Minimal Duration
Isoniazid	900 mg	Once daily for 8 weeks or 5 times per week for 8 weeks (DOT)	Isoniazid	900 mg	Once daily for 18 weeks or 5 times per week for 18 weeks (DOT) or twice weekly for 18 weeks
Rifampin	600 mg		Rifampin	600 mg	
Pyrazinamide†	1500 mg				
Ethambutol‡	1200 mg		Isoniazid	900 mg	Once weekly for 18 weeks
			Rifapentine	600 mg	
Isoniazid	900 mg	Once daily for 2 weeks then twice weekly for 6 weeks or 5 times per week for 2 weeks, then twice weekly for 6 weeks (DOT)	Isoniazid	900 mg	Twice weekly for 18 weeks
Rifampin	600 mg		Rifampin	600 mg	
Pyrazinamide†	1500 mg				
Ethambutol‡	1200 mg		Isoniazid	900 mg	Once weekly for 18 weeks
			Rifapentine	600 mg	

DOT, directly observed therapy.
†Pyrazinamide dose is 1500 mg for daily or 5 times weekly dosing, 2500 mg for 3 times weekly dosing and 3000 mg for twice weekly dosing (70-kg person).
‡Ethambutol dose is 1200 for daily or 5 times weekly dosing, 2000 mg for 3 times weekly dosing, and 2800 mg for twice weekly dosing (70-kg person).

Continued

Table 5-26 **Treatment Regimens For Patients with Pulmonary Tuberculosis Caused by Drug-Susceptible Organisms—cont'd**

	Initiation Phase			Continuation Phase		
Agents	Typical Dose	Schedule and Minimal Duration		Agents	Typical Dose	Schedule and Minimal Duration
Isoniazid	900 mg	3 times per week for 8 weeks (DOT)		Isoniazid	900 mg	3 times per week for 18 weeks
Rifampin	600 mg			Rifampin	600 mg	
Pyrazinamide[†]	1500 mg					
Ethambutol[‡]	1200 mg					
Isoniazid	900 mg	Once daily for 8 weeks or		Isoniazid	900 mg	Once daily for 31 weeks or
Rifampin	600 mg	5 times per week for 8 weeks (DOT)		Rifampin	600 mg	5 times per week for 31 weeks (DOT) or twice weekly for 31 weeks
Ethambutol[‡]	1200 mg					

      (c) EMB 15 mg/kg (max 2500 mg).

      (d) PZA.

         i. Patients lighter than 50 kg: 1.5 g.

         ii. Patients 51 to 74 kg: 2 g.

         iii. Patients heavier than 75 kg: 2.5 g.

   (2) Then INH plus rifampin daily for 4 months.

4. Treatment guidelines.

  a. Never add a single drug to a failing regimen.

  b. Never treat TB with only one drug.

  c. Monitor for clinical toxicity (especially hepatitis).

   (1) Patient and physician awareness that anorexia, nausea, right upper quadrant pain, and unexplained malaise require immediate cessation of treatment.

   (2) Evaluation of liver function tests: Minimal serum glutamic pyruvic transaminase (SGPT) elevations without symptoms is generally transient and not clinically significant.

  d. Treatment for 12 months is often required for bone and renal TB.

  e. Prolonged treatment is often required for central nervous system and pericardial TB.

  f. Drug resistance (multiple drug resistance) should be referred to a specialty setting.

  g. Follow-up.

   (1) Monthly follow-up by a physician experienced in TB treatment.

   (2) Confirm chest x-ray regression at 2 to 3 months.

5. Preventive treatment for PPD conversion only (infection without disease).

  a. Must be certain that the chest x-ray examination is negative and the patient has no symptoms of TB.

  b. INH 300 mg daily for 6 to 12 months and for at least 12 months if the patient is HIV-positive.

  c. Most important groups.

   (1) Close contact of a patient with active TB.

   (2) Recent converter.

   (3) Old TB on chest x-ray examination.

   (4) Medical risk factors (e.g., corticosteroid use).

   (5) Immigrant from a high-risk foreign country.

   (6) Homeless person.

6. Chronic stable positive PPD (several years): INH prophylaxis is not recommended for geriatric patients because INH toxicity outweighs benefit.

7. Use of preventive therapy for suspected INH-resistant organisms is unclear.

SUGGESTED READINGS

American Thoracic Society: Diagnostic standards and classification of tuberculosis in adults and children. *Am J Respir Crit Care Med* 161:1376-1395, 2000.

Kanaya AM, Glidden DV, Chambers HF: Identifying pulmonary tuberculosis in patients with negative sputum smear results. *Chest* 120(2):349-355, 2001.

Karcic AA et al: An elderly woman with chronic knee pain and abnormal chest radiography. *Postgrad Med* 77(911):606-607, 2001.

Mulder K: Tuberculosis: A case history. *Lancet* 358(9283):766, 2001.

Potter B, Rindfleish K, Kraus CK: Management of active tuberculosis. *Am Fam Physician* 72:2225-2232, 2005.

Small P, Fujiwara P: Management of tuberculosis in the United States. *N Engl J Med* 345:189-200, 2001.

Tudo G, Gonzalez J, Gatell JM, et al: Detection of unsuspected cases of nosocomial transmission of tuberculosis by use of a molecular typing method. *Clin Infec Dis* 33(4):453-459, 2001.

URINARY TRACT INFECTION

Philip J. Aliotta, with revisions by Tom J. Wachtel

Definition

Urinary tract infection (UTI) is a term that covers a range of clinical entities that have in common a positive urine culture.

1. The usual threshold for positivity is growth of more than 100,000 colony forming units (CFU) per milliliter from a midstream-catch urine sample.
2. In symptomatic patients, infection is diagnosed from a smaller number of bacteria (between 100 and 10,000 CFU/mL of midstream urine).

Classification

1. First infection: The first documented UTI tends to be uncomplicated and is easily treated.
2. Unresolved bacteriuria.
   a. UTI in which the urinary tract is not sterilized with therapy.
   b. Main causes.
      (1) Bacterial resistance.
      (2) Patient noncompliance.
      (3) Mixed bacterial infections.
      (4) Rapid reinfection.
      (5) Azotemia.
      (6) Infected stones.
      (7) Papillary necrosis.
3. Bacterial persistence.
   a. UTI in which the urine cultures become sterile during therapy, but a persistent source of infection from a site within the urinary tract gives rise to reinfection by the same organism.
   b. Causes.
      (1) Infected stone.
      (2) Chronic bacterial prostatitis.
      (3) Atrophic infected kidney.
      (4) Vesicovaginal or enterovesical fistulas.
      (5) Obstructive uropathy.
4. Reinfection: UTI in which a new infection occurs with new pathogens at variable intervals after a previous infection has been eradicated.
5. Relapse.
   a. The less common form of recurrent infection.
   b. It occurs within 2 weeks of treatment when the same organism reappears in the same site as the previous infection.
   c. Relapsing infections of the urinary tract most commonly occur in pyelonephritis, kidney obstruction from a stone, and prostatitis.

Epidemiology

1. More common in women.
2. In adults 65 years and older, at least 10% of men and 20% of women have bacteriuria. The number is even higher in the nursing home population.

Pathogenesis

1. Four major pathways.
   a. Ascending from the urethra.
   b. Lymphatic.
   c. Hematogenous.
   d. Direct extension from another organ (e.g., prostate).
2. Risk factors.
   (a) Neurologic diseases.
   (b) Renal failure.
   (c) Diabetes.
   (d) Anatomic abnormalities.
      (1) Bladder outlet obstruction.
      (2) Urethral stricture.
      (3) Vesicoureteral reflux.
      (4) Fistula.
      (5) Urinary diversion.
      (6) Infected stones.
   (e) Older age.
   (f) Instrumentation.
   (g) Poor patient compliance.
   (h) Poor hygiene.
   (i) Infrequent voider.
   (j) Douches.
   (k) Catheters.
3. Catheters.
   a. All patients who require a long-term Foley catheter eventually develop significant levels of bacteriuria.
   b. Treatment is reserved for patients who become symptomatic (leukocytosis, fever, chills, malaise, anorexia, etc.).
   c. Prophylactic antibiotics to treat patients who have chronic catheters are not recommended because they increase the risk of acquiring bacteria that are or become resistant to antibiotic therapy.
4. Once bacteria reach the urinary tract, three factors determine whether the infection occurs.
   a. Virulence of the microorganism.
   b. Inoculum size.
   c. Adequacy of the host defense mechanism.
5. Urinary pathogens.
   a. In more than 95% of UTIs, the infecting organism is a member of the Enterobacteriaceae family, is an *Enterococcus* species, or is *Pseudomonas aeruginosa*.
   b. The isolation of two or more bacterial species from a urine culture generally signifies a contaminated specimen, unless the patient has an indwelling catheter, a urinary diversion, or a chronic complicated infection.

6. Defense mechanisms against cystitis.
   a. Low pH and high osmolarity.
   b. Mucopolysaccharide glycosaminoglycan protective layer.
   c. Normal bladder that empties completely and has no incontinence.
   d. Estrogen.

Clinical Findings

1. UTI presentation is inconsistent and clinical symptoms cannot be relied upon to diagnose UTI accurately or to localize the site of infection. Patients complain of:
   a. Urinary frequency and urgency.
   b. Dysuria.
   c. New urinary incontinence (usually urge incontinence).
   d. Suprapubic pain.
   e. Gross or microscopic hematuria.
   f. Sepsis (urosepsis).
   g. Acute or subacute change in mental status (delirium).
2. Acute pyelonephritis.
   a. Manifests with:
      (1) Fever.
      (2) Flank or abdominal pain.
      (3) Chills.
      (4) Malaise.
      (5) Vomiting.
      (6) Diarrhea.
   b. Complications.
      (1) Renal abscess.
      (2) Perinephric abscess.
      (3) Emphysematous pyelonephritis.
      (4) Pyonephrosis.

Differential Diagnosis

1. Vaginitis.
2. Prostatitis.
3. Overactive bladder.
4. Interstitial cystitis.
5. Obstructive uropathy.
6. Kidney stones.
7. Urologic malignancy (e.g., bladder cancer).
8. Fistulas.

Work-up

1. Laboratory tests.
   a. Urinalysis with microscopic evaluation of clean-catch urine for bacteria and pyuria.
   b. Urine culture and sensitivity.
   c. CBC with differential (may show leukocytosis).
2. Imaging studies.
   a. Warranted only if renal infection or genitourinary abnormality is suspected.
   b. Kidney, ureter, and bladder (KUB), renal sonogram, intravenous pyelogram (IVP), CT scan.

  c. Cystoscopy with occasional retrograde pyelography to rule out obstructive uropathy; stenting the obstruction is possibly required.

Treatment

1. Hydration.
2. Pelvic hygiene.
3. Antibiotics.
4. Conventional therapy of 7 days.
   a. Shorter-term therapy is not appropriate for geriatric patients.
   b. Agents of choice.
      (1) Amoxicillin with or without clavulanate.
      (2) Cephalosporins.
      (3) Fluoroquinolones.
      (4) Nitrofurantoin.
      (5) Trimethoprim with sulfonamide.
5. For pyelonephritis or urosepsis.
   a. Hospitalization and IV antibiotics (aminoglycoside plus cephalosporin) until the patient is afebrile and stable. followed by oral agents (based on sensitivity) for 2 weeks.
   b. Moderate forms of pyelonephritis have been successfully treated with fluoroquinolone therapy for 21 days, without requiring hospitalization.
   c. Most important, complicating factors such as obstructive uropathy or infected stones must be identified and treated. In men, consider comorbid or underlying prostatitis.
6. Recurrent UTI.
   a. Management options include continuous antibiotic prophylaxis, intermittent self-treatment, or postcoital prophylaxis.
   b. Prophylaxis is considered for women who experience two or more symptomatic UTIs over a 6-month period or three or more episodes over a 12-month period.
7. Asymptomatic bacteriuria.
   a. Occurs in both anatomically normal and abnormal urinary tracts.
   b. This can clear spontaneously, persist, or lead to symptomatic kidney infection.
   c. Treatment is not recommended except in patients with stones, obstructive uropathy, parenchymal renal disease, and diabetes mellitus.

SUGGESTED READINGS

Bent S, Nallamothu BK, Simel DL, et al: Does this woman have an acute uncomplicated urinary tract infection? JAMA 287:2701-2710, 2002.

Gomolin IH, Siami PF, Reuning-Scherer J, et al: Efficacy and safety of ciprofloxacin oral suspension versus trimethoprim–sulfamethoxazole oral suspension for treatment of older women with acute urinary tract infection. J Am Geriatr Soc 49:1606-1613, 2001.

Gupta K, Hooton TM, Stamm WE: Increasing antimicrobial resistance and the management of uncomplicated community-acquired urinary tract infections. Ann Int Med 135:41-50, 2001.

Kamel HK: Managing urinary tract infections: Guide for nursing home practitioners. Ann Long-Term Care 13:25-30, 2005.

Levy SB: Multidrug resistance—a sign of the times, N Engl J Med 338:1376-1378, 1998.

VANCOMYCIN-RESISTANT ENTEROCOCCI

Tom J. Wachtel

Definition

Two enterococcal species, *Enterococcus faecalis* and *Enterococcus faecium* are seen in clinical practice. *E. faecalis* accounts for 80% of isolates. Among vancomycin-resistant enterococci (VRE), 90% of the isolates are *E. faecium*.

Epidemiology

1. Identified as a problem in the United States since 1989.
2. Vancomycin resistance is associated with aminoglycosides and ampicillin.
3. Patient-to-patient transmission.
   a. Direct contact.
   b. Indirect contact.
      (1) Hands of health care personnel.
      (2) Patient care equipment such as electronic thermometers and environmental surfaces.
4. Most hospitals in the United States have encountered VRE.
5. Enterococci rank second or third in frequency as causes of nosocomial infections in the United States.

Clinical Findings

1. Asymptomatic colonization. Enterococci, which are gram-positive cocci, are part of the normal gastrointestinal flora and can also be found in the mouth, vagina, and perineal skin.
2. Nosocomial UTI.
3. Infected pressure ulcer or surgical wound.
4. Nosocomial pneumonia.
5. Bacteremia/sepsis.
6. Other.
7. Risk factors for VRE colonization or infection.
   a. Serious illness.
   b. Advanced age.
   c. Immunosuppression.
   d. Intensive care unit residence.
   e. Prior surgery.
   f. Renal insufficiency.
   g. Long hospital stay (7 days or more).
   h. Presence of a urinary or vascular catheter.
   i. Use of antibiotics, especially third-generation cephalosporins, vancomycin, and drugs for anaerobes.
8. Patients colonized with VRE may remain so for many years.

Pathogenesis

1. Resistance to vancomycin can be classified as three phenotypes.
   a. Strains with van A resistance show a high level of resistance to vancomycin (minimum inhibitory concentrations [MICs] ≥ 64 µg/mL) and resistance to another glycopeptide, teicoplanin (MICs ≥ 16 µg/mL).
   b. Isolates with van B resistance are resistant to vancomycin (MICs from 4 µg/mL-1000 µg/mL or higher) but remain susceptible to teicoplanin.

   c. Strains with van C resistance have a low level of resistance to vancomycin (MICs of 4-32 µg/mL) and are susceptible to teicoplanin.

2. VRE is usually also resistant to ampicillin, oxacillin, cephalosporins, aminoglycosides, sulfa-trimethoprim, clindamycin, and the fluoro-quinolones.

Treatment

1. Simple colonization is not treated with antibiotics.
2. Linezolid (Zyvox).
   a. Linezolid is the drug of choice for many VRE infections.
   b. It is active against both *E. faecium* and *E. faecalis*, but resistant strains have been identified.
   c. The drug is bacteriostatic and available for use IV and orally with almost 100% bioavailability.
   d. The dosage is 600 mg IV or PO bid for 2 to 4 weeks.
   e. Bone marrow suppression and thrombocytopenia can occur in one third of patients receiving the drug.
   f. The drug should be avoided if the platelet count initially is less than 50,000.
   g. Weekly CBC is appropriate during treatment.
3. Daptomycin (Cubicin).
   a. Daptomycin is bactericidal for VRE but not yet approved for treatment of VRE infections.
   b. The dose is 4 mg/kg IV infusion qd (over 30 min) for 7 to 14 days.
   c. Renal adjustment is required.
4. Dalfopristin-quinupristin (Synercid).
   a. Dalfopristin-quinupristin, a streptogramin antibiotic, may be effective against some strains of *E. faecium*, but not *E. faecalis*.
   b. The dose is 7.5 mg/kg IV q8h for 7 to 14 days.
5. Chloramphenicol IV has been used with some success.
6. Nitrofurantoin or fosfomycin may be used for lower UTIs resulting from VRE.
7. Surgical debridement with drainage of an abscess and removal of a Foley catheter or IV catheter should be carried out when they have a role in VRE infection.

Infection Control

1. Patients colonized and/or infected with VRE are to be placed on gown and glove isolation.
   a. The gown and glove isolation sign should be placed in clear view at the entrance to the patient's room.
   b. No one should enter the room for any purpose without wearing gowns and gloves.
   c. Remove gloves and gown before leaving the room and wash hands with antiseptic soap.
   d. Shoe covers are not required.
   e. Masks are indicated only if the VRE organism is in the sputum.
2. Patients should be placed in private rooms or be cohorted with other patients who are VRE positive. VRE-positive patients must be in a private room if they have fecal incontinence, are unable to contain feces,

or have an exposed foreign body, open wounds, or urinary incontinence with urine colonized and/or infected with VRE.

3. Assign equipment, such as the stethoscope, BP cuff, and thermometer, to a single patient with VRE or a cohort of VRE patients.

4. Continue VRE isolation until three stool or other cultures obtained at weekly intervals are negative.

5. Establish a system to identify patients with VRE so that they can be placed in isolation on readmission to the hospital.

6. Judicious use of vancomycin has been reported to decrease the risk of colonization and infection with VRE. Appropriate indications for vancomycin are:

   a. Treatment of infections caused by MRSA, *S. epidermidis,* and enterococci in a penicillin-allergic patient.

   b. Treatment of infections caused by gram-positive organisms in patients with a life-threatening penicillin allergy.

   c. Treatment of antibiotic-associated colitis when metronidazole fails (second-line treatment).

   d. Prophylaxis for endocarditis in patients at high risk for infection.

   e. Surgical prophylaxis in patients with a history of life-threatening penicillin allergy.

SUGGESTED READINGS

Bonilla HF, Zervos MA, Lyons MJ, et al: Colonization with vancomycin-resistant *Enterococcus faecium:* Comparison of a long-term care unit with an acute-care hospital. *Infect Control Hosp Epidemiol* 18:333-339, 1997.

Centers for Disease Control and Prevention: Recommendations for preventing the spread of vancomycin resistance: Recommendations of the Hospital Infection Control Practices Advisory Committee (HICPAC). *MMWR Recomm Rep* 44:1-13, 1995.

Gantz NM: Vancomycin-resistant enterococci. In Gantz NM, Brown RB, Berk SL, Myers JW (eds): *Manual of clinical problems in infectious disease*, ed 5. Philadelphia, Lippincott William & Wilkins, 2006, pp 272-276.

Harbath S, Cosgrove S, Carmeli Y: Effects of antibiotics on nosocomial epidemiology of vancomycin-resistant enterococci. *Antimicrob Agents Chemother* 46:1619-1628, 2002.

Kauffman CA: Therapeutic and preventative options for the management of vancomycin-resistant enterococcal infections. *J Antimicrob Chemo* 51(suppl S3): iii23-iii30, 2003.

Murray BE: Vancomycin-resistant enterococcal infections. *N Engl J Med* 342: 710-721, 2000.

Muto CA, Jernigan JA, Ostrowsky BE, et al: SHEA guideline for preventing nosocomial transmission of multidrug-resistant strains of *Staphylococcus aureus* and enterococcus. *Infect Control Hosp Epidemiol* 24:362-386, 2003.

Perencevich EN, Fisman DN, Lipsitch M, et al: Projected benefits of active surveillance for vancomycin-resistant enterococci in intensive care units. *Clin Infec Dis* 38:1108-1115, 2004.

Richards CL: Preventing antimicrobial-resistant bacterial infections among older adults in long-term care facilities. *J Am Dir Assoc* 6:144-151, 2005.

Rici LB: Antimicrobial resistance in gram-positive bacteria. *Am J Med* 119:S11-S19, 2006.

Tacconelli E, Karchmer AW, Yokoe D, D'Agata EM: Preventing the influx of vancomycin-resistant enterococci into health care institutions, by use of a simple validated prediction rule. *Clin Infect Dis* 39:964-970, 2004.

Zirakzadeh A, Patel R: Vancomycin-resistant enterococci: Colonization, infection, detection and treatment. *Mayo Clin Proc* 84:529-536, 2006.

5.9 Nephrology, Urology, and Gynecology

BENIGN PROSTATIC HYPERPLASIA
Fred F. Ferri and Tom J. Wachtel

Definition
Benign prostatic hyperplasia (BPH) is the benign growth of the prostate, generally originating in the periureteral and transition zones, with subsequent irritative and obstructive voiding.

Epidemiology
1. All prostates increase in size with age, with substantial individual variability.
2. About 80% percent of men have clinical evidence of BPH by age 80.
3. Medical or surgical interventions for symptoms related to BPH are performed on more than 20% of men by age 75 years.
4. Transurethral resection of the prostate (TURP) is the tenth most common operative procedure in the United States (>400,000/yr).
5. From 10% to 30% of men with BPH also have occult prostate cancer.

Clinical Findings
1. Symptoms.
   a. Irritative symptoms are usually the first to manifest.
   b. The hallmark is urgency; the patient has progressively less time between the first sensation of bladder fullness and an irresistible urge to void. "When I have to go, I need to go now."
   c. These symptoms progress in association with reduced urinary flow, especially in the morning.
   d. In time, obstructive symptoms take center stage, with difficulty initiating flow (hesitancy), dribbling during micturition, incomplete emptying of the bladder resulting in double voiding (need to urinate again a few minutes after voiding), and postvoid dribbling or incontinence.
   e. Eventually, obstructive symptoms can lead to urinary retention.
2. Digital rectal examination (DRE) reveals enlargement of the prostate. Areas of firmness (nodular or diffuse), asymmetry, or focal enlargement raise the possibility of malignancy.
3. Correlation between size of prostate and symptoms is poor. BPH may be asymptomatic if the prostate does not encroach on the urethral lumen.
4. See Table 5-27 for the impact of lower urinary tract symptoms (LUTS) on the patient.

Etiology
1. Causes are multifactorial.
2. A functioning testicle is necessary for development of BPH, as evidenced by the total absence of prostate in persons with congenital absence of the enzyme 5α-reductase.

Differential Diagnosis
1. Prostatitis.
2. Prostate cancer.

Table 5-27 **International Prostate Symptom Score (I-PSS)**

Symptom		Score					
	Not at All	Less than 1 Time in 5	Less than Half the Time	About Half the Time	More than Half the Time	Almost Always	Total Score
Incomplete emptying: Over the past month, how often have you had a sensation of not emptying your bladder completely after you finished urinating?	0	1	2	3	4	5	
Frequency: Over the past month, how often have you had to urinate again 2 hours after you finished urinating?	0	1	2	3	4	5	
Intermittency: Over the past month, how often have you found you stopped and started again several times when you urinated?	0	1	2	3	4	5	
Urgency: Over the past month, how often have you found it difficult to postpone urination?	0	1	2	3	4	5	

	None	1 Time	2 Times	3 Times	4 Times	5 or More Times
Weak stream: Over the past month, how often have you had a weak urinary stream?	0	1	2	3	4	5
Straining: Over the past month, how often have you had to push or strain to begin urination?	0	1	2	3	4	5
Nocturia: Over the past month, how many times did you most typically get up to urinate from the time you went to bed at night until the time you got up in the morning?	0	1	2	3	4	5

Total I-PSS score =

3. Strictures (urethral).
4. Medication interfering with the muscle fibers in the prostate and also with bladder function.

Work-up

1. Symptom assessment as described earlier (may use American Urological Association or Symptom Index for BPH; see Table 5-27).
2. Laboratory tests.
   a. Prostate-specific antigen (PSA) to screen for prostate cancer.
      (1) PSA is a protease secreted by epithelial cells of the prostate.
      (2) It is elevated in 30% to 50% of patients with BPH.
      (3) It also increases with age independent of prostate size.
      (4) PSA testing (and DRE) should be offered to any asymptomatic man older than 50 years of age with a life expectancy of 10 years.
      (5) PSA testing can also be offered to 40-year-old men at higher risk of prostatic cancer (e.g., first-degree relatives with prostate cancer; black men).
      (6) Measurement of free PSA is useful to assess the probability of prostate cancer.
         (a) In patients with normal DRE and total PSA between 4 and 10 ng/mL, the global risk of prostate cancer is 25%.
         (b) If the free PSA is >25%, the risk of prostate cancer decreases to 8%.
         (c) If the free PSA is <10%, the risk of cancer increases to 56%.
      (7) Another approach is to measure PSA velocity.
         (a) Repeat PSA measurement is obtained every 3 months to assess the rate of increase.
         (b) PSA should increase by less than 0.85 ng/mL per year and should take at least 4 years to double.
   b. Usefulness of the test.
      (1) Testing for PSA has been shown to increase the detection rate for prostate cancer and tends to detect cancer at an earlier stage.
      (2) The PSA test does not discriminate well between patients with BPH and those with prostate cancer, particularly if the cancers are pathologically localized and curable.
   d. Urinalysis, urine culture, and sensitivity to rule out infection (if suspected).
   e. BUN and creatinine to rule out postrenal insufficiency.
3. Imaging studies and other urologic studies.
   a. Transrectal ultrasound may be indicated in patients with palpable nodules or significant elevation of PSA. It is also useful for estimating prostate size.
   b. Urine flowmetry may be used to determine the relative impact of obstruction on urine flow (not routine).
   c. Pressure flow studies, although invasive, are useful in occasional patients for whom a distinction between prostatic obstruction and impaired detrusor contractility might affect the choice of therapy.
   d. Postvoid residual (PVR) urine measurement can identify patients who should not receive anticholinergic drugs (PVR >100 mL).
   e. Cystoscopy is an option during later evaluation if invasive treatment is planned.

Treatment

1. Medical therapy.
   a. Nonpharmacologic therapy.
      (1) Caffeine or any other foods that can exacerbate symptoms should be avoided.
      (2) Medications that can exacerbate symptoms are contraindicated in anyone with a PVR greater than 100 mL.
         (a) Most cold and allergy remedies.
         (b) Anticholinergic drugs (e.g., antihistamines) decrease detrusor contractility.
         (c) Sympathomimetics (e.g., decongestants) increase bladder outlet pressure.
      (3) To reduce nocturia, do not drink much after 4:00 PM.
      (4) Avoid diuretic therapy.
      (5) The dietary supplement saw palmetto is effective in relieving BPH symptoms in some patients with mild obstruction.
   b. Pharmacologic therapy.
      (1) Asymptomatic patients with prostate enlargement caused by BPH generally do not require treatment. Patients with mild to moderate symptoms are candidates for pharmacologic treatment.
      (2) α1-Adrenergic blockers.
         (a) α1-Adrenergic blockers (e.g., tamsulosin, alfluzosin, doxazosin, prazosin, and terazosin) relax smooth muscle of the bladder neck and prostate and can increase urinary flow rate.
         (b) They have no effect on the size of the prostate.
         (c) α1-Adrenergic blockers are useful in symptomatic patients to relieve LUTS by causing relaxation of smooth muscle tone in the prostatic capsule and urethra/bladder neck.
         (d) Tamsulosin and alfluzosin are more specific to bladder α_1-receptors and do not cause (much) hypotension.
         (e) Prazosin, doxazosin, and terazosin are nonspecific α_1-blockers and are used to treat hypertension, particularly in men with symptomatic BPH. They can cause (postural) hypotension.
         (f) α1-Adrenergic blockers are the most effective medical pharmacologic therapy for BPH-associated LUTS.
         (g) Dosing.
            i. Tamsulosin (Flomax) 0.4 to 0.8 mg qd.
            ii. Alfluzosin (Uroxastral) 10 mg qd.
            iii. Prazosin 1 mg tid titrated to 5 to 10 mg tid.
            iv. Doxazosin 1, 2, 5, or 10 mg qd.
            v. Terazosin 1, 2, 4, or 8 mg qd.
      (3) Hormonal manipulation.
         (a) Finasteride and dutasteride are 5α-reductase inhibitors that block conversion of testosterone to dihydrotestosterone.
         (b) They can reduce the size of the prostate by up to 30%.
         (c) Treatment requires 6 months or more for maximal effect.
         (d) 5α-Reductase inhibitors cut PSA levels in half. Therefore, the measured PSA level should be doubled to interpret the result in a patient using such treatment.

(e) Dosing.
  i. Finasteride (Proscar): 5 mg qd.
  ii. Dutasteride (Avodart): 0.5 mg qd.

2. Bladder catheterization.
  a. Patients with BPH who experience acute urinary retention should be treated with bladder catheterization, an α_1-blocker, a 5α-reductase agent, and probably an antibiotic if there is any likelihood of bacterial prostatitis acting as precipitant.
  b. If early attempt (e.g., 2 days) at removing the catheter does not result in restoration of micturition, the catheter is left in place for 4 to 6 weeks.
  c. If, at the end of that interval, the patient is still unable to urinate after the removal of the catheter, a surgical procedure is preferable to a long-term indwelling catheter.

3. Surgical therapy.
  a. Types of surgery.
    (1) Transurethral prostatectomy.
      (a) TURP is the most commonly used surgical procedure for patients with BPH and LUTS.
      (b) The increase in the use of pharmacologic management has resulted in a more than 30% reduction in the total number of TURPs.
      (c) The decision to consider surgery should be based on how bothersome the urologic symptoms are for a given patient (see Table 5-27), and then those symptoms should be weighed against the potential complications of surgery (e.g., incontinence).
      (d) Open prostatectomy is typically performed on symptomatic patients with a very large prostate. Surgery can result in significant complications (e.g., incontinence, infection).
      (e) Prostate volume reduction procedures are considered more effective than the less-invasive interventions, and the effect is more durable.
      (f) Transurethral incision of the prostate (TUIP) is appropriate for patients whose estimated resection tissue weight is 30 g or less. TUIP can be performed in an ambulatory setting or during a 1-day hospitalization.
      (g) Laser therapy for BPH is a less-invasive alternative to TURP. However, TURP is moderately more effective than laser therapy in relieving symptoms of BPH.
      (h) Balloon dilation of the prostatic urethra is less effective than surgery for relieving symptoms but is associated with fewer complications. It is a reasonable treatment option for patients with smaller prostates and no middle lobe enlargement.
      (i) Emerging technologies for treating BPH include coils, stents, thermal therapy, and hyperthermia. Some appear promising; however, long-term effectiveness has not yet been demonstrated.
  b. Results.
    (1) With appropriate therapy, symptoms improve or stabilize in more than 70% of patients with BPH.

(2) There is no evidence that prostate surgery prevents urinary tract infection (UTI), prostitis, or urosepsis.

SUGGESTED READING

Dull P, Reagan RW Jr, Bahnson RR: Managing benign prostatic hyperplasia. *Am Fam Physician* 66:77-84, 2002.

ELECTROLYTES AND ACID–BASE DISORDERS

Tom J. Wachtel

Sodium

1. Hyponatremia (serum Na <135 mEq/L) occurs when total body water is in relative excess to body Na. Total body water may be low, normal, or high.
   a. Symptoms.
      (1) Confusion.
      (2) Lethargy.
      (3) Anorexia.
      (4) Cramps.
      (5) Rapid sodium drop can cause seizures.
   b. Causes.
      (1) Hypovolemia.
         (a) Extrarenal sodium loss (urinary Na <10 mM/L).
            i. Diaphoresis.
            ii. Vomiting or diarrhea, or both.
            iii. Pancreatitis.
         (b) Renal loss (urinary Na >20 mM/L).
            i. Renal failure.
            ii. Diuretics.
            iii. Addison's disease.
            iv. Salt-losing nephropathy.
      (2) Isovolemia.
         (a) Water intoxication (urinary Na <10 mM/L).
         (b) Water retention (urinary Na >20 mM/L): Syndrome of inappropriate secretion of antidiuretic hormone (urinary osmolarity greater than serum osmolarity).
         (c) Sodium loss greater than water loss (urinary Na >20 mM/L) with water intake compensation.
            i. Addison's disease.
            ii. Salt-losing nephropathy.
            iii. Hypothyroidism.
      (3) Hypervolemia or edematous states (urinary Na <10 mM/L).
         (a) CHF.
         (b) Cirrhosis.
         (c) Nephrotic syndrome.
2. Hypernatremia (serum Na >150 mEq/L) occurs in the setting of a greater deficit of total body water relative to Na.
   a. Symptoms.
      (1) Confusion.
      (2) Muscle twitching.
      (3) Seizures.
      (4) Coma.

b. Causes.
  (1) Hypovolemia (water loss greater than sodium loss).
    (a) Extrarenal water loss.
      i. Diaphoresis.
      ii. Vomiting or diarrhea or both.
      iii. Pancreatitis.
    (b) Renal water loss.
      i. Renal failure.
      ii. Diuretics.
      iii. Osmotic diuresis (e.g., hyperglycemia).
  (2) Isovolemia: diabetes insipidus.
  (3) Hypervolemia (gain of sodium greater than water).
    (a) Primary hyperaldosteronism.
    (b) Cushing's syndrome.
    (c) Hypertonic solution administration.

Potassium

1. Hypokalemia (serum K <3.5 mEq/L).
  a. Symptoms.
    (1) Muscle weakness.
    (2) Cramps.
    (3) Ileus.
    (4) ECG changes (U waves, increased Q-T interval, flat T waves).
    (5) With severe hypokalemia, flaccid paralysis and cardiac arrest.
  b. Causes.
    (1) Gastrointestinal potassium losses (vomiting, diarrhea, villous adenoma, ureterosigmoidostomy).
    (2) Renal losses.
      (a) Metabolic acidosis.
      (b) Diuretics (thiazides, loop diuretics).
      (c) Excessive mineralocorticoid effect.
        i. Primary hyperaldosteronism.
        ii. Secondary hyperaldosteronism.
        iii. Cushing's syndrome and exogenous steroids.
        iv. Licorice ingestion.
      (d) Renal tubular acidosis and Liddle's syndrome.
      (e) Hypomagnesemia.
    (3) Potassium shift into cells.
      (a) Insulin effect.
      (b) Alkalosis.
      (c) Hypokalemic periodic paralysis (may be associated with Graves' disease).
2. Hyperkalemia (serum K >5.5 mEq/L).
  a. Symptoms.
    (1) ECG changes (peaked T waves, diminished R wave, oxide QRS, loss of P wave, sine wave).
    (2) Arrhythmias.
    (3) All cardiac symptoms are exaggerated by decreased Na and Ca, increased Mg, acidosis, and digitalis.
  b. Causes.

(1) Inadequate excretion.
    (a) Renal disease.
    (b) Addison's disease.
    (c) Potassium-sparing diuretics, angiotensin converting enzyme (ACE) inhibitors.
(2) Potassium shift from intracellular to extracellular space.
    (a) Crush injury.
    (b) Acidosis.
    (c) Hyperkalemic periodic paralysis.
(3) Excessive intake.
(4) Artifactual (in vitro hemolysis and poor venipuncture technique).

Metabolic Acidosis (pH <7.35)

1. Low serum bicarbonate caused by addition of acids (increased anion gap acidosis: $Na [Cl + HCO_3] > 12$ mEq/L) or loss of HCO_3 (normal anion gap acidosis).
   a. Loss of HCO_3 (normal anion gap acidosis).
2. Anion gap acidosis.
   a. Diabetic ketoacidosis.
   b. Renal failure.
   c. Lactic acidosis.
   d. Alcoholic ketoacidosis.
   e. Starvation ketosis.
   f. Salicylate poisoning.
   g. Methanol poisoning.
   h. Ethylene glycol poisoning.
3. Non-anion gap acidosis.
   a. Diarrhea.
   b. Renal tubular acidosis.
   c. Enterostomy.
   d. Ureterosigmoidostomy.
   e. Hyperalimentation.
   f. Acetazolamide.
   g. Ammonium chloride, lysine HCl, arginine HCl.

Metabolic Alkalosis (pH >7.45)

1. High serum bicarbonate caused by loss of acid (NaCl responsive, low urine chloride <10 mEq/L) or by hyperaldosteronism or hypokalemia (NaCl resistant, high urine chloride >20 mEq/L).
2. NaCl responsive.
   a. Gastrointestinal losses.
      (1) Vomiting.
      (2) Nasogastric suction.
      (3) Chloride-wasting diarrhea.
      (4) Villous adenoma (colon).
   b. Diuretic therapy.
   c. Posthypercapnia.
   d. Penicillin, carbenicillin.
3. NaCl resistant.
   a. Hyperaldosteronism.

b. Cushing's syndrome.
c. Licorice.
d. Bartter's syndrome.
e. Refeeding alkalosis.
f. Alkali ingestion.

Respiratory Acidosis

1. CO_2 retention caused by ventilating failure.
2. Symptoms.
   a. Confusion.
   b. Lethargy.
3. Causes.
   a. COPD.
   b. Sedative overdose.
   c. Stroke.
   d. Airway obstruction.
   e. Neuromuscular diseases.

Respiratory Alkalosis

1. CO_2 loss caused by hyperventilation.
2. Symptoms.
   a. Tetany.
   b. Seizures.
   c. Syncope.
   d. Arrhythmias.
3. Causes.
   a. Anxiety, panic disorder.
   b. Lung diseases (e.g., asthma, pneumonia).
   c. Sepsis.
   d. Salicylate poisoning.
   e. Hepatic failure.
   f. Hyperestrogenemia.
   g. Central nervous system lesions.

HEMATURIA

Michael P. Gerardo and Tom J. Wachtel

Definitions

1. Hematuria is blood in the urine.
2. Hematuria is classified as either microscopic or gross.
3. In microscopic hematuria, two or more RBCs per high-power field are identified in a centrifuged urine specimen.
4. In gross hematuria, the blood is visualized by the naked eye. If the RBC per high-power field is greater than 20, a tint to the urine can be visible.

Epidemiology

1. In patients older than 50 years, the prevalence is estimated at 13%.
2. Prevalence is slightly higher in women.

Clinical Findings

1. Lower urinary tract symptoms (LUTS)
   a. Urgency.
   b. Frequency.

   c. Nocturia.
   d. Dribbling.
   e. Hesitancy.
   f. Dysuria.
2. Renal colic, recent or past, or history of kidney stones.
3. Fever.
4. Weight loss.
5. Coagulopathy.
6. Family history of renal disease.
7. Systemic illness.
8. Mass of bimanual exam of the abdomen.
9. Costovertebral angle tenderness.
10. Abnormal prostate on rectal exam.

Etiology

1. To identify the cause of hematuria, the physician should differentiate between a glomerular (medical) or nonglomerular (urologic) source of bleeding.
   a. Glomerular hematuria is suggested by the presence of proteinuria or granular casts.
   b. Isolated hematuria suggests nonglomerular hematuria.
2. The three most common causes of glomerular hematuria.
   a. IgA nephropathy (hematuria, hypertension, rising creatinine).
   b. Thin basement membrane disease (hematuria, no extrarenal manifestations, rarely renal failure).
   c. Hereditary nephritis (hematuria, rising creatinine, <2 g proteinuria, sensorineural deafness).
3. Nonglomerular causes of hematuria.
   a. Lesions in either the kidney or upper urinary tract.
     (1) Neoplasm.
     (2) Nephrolithiasis.
     (3) Cystic disease.
     (4) Papillary necrosis.
   b. Lower urinary tract lesions, chiefly including infectious or neoplastic diseases of the bladder, urethra, and prostate, can result in hematuria.
   c. Metabolic defects (hypercalciuria or hyperuricosuria).
   d. Urologic cancer.
     (1) Gross hematuria suggests a urologic cause of bleeding and is associated with a much higher risk of urologic cancer.
     (2) The suspicion of neoplasm increases with age, with no specific age threshold.
     (3) Risk factors for bladder cancer.
       (a) Age greater than 65 years.
       (b) Cigarette smoking.
       (c) Occupational exposure to chemicals (leather, dye, rubber, or tire manufacturing).
       (d) Heavy phenacetin use.
       (e) Previous cyclophosphamide treatment.
       (f) Aristolochic acid (found in some weight loss medications).
       (g) Exposure to schistosomiasis.

4. Some clinicians recommend that patients who develop hematuria during anticoagulation therapy should undergo an evaluation of the cause of hematuria. However, if the patient was over-anticoagulated at the time of hematuria, most would correct the coagulopathy to therapeutic goal and reevaluate the urine.

Differential Diagnosis

1. False positive tests can result from substances other than hemoglobin such as myoglobin, vitamin C, beets, and rhubarb.
2. A urinalysis dipstick that is positive for "blood" but not associated with RBC on microscopic urinalysis is not hematuria.

Work-up

1. Laboratory tests.
   a. Initially, a repeat urinalysis should be obtained in a few weeks.
      (1) If microscopic hematuria is absent on a repeat test, or if the cause of hematuria is a UTI or prostatitis, no further evaluation is warranted.
      (2) If hematuria is present on repeat testing, a basic chemistry and microscopy are obtained from the patient.
   b. Combination of dysmorphic red cells and red cell casts suggests glomerular disease.
   c. An elevated creatinine suggests a renal source of the bleeding.
   d. A urine dipstick that is positive for protein should then be followed by the spot protein-to-creatinine ratio (P/Cr) or a 24-hour urine protein. A P/Cr greater than 0.3 or protein more than 300 mg/24 hours suggests a glomerular source of bleeding.
   e. Anatomic evaluation is appropriate in all patients with nonglomerular hematuria.
2. Imaging and other studies.
   a. Glomerular: No imaging studies differentiate between the glomerular diseases.
   b. Nonglomerular.
      (1) Upper urinary tract.
         (a) In patients suspected of stone disease, a CT scan without contrast is appropriate.
         (b) If there is no suspicion of stone disease, CT urography is obtained first without contrast followed by imaging with contrast dye.
         (c) Ultrasound and excretory urography most often are followed by additional imaging and therefore are not considered cost-saving tests. If a CT scan cannot be performed (unavailable, contrast hypersensitivity, renal failure, pregnancy), ultrasound is the most reasonable alternative test.
      (2) Lower urinary tract: Cystoscopy is indicated in all patients with risk factors for bladder cancer, gross hematuria, or a urine cytology showing neoplastic cells and in whom a source of hematuria is not identified with upper urinary tract imaging.

Treatment

1. Nonglomerular hematuria.

a. Treat any infection with appropriate antibiotic therapy (see "Urinary Tract Infection" and "Prostatitis").

b. Treat renal colic (nephrolithiasis) with hydration and narcotic analgesia (see "Kidney Stones" later).

c. The treatment of renal and bladder cancer is mostly surgical and carried out by urologists.

d. Prostate cancer can be treated surgically, medically, or with radiation.

e. A risk-to-benefit analysis, including goals of care and quality of life expectations, should be discussed with the patient before any surgical intervention for neoplastic disease.

f. Patients with urologic cancer in whom surgery is not performed and in whom the hematuria results in a progressive anemia might require intermittent RBC transfusion therapy.

g. Isolated urologic microscopic hematuria can be monitored every 3 months for 1 year, yearly for 3 years, and episodically thereafter.

2. Glomerular hematuria.

a. When microscopic hematuria accompanies either proteinuria or renal insufficiency, a nephrology consult is warranted. Glucocorticoid therapy is appropriate for certain types of gomerulonephritis.

b. Management of hypertension and proteinuria should include ACE-inhibitor or angiotensin receptor blocker therapy.

c. Isolated glomerular hematuria requires repeating testing for proteinuria and renal insufficiency at 6 months and then annually if stable.

Comments

1. The United States Preventative Task Force does not recommend routine screening for hematuria due to lack of evidence for effectiveness.

2. A diagnosis of nephrolithiasis does not rule out the possibility of an associated urologic malignancy.

3. A finding of hematuria in a patient with a recent urinary catheterization should be discarded; urinalysis should be repeated in 2 to 3 weeks.

SUGGESTED READINGS

Brehmer M: Imaging for microscopic haematuria. *Curr Opin Urol* 12:155-159, 2002.

Cohen, RA, Brown, RS: Microscopic hematuria. *N Engl J Med* 348:2330-2338, 2003.

Jaffe JS, Ginsberg PC, Gill R, Harkaway RC: A new diagnostic algorithm for the evaluation of microscopic hematuria. *Urology* 57:889-894, 2001.

Khadra M, Pickard R, Charlton M: A prospective analysis of 1930 patients with hematuria to evaluate current diagnostic practice. *J Urol* 163:524-527, 2000.

McDonald MM, Swagerty D, Swetzel L: Assessment of microscopic hematuria in adults. *Am Fam Physician* 73:1748-1754, 2006.

KIDNEY STONES

Tom J. Wachtel and Fred F. Ferri

Definition

1. Urolithiasis is the presence of calculi within the urinary tract.

2. The four major types of urinary stones are:
   a. Calcium oxalate or phosphate (70%).
   b. Uric acid (10%).

    c. Struvite (10%).

    d. Cystine (3%).

3. Stones may be mixed.

Epidemiology

1. Urinary stone disease afflicts 250,000 to 750,000 Americans a year.
2. Male-to-female ratio is 1.5:1 after the sixth decade.
3. Incidence of symptomatic nephrolithiasis is greatest during the summer (resulting from increased risk of dehydration and concentrated urine).

Stone Characteristics

1. Calcium oxalate.
    a. Radiodense.
    b. Size: Small (<2 cm).
    c. Color: Shades of gray.
    d. Etiology.
        (1) Hyperparathyroidism.
        (2) Idiopathic hypercalciuria.
        (3) Hyperoxaluria.
        (4) Hyperuricosuria.
        (5) Hypocitraturia.
2. Calcium phosphate (rare).
    a. Radiodense.
    b. Etiology: Renal tubular acidosis.
3. Uric acid.
    a. Radiolucent.
    b. Size: Small to staghorn.
    c. Color: Orange.
    d. Etiology: Hyperuricosuria.
4. Struvite.
    a. Radiodense.
    b. Size: Small to staghorn.
    c. Color: Brown.
    d. Etiology: Urinary infection with urease-splitting organism (e.g., *Proteus*, *Klebsiella*, *Pseudomonas*, and *Enterococcus* species).
5. Cystine.
    a. Radiodense.
    b. Size: Small to staghorn.
    c. Onset: Long before middle age.
    d. Color: Yellow.
    e. Etiology: Cystinuria.

Clinical Presentation

1. Renal colic.
    a. Sudden onset of severe costovertebral angle or flank pain that radiates around the flank anteriorly toward the groin and is associated with the descent of a urinary calculus through a ureter.
    b. Nausea, vomiting, urinary frequency, and dysuria may be associated with the pain.
    c. Pain persists until the stone passes into bladder or is removed.
    d. Gross or microscopic hematuria may be present.

2. Recurrent UTI.
3. Hematuria.
4. Obstructive uropathy that might remain silent.
5. Incidental radiologic findings.
6. Passage of gravel through the urethra.

Etiology

1. Increased absorption of calcium in the small bowel: Type I absorptive hypercalciuria (independent of calcium intake).
2. Idiopathic hypercalciuria nephrolithiasis is the most common diagnosis for patients with calcium stones. The diagnosis is made only if there is no hypercalcemia and no known cause for hypercalciuria.
3. Increased vitamin D synthesis (e.g., secondary to renal phosphate loss): Type III absorptive hypercalciuria.
4. Renal tubular malfunction with inadequate reabsorption of calcium and resulting hypercalciuria.
5. Heterozygous mutations in the *NPT2a* gene result in hypophosphatemia and urinary phosphate loss.
6. Hyperparathyroidism with resulting hypercalcemia and secondary calciuria.
7. Elevated uric acid level (metabolic defects, dietary excess, chemotherapy for malignancies).
8. Chronic diarrhea (e.g., inflammatory bowel disease) with increased oxalate absorption.
9. Type I (distal tubule) renal tubular acidosis (<1% of calcium stones).
10. Chronic infections with urease-producing organisms (e.g., *Proteus, Providencia, Pseudomonas,* and *Klebsiella* species). Struvite, or magnesium ammonium phosphate crystals, are produced when the urinary tract is colonized by bacteria, producing elevated concentrations of ammonia.
11. Abnormal excretion of cystine.

Diagnostic Evaluation

The chemical composition of the stone and the pathophysiology of the stone formation must be defined in order to propose a preventive treatment. This is important because more than half of all patients who pass one stone will pass another.

1. Laboratory studies.
    a. Urinalysis. Table 5-28 shows characteristics of nephroliths.
    b. Stone analysis if the stone available.

Table 5-28 **Characteristics of Kidney Stones**		
Type of Stone	**Urine pH**	**Shape of Crystal**
Calcium oxalate	Acid to neutral	Envelope
Uric acid	Acid	Plates, prism, clumps, needles, or fan
Struvite	Alkaline	Coffin lid
Cystine	Acid	Hexagonal

c. Metabolic workup. (If the stone is not available, it is most likely calcium oxalate.)
  (1) Calcium oxalate stone.
    (a) Serum calcium, phosphorus, and alkaline phosphatase.
    (b) Parathormone level if serum calcium is high and phosphorus is low.
    (c) Twenty-four-hour urine collection on normal diet.
      i. Creatinine.
      ii. Calcium (normal urinary calcium <250 mg/24h in women and <300 mg/24 h in men).
      iii. Oxalate (normal <150 mg/24 h).
    (d) Effect of a low-calcium diet on 24-hour urinary calcium can diagnose idiopathic hypercalciuria that does not respond to diet.
    (e) If hypercalcemia is present, consider the various causes, such as hyperparathyroidism, malignancy, sarcoidosis, milk-alkali syndrome, Paget's disease, immobilization, hyperthyroidism, vitamin D toxicity.
  (2) Uric acid stone.
    (a) Serum uric acid.
    (b) Twenty-four-hour urine collection for creatinine and uric acid (normal urinary uric acid <750 mg/24 h).
  (3) Struvite stone.
    (a) No metabolic studies.
    (b) Urinalysis and urine culture with sensitivity.
  (4) Cystine stone: Urine cystine screen.
2. Imaging studies.
  a. Plain films of the abdomen can identify radiopaque stones (calcium, mixed stones).
  b. A renal sonogram may be helpful.
  c. Intravenous pyelogram demonstrates the size and location of the stone as well as the degree of obstruction.
  d. Unenhanced helical CT.
    (1) Unenhanced (noncontrast) helical CT scan does not require contrast media and can visualize the calculus (identified by the rim sign or halo representing the edematous ureteral wall around the stone).
    (2) It is fast and accurate (sensitivity, 95% to 100%; specificity, 94% to 96%).
    (3) It readily identifies all stone types in all locations.
    (4) This modality is being used increasingly in the initial assessment of renal colic.

Treatment
Management of Renal Colic
1. Diagnosis.
  a. About 90% of all kidney stones are radiopaque and theoretically visible on a plain x-ray.
  b. Sonography or intravenous pyelogram may be required.
2. Pain control: Narcotic analgesics are typically required.
3. Stone removal.

a. Spontaneous passage can be expected of stones smaller than 0.5 cm and is possible for stones 0.5 to 0.7 cm.

b. Treatment at home is reasonable for stones smaller than 0.7 cm for which spontaneous passage is likely.

c. Patient should strain all urine to recover the stone, which should then be analyzed for its chemical composition.

d. Stones that progress and then become lodged in the distal ureter (below the pelvic brim on x-ray) can be moved ureteroscopically with a basket or disrupted by lithotripsy.

e. A stone lodged in the upper ureter can be pushed back into the renal pelvis endoscopically and disrupted later by lithotripsy.

   (1) If lithotripsy fails or if the stone is larger than 2 cm, percutaneous nephrolithotomy is performed.

   (2) Surgical (i.e., open) ureterolithotomy is indicated only after all else fails.

f. In 1997, the American Urological Association issued the following guidelines for the treatment of ureteral stones:

   (1) Proximal ureteral stones less than 1 cm in diameter.

      (a) Extracorporeal shock wave lithotripsy (ESWL).

      (b) Percutaneous nephroureterolithotomy.

      (c) Ureteroscopy.

   (2) Proximal ureteral stones larger than 1 cm in diameter.

      (a) ESWL.

      (b) Percutaneous nephroureterolithotomy.

      (c) Ureteroscopy.

      (d) Placement of a ureteral stent should be considered if the stone is causing high-grade obstruction.

   (3) Distal ureteral stones less than 1 cm in diameter.

      (a) Most of these pass spontaneously.

      (b) If not, ESWL and ureteroscopy are two accepted modes of therapy.

   (4) Distal ureteral stones larger than 1 cm in diameter.

      (a) Watchful waiting.

      (b) ESWL.

      (c) Ureteroscopy following stone fragmentation.

Preventive Treatment

1. Stones will recur in approximately 50% of patients within 5 years if no medical treatment is provided.

2. General measures.

   a. Increase fluid intake (3 L/24 h).

   b. Avoid dehydration.

3. Calcium stone formers.

   a. Surgical treatment of primary hyperparathyroidism if present.

   b. Treatment of underlying cause of hypercalcemia if relevant.

   c. Low-calcium diet unless diagnosis is idiopathic hypercalciuria.

   d. Hyperoxaluria.

      (1) Low-oxalate diet (avoid tea, spinach, rhubarb).

      (2) Treat ileal disease if present.

      (3) Consider pyridoxine deficiency.

e. Thiazide diuretic (e.g., hydrochlorothiazide 25 to 50 mg bid) is the drug of choice to manage hypercalciuria.

f. Citrate (e.g., Polycitra) inhibits calcium stone formation and alkalinizes urine.

4. Uric acid stones (or calcium or mixed stone formers with hyperuricosuria).

a. Avoid purine-rich foods (e.g., liver, kidney, cold cuts).

b. Alkalinize urine (with citrate).

c. Allopurinol (Zyloprim) titrated upward from 200 mg qd to reduce urinary uric acid to below 600 mg/24 h.

d. Avoid uricosuric drugs (e.g., probenecid).

5. Struvite stones: Referral to urology for complete stone removal combined with specific antibiotics is the treatment of choice.

6. Cystine stones.

a. Alkalinize urine with citrate.

b. D-Penicillamine: 4 g/day until stone is dissolved, then 1 d/day maintenance.

c. ACE inhibitors.

SUGGESTED READINGS

Borghi L, Schianchi T, Meschi T, et al: Comparison of two diets for the prevention of recurrent stones in idiopathic hypercalciuria. *N Engl J Med* 346:77-84, 2002.

Moe OW: Kidney stones. Pathophysiology and medical management. *Lancet* 367: 333-344, 2006.

Worster A, Preyra I, Weaver B, Haines T: The accuracy of noncontrast helical computed tomography versus intravenous pyelography in the diagnosis of suspected acute urolithiasis: A meta-analysis, *Ann Intern Med* 40:280-286, 2002.

PROSTATITIS

Tom J. Wachtel

Definition

Prostatitis refers to inflammation of the prostate gland. There are four major categories:

1. Acute bacterial prostatitis.
2. Chronic bacterial prostatitis.
3. Nonbacterial prostatitis.
4. Prostatodynia.

Epidemiology

1. About 50% of men experience symptoms of prostatitis in their lifetime.
2. Acute bacterial prostatitis is uncommon.
3. The relative prevalence of the other three entities among men with inflammatory prostatic symptoms is:

a. Chronic bacterial prostatitis: 5% to 10%.

b. Nonbacterial prostatitis:10% to 65%.

c. Prostatodynia: 30% to 80%.

4. The figures are imprecise because nonbacterial prostatitis and prostatodynia are very difficult to differentiate.

Clinical Findings

1. Acute bacterial prostatitis.

a. Sudden or rapidly progressive onset of:

(1) Dysuria.

    (2) Frequency.

    (3) Urgency.

    (4) Nocturia.

    (5) Perineal pain that can radiate to the back, the rectum, or the penis.

  b. Hematuria or a purulent urethral discharge can occur.

  c. Occasionally, urinary retention complicates the course.

  d. Fever, chills, and signs of sepsis can also be part of the clinical picture.

  e. On rectal examination, the prostate is typically tender.

2. Chronic bacterial prostatitis.

  a. May be asymptomatic when the infection is confined to the prostate.

  b. Can manifest as an increase in severity of baseline symptoms of BPH.

  c. When cystitis is also present, urinary frequency, urgency, and burning may be reported.

  d. Hematuria may be a presenting complaint.

  e. In elderly men, new onset of urinary incontinence may be noted.

3. Nonbacterial prostatitis and prostatodynia.

  a. Present similarly with symptoms of bladder irritation (urinary frequency, urgency, dysuria, increase in nocturia episodes) and perineal discomfort.

  b. The term *prostatodynia* is usually applied to patients with normal prostate (i.e., no BPH).

  c. The severity of the symptoms varies, but they tend to be more bothersome in prostatodynia.

Etiology

1. Acute bacterial prostatitis.

  a. Acute, usually gram-negative infection of the prostate gland.

    (1) Generally associated with cystitis.

    (2) Resulting from the ascent of bacteria in the urethra.

  b. Occasionally, the route of infection is hematogenous or a lymphatogenous spread of rectal bacteria.

  c. The condition is seen in young or middle-aged men.

2. Chronic bacterial prostatitis.

  a. Often asymptomatic.

  b. Exacerbation of symptoms of BPH caused by the same mechanism as in acute bacterial prostatitis.

3. Nonbacterial prostatitis.

  a. Refers to symptoms of prostatic inflammation associated with the presence of white blood cells in prostatic secretions with no identifiable bacterial organism.

  b. Chlamydia infection may be etiologically implicated in some cases.

4. Prostatodynia.

  a. Refers to symptoms of prostatic inflammation with no or few white blood cells in the prostate secretion.

  b. Spasm in the bladder neck or urethra is felt to be the cause of symptoms.

Differential Diagnosis

1. BPH with LUTS.

2. Prostate cancer.

3. Also see differential diagnosis of hematuria earlier.

Work-up

1. Rectal examination.
   a. Tender prostate is most suggestive of acute bacterial prostatitis.
   b. Enlarged prostate is common in chronic bacterial prostatitis.
   c. Normal prostate is consistent with chronic bacterial and nonbacterial prostatitis and is typical in prostatodynia.
2. Expression of prostatic secretions by prostate massage is contraindicated in acute bacterial prostatitis but is appropriate in the other three situations.
3. Laboratory tests.
   a. Urinalysis.
   b. Urine culture and sensitivity.
   c. Bacterial localization studies can be performed but are cumbersome and impractical in most clinical settings.
   d. Cell count and culture of expressed prostatic secretions.
   e. The yield of a urine culture may be increased if the specimen is obtained after a prostatic massage.
   f. PSA is not used to diagnose prostatitis; however, a rapid rise over baseline should raise the possibility of prostatitis even in the absence of symptoms. In such cases, a follow-up PSA after treatment of prostatitis is appropriate.
   g. CBC and blood cultures if fever, chills, or signs of sepsis exist.
   h. If hematuria is present, a work-up to rule out a urologic malignancy should be considered if the hematuria does not clear after treatment of prostatitis.

Treatment

1. Acute bacterial prostatitis.
   a. Culture-guided antibiotic therapy for 4 weeks (beginning with a few days of IV antibiotics if the infection is serious or if the patient is bacteremic).
   b. Select an antibiotic that provides good prostatic tissue penetration.
      (1) Penicillins and cephalosporins are poor choices.
      (2) Best drugs are trimethoprim–sulfamethoxazole (TMP-SMX), tetracyclines, and quinolones provided that the bacteria are sensitive to them.
2. Chronic bacterial prostatitis.
   a. TMP-SMX is the first-line choice for 4 weeks if the organism is sensitive.
   b. Second-line choice for treatment failure or organisms resistant to TMP-SMX is a fluoroquinolone.
   c. A patient with refractory infection or with multiple relapses may be offered long-term suppressive therapy.
3. Nonbacterial prostatitis and prostatodynia.
   a. No specific treatment.
   b. Antibiotics are not effective.
   c. A trial of treatment with an α-adrenergic blocker (terazosin, doxazosin, tamsulosin, or alfuzosin) may be considered.
   d. Any underlying bladder pathology should be ruled out by cystoscopy and treated if identified.

SUGGESTED READINGS

Fowler JE: Prostatitis. In Gillenwater JY, Grayhack JT, Howards SS, Duckett JW (eds): *Adult and pediatric urology*. St. Louis, Mosby, 1996.

McNaughton Collins M, MacDonald R, Wilt TJ: Diagnosis and treatment of chronic abacterial prostatitis: A systematic review. *Ann Intern Med* 133:367-381, 2000.

ACUTE RENAL FAILURE

Fred F. Ferri and Tom J. Wachtel

Definition

Acute renal failure (ARF) is the rapid impairment in renal function resulting in retention of products in the blood that are normally excreted by the kidneys.

Epidemiology

1. ARF requiring dialysis develops in 5/100,000 persons annually.
2. More than 10% of intensive care unit patients develop ARF.
3. More than 40% of hospital ARF is iatrogenic.
4. ARF occurs in 20% of patients with moderate sepsis and more than 50% of patients with septic shock and positive blood cultures.

Clinical Findings

1. Weakness, anorexia, generalized malaise, nausea.
2. Back pain, muscle cramps.
3. Skin pallor, ecchymoses.
4. Peripheral edema.
5. Oliguria (however, patients can have nonoliguric renal failure), anuria.
6. Tachypnea, tachycardia.
7. Delirium, lethargy, myoclonus, fasciculations, seizures.
8. The physical examination should focus on volume status.

Etiology

The kidneys ultrafilter blood, secrete and absorb the filtrate in the renal tubules, and eliminate urine through the ureters, bladder, and urethra. ARF results from a problem at any stage of this process. *Prerenal azotemia* occurs because of a decrease in blood delivered to the kidney. *Renal azotemia* results from a malfunction within the renal parenchyma. *Postrenal azotemia* results from an obstruction of urinary flow.

1. Prerenal: Inadequate renal perfusion (most common category: 60%).
   a. Fluid volume loss (diarrhea, diuresis).
   b. Impaired cardiac output.
   c. Renal vasoconstriction (nonsteroidal antiinflammatory medications [NSAIDS], ACE inhibitors).
   d. Decreased systemic vascular resistance as seen in sepsis, pancreatitis, cirrhosis, and afterload-reducing drugs.
   e. Decreased oncotic vascular volume support: Nephrosis, severe catabolic states.
   f. Hepatorenal syndrome: Labeled *prerenal* because when the involved kidney is transplanted into a normal host, it functions normally.
2. Intrinsic renal.
   a. Acute tubular necrosis (ATN).
      (1) Perfusional deficits.
         (a) Prolonged prerenal failure.

      (b) Shock.
      (c) Hypovolemia.
      (d) Sepsis.
      (e) Pancreatitis.
      (f) Low-output states.
      (g) Coronary artery bypass graft surgery.
      (h) Aortic aneurysm repair.
    (2) Pigment nephropathy.
      (a) Myoglobinuria (rhabdomyolysis).
      (b) Hemoglobinuria.
    (3) Contrast-agent toxicity.
    (4) Drug toxicity.
      (a) Aminoglycosides.
      (b) Cisplatinum.
      (c) Pentamidine.
      (d) Lithium.
      (e) Amphotericin.
    (5) Crystal-induced ATN.
      (a) Acyclovir.
      (b) Sulfonamides.
      (c) Methotrexate.
      (d) Oxalate from ethylene glycol ingestion.
      (e) High dose of vitamin C.
    (6) Uric acid deposition in the tumor lysis syndrome.
  b. Acute and subacute glomerulonephropathies (GN).
    (1) Poststreptococcal glomerulonephritis.
    (2) Membranous nephropathy.
    (3) Membranoproliferative nephropathy.
    (4) Rapidly progressive GN (50% loss of renal function in 3 months).
  c. Drug-induced interstitial nephritis.
    (1) Penicillins, cephalosporins.
    (2) TMP-SMX.
    (3) Rifampin.
    (4) NSAIDs.
    (5) Diuretics.
    (6) Cimetidine, allopurinol, amphetamines, sulfinpyrazone.
  d. ARF secondary to vascular disorders.
    (1) Atheromatous emboli (e.g., following cardiac catheterization).
    (2) Major renal vascular occlusive disease (e.g., thromboembolism associated with atrial fibrillation).
    (3) Disseminated coagulopathy with ARF.
      (a) Hemolytic-uremic syndrome.
      (b) Thrombotic thrombocytopenic purpura.
      (c) Malignant hypertension.
3. Postrenal.
  a. Urethral obstruction (prostatic hypertrophy, urethral stricture).
  b. Bladder calculi or neoplasms.
  c. Pelvic or retroperitoneal neoplasms.
  d. Bilateral ureteral obstruction (neoplasm, calculi).
  e. Retroperitoneal fibrosis.

Work-up

1. The first step is to distinguish among prerenal, intrarenal, and postrenal causes by reviewing recent clinical events and drug therapy. The clinical evaluation should include:
   a. Orthostatic changes.
   b. Daily weights.
   c. Urinary output (in particular, anuria).
   d. Fluid loss.
   e. Heart failure.
   f. Vascular catheterization within the last month.
   g. Systemic diseases that can cause glomerulonephritis (e.g., lupus) or intestinal disease (e.g., myeloma).
   h. Past renal disease.
   i. Medications.
   j. Uremic symptoms (confusion, itching, pericarditis, asterixis).
   k. Rule out urinary retention (bladder catheterization).
2. Laboratory tests (Tables 5-29 and 5-30).
   a. Elevated serum creatinine.
      (1) The rate of rise of creatinine is approximately 1 mg/dL per day in complete renal failure.
      (2) A more rapid rise is only seen with rhabdomyolysis.
   b. Elevated BUN.
      (1) BUN/creatinine ratio is greater than 20:1 in prerenal azotemia, postrenal azotemia, and acute glomerulonephritis.
      (2) It is less than 20:1 in acute interstitial nephritis and acute tubular necrosis.
   c. Electrolytes (potassium, phosphate) are elevated; bicarbonate level and calcium are decreased.
   d. CBC can reveal anemia because of decreased erythropoietin production, hemoconcentration, or hemolysis.
   e. Urinalysis can reveal:
      (1) "Hematuria" (GN, rhabdomyolysis).
      (2) Proteinuria (nephrotic syndrome).
      (3) Casts (e.g., granular casts in ATN, RBC casts in acute GN, white blood cell casts in acute interstitial nephritis).
      (4) Eosinophiluria (acute interstitial nephritis).
   f. Urinary sodium and urinary creatinine should also be obtained to calculate the fractional excretion of sodium (FE_{Na}).

$$[FE_{Na} = (Urine\ Na/Plasma\ Na) \times (Plasma\ creatinine/Urine\ creatinine) \times 100]$$

   (1) The FE_{Na} is less than 1 in prerenal failure.
   (2) The FE_{Na} is greater than 1 in intrinsic renal failure in patients with urine output less than 400 mL/day.
   g. Urinary osmolarity (see Table 5-30).
      (1) Osmolarity is 250 to 300 mOsm/kg in ATN.
      (2) Osmolarity is less than 400 mOsm/kg in postrenal azotemia.
      (3) Osmolarity is greater than 500 mOsm/kg in prerenal azotemia and acute glomerulonephritis.
   h. Additional useful studies.
      (1) Blood cultures for patients suspected of sepsis.

Table 5-29 Serum and Radiographic Abnormalities in Renal Failure

Test	Prerenal	Postrenal (Acute)	Intrinsic Renal (Acute)	Intrinsic Renal (Chronic)
BUN	↑10:1 > Cr	↑ 20-40/d	↑ 20-40/d	Stable, ↑ varies with protein intake
Serum creatinine	N/moderate ↑	↑ 2-4/d	↑ 2-4/d	Stable ↑ (production equals excretion)
Serum potassium	N/moderate ↑	↑ varies with urinary volume	↑↑ (particularly when patient is oliguric) ↑↑↑ with rhabdomyolysis	Normal until end stage, unless tubular dysfunction (type 4 RTA)
Serum phosphorus	N/moderate ↑	Moderate ↑↑↑ with rhabdomyolysis	↑ Poor correlation with duration of renal disease	Becomes significantly elevated when serum creatinine level surpasses 3 mg/dL
Serum calcium	N	N/↑ with PO_4^{3-} retention	↑ (poor correlation with duration of renal failure)	Usually ↓
Renal size By ultrasound FE_{Na}*	N/↑ <1	↑ and dilated calyces <1->1	N/↑ >1	↓ and with ↑ echogenicity FE_{Na}* >1

*FE_{Na} = [(Urine Na × Serum Cr) / (Urine Cr × Serum Na)] × 100
↑, Increase; ↓, decrease; ↑↑, large increase; BUN, blood urea nitrogen; Cr, creatinine; FE_{Na}, fractional excretion of sodium; N, normal; P, plasma; RTA, renal tubular acidosis.
From Kiss B: Renal failure. In Ferri FF (ed): *Practical guide to the care of the medical patient*, ed 6. St Louis, Mosby, 2004.

Table 5-30 Urinary Abnormalities in Renal Failure				
Test	Prerenal	Postrenal (Acute)	Intrinsic Renal (Acute)	Intrinsic Renal (Chronic)
Urinary volume	↓	Absent-to-wide fluctuation	Oliguric or nonoliguric	1000 mL+ until end stage
Urinary creatinine	↑ (U/P Cr ±40)	↓ (U/P Cr ±20)	↓ (U/P Cr <20)	↓ (U/P Cr <20)
Osmolarity	↑ (±400 mOsm/kg)	(<350 mOsm/kg)	(<350 mOsm/kg)	(<350 mOsm/kg)
Degree of proteinuria	Minimum	Absent	Varies with cause of renal failure: Modest with ATN Nephrotic range common with acute glomerulopathies, usually <2 g/24 h with interstitial disease	Varies with cause of renal disease (1-2 g/d to nephrotic range)
Urinary sediment	Negative, or occasional hyaline cast	Negative, or hematuria with stones or papillary necrosis Pyuria with infectious prostatic disease	ATN: muddy brown Interstitial nephritis: lymphocytes, eosinophils (in stained preparations), and WBC casts RPGN: RBC casts Nephrosis: oval fat bodies	Broad casts with variable renal "residual" acute findings

↑, Increased; ↓, decreased; ATN, acute tubular necrosis; Cr, creatinine; RBC, red blood cell; RPGN, rapidly progressive glomerulonephritis; U/P, urine/plasma; WBC, white blood cell.
From Kiss B: Renal failure. In Ferri FF (ed): *Practical guide to the care of the medical patient*, ed 6. St Louis, Mosby, 2004.

  (2) Liver function tests, immunoglobulins, and protein electrophoresis in patients suspected of myeloma.
  (3) Creatinine kinase in patients with suspected rhabdomyolysis.
3. Imaging studies.
   a. Chest x-ray is useful to evaluate for CHF and for pulmonary renal syndromes (Goodpasture's syndrome, Wegener's granulomatosis).
   b. Ultrasound of the kidneys is used to evaluate for kidney size (useful to distinguish ARF from chronic renal failure [CRF]), to evaluate for the presence of obstruction, and to evaluate renal vascular status (with Doppler evaluation).
   c. Anterograde and/or retrograde pyelogram can be used for ruling out obstruction, which is useful in patients at high risk for obstruction.
4. Kidney biopsy.
   a. Renal biopsy may be indicated in patients with intrinsic renal failure when considering specific therapy.
   b. Major uses of renal biopsy are:
      (1) Differential diagnosis of the nephrotic syndrome.
      (2) Separation of lupus vasculitis from other vasculitis.
      (3) Separation of lupus membranous GN from idiopathic membranous GN.
      (4) Confirmation of hereditary nephropathies on the basis of ultrastructure.
      (5) Diagnosis of rapidly progressing glomerulonephritis.
      (6) Separation of allergic interstitial nephritis from ATN.
      (7) Separation of primary glomerulonephritis syndromes.
   c. The biopsy may be performed percutaneously or by open method.
      (1) The percutaneous approach is favored and generally yields adequate tissue in more than 90% of cases.
      (2) Open biopsy is generally reserved for uncooperative patients, those with solitary kidney, and patients at risk for uncontrolled bleeding.

Treatment

1. Prerenal.
   a. Correct hypovolemia if present; treat heart failure.
   b. Halt medications that could worsen the renal insufficiency (diuretics, NSAIDs, ACE inhibitors).
2. Renal.
   a. Halt medications that may be nephrotoxic.
   b. Treat pyelonephritis if present.
   c. If renal vascular disease is a possibility, consider obtaining a renal scan.
   d. Steroids are appropriate for certain types of GN.
   e. With euvolemic patients, fluid intake should equal urinary and other losses, allowing insensible losses of 300 to 500 mL/day.
   f. During recovery, urine volumes will increase markedly with each day, so observe for dehydration.
   g. Hemodialysis or peritoneal dialysis may be necessary on a temporary or permanent basis. General indications for initiation of dialysis are:
      (1) Florid symptoms of uremia (encephalopathy, pericarditis).
      (2) Severe volume overload.

(3) Severe acid-base imbalance.

(4) Significant derangement in electrolyte concentrations (e.g., hyperkalemia, hyponatremia).

3. Postrenal.
   a. Bladder catheterization is usually necessary.
      (1) A residual volume of more than 100 mL suggests obstruction.
      (2) Ultrasonography can be used to investigate the ureter or renal pelvis for hydronephrosis.
      (3) Ureteral stents or percutaneous nephrostomy following urologic consultation.
   b. Partial obstruction may yield variable daily urinary volumes (500 mL to 4 L/day). During recovery, urinary volumes increase gradually.
   c. Polyuria and dehydration can occur after relief of obstruction.

4. In general, monitor clinical biochemical status, particularly serum potassium, and adjust doses of renally excreted medications.

Prognosis

1. Prognosis is variable depending on the etiology of the renal failure, degree of renal failure, multiorgan involvement, and patient's age.
2. Renal function recovery (ability to discontinue dialysis) varies from 50% to 75% in survivors of ARF.
3. Overall mortality rate in ARF is nearly 50%, varying from 60% in patients with ATN to 35% in patients with prerenal or postrenal ARF.
4. The combination of ARF and sepsis is associated with a 70% mortality rate.

SUGGESTED READINGS

Albright RC Jr: Acute renal failure: A practical update. *Mayo Clin Proc* 76:67-74, 2001.

Merten GJ, Burgess WP, Gray LV, et al: Prevention of contrast-induced nephropathy with sodium bicarbonate: A randomized controlled trial. *JAMA* 291:2328-2334, 2004.

Nally JV Jr: Acute renal failure in hospitalized patients. *Cleve Clin J Med* 69:569-574, 2002.

Schiffl H, Lang SM, Fischer R: Daily hemodialysis and the outcome of acute renal failure. *N Engl J Med* 346:305-310, 2002.

Schrier RW, Wang W: Acute renal failure and sepsis. *N Engl J Med* 351:159-169, 2004.

Uchino S, Kellum JA, Bellomo R, et al: Acute renal failure in critically ill patients. *JAMA* 294:813-818, 2005.

CHRONIC RENAL FAILURE

Fred F. Ferri, with revisions by Tom J. Wachtel

Definition

Chronic renal failure (CRF) is a progressive decrease in renal function (CFR <60 mL/min for ≥3 months) with subsequent accumulation of waste products in the blood, electrolyte abnormalities, and anemia. It can lead to end-stage renal disease (ESRD).

Epidemiology

1. The number of patients with ESRD is increasing at the rate of 7% to 9%/year in the United States. Each year, 2/10,000 persons develop end-stage CRF.
2. In the United States, more than 250,000 persons a year receive dialysis treatment for ESRD.

Clinical Findings

1. The clinical presentation varies with the degree of renal failure and its underlying etiology.
   a. Common symptoms are:
      (1) Generalized fatigue.
      (2) Nausea.
      (3) Anorexia.
      (4) Pruritus.
      (5) Insomnia.
      (6) Taste disturbances.
   b. Urine output is variable.
2. Skin pallor, ecchymoses.
3. Heart failure related to volume overload and/or anemia.
4. Edema.
5. Hypertension.
6. Confusion delirium.
7. Emotional lability and depression.

Etiology

1. Diabetes (37%).
2. Hypertension (30%).
3. Chronic GN (12%).
4. Polycystic kidney disease.
5. Tubular interstitial nephritis (e.g., drug hypersensitivity, analgesic nephropathy), obstructive nephropathies (e.g., nephrolithiasis, prostatic disease).
6. Vascular diseases.
   a. Renal artery stenosis.
   b. Hypertensive nephrosclerosis.

Work-up

1. Laboratory tests.
   a. Reduced creatinine clearance in mL/min calculated by the Cockcroft-Gault formula.

   $$\text{Creatinin clearance in mL/min} = \frac{(140 - \text{age}) \times (\text{lean weight in kg})}{\text{Serum creatinine} - 72}$$

   b. Urinalysis can reveal proteinuria, RBC casts.
   c. Serum chemistry.
      (1) Elevated BUN and creatinine.
      (2) Hyperkalemia.
      (3) Hyperuricemia.
      (4) Hypocalcemia.
      (5) Hyperphosphatemia.
      (6) Hyperglycemia.
      (7) Low bicarbonate.
   d. Measure urinary protein excretion. The finding of a ratio of protein to creatinine higher than 1000 mg/g suggests the presence of glomerular disease.
   e. Special studies.
      (1) Serum and urine immunoelectrophoresis (in suspected multiple myeloma).

(2) Antinuclear antibody (in suspected SLE).
  f. The glomerular filtration rate (GFR) is the best overall indicator of kidney function. It can be estimated using prediction equations that take into account the serum creatinine level and some or all of specific variables (body size, age, sex, race). The creatinine clearance is generally considered an adequate proxy for GFR.
2. Imaging studies.
  a. Ultrasound of kidneys to measure kidney size and to rule out obstruction.
  b. Kidney biopsy is generally not performed in patients with small kidneys or with advanced disease.

Treatment

1. Nonpharmacologic therapy.
  a. Provide adequate nutrition and calories. Referral to a dietitian for nutritional therapy for patients with GFR less than 50 mL/1.73 m^2 is recommended and is now a covered service by Medicare.
  b. Restrict sodium (approximately 100 mM/day), potassium ($\leq$60 mM/day), and phosphate (<800 mg/day).
  c. Restrict fluid if significant edema is present.
  d. Protein restriction ($\leq$0.8 g/kg/day) can slow deterioration of renal function; however, recent studies have not confirmed this benefit. There is insufficient evidence to recommend for or against routine restriction of protein intake.
  e. Resistance exercise training can preserve lean body mass, nutritional status, and muscle function in patients with moderate chronic kidney disease.
  f. Avoid radiocontrast agents.
  g. Adjust drug doses to correct for prolonged half-lives.
2. Pharmacologic therapy.
  a. ACE inhibitors, ARBs, and nondihydropyridine CCBs (e.g., verapamil) are useful in reducing proteinuria and slowing the progression of chronic renal disease, especially in hypertensive diabetic patients. A systolic BP between 110 and 129 mm Hg may be beneficial in patients with urine protein excretion higher than 1.0 g/day.
  b. Erythropoietin for anemia: 2000 to 3000 U three times a week IV/SC to maintain hematocrit (Hct) at 30% to 33%.
  c. Diuretics for significant fluid overload (loop diuretics are preferred, thiazides are ineffective) when creatinine clearance is less than 20 mg/min.
  d. Correction of electrolyte abnormalities (e.g., calcium chloride, glucose, sodium polystyrene sulfonate for hyperkalemia).
  e. Sodium bicarbonate in patients with severe metabolic acidosis.
  f. Lipid-lowering agents in patients with dyslipidemia; target low-density lipoprotein (LDL) cholesterol is 100 mg/dL.
  g. Control of renal osteodystrophy with calcium supplementation and vitamin D.
    (1) Starting dose of calcium carbonate is 0.5 g with each meal, increased until the serum phosphorus concentration is normalized (most patients require 5 to 10 g/day).

(2) Calcitriol 0.125 µ/day PO is effective in increasing serum calcium concentration.

(3) Paricalcitol, a new vitamin D analogue, has been reported more effective than calcitriol in lessening the elevations in serum calcium and phosphorus levels.

(4) Sevelamer (Renagel) is a phosphate binder prescribed to reduce serum phosphate levels.

3. Other therapy.
   a. Initiate hemodialysis or peritoneal dialysis.
      (1) Urgent indications.
         (a) Uremic pericarditis.
         (b) Neuropathy.
         (c) Neuromuscular abnormalities.
         (d) CHF.
         (e) Hyperkalemia.
         (f) Seizures.
      (2) Elective indications.
         (a) Creatinine clearance 10 to 15 mL/min.
         (b) Progressive anorexia.
         (c) Weight loss.
         (d) Reversal of sleep pattern.
         (e) Pruritus.
         (f) Uncontrolled fluid gain with hypertension and signs of CHF.
   b. Kidney transplantation.
      (1) Kidney transplantation in selected patients improves survival.
      (2) The 2-year kidney graft survival rate for living related donor transplantations is greater than 80%.
      (3) The 2-year graft survival rate for cadaveric donor transplantation is approximately 70%.

SUGGESTED READINGS

Jafar TH, Stark PC, Schmid CH, et al: Progression of chronic kidney disease: The role of blood pressure control, proteinuria, and angiotensin-converting enzyme inhibition. Ann Intern Med 139:244-252, 2003.

Johnson CA, Levey AS, Coresh J, et al: Clinical practice guidelines for chronic kidney disease in adults: Part I. Definition, disease stages, evaluation, treatment, and risk factors. Am Fam Physician 70:869-876, 2004.

Kinchen KS, Sadler J, Fink N, et al: The timing of specialist evaluation in chronic kidney disease and mortality. Ann Intern Med 137:479-486, 2002.

Levey AS: Clinical practice. Nondiabetic kidney disease. N Engl J Med 347:1505-1511, 2002

Levey AS, Coresh J, Balk E, et al: National Kidney Foundation practice guidelines for chronic kidney disease: Evaluation, classification and stratification. Ann Intern Med 139:137-147, 2003.

Yu HT: Progression of chronic renal failure. Arth Intern Med 163:1417-1429, 2003.

VAGINAL BLEEDING

Tom J. Wachtel

Definition

Postmenopausal gynecologic bleeding is any bleeding occurring after menopause (defined as the cessation of menses for 12 months). It can be an early sign of endometrial cancer (10%) and therefore requires evaluation.

Epidemiology

1. Incidence in the first year immediately after menopause: 409/1000 woman-years.
2. Incidence more than 3 years after menopause: 42/1000 woman-years.

Clinical Findings

1. Vaginal bleeding in a postmenopausal woman.
2. Risk factors for endometrial cancer.
   a. Obesity.
   b. Chronic anovulation.
   c. Nulliparity.
   d. Diabetes.
   e. Tamoxifen use.
   f. Personal history of breast or ovarian cancer.
   g. Family history of breast, ovarian, or endometrial cancer and perhaps colon cancer.
   h. Unopposed estrogen use in a patient with a uterus.

Etiology

1. Polyps (12%).
2. Atrophy due to hypoestrogenism (59%).
3. Hormone therapy (7%).
4. Endometrial hyperplasia (10%).
5. Endometrial cancer (10%).
6. Uterine leiomyomas (fibroids).
7. Adenomyosis.
8. Cervical or vaginal cancer.
9. Endometritis, salpingitis, vaginitis.
10. Disease of other pelvic organs.
11. Anticoagulant therapy.
12. Radiation therapy to the pelvic region.

Work-up

1. Cervical cytology (Pap smear).
2. Biopsy of visible lesions.
3. Transvaginal sonography.
   a. Endometrial cancer in postmenopausal women can be ruled out if the endometrium is less than 4 mm thick and homogeneous on transvaginal sonography.
   b. Sonography is 96% sensitive for detection of endometrial cancer if the endometrial stripe is greater than 5 mm (i.e., low probability of a false-negative test).
4. Endometrial biopsy can detect >99% of endometrial cancers in postmenopausal women with vaginal bleeding.
5. Hysteroscopy with dilation and curettage.
   a. Hysteroscopy directly visualizes the endometrial cavity.
   b. Biopsy or excision of lesions is then performed under direct visualization.

c. The probability of endometrial cancer after a negative hysteroscopy is 0.4% to 0.5%.

Treatment

Directed at the underlying cause.

Endometrial cancer is treated primarily with hysterectomy and bilateral salpingo-oophorectomy.

SUGGESTED READINGS

Astrup K, Olivarius Nde F: Frequency of spontaneously occurring postmenopausal bleeding in the general population. *Acta Obstet Gynecol Scand* 83:203-207, 2004.

Cheng RF: Evaluation of postmenopausal bleeding. *Women's Health in Primary Care* 15-22, 2006.

Clark TJ, Voit D, Gupta JK, et al: Accuracy of hysteroscopy in the diagnosis of endometrial cancer and hyperplasia: A systematic quantitative review. *JAMA* 228:1610-1621, 2002.

Dijkhuizen FP, Mol BW, Brolmann HA, Heintz AP: The accuracy of endometrial sampling in the diagnosis of patients with endometrial carcinoma and hyperplasia: A meta-analysis. *Cancer* 89:1765-1772, 2000.

Gull B, Carlsson S, Karlsson B, et al: Transvaginal ultrasonography of the endometrium in women with postmenopausal bleeding: Is it always necessary to perform an endometrial biopsy? *Am J Obstet Gynecol* 182:509-515, 2000.

Smith-Bindman R, Kerlikowske K, Feldstein VA, et al: Endovaginal ultrasound to exclude endometrial cancer and other endometrial abnormalities. *JAMA* 280:1510-1517, 1998.

5.10 Hematology and Oncology

ANEMIA

Tom J. Wachtel

Definition

1. Anemia is a reduction in circulating RBC mass to less than 14 g/dL (Hct <42%) in men and postmenopausal women.
2. Anemia is not part of normal aging, but it is more prevalent in geriatric patients.

Etiology

Decreased RBC Production (Low Reticulocyte Index)

1. Anemias with low mean corpuscular volume (MCV) (microcytic anemias).
   a. Iron deficiency.
   b. Anemia of chronic inflammation.
   c. Thalassemia.
   d. Sideroblastic anemia.
2. Anemias with high MCV (macrocytic anemias).
   a. Megaloblastic anemia.
      (1) Vitamin B_{12} deficiency (prevalence 2% in persons older than 60 years).
      (2) Folic acid deficiency.
      (3) Drugs.
   b. Alcoholism.
   c. Myelodysplastic syndromes.

d. Hypothyroidism.
e. Chronic liver disease.
3. Anemias with normal MCV in the majority of cases (normocytic anemias).
   a. Aplastic anemia.
   b. Anemia of chronic inflammation.
   c. Anemia of chronic renal insufficiency.
   d. Sideroblastic anemia.
   e. Anemia associated with marrow infiltration (myelophthisis).
   f. Chronic liver disease.

Increased RBC Destruction (Appropriate, i.e. Elevated, Reticulocyte Index)

1. Bleeding.
2. Hemolytic anemias.
   a. Hereditary.
      (1) Abnormalities of RBC interior.
          (a) Hemoglobinopathies (e.g., sickle cell, thalassemia).
          (b) Enzyme deficiencies (e.g., glucose-6-phosphate dehydrogenase [G6PD] deficiency).
      (2) Membrane abnormalities (e.g., hereditary spherocytosis).
   b. Acquired.
      (1) Splenomegaly.
      (2) Immune mediated immunohemolytic anemias).
          (a) Warm antibody.
              i. Idiopathic.
              ii. Lymphoproliferative disorders: chronic lymphocytic leukemia, non-Hodgkin's lymphomas, Hodgkin's disease.
              iii. SLE.
              iv. Drugs: α-methyldopa type, penicillin type (hapten), quinidine-type (innocent bystander).
          (b) Cold antibody.
              i. Cold agglutinin disease: acute (*Mycoplasma* infection, infectious mononucleosis) or chronic (idiopathic lymphoma).
              ii. Paroxysmal cold hemoglobinuria: idiopathic or secondary to acute viral infections (e.g., measles and mumps) or tertiary syphilis.
      (3) Intravascular trauma.
          (a) Marcher's hemoglobinuria (secondary to external impact).
          (b) Cardiac valve prosthesis.
          (c) Microangiopathic hemolytic anemia (secondary to fibrin deposition in microvasculature): malignant hypertension, renal allograft rejection, disseminated cancer, large hemangiomas, thrombotic thrombocytopenic purpura (TTP), hemolytic uremic syndrome, and disseminated intravascular coagulation.
      (4) Direct toxic effect.
          (a) Infections (e.g., malaria, *Clostridium perfringens*, babesiosis).
          (b) Physical agents (e.g., extensive burns).

      (c) Chemicals (e.g., copper toxicity).
    (5) Membrane abnormalities.
      (a) Spur cell anemia (advanced cirrhosis).
      (b) Paroxysmal nocturnal hemoglobinuria.

Work-up

1. History.
   a. Symptoms depend on etiology, degree, and rapidity of onset.
     (1) Gradual onset.
      (a) Symptoms are related to tissue hypoxia (e.g., fatigue, headache, dyspnea, lightheadedness, angina).
      (b) Gradual onset suggests a chronic process (e.g., vitamin B_{12} deficiency, malignancy).
     (2) Rapid onset.
      (a) May result in sudden hemodynamic instability.
      (b) Sudden onset suggests hemolysis or acute hemorrhage.
   b. Associated symptoms.
     (1) Blood loss.
      (a) Melena.
      (b) Hematochezia.
      (c) Hematuria.
      (d) Menorrhagia.
     (2) Hemolysis.
      (a) Jaundice.
      (b) Darkening of urine.
     (3) Vitamin B_{12} deficiency.
      (a) Paresthesias.
      (b) Ataxia.
      (c) Confusion.
   c. Drug and toxin exposures.
     (1) Alcohol.
     (2) Alkylating agents.
     (3) Benzene.
     (4) Colchicine.
     (5) Isoniazid.
     (6) Lead.
     (7) Quinidine.
     (8) Methotrexate.
     (9) Phenytoin.
     (10) Sulfa compounds.
     (11) Trimethoprim.
     (12) Zidovudine.
   d. Family and ethnic history.
     (1) Sickle cell disease.
     (2) Thalassemia.
     (3) Other hereditary hemolytic anemias.
   e. Other past medical history.
     (1) Renal failure.
     (2) Endocrine disorders.
     (3) Inflammatory disorders.

      (4) Chronic infections.
      (5) Cholelithiasis at an early age (may suggest a hereditary hemolytic anemia).
      (6) Valve replacement.
2. Physical exam.
  a. General appearance: assess nutritional status.
  b. Vital signs.
    (1) Tachycardia.
    (2) Hypotension in acute blood loss.
  c. Skin.
    (1) Pallor.
    (2) Jaundice (hemolysis).
    (3) Petechiae or purpura (thrombocytopenia).
    (4) Spider angiomas or palmar erythema (liver disease).
  d. Mouth: glossitis (pernicious anemia, Plummer-Vinson syndrome).
  e. Cardiac: prosthetic valve (traumatic hemolysis).
  f. Abdomen.
    (1) Splenomegaly.
    (2) Infiltrative disorders.
    (3) Hemolytic disorders.
    (4) Megaloblastic anemias.
    (5) Liver disease.
  g. Rectal: occult or gross blood in the stool.
  h. Lymphadenopathy.
    (1) Infiltrative disease.
    (2) Infections.
    (3) Collagen vascular disease.
  i. Neurologic.
    (1) Impaired vibratory and position sense and/or impaired cognition suggestive of vitamin B_{12} deficiency.
    (2) Acute mental status changes and/or neurologic deficits seen in TTP.
3. Laboratory.
  a. Hemoglobin (Hgb) and Hct estimate RBC mass.
  b. Reticulocyte count.
    (1) Indicator of bone marrow response to anemia.
    (2) Reticulocyte index (RI) corrects for degree of anemia.
      (a) RI higher than 2.5% suggests increased RBC destruction.
      (b) RI lower than 2.5% suggests decreased RBC production.
  c. MCV.
    (1) Classifies anemia as microcytic, macrocytic, or normocytic.
    (2) Should be interpreted in the context of an evaluation of a peripheral smear, because:
      (a) Small and large cells may be present simultaneously, resulting in a normal MCV (see "Red-cell distribution").
      (b) MCV may be elevated by reticulocytes, which are larger than mature RBCs.
  d. Red-cell distribution width (RDW).
    (1) A measure of anisocytosis or RBCs of variable size (e.g., multifactorial anemia).

  (2) May be useful in differentiating anemias sharing similar MCV ranges (e.g., thalassemia and iron deficiency are both characterized by low MCV, the former with normal RDW, the latter often with increased RDW).
  (3) Elevated before MCV becomes abnormal in early iron, folic acid, and vitamin B_{12} deficiency.
  e. Peripheral smear.
    (1) RBC morphology.
      (a) Size.
        i. Microcytosis.
        ii. Macrocytosis.
        iii. Anisocytosis.
      (b) Shape.
        i. Spherocytes (hereditary spherocytosis, immunohemolytic anemia).
        ii. Teardrop cells (myeloproliferative diseases, pernicious anemia, thalassemia).
        iii. Schistocytes (traumatic and microangiopathic hemolysis).
        iv. Sickle cells (sickle cell disease).
        v. Target cells (liver disease, sickle cell disease, thalassemias, HbC).
      (c) Color.
        i. Hypochromia iron deficiency, sideroblastic anemias.
        ii. Hyperchromia in megaloblastic anemia, spherocytosis.
    (2) WBC and platelet abnormalities.
      (a) WBC hypersegmentation: megaloblastic anemias.
      (b) Immature WBC forms: marrow infiltrative disorder.
      (c) Large or increased numbers of platelets: myeloproliferative disorders.
    (3) Other abnormalities.
      (a) Basophilic stippling.
        (1) Lead poisoning.
        (2) Thalassemias.
        (3) Hemolysis.
      (b) Nucleated RBCs.
        (1) Marrow infiltrative disorders.
        (2) Hemolysis.
        (3) Megaloblastic anemias.
      (c) Howell-Jolly bodies (nuclear fragments).
        (1) Hemolytic and megaloblastic anemias.
        (2) Functional or anatomic asplenia.
      (d) Rouleaux formation.
        (1) Multiple myeloma.
        (2) Waldenström's macroglobulinemia.

Further Evaluation

1. Microcytic anemia.
  a. Serum ferritin.
    (1) Serum ferritin less than 12 μg/dL (normal 12-300) indicates iron deficiency.

(2) Because serum ferritin is an acute-phase reactant, the level may be normal or increased in inflammatory states, liver disease, infection, or malignancy.

(3) Serum ferritin greater than 200 μg/dL generally indicates adequate iron stores.

(4) It is normal or increased in sideroblastic anemia and thalassemias.

b. Serum iron (Fe) and total iron-binding capacity (TIBC) (Fe/TIBC ratio is called *transferrin saturation*).

(1) Fe and TIBC in iron-deficiency anemia.

(a) Fe is usually decreased and TIBC is usually elevated in iron-deficiency anemia (rise in TIBC occurs before drop in Fe).

(b) Transferrin saturation is less than 10% in iron deficiency.

(c) These changes occur later than does the decline in serum ferritin.

(2) Both Fe and TIBC are decreased in anemia of chronic inflammation (transferrin saturation usually >10%).

(3) Fe and TIBC are normal or increased in sideroblastic anemias and thalassemia.

c. Hemoglobin electrophoresis is the definitive diagnostic test for heterozygous β-thalassemia (increased HbA2).

d. General.

(1) Any man or postmenopausal woman with iron-deficiency anemia is assumed to have a gastrointestinal (GI) malignancy until proved otherwise.

(2) Iron-deficiency anemia.

(a) Decline in MCV is usually proportional to the degree of anemia.

(b) Mild microcytic anemia with MCV decreased out of proportion to degree of anemia (once iron deficiency is ruled out), in which HbA2 is normal, is consistent with heterozygous α-thalassemia (normal Hb electrophoresis).

(3) To determine if a patient with a chronic inflammatory disease (e.g., rheumatoid arthritis) has become iron deficient, it may be necessary to either give a trial of iron therapy or check marrow iron stores.

(4) Bone marrow aspiration and biopsy.

(a) Bone marrow aspiration and biopsy are indicated in the evaluation of any unexplained anemia.

(b) This is the definitive way to diagnose iron deficiency and the only way to diagnose sideroblastic anemia (i.e., by finding ringed sideroblasts).

2. Macrocytic anemias.

a. TSH level, liver function tests.

b. Reticulocyte count, because reticulocytosis can cause spurious elevation of the MCV.

c. History of drug and toxin exposures.

d. Serum B12 and RBC folate levels.

(1) Serum folate is not a reliable indicator of tissue folate levels, because it can reflect recent changes in dietary intake.

(2) Severe B12 deficiency can cause falsely low levels of RBC folate, despite adequate folate intake.

(3) Severe deficiency of either vitamin causes megaloblastic changes in intestinal epithelial cells, which can lead to malabsorption of the other vitamin.

e. Antiparietal cell antibody test is positive in 70% of pernicious anemia patients.

f. Anti-intrinsic factor antibody test is positive in 50% of pernicious anemia patients.

g. Schilling test if the patient is B_{12} deficient, to investigate the cause (e.g., pernicious anemia, bacterial overgrowth, or ileal disease).

h. Bone marrow aspiration and biopsy if macrocytic anemia remains unexplained (to look for a myelodysplastic syndrome), especially if other cell lines are also affected.

i. Neurologic symptoms of B_{12} deficiency can occur in the absence of anemia (especially in patients with normal or supranormal levels of folate intake) and might not remit completely with treatment.

3. Normocytic anemias.

a. If the patient is not known to have an underlying systemic disease (e.g., chronic infection or inflammation) that would explain the anemia, one should search for one of these conditions as well as:

(1) Renal disease.

(2) Endocrine disease (e.g., hypothyroidism, hypogonadism, Addison's disease).

(3) Liver disease.

(4) Possible occult malignancy.

b. If such a condition is found:

(1) Treat the underlying disorder.

(2) Also look for other factors that may be exacerbating the anemia (e.g., blood loss, nutritional deficiency).

c. If the anemia remains unexplained, bone marrow aspiration and biopsy should be considered (looking for aplasia as well as marrow-infiltrative disorders), especially if the WBC and platelet counts are also reduced.

4. Hemolytic anemias.

a. Coombs' test should be done in all patients with suspected hemolysis. Both direct and indirect Coombs' tests detect the presence of anti-RBC antibodies circulating in the patient's serum.

b. Other tests.

(1) Elevated total bilirubin, elevated lactate dehydrogenase (LDH), and decreased or absent haptoglobin can be helpful in establishing the presence of hemolysis but are not helpful in establishing the cause.

(2) Other evaluation depends on the results of the initial evaluation.

(a) Patients with a Coombs'-positive hemolytic anemia might require antinuclear antibody, CT scan of chest and abdomen, bone marrow aspiration and biopsy (to rule out lymphoma), and *Mycoplasma* titers.

(b) Acid hemolysis or sucrose lysis test to rule out paroxysmal nocturnal hemoglobinuria in the setting of recurrent venous thrombosis and/or mild pancytopenia.

(c) Platelets, BUN/creatinine, prothrombin time/partial thromboplastin time (PT/PTT), fibrin degradation products, and fibrinogen in a patient with schistocytes on peripheral smear (to rule out disseminated intravascular coagulation, TTP).

(d) G6PD level in a patient who has had a hemolytic episode (with Heinz bodies on peripheral smear) after exposure to certain drugs (e.g., sulfonamides, nitrofurantoin, antimalarials) or consuming fava beans.

Treatment

1. Iron deficiency anemia.
   a. When a diagnosis of iron-deficiency anemia is made, some effort should be made to try to locate the suspected site of iron loss (e.g., colonoscopy, esophagogastroduodenoscopy [EGD]).
   b. Patients should be instructed to consume foods containing large amounts of iron, such as liver, red meat, and legumes.
   c. Treatment consists of ferrous sulfate 325 mg PO qd for at least 6 months. Calcium supplements can decrease iron absorption; therefore, these two medications should be staggered.
   d. Patients should be instructed to continue their iron supplements for at least 6 months or longer to correct depleted body iron stores.
   e. Reticulocyte count will peak in 5 to 10 days. Hb will rise over 1 to 2 months. Failure to respond is consistent with intestinal malabsorption (e.g., celiac disease).
   f. Therapy is usually required for at least 6 months.
   g. Transfusion of packed RBCs is indicated in patients with severe symptomatic or life-threatening anemia (e.g., angina).
2. Megaloblastic anemias.
   a. Folate deficiency.
      (1) Folic acid deficiency is treated with folic acid 1 mg PO daily until the deficiency is corrected.
      (2) Treatment may be indefinite in patients with high baseline requirements (e.g., patients with chronic hemolytic anemias and patients on hemodialysis).
   b. Vitamin B_{12} deficiency.
      (1) Nutritional deficiency.
         (a) Oral cobalamin 1000 mg PO qd.
         (b) This is a safe, effective, and inexpensive alternative in patients with inadequate dietary intake, provided normal cobalamin levels are ensured.
      (2) Pernicious anemia.
         (a) Vitamin B_{12} deficiency is corrected with cyanocobalamin.
            i. Initial dose is typically 1000 mcg IM daily for 7 days, then weekly for 1 to 2 months, then every month indefinitely unless a reversible cause is found.
            ii. Reticulocyte count usually peaks in 1 week, and Hb rises over 6 to 8 weeks.
         (b) Avoid folic acid supplementation without vitamin B_{12} supplementation.
         (c) When hematologic parameters have returned to the normal range:
            i. Intranasal cyanocobalamin may be used in place of IM cyanocobalamin.

      ii. The initial dose of intranasal cyanocobalamin (Nascobal) is one spray (500 µg) in one nostril once per week.

      iii. Monitor response and increase dose if serum B_{12} levels decline.

      iv. Consider return to IM vitamin B_{12} supplementation if decline persists.

   (d) Self-injection of vitamin B_{12} may be taught in selected patients.

   (e) Oral cobalamin (1000 µg/day) has been found effective in mild cases of pernicious anemia because about 1% of an oral dose is absorbed by passive diffusion, a pathway that does not require intrinsic factor.

   (f) Consider GI referral for endoscopy upon diagnosis of pernicious anemia and surveillance endoscopy every 5 years to rule out gastric carcinoma, particularly if associated iron deficiency is present.

3. Anemia of chronic disease or inflammation.
   a. Treat the underlying condition.
   b. Prevent exacerbating factors, such as nutritional deficiencies and marrow-suppressive drugs.
   c. Consider erythropoietin (Epo).
     (1) Epo 12.5 to 250 U/kg SC three times per week can correct the anemia associated with chronic inflammatory disorders.
     (2) It should be considered in patients with symptoms of severe anemia or Hb less than 10 g/dL.
     (3) Response is not dependent on patient's endogenous Epo level.

4. Anemia from chronic renal insufficiency.
   a. This anemia is attributed primarily to decreased endogenous Epo production.
   b. Epo therapy is indicated in both predialysis and dialysis patients who are symptomatic.
   c. Benefits.
     (1) Increased energy.
     (2) Enhanced appetite.
     (3) Better sleep.
     (4) Improved cognitive function.
     (5) Elimination of RBC transfusions.
     (6) Reduction of iron overload.
   d. Administration of Epo may be IV in hemodialysis patients.
   e. Most patients increase their Hct by 10 points or to a level greater than 32% within 12 weeks of therapy.
   f. Initial dosage is 50 to 100 U/kg two to three times per week until the Hct reaches 32%, at which point the dose is adjusted to maintain the Hct.
   g. Inadequate responses can occur with coexisting iron deficiency; therefore, many patients benefit from iron supplementation.

5. Sideroblastic anemia.
   a. Eliminate potential precipitants (e.g., isoniazid, alcohol, lead).
   b. Empirical trial of pyridoxine 50 to 200 mg daily, although response rate is low.

   c. Supportive therapy in idiopathic acquired cases: refractory anemia with ringed sideroblasts, which is one of the myelodysplastic syndromes.
     (1) Transfusions as needed.
     (2) Avoiding marrow-suppressive drugs.
     (3) Avoiding nutritional deficiencies.
   d. Epo 100 to 300 U/kg SC three times per week.
     (1) May be useful in decreasing RBC transfusion requirements in approximately 20% of patients.
     (2) More likely effective when the serum Epo level is low.
   e. Organ dysfunction resulting from iron overload can necessitate periodic phlebotomy.
   f. In advanced cases, desferoxamine 40 mg/kg per day IV is given.
6. Autoimmune hemolytic anemia.
   a. Discontinue any potentially offensive drugs.
   b. Avoid cold exposure in patients with cold antibody.
   c. Give prednisone 1 to 2 mg/kg per day in divided doses initially in warm antibody autoimmune hemolytic anemia. Corticosteroids are generally ineffective in cold antibody autoimmune hemolytic anemia.
   d. Perform splenectomy in patients responding inadequately to corticosteroids when RBC sequestration studies indicate splenic sequestration.
   e. Give danazol, usually used in conjunction with corticosteroids (may be useful in warm antibody autoimmune hemolytic anemia).
   f. Immunosuppressive drugs (azathioprine, cyclophosphamide) may be useful in warm antibody autoimmune hemolytic anemia but are indicated only after both corticosteroids and splenectomy (unless surgery is contraindicated) have failed to produce an adequate remission.
   g. Plasmapheresis/exchange transfusion is used for severe life-threatening cases only.

SUGGESTED READINGS

Alcindor T, Bridges KR: Sideroblastic anemias. Br J Haematol 116:733-743, 2002.

Ble A, Fink JC, Woodman RC et al: Renal function, erythropoietin and anemia of older persons. Arch Intern Med 165:2222-2227, 2005.

Dhaliwal G, Cornett PA, Tierney LM Jr: Hemolytic anemia. Am Fam Physician 69:2599-2606, 2004.

Dharmarajan TS, Pais W, Norkus EP: Does anemia matter? Anemia, morbidity and mortality in older adults: Need for greater recognition. Geriatrics 60:22-29, 2005.

Spivak JL: Anemia in the elderly. Arch Intern Med 165:2187-2189, 2005.

Steensma DP, Bennett JM: The Myelodysplastic syndromes: diagnostic and treatment. Mayo Clin Proc 81:104-130, 2006.

Tefferi A: Anemia in adults: A contemporary approach to diagnosis, Mayo Clin Proc 78:1274-1280, 2003.

Zakai NA, Katz R, Hirsch C, et al: A prospective study of anemia status, hemoglobin concentration and mortality in an elderly cohort. Arch Intern Med 165:2214-2220, 2005.

COLON CANCER

Fred F. Ferri and Tom J. Wachtel

Definition

Colorectal cancer is a neoplasm arising from the luminal surface of the large bowel.

Epidemiology

1. Incidence.
   a. Colorectal cancer is the second leading cause of cancer death in the United States (>135,000 new cases and >50,000 deaths/year).
   b. Colorectal cancer accounts for 14% of all cases of cancer (excluding skin malignancies) and 14% of all cancer deaths every year.
   c. Peak incidence is in the seventh decade of life.
2. Location.
   a. About 50% of rectal cancers are within reach of the examiner's finger.
   b. About 50% of colon cancers are within reach of the flexible sigmoidoscope.
   c. From 40% to 42% are found in the descending colon.
   d. From 30% to 33% are found in the rectosigmoid and rectum.
   e. From 25% to 30% are found in the cecum and ascending colon.
   f. From 10% to 13% are found in the transverse colon.
3. Risk factors.
   a. Hereditary polyposis syndromes.
      (1) Familial polyposis (high risk).
      (2) Gardner's syndrome (high risk).
      (3) Turcot's syndrome (high risk).
      (4) Peutz-Jeghers syndrome (low to moderate risk).
   b. Inflammatory bowel disease, both ulcerative colitis and Crohn's disease.
   c. Family history of "cancer family syndrome."
   d. Heredofamilial breast cancer and colon cancer.
   e. History of previous colorectal carcinoma.
   f. History of irradiation for gynecologic cancer.
   g. First-degree relatives with colorectal carcinoma.
   h. Possible dietary factors (diet high in fat or meat, beer drinking, reduced vegetable consumption).
   i. Previous endometrial or ovarian cancer, particularly when diagnosed at an early age.
   j. History of adenomatous polyp.
   k. Hereditary nonpolyposis colon cancer (HNPCC).
      (1) Autosomal-dominant disorder characterized by early age of onset (mean age of 44 years) and:
         (a) Right-sided or proximal colon cancers.
         (b) Synchronous and metachronous colon cancers.
         (c) Mucinous and poorly differentiated colon cancers.
      (2) It accounts for 1% to 5% of all cases of colorectal cancer.
4. Mitigation of risk factors.
   a. Chemoprophylaxis with aspirin (81 mg/day) reduces the incidence of colorectal adenomas in persons at risk.
   b. Hormone replacement therapy reduces the incidence of colon cancer in women.

Etiology

1. Colorectal cancer can arise through two mutational pathways:
   a. Microsatellite instability.
   b. Chromosomal instability.
2. Germline genetic mutations are the basis of inherited colon cancer syndromes.

3. An accumulation of somatic mutations in a cell is the basis of sporadic colon cancer.

Clinical Findings

1. History.
   a. Change in bowel habits.
   b. Unexplained abdominal pain.
   c. Lower GI bleeding (red blood).
   d. Painful defecation (tenesmus).
   e. Jaundice.
   f. Screening.
2. Physical examination.
   a. Physical examination may be completely unremarkable.
   b. DRE can detect approximately 50% of rectal cancers.
   c. Palpable abdominal masses can indicate metastasis or complications of colorectal carcinoma (abscess, intussusception, volvulus).
   d. Abdominal distention and tenderness suggest colonic obstruction.
   e. Hepatomegaly can indicate hepatic metastasis.
   f. The clinical presentation of colorectal malignancies is initially vague and nonspecific (weight loss, anorexia, malaise). It is useful to divide colon cancer symptoms into those usually associated with the right colon and those commonly associated with the left colon, because the clinical presentation varies with the location of the carcinoma.
      (1) Right colon.
         (a) Anemia (iron deficiency secondary to chronic blood loss).
         (b) Dull, vague, and uncharacteristic abdominal pain may be present or the patient may be completely asymptomatic.
         (c) Rectal bleeding is often missed because blood is mixed with feces.
         (d) Obstruction and constipation are unusual because of large lumen and more liquid stools.
      (2) Left colon.
         (a) Change in bowel habits (constipation, diarrhea, tenesmus, pencil-thin stools).
         (b) Rectal bleeding (bright red blood coating the surface of the stool).
         (c) Intestinal obstruction is common because of the small lumen.
         (d) Early diagnosis of patients with surgically curable disease (Dukes' A, B).
            i. Early diagnosis is necessary because survival time is directly related to the stage of the carcinoma at the time of diagnosis.
            ii. The most important tool for screening colon cancer is colonoscopy every 5 to 10 years beginning at age 50 (or earlier in high-risk persons).
            iii. The residual value of rectal exam and stool for occult blood (recommended yearly) is unclear in patients who undergo regular colonoscopy.

Differential Diagnosis

1. Diverticular disease.

2. Strictures.
3. Inflammatory bowel disease.
4. Infectious or inflammatory lesions.
5. Adhesions.
6. Metastatic carcinoma (prostate, sarcoma).
7. Extrinsic masses (cysts, abscesses).

Classification

Dukes' and International Union Against Cancer (UICC) classification for colorectal cancer.

1. Confined to the mucosa or submucosa (I).
2. Invasion of muscularis propria (II).
3. Local node involvement (III).
4. Distant metastasis (IV).

Work-up

1. Laboratory tests.
   a. Positive fecal occult blood test.
   b. Microcytic anemia.
   c. Elevated plasma carcinoembryonic antigen (CEA).
      (1) CEA should not be used as a screening test for colorectal cancer because it can be elevated in patients with many other conditions (smoking, inflammatory bowel disease, alcoholic liver disease).
      (2) A normal CEA does not exclude the diagnosis of colorectal cancer.
   d. Liver function tests.
   e. Newer modalities for early detection of colorectal neoplasms include detection of mutations in the adenomatous polyposis coli (APC) gene from stool samples. This test is still experimental.
2. Imaging studies.
   a. Colonoscopy with biopsy (primary assessment tool).
   b. CT scan of abdomen to assist in preoperative staging.
   c. Chest x-ray examination to look for evidence of metastatic disease.
   d. Air-contrast barium enema only in patients refusing colonoscopy or unable to tolerate colonoscopy.

Treatment

1. Surgical resection.
   a. About 70% of colorectal cancers are resectable for cure at presentation.
   b. About 45% of patients are cured by primary resection.
2. Radiation therapy is a useful adjunct to fluorouracil and levamisole therapy for stage II or III rectal cancers.
3. Adjuvant chemotherapy.
   a. Levamisole and 5-fluorouracil (5-FU).
      (1) A combination of 5-FU and levamisole substantially increases cure rates for patients with stage III colon cancer.
      (2) It should be considered standard treatment for all stage III patients and selected patients with high-risk stage II colon cancer.
   b. Leucovorin (folinic acid).
      (1) Leucovorin enhances the effect of fluorouracil and is given together with it (FL).

(2) When given as adjuvant therapy after a complete resection in stage III disease, FL increases overall 5-year survival from 51% to 64%.

(3) The use of adjuvant FL in stage II disease (no involvement of regional nodes) is controversial.

    (a) The 5-year overall survival is 80% for treated or untreated patients.

    (b) The addition of FL only increases the probability of 5-year disease-free interval from 72% to 76%.

(4) For patients with standard-risk stage III tumors (e.g., involvement of one to three regional lymph nodes), FL alone or FL with oxaliplatin (Eloxatin, an inhibitor of DNA synthesis) are both reasonable choices.

(5) In general, reversible peripheral neuropathy is the main side effect of FL plus oxaliplatin.

  c. Irinotecan (Camptosar).

    (1) Irinotecan is a potent inhibitor of topoisomerase I, a nuclear enzyme involved in the unwinding of DNA during replication.

    (2) It can be used to treat metastatic colorectal cancer refractory to other drugs, including 5-FU.

    (3) It may offer a few months of palliation but is expensive and associated with significant toxicity.

  d. Oxaliplatin.

    (1) Oxaliplatin can be used in combination with FL for patients with metastatic colorectal cancer whose disease has recurred or progressed despite treatment with FL plus irinotecan.

    (2) FL plus oxaliplatin should be considered for high-risk patients with stage III cancers (e.g., >3 involved regional nodes [N2] or tumor invasion beyond the serosa [T4 lesion]).

4. Monoclonal antibodies.

    (1) The monoclonal antibodies cetuximab (Erbitux) and bevacizumab (Avastin) have been approved by the FDA for advanced colorectal cancer.

    (2) Bevacizumab.

      (a) Bevacizumab is an angiogenesis inhibitor that binds and inhibits the activity of human vascular endothelial growth factor.

      (b) The addition of bevacizumab to FL in patients with advanced colorectal cancer has been reported to increase the response rate from 17% to 40%.

    (3) Cetuximab is an epidermal growth factor receptor (EGFR) blocker that inhibits the growth and survival of tumor cells that overexpress EGFR.

      (a) Cetuximab has synergism with irinotecan.

      (b) Adding cetuximab to irinotecan in patients with advanced disease resistant to irinotecan increases the response rate from 10% when cetuximab is used alone to 22% with combination of cetuximab and irinotecan.

5. In patients who undergo resection of liver metastases from colorectal cancer, postoperative treatment with a combination of hepatic arterial infusion of floxuridine and IV fluorouracil improves the outcome at 2 years.

Follow-up

1. Physician visits.
   a. Focus on the clinical and disease-related history.
   b. Directed physical examination guided by this history.
   c. Coordination of follow-up.
   d. Counseling every 3 to 6 months for the first 3 years, then decreased frequency thereafter for 2 years.
2. Colonoscopy yearly for the initial 2 years, then every 3 years.
3. CEA.
   a. CEA level should be obtained at baseline.
   b. If CEA is elevated, it can be used postoperatively as a measure of completeness of tumor resection or to monitor tumor recurrence.
   c. If CEA is used to monitor tumor recurrence, it should be obtained every 3 to 6 months for up to 5 years.
   d. The role of CEA for monitoring patients with resected colon cancer has been questioned because of the small number of cures attributed to CEA monitoring despite the substantial cost in dollars and physical and emotional stress associated with monitoring.

Prognosis

1. The 5-year survival varies with the stage of the carcinoma.
   a. Dukes' A 5-year survival is >80%.
   b. Dukes' B 5-year survival is 60%.
   c. Dukes' C 5-year survival is 20%.
   d. Dukes' D 5-year survival is 3%.
2. Overall 5-year disease-free survival is approximately 50% for colon cancer.
3. In patients with Dukes' C (stage III) colorectal cancer there is improved 5-year survival among women treated with adjuvant chemotherapy (53% with chemotherapy vs. 33% without) and among patients with right-sided tumors treated with adjuvant chemotherapy.

SUGGESTED READINGS

Andre T, Boni C, Mounedji-Boudiaf L, et al: Oxaliplatin, fluorouracil, and leucovorin as adjuvant treatment for colon cancer, *N Engl J Med* 350:2343-2351, 2004.

Baron JA, Cole BF, Sandler RS, et al: A randomized trial of aspirin to prevent colorectal adenomas. *N Engl J Med* 348:891-899, 2003.

Cunningham D, Humblet Y, Siena S, et al: Cetuximab monotherapy and cetuximab plus irinotecan in irinotecan-refractory metastatic colon cancer. *N Engl J Med* 351:337-345, 2004.

Hurwitz H, Fehrenbacher L, Novotny W, et al: Bevacizumab plus irinotecan, fluorouracil, and leucovorin for metastatic colon cancer. *N Engl J Med* 350:2335-2342, 2004.

Mayer R: Two steps forward in the treatment of colorectal cancer. *N Engl J Med* 350:2406-2408, 2004.

Pfister D, Benson AB 3rd, Somerfield MR: Clinical practice. Surveillance strategies after curative treatment of colorectal cancer. *N Engl J Med* 350:2375-2382, 2004.

DISEASES OF THE BREAST

Tom J. Wachtel

Benign Tumors

1. Fibroadenoma.

     a. Fibroadenoma is the most common cause of a unilateral discrete mass in the 15- to 35-year age group.

       (1) Peak incidence is 20 to 25 years of age.

       (2) It is rare in elderly women.

     b. Multiple lesions are found in 10% to 15% of cases.

     c. Symptoms are painless mass, no discharge.

     d. Examination finds firm, smooth, nontender, circumscribed tumor.

     e. Mammography is usually diagnostic.

     f. Treatment is excisional biopsy.

     g. Prognosis: Not associated with breast cancer risk.

2. Intraductal papilloma.

     a. Occurs at any age.

     b. Symptom is recurrent serosanguineous nipple discharge.

     c. Examination finds no palpable lesion, but nipple discharge can be expressed.

     d. Mammography is undependable.

     e. Treatment is biopsy to exclude intraductal cancer.

     f. Prognosis: Slightly increased risk of breast cancer.

3. Simple cyst.

     a. Occurs during menstruating years, rare but occasionally is seen in postmenopausal women.

     b. Symptom is a painful lump that varies in size and pain throughout the menstrual cycle.

     c. Examination shows a circumscribed, firm, tender lesion that varies in size with serial examinations.

     d. Mammography is unreliable, but ultrasonography may be diagnostic.

     e. Treatment is observation or biopsy.

     f. Prognosis: Simple cysts are not associated with breast cancer.

4. Other benign lesions.

     a. Fat necrosis.

     b. Mammary duct ectasia.

     c. Hamartomas.

     d. Radial scars.

     e. Granular cell tumors.

     f. Cystosarcoma phyllodes (but 25% are malignant).

Fibrocystic Changes

1. Not a disease; fibrocystic changes are present in varying degrees in 90% of all women.

2. Symptoms.

     a. Dull ache in areas of most nodularity.

     b. Most severe during premenstrual phase of cycle.

3. Examination finds lumpy breasts with tender movable masses that vary over the cycle.

4. Mammography is often difficult to interpret.

5. Treatment.

     a. Close observation by patient with breast self-exams and by physician with regular physical exams (at least yearly after age 40).

     b. Yearly mammography (beginning at age 35 to 40).

c. Danazol and tamoxifen can be used for pain control.
6. Prognosis.
   a. Association with breast cancer depends on other breast cancer risk factors (e.g., family history) and on the degrees of hyperplasia and atypia on biopsy if one is done.
   b. The 40% lifetime risk of breast cancer in patients with atypical hyperplasia and a positive family history can justify consideration of prophylactic simple bilateral mastectomy with breast reconstruction.

Breast Cancer

Epidemiology

1. Lifetime cumulative incidence.
   a. One in nine women.
   b. Increasing incidence with age.
2. About 205,000 new cases per year in the United States and 40,000 annual deaths.
3. Risk factors.
   a. Age older than 50 years.
   b. Personal history of prior breast cancer.
   c. Personal history of endometrial or ovarian cancer.
   d. First-degree relative with breast cancer, especially bilateral or premenopausal.
   e. Upper socioeconomic class.
   f. Fibrocystic breast changes with atypical hyperplasia (lower risk with simple hyperplasia).
   g. Genetic phenotypes *BRCA1* or *BRCA2* increase lifetime risk to 85%.
   h. Role of postmenopausal estrogen replacement is not established but probably increases risk by 30%.
   i. About 1% of all breast cancers occur in men.

Clinical Features

1. Screening.
   a. Breast self-exam monthly.
   b. Physical exam by physician every 3 years to age 40 years and yearly thereafter.
   c. Mammography.
      (1) Baseline at age 35 years.
      (2) Every 2 years from age 40 to 50 years.
      (3) Yearly after age 50 years, with no defined upper age limit.
2. Evaluation of a breast mass.
   a. In women older than 30 years, mammography is always the first step in management.
   b. Other indications for diagnostic mammography include:
      (1) Breast pain.
      (2) Skin thickening.
      (3) Nipple retraction.
      (4) Nipple discharge.
      (5) Nipple eczema.
      (6) Axillary lymphadenopathy.

   c. For a palpable breast mass, a fine needle aspirate or a core needle biopsy should be done.

     (1) Accuracy is 90%.

     (2) If aspirate or biopsy is benign, scrupulous follow-up is advised (see screening earlier).

   d. For a nonpalpable suspicious lesion found on mammography, a sterotactic-guided fine-needle aspiration should be performed. If sterotactic needle aspiration is negative, it should be repeated or patient should undergo open biopsy.

   e. If aspirate or biopsy is positive for breast cancer, patient should undergo surgical staging.

Pathologic Findings

1. Ductal carcinoma in situ.
   a. About 20% of all cancer.
   b. About 2% risk per year of developing invasive cancer.
2. Lobular carcinoma in situ.
   a. About 2% of cancers.
   b. About 1% risk per year of developing invasive cancer.
3. Infiltrating ductal cancer is the most common invasive cancer: 65%.
4. Infiltrating lobular cancer: 5%.
5. Medullary cancer: 5%.
6. Mucinous cancer: 2%.
7. Tubular cancer: 1%.
8. Others: 2%.

Staging

1. Work-up.
   a. In situ cancers: Consider four-quadrant random biopsies to confirm in situ stage (controversial).
   b. Invasive cancer: two staging modalities.
      (1) Modified radical mastectomy with axillary dissection.
      (2) Lumpectomy with axillary node sampling.
   c. All cancers.
   d. Estrogen and progesterone receptor status of cancer must be done.
   e. Flow cytometry may be a useful prognosticator.
   f. Other.
      (1) A complete physical exam routinely.
      (2) CBC routinely.
      (3) Aspartate aminotransferase (AST) routinely.
      (4) Alkaline phosphatase routinely.
      (5) Chest x-rays routinely.
      (6) A bone scan is indicated only in patients with relevant symptoms, although some clinicians advise a baseline bone scan in all patients with confirmed invasive cancer.
2. Stage.
   a. Tumor.
      (1) T_o: No evidence of primary breast tumor.
      (2) T_{is}: Carcinoma in situ.
      (3) T_1: Tumor smaller than 2 cm in greatest dimension.
         (a) Not fixed to pectoral muscle.

    (b) Fixed to pectoral muscle.
  (4) T_2: Tumor 2 to 5 cm in greatest dimension.
    (a) Not fixed to pectoral muscle.
    (b) Fixed to pectoral muscle.
  (5) T_3: Tumor larger than 5 cm in greatest dimension.
    (a) Not fixed to pectoral muscle.
    (b) Fixed to pectoral muscle.
  (6) T_4: Tumor fixed to chest wall or involving skin.
 b. Lymph nodes.
  (1) N_0: No regional lymph nodes.
  (2) N_1: Palpable, movable, ipsilateral lymph nodes.
  (3) N_2: Palpable, fixed, ipsilateral lymph nodes.
  (4) N_3: Ipsilateral internal mammary lymph nodes.
 c. Metastases.
  (1) M_0: none.
  (2) M_1: distant metastases are present.

Treatment Guidelines

1. Ductal carcinoma in situ.
  a. Diffuse disease confirmed by four-quadrant biopsies. Simple mastectomy.
  b. Localized disease.
    (1) Simple mastectomy.
    (2) Breast-conserving surgical excision of lesion with clear microscopic margins followed by radiation.
  c. Consider tamoxifen 20 mg daily for 5 or more years.
2. Lobular carcinoma in situ: Close follow-up or bilateral simple mastectomy (usually with breast reconstruction).
3. Invasive breast cancer, early disease (stages T_1 and T_2) (currently 80% of all new breast cancers).
  a. Step 1: Definitive local treatment.
    (1) Stage T_{1a} or T_{2a}.
      (a) Preferred option is breast-conserving surgery (lumpectomy) with axillary node dissection followed by radiation.
      (b) Alternate option is modified radical mastectomy.
    (2) Stage T_{1b} or T_{2b}: Modified radical mastectomy.
  b. Step 2.
    (1) Pathologic staging.
    (2) Estrogen receptor (ER) and progesterone receptor (PgR) status.
    (3) Flow cytometry.
  c. Step 3: Adjuvant therapy.
    (1) $T_{1a} N_0$ with tumor smaller than 1 cm or too small for ER and PgR assay, one of the following:
      (a) Observation.
      (b) Tamoxifen 10 to 20 mg daily for 5 years.
      (c) Aromatase inhibitors.
        i. Anastrozole (Arimedex) 1 mg qd.
        ii. Letrozole (Femara) 2.5 mg qd.
        iii. Exemestane (Aromasin) 25 mg qd.
    (2) $T_{1a} N_0$ with ER^+ or PgR^+, one of the following:
      (a) Observation (low risk tumor by flow cytometry).

(b) Combined chemotherapy and/or tamoxifen or aromatase inhibitor (high-risk tumor by flow cytometry).

(3) T_{2a} N_0 with ER$^+$ or PgR$^+$ or T_{1a}/T_{2a} N_0 with ER$^-$ and PgR$^-$, one or both of the following:

(a) Combined chemotherapy.

(b) Tamoxifen or aromatase inhibitor.

(4) T_1 or T_2 N_1 with ER$^+$ or PgR$^+$ and premenopausal.

(a) Combined chemotherapy.

(b) Tamoxifen or aromatase inhibitor may be added.

(5) T_1 or T_2 N_1 with ER$^+$ or PgR$^+$ and postmenopausal-Rx:

(a) Tamoxifen or aromatase inhibitor.

(b) Combined chemotherapy may be added.

(6) T_1 or T_2 N_1 with ER$^-$ and PgR$^-$: Combined chemotherapy.

d. Treatment in advanced age (e.g., 85 years or older) has not been standardized.

(1) Lumpectomy followed by tamoxifen is often recommended.

(2) Radiation may be omitted.

4. Invasive advanced breast cancer.

a. Stage T_3.

(1) Preoperative debulking systemic chemotherapy followed by simple mastectomy (axillary node sampling is controversial) followed by chemotherapy.

(2) If complete tumor resection is not possible, treatment is palliative.

b. Stage T_4: Palliative treatment.

Prognosis

1. Favorable prognostic factors.

(1) Older age.

(2) Postmenopausal status.

(3) Small tumor size.

(4) Absent axillary lymph node involvement.

(5) High steroid hormone receptor content.

(6) Good tissue differentiation (by flow cytometry).

(7) Absent intratumor lymphatic invasion on pathologic examination.

(8) Absent metastases.

2. Survival statistics by lymph node involvement are shown in Table 5-31.

Gynecomastia (Breast Enlargement In Men)

1. Causes.

a. Drugs.

(1) Estrogens and gonadotropins.

Table 5-31 **Breast Cancer Survival by Lymph Node Involvement**

Lymph Node Involvement	5-year Survival	10-year Survival
None	78%	65%
<3 positive lymph nodes	62%	37%
>4 positive lymph nodes	32%	13%

      (2) Testosterone inhibitors.
        (a) Cimetidine.
        (b) Spironolactone.
        (c) Metronidazole.
        (d) Ketoconazole.
        (e) Antitumor agents.
      (3) Digitalis.
      (4) Others.
        (a) Isonicotinic acid hydrazide.
        (b) Methyldopa.
        (c) Narcotics.
        (d) Benzodiazepines.
        (e) Tricyclic antidepressants.
        (f) Penicillamine.
    b. Increased estrogen secretion.
      (1) Liver disease.
      (2) Choriocarcinoma and other hCG-producing tumors.
      (3) Adrenal cancer.
      (4) Thyrotoxicosis.
      (5) Hermaphoditism.
    c. Decreased testosterone secretion.
      (1) Castration.
      (2) Orchitis.
      (3) Renal failure.
      (4) Various congenital defects (e.g., Klinefelter's syndrome, testicular feminization).
    d. Idiopathic.

SUGGESTED READINGS

Baum M, Budzar AU, Cuzick J, et al: ATAC Trialists' Group: Anastrozole alone or in combination with tamoxifen versus tamox alone for adjuvant treatment of post-menopausal women with early breast cancer: first results of ATAC randomized trial, Lancet 359:2131-2139, 2002.

Boyd NF, Dite GS, Stone J, et al: Heritability of mammographic density, a risk factor for breast cancer, N Engl J Med 347:886-894, 2002.

Hellekson KL: NIH statement on adjuvant therapy for breast cancer. Am Fam Physician 63:1857-1858, 2001.

Hughes K, Schnaper LA, Berry D, et al: Lumpectomy plus tamoxifen with or without irradiation in women 70 years of age or older with early breast cancer. N Eng J Med 351:971-977:2004.

Humphrey LL et al: Breast cancer screening: A summary of the evidence for the U.S. Preventive Services Task Force. Ann Intern Med 137:347-360, 2002.

Marchbanks PA, McDonald JA, Wilson HG, et al: Oral contraceptives and the risk of breast cancer. N Engl J Med 346:2025-2032, 2002.

Miller AB, To T, Baines CJ, Wall C: The Canadian National Breast Screening Study-1: Breast cancer mortality after 11 to 16 years of follow-up. A randomized screening trial of mammography in women age 40 to 49 years. Ann Intern Med 137:305-312, 2002.

Pruthi S: Detection and evaluation of palpable breast mass. Mayo Clin Proc 76: 641-647, 2001.

Rebbeck TR, Lynch HT, Neuhausen SL, et al: Prophylactic oophorectomy in carriers of BRCA1 or BRCA2 mutations. N Engl J Med 346:1616-1622, 2002.

U.S. Preventive Services Task Force: Chemoprevention of breast cancer. Recommendations and rationale. Ann Intern Med 137:56-58, 2002.

ESSENTIAL THROMBOCYTOSIS

Tom J. Wachtel

1. Clinical features: Bleeding is more common than thrombotic events.
2. Laboratory findings.
   a. CBC: Platelets more than 500,000/mL.
   b. Bone marrow shows increased megakaryocytes.
3. Treatment.
   a. Palliative chemotherapy or hydroxyurea to control symptoms (e.g., bleeding). or initiated preventively when platelets are 1,000,000. This treatment does not prolong survival.
   b. Anagrelide can be used as well, but it is less effective than hydroxyurea.
4. Prognosis: Median survival time is 10 to 15 years..

SUGGESTED READINGS

Barbui T, Finazzi G: When and how to treat essential thrombocythemia. *N Eng J Med* 353:85-86, 2005.

Harrison CN, Campbell PJ, Buck G, et al: Hydroxyurea compared with Anagrelide in high risk essential thrombocythemia. *N Engl J Med* 353:33-45, 2005.

IMMUNE THROMBOCYTOPENIC PURPURA

Fred F. Ferri

Definition

Immune thrombocytopenic purpura (ITP) is an autoimmune disorder characterized by a low platelet count and leading, if severe enough, to mucocutaneous bleeding (purpura) and potential cerebral hemorrhage.

Epidemiology

1. Prevalence.
   a. Approximately 5 to 10 cases/100,000 persons.
   b. About 72% of patients are female.
2. Incidence is 100 cases/1,000,000 persons per year.
3. Presentation.
   a. Manifestation is often insidious.
   b. The patient might have a history of purpura.
   c. Many cases are diagnosed incidentally by routine laboratory tests that include platelet counts.
4. The physical examination may be entirely normal.
   a. Patients with severe thrombocytopenia can have petechiae, purpura, epistaxis, or heme-positive stool from GI bleeding.
   b. Splenomegaly is unusual. Its presence should alert to the possibility of other causes of thrombocytopenia.

Etiology

Increased platelet destruction caused by autoantibodies to platelet-membrane antigens.

Differential Diagnosis

1. Falsely low platelet count resulting from ethylenediaminetetraacetic acid (EDTA)-dependent or cold-dependent agglutinins.
2. Viral infections.

3. Drug-induced thrombocytopenia (e.g., heparin, quinidine, sulfonamides).
4. Hypersplenism resulting from liver disease.
5. Myelodysplastic and lymphoproliferative disorders.
6. Hypothyroidism.
7. SLE, TTP, hemolytic-uremic syndrome.

Work-up

1. Laboratory tests.
   a. CBC, platelet count, and peripheral smear.
      (1) Platelets are decreased in number but are normal in size or may appear larger than normal.
      (2) RBCs and WBCs have a normal morphology.
   b. Additional tests may be ordered to exclude other etiologies of the thrombocytopenia when clinically indicated.
      (1) HIV infection.
      (2) Antinuclear antibody.
      (3) TSH.
      (4) Liver enzymes.
      (5) Bone marrow examination.
   c. The direct assay for measuring platelet-bound antibodies has an estimated positive predictive value of 80%. A negative test does not rule out the diagnosis.
2. Imaging studies: CT scan of abdomen in patients with splenomegaly to exclude other disorders causing thrombocytopenia.

Treatment

Treatment varies with the platelet count and bleeding status.

1. Nonpharmacologic therapy.
   a. Measures to prevent injury (e.g., falls) or bruising.
   b. Avoid medications that increase the risk of bleeding (e.g., aspirin and NSAIDs).
   c. Observation with frequent monitoring of platelet count is needed in asymptomatic patients with platelet counts higher than 30,000/mm^3.
2. Pharmacologic therapy.
   a. Methylprednisolone 30 mg/kg/day IV infused over 20 to 30 min (maximum dose of 1 g/day for 2 or 3 days) plus IVIg (1 g/kg/day for 2 or 3 days) and infusion of platelets should be given to patients who have neurologic symptoms, have internal bleeding, or are undergoing emergency surgery.
   b. Prednisone 1 to 2 mg/kg PO qd, continued until the platelet count is normalized, then slowly tapered off, is indicated in adults with platelet counts lower than 20,000/mm^3 and those who have counts lower than 50,000/mm^3 and significant mucous membrane bleeding. Response rates range from 50% to 75%, and most responses occur within the first 3 weeks.
   c. Rituximab, a monoclonal antibody directed against the CD20 antigen, has been reported useful for ITP patients resistant to conventional treatment and can help prevent serious bleeding.
   d. A regimen of cyclophosphamide, vincristine, and prednisone (CVP) has been partially effective in chronic ITP.

3. Other therapy.
   a. Platelet transfusion is appropriate only in case of life-threatening hemorrhage.
   b. Splenectomy.
      (1) Splenectomy should be considered in patients with platelet count less than 30,000/mm³ after 6 weeks of medical treatment or after 6 months if more than 10 to 20 mg of prednisone per day is required to maintain a platelet count greater than 30,000/mm³.
      (2) Appropriate immunizations (e.g., pneumococcal vaccine) should be administered before splenectomy.
4. Monitoring of platelet count and symptom review in patients with chronic ITP are recommended to detect and prevent significant bleeding.

Prognosis

1. The course of the disease is chronic, and only 5% of patients have spontaneous remission.
2. The principal cause of death from ITP is intracranial hemorrhage (5%).

SUGGESTED READINGS

Cheng Y, Wong RS, Soo YO, et al: Initial treatment of immune thrombocytopenic purpura with high dose dexamethasone. *N Engl J Med* 349:831-836, 2003.

Cines DB, Blanchette VS: Immune thrombocytopenic purpura. *N Engl J Med* 346:995-1000, 2002.

Shanafelt TD, Madueme HL, Wolf RC, Terreri A: Rituximab for immune cytopenia in adults: Idiopathic thrombocytopenic purpura, autoimmune hemolytic anemia, and Evans syndrome. *Mayo Clin Proc* 78:1340-1346, 2003.

Zheng X, Pallera AM, Goodnough LT, et al: Remission of chronic ITP after treatment with cyclophosphamide and rituximab. *Ann Intern Med* 138:105-108, 2003.

CHRONIC LYMPHOCYTIC LEUKEMIA

Fred F. Ferri

Definition

Chronic lymphocytic leukemia (CLL) is a lymphoproliferative disorder characterized by proliferation and accumulation of mature-appearing neoplastic lymphocytes.

Epidemiology

1. Most frequent form of leukemia in Western countries (10,000 new cases/year in the United States).
2. Generally occurs in middle-aged and elderly patients (median age of 65 years).
3. Male-to-female ratio is 2:1.

Clinical Findings

1. Lymphadenopathy, splenomegaly, and hepatomegaly in the majority of patients.
2. Variable clinical presentation according to the stage of the disease.
3. Abnormal CBC: Many cases are diagnosed on the basis of laboratory results obtained after routine physical examination.
4. Some patients come to medical attention because of weakness and fatigue (secondary to anemia) or lymphadenopathy.

Etiology

Unknown.

Differential Diagnosis

1. Hairy cell leukemia.
2. Adult T cell lymphoma.
3. Prolymphocytic leukemia.
4. Viral infections.
5. Waldenström's macroglobulinemia.

Work-up

1. Laboratory tests.
   a. Proliferative lymphocytosis (≥15,000/dL) of well-differentiated lymphocytes is the hallmark of CLL.
   b. Hypogammaglobulinemia and elevated LDH may be present at the time of diagnosis.
   c. Anemia or thrombocytopenia, if present, indicates poor prognosis.
   d. Bone marrow aspirate.
      (1) There is monotonous replacement of the bone marrow by small lymphocytes.
      (2) Marrow contains at least 30% well-differentiated lymphocytes.
   e. Chromosome analysis.
      (1) Trisomy-12 is the most common chromosomal abnormality, followed by 14Q+, 13 q, and 11 q.
      (2) These all indicate a poor prognosis.
   f. New laboratory techniques (CD 38, fluorescence in situ hybridization) can identify patients with early-stage CLL at higher risk of rapid disease progression.
2. Staging protocols.
   a. Rai and colleagues divided CLL into five clinical stages.
      (1) Stage 0.
         (a) Characterized by lymphocytosis only (≥15,000/mm^3 on peripheral smear, bone marrow aspirate ≥40% lymphocytes).
         (b) The coexistence of lymphocytosis and other factors increases the clinical stage.
      (2) Stage 1: Lymphadenopathy.
      (3) Stage 2: Lymphadenopathy/hepatomegaly.
      (4) Stage 3: Anemia (Hb <11 g/mm^3).
      (5) Stage 4:Thrombocytopenia (platelets <100,000/mm^3).
   b. Another well-known staging system developed by Binet divides chronic lymphocytic leukemia into three stages.
      (1) Stage A.
         (a) Hb at least 10g/dL.
         (b) Platelets at least 100,000/mm^3.
         (c) Fewer than three areas involved.
            i. The cervical, axillary, and inguinal lymph nodes, either unilaterally or bilaterally.
            ii. The spleen.
            iii. The liver.
      (2) Stage B.
         (a) Hb at least 10 g/dL.

    (b) Platelets at least 100,000/mm^3.
    (c) Three or more areas involved.
  (3) Stage C.
    (a) Hb less than 10 g/dL.
    (b) Low platelets (<100,000/mm^3).
    (c) Both Hb and low platelets independent of the areas involved.

Treatment

1. Treatment goals are relief of symptoms and prolongation of life.
2. Observation is appropriate for patients in Rai stage 0 or Binet stage A.
3. Symptomatic patients in Rai stages I and II or Binet stage B.
   a. Chlorambucil.
   b. Local irradiation for isolated symptomatic lymphadenopathy and lymph nodes that interfere with vital organs.
4. Fludarabine.
   a. Fludarabine is an effective treatment for CLL that does not respond to initial treatment with chlorambucil.
   b. Recent reports indicate that when used as the initial treatment for CLL, fludarabine yields higher response rates and a longer duration of remission and progression-free survival than chlorambucil.
   c. Overall survival, however, is not enhanced.
5. Rai stages III and IV, Binet stage C.
   a. Chlorambucil chemotherapy with or without prednisone.
   b. Fludarabine, CAP (cyclophosphamide, Adriamycin, prednisone), or cyclophosphamide, doxorubicin, vincristine, and prednisone (mini-CHOP) can be used in patients who respond poorly to chlorambucil.
   c. Splenic irradiation can be used in selected patients with advanced disease.
6. Treatment of complications.
   a. Hypogammaglobulinemia.
      (1) Hypogammaglobulinemia is common in CLL and is the chief cause of infections.
      (2) Immune globulin (250 mg/kg IV every 4 weeks) can prevent infections but has no effect on survival.
      (3) Infections should be treated with broad-spectrum antibiotics.
      (4) Patients should be monitored for opportunistic infections.
   b. Recombinant hematopoietic cofactors (e.g., granulocyte-macrophage colony-stimulating factor and granulocyte colony-stimulating factor) may be used to control neutropenia related to treatment.
   c. Erythropoietin may be useful to treat anemia that is unresponsive to other measures.

Prognosis

1. The patient's prognosis is directly related to the clinical stage (e.g., the average survival in patients in Rai stage 0 or Binet stage A is >120 months; for RAI stage 4 or Binet stage C, survival is approximately 30 months).
2. Overall 5-year survival is 60%.

SUGGESTED READING

Shanafelt TD, Call TG: Current approach to diagnosis and management of chronic lymphocytic leukemia. *Mayo Clin Proc* 79:388-398, 2004.

LUNG CANCER

Fred F. Ferri and Tom J. Wachtel

Definition

A primary lung neoplasm is a malignancy arising from lung tissue. The World Health Organization distinguishes 12 types of pulmonary neoplasms. Among them, the major types are squamous cell carcinoma, adenocarcinoma, small cell carcinoma, and large cell carcinoma. However, the crucial difference in the diagnosis of lung cancer is between small cell and non–small cell types, because the therapeutic approach is different.

Selected characteristics of lung carcinomas:

1. Adenocarcinoma.
   a. Represents 35% of lung carcinomas.
   b. Commonly located in midlung and periphery.
   c. Initial metastases are to lymphatics.
   d. Commonly associated with peripheral scars.
2. Squamous cell (epidermoid).
   a. Represents 20% to 30% of lung cancers.
   b. Central location.
   c. Metastasis by local invasion.
   d. Frequent cavitation and obstructive phenomena.
3. Small cell (oat cell).
   a. Represents 20% of lung carcinomas.
   b. Central location.
   c. Metastasis through lymphatics.
   d. Associated with lesion of the short arm of chromosome 3.
   e. High cavitation rate.
4. Large cell.
   a. Represents 15% to 20% of lung carcinomas.
   b. Commonly located in the periphery.
   c. Metastasis to central nervous system (CNS) and mediastinum.
   d. Rapid growth rate with early metastasis.
5. Bronchoalveolar.
   a. Represents 5% of lung carcinomas.
   b. Commonly located in the periphery.
   c. May be bilateral.
   d. Initial metastasis through lymphatic, hematogenous, and local invasion.
   e. No correlation with cigarette smoking.
   f. Cavitation rate.

Epidemiology

1. Lung cancer is responsible for more than 30% of cancer deaths in men and more than 25% of cancer deaths in women.
2. Tobacco smoking is implicated in 85% of cases.
3. There are more than 180,000 new cases of lung cancer yearly in the United States, most occurring in persons older than 50 years.

Clinical Findings

1. Weight loss, fatigue, fever, anorexia, dysphagia.
2. Cough, hemoptysis, dyspnea, wheezing.
3. Chest, shoulder, and bone pain.

4. Paraneoplastic syndromes.
    a. Eaton-Lambert syndrome: Myopathy involving proximal muscle groups.
    b. Endocrine manifestations.
        (1) Hypercalcemia.
        (2) Ectopic ACTH.
        (3) Syndrome of inappropriate antidiuretic hormone (SIADH)
    c. Neurologic.
        (1) Subacute cerebellar degeneration.
        (2) Peripheral neuropathy.
        (3) Cortical degeneration.
    d. Musculoskeletal.
        (1) Polymyositis.
        (2) Clubbing.
        (3) Hypertrophic pulmonary osteoarthropathy.
    e. Hematologic or vascular.
        (1) Migratory thrombophlebitis.
        (2) Marantic thrombosis.
        (3) Anemia.
        (4) Thrombocytosis.
        (5) Thrombocytopenia.
    f. Cutaneous.
        (1) Acanthosis nigricans.
        (2) Dermatomyositis.
5. Pleural effusion (10% of patients), recurrent pneumonias (secondary to obstruction), localized wheezing.
6. Superior vena cava syndrome.
    a. Obstruction of venous return of the superior vena cava is most commonly caused by bronchogenic carcinoma or metastasis to paratracheal nodes.
    b. The patient usually complains of headache, nausea, dizziness, visual changes, syncope, and respiratory distress.
    c. Physical examination reveals distention of thoracic and neck veins, edema of face and upper extremities, facial plethora, and cyanosis.
7. Horner's syndrome.
    a. Constricted pupil, ptosis, facial anhidrosis caused by spinal cord damage between C8 and T1 secondary to a superior sulcus tumor (bronchogenic carcinoma of the extreme lung apex).
    b. A superior sulcus tumor associated with ipsilateral Horner's syndrome and shoulder pain is known as Pancoast's tumor.

Etiology

1. Tobacco abuse.
2. Environmental agents (e.g., radon).
3. Industrial agents (e.g., ionizing radiation, asbestos, nickel, uranium, vinyl chloride, chromium, arsenic, coal dust).

Differential Diagnosis

1. Pneumonia.
2. Tuberculosis (TB).
3. Metastatic carcinoma to the lung.

  4. Lung abscess.
  5. Granulomatous disease.
  6. Carcinoid tumor.
  7. Mycobacterial and fungal diseases.
  8. Sarcoidosis.
  9. Viral pneumonitis.
  10. Benign lesions that simulate thoracic malignancy.
      a. Lobar atelectasis.
         (1) Pneumonia.
         (2) TB.
         (3) Chronic inflammatory disease.
         (4) Allergic bronchopulmonary aspergillosis.
      b. Multiple pulmonary nodules.
         (1) Septic emboli.
         (2) Wegener's granulomatosis.
         (3) Sarcoidosis.
         (4) Rheumatoid nodules.
         (5) Fungal disease.
         (6) Multiple pulmonary arteriovenous fistulas.
      c. Mediastinal adenopathy.
         (1) Sarcoidosis.
         (2) Lymphoma.
         (3) Primary TB.
         (4) Fungal disease.
         (5) Silicosis.
         (6) Pneumoconiosis.
         (7) Drug-induced (e.g., phenytoin, trimethadione).
      d. Pleural effusion.
         (1) CHF.
         (2) Pneumonia with parapneumonic effusion.
         (3) TB.
         (4) Viral pneumonitis.
         (5) Ascites.
         (6) Pancreatitis.
         (7) Collagen-vascular disease.

Work-up

Work-up generally includes chest x-ray, CT scan of chest, positron emission tomography (PET) scan, and tissue biopsy.
  1. Imaging studies.
     a. Chest x-ray.
        (1) The radiographic presentation often varies with the cell type.
        (2) Pleural effusion, lobar atelectasis, and mediastinal adenopathy can accompany any cell types.
     b. CT scan of the chest to evaluate mediastinal and pleural extension of suspected lung neoplasms.
     c. PET with ^{18}F-fluorodeoxyglucose (18 FDG-PET), a metabolic marker of malignant tissue, is superior to CT scan in detecting mediastinal and distant metastases in non–small cell lung cancer. It is useful for preoperative staging of non–small cell lung cancer.

2. Biopsy modalities for tissue diagnosis.
   a. Biopsy of any suspicious lymph nodes (e.g., supraclavicular node).
   b. Flexible fiberoptic bronchoscopy: Brush and biopsy specimens are obtained from any visualized endobronchial lesions.
   c. Transbronchial needle aspiration.
      (1) Done via a special needle passed through the bronchoscope.
      (2) This technique is useful to sample mediastinal masses or paratracheal lymph nodes.
   d. Transthoracic fine-needle aspiration biopsy with fluoroscopic or CT scan guidance to evaluate peripheral pulmonary nodules.
   e. Mediastinoscopy and anteromedial sternotomy in suspected tumor involvement of the mediastinum.
   f. Pleural biopsy in patients with pleural effusion.
   g. Thoracentesis of pleural effusion and cytologic evaluation of the obtained fluid can confirm diagnosis.

Staging

1. The international staging system is the most widely accepted staging system for non–small cell lung cancer.
   a. In this system, stage 1 (N0 [no lymph node involvement]) and stage 2 (N1 [spread to ipsilateral bronchopulmonary or hilar lymph nodes]) include localized tumors for which surgical resection is the preferred treatment.
   b. Stage 3 is subdivided into 3A (potentially resectable) and 3B. The surgical management of stage 3A disease (N2 [involvement of ipsilateral mediastinal nodes]) is controversial. Only 20% of N2 disease is considered minimal disease (involvement of only one node) and technically resectable.
   c. Stage 4 indicates metastatic disease.
2. In patients with small cell lung cancer, a more practical accepted staging system is the one developed by the Veterans Administration Lung Cancer Study Group (VALG). This system contains two stages.
   a. Limited stage: Disease confined to the regional lymph nodes and to one hemithorax (excluding pleural surfaces).
   b. Extensive stage: Disease spread beyond the confines of limited-stage disease.

Treatment
Non–Small Cell Carcinoma

1. Surgery.
   a. Indications.
      (1) Surgical resection is indicated in patients with limited disease (not involving mediastinal nodes, ribs, pleura, or distant sites). This represents approximately 15% to 30% of diagnosed cases.
      (2) Mediastinoscopy or anterior mediastinotomy in patients being considered for possible curative lung resection may be appropriate.
      (3) A Dutch trial revealed a 51% relative reduction in futile thoracotomies for patients with suspected non–small cell lung cancer who underwent preoperative assessment with PET with the tracer 18 FDG-PET in addition to conventional work-up.

(4) Biopsy of any accessible suspect lesions may also be needed.
b. Preoperative evaluation.
  (1) Includes review of cardiac status (e.g., recent myocardial infarction, major arrhythmias).
  (2) Laboratory evaluation.
    (a) CBC, electrolytes, platelets.
    (b) Calcium, phosphorus.
    (c) Glucose.
    (d) Renal and liver function studies.
    (e) Arterial blood gases.
    (f) Skin tests for TB.
    (g) Evaluation of pulmonary function (to determine if the patient can tolerate any loss of lung tissue).
  (3) Pneumonectomy is possible if the patient has a preoperative FEV_1 at least 2L or if the maximum voluntary ventilation is more than 50% of predicted capacity.
c. Preoperative chemotherapy should be considered in patients with more advanced disease (stage 3A) who are being considered for surgery, because it increases the median survival time in patients with non–small cell lung cancer compared with the use of surgery alone.

2. Radiation.
  a. Radiation therapy can be used alone or in combination with chemotherapy.
  b. It is used primarily for treatment of CNS and skeletal metastases, superior vena cava syndrome, and obstructive atelectasis.
  c. Although thoracic radiation therapy is generally considered standard therapy for stage 3 disease, it has limited effect on survival.
  d. Palliative radiation therapy should be delayed until symptoms occur because immediate therapy offers no advantage over delayed therapy and results in more adverse events from the radiation therapy.

3. Chemotherapy.
  a. Various combination regimens are available. Current drugs of choice include:
    (1) Paclitaxel plus either carboplatin or cisplatin.
    (2) Cisplatin plus vinorelbine.
    (3) Gemcitabine plus cisplatin.
    (4) Carboplatin or cisplatin plus docetaxel.
  b. The overall results are disappointing, and none of the standard regimens for non–small cell lung cancer is clearly superior to the others.
  c. Gefitinib (Iressa), an inhibitor of EGFR tyrosine kinase, is an oral preparation currently undergoing clinical trials for advanced non–small cell lung cancer.

4. Addition of chemotherapy to radiation therapy.
  a. Chemotherapy added to radiation therapy improves survival in patients with locally advanced, unresectable non–small cell lung cancer.
  b. The absolute benefit is relatively small, however, and should be balanced against the increased toxicity associated with the addition of chemotherapy.

Small Cell Lung Cancer

Staging work-up.

1. CT scan of liver and brain.
2. Radionuclide scans of bone in all patients with small cell carcinoma of the lung and patients with non–small cell lung neoplasms suspected of involving these organs.
3. Bone marrow aspiration and biopsy only in selected patients with small cell carcinoma of the lung. In the absence of an increased LDH or cytopenia, routine bone marrow examination is not recommended.
   a. Limited stage disease: Standard treatments include thoracic radiation therapy and chemotherapy (cisplatin and etoposide).
   b. Extensive stage disease: Standard treatments include combination chemotherapy (cisplatin or carboplatin plus etoposide or combination of irinotecan and cisplatin).
   c. Prophylactic cranial irradiation for patients in complete remission to decrease the risk of CNS metastasis.

Prognosis

1. The 5-year survival of patients with non–small cell carcinoma when the disease is resectable is approximately 30%.
2. Median survival time in patients with limited stage disease and small cell lung cancer is 15 months; in patients with extensive stage disease, it is 9 months.

SUGGESTED READINGS

Kris MG, Herbst RS, Lynch TJ Jr, et al: Efficacy of gefitinib, an inhibitor of the epidermal growth factor receptor tyrosine kinase, in symptomatic patients with non–small cell lung cancer. *JAMA* 290:2149-2158, 2003.

Lardinois D et al: Staging of non–small cell lung cancer with integrated positron-emission tomography and computed tomography. *N Engl J Med* 348:2500-2507, 2003.

Schiller JH, Harrington D, Belani CP, et al: Comparison of four chemotherapy regimens for advanced non–small cell lung cancer. *N Engl J Med* 346:92-98, 2002.

Spira A, Ettinger DS: Multidisciplinary management of lung cancer. *N Engl J Med* 350:379-392, 2004.

HODGKIN'S DISEASE

Fred F. Ferri and Tom J. Wachtel

Definition

Hodgkin's disease is a malignant disorder of lymphoreticular origin. It is characterized histologically by the presence of multinucleated giant cells (Reed–Sternberg cells) usually originating from B lymphocytes in germinal centers of lymphoid tissue.

Epidemiology

1. There is a bimodal age distribution (15 to 34 years and older than 50 years).
2. Overall incidence of Hodgkin's disease in the United States is approximately 4:100,000.

Clinical Findings

1. Lymphadenopathy.
2. Splenomegaly (40%), hepatomegaly (10%).

3. Respiratory symptoms (cough, dyspnea).
4. Pleural effusion.
5. B symptoms: Fever, night sweats, weight loss.
6. Pruritus (not a B symptom).

Work-up

1. Lymph node biopsy (frequency of histologic type).
   a. Lymphocytic predominance (10%) has an excellent prognosis.
   b. Nodular sclerosis (55%) has an excellent prognosis.
   c. Mixed cellularity (30%) is associated with abundant Reed-Sternberg cells and has a good prognosis.
   d. Lymphocytic depletion (5%) is associated with abundant Reed-Sternberg cells and has a poor prognosis.
2. Staging.
   a. Laboratory evaluation.
      (1) CBC.
      (2) Sedimentation rate.
      (3) BUN.
      (4) Creatinine.
      (5) Alkaline phosphatase.
      (6) ALT.
      (7) Calcium.
      (8) Albumin.
      (9) LDH.
      (10) Uric acid.
   b. Chest x-ray study followed by chest CT scan if chest x-ray film is suspicious.
   c. Abdominal CT scan.
   d. Bone marrow examination.
   e. Lymphangiography.
   f. Staging laparotomy and splenectomy unless the disease is obviously advanced. Give pneumonia vaccine (Pneumovax) before surgery.

Ann Arbor Staging Classification

1. Stage I: Involvement of a single lymph node region.
2. Stage II: Two or more lymph node regions on the same side of the diaphragm.
3. Stage III: Lymph node involvement on both sides of diaphragm, including spleen.
4. Stage IV: Diffuse involvement of extranodal sites.
5. Suffix A: No systemic symptoms.
6. Suffix B: Presence of fever, night sweats, or unexplained weight loss of 10% (body weight) or more over 6 months.
7. Suffix X Indicates bulky disease: Greater than one third widening of mediastinum or greater than 10 cm maximum dimension of nodal mass on a chest film.

Treatment

1. Stage I and II.
   a. Radiation therapy alone unless a large mediastinal mass is present (mediastinal to thoracic ratio ≥1.3).

b. In the latter case, a combination of chemotherapy and radiation therapy is indicated.

2. Stage IB or IIB: Total nodal irradiation is often used, although chemotherapy is performed in many centers.

3. Stage IIIA: Treatment is controversial. It varies with the anatomic substage after splenectomy.

   a. III_1A and minimal splenic involvement: Radiation therapy alone may be adequate.

   b. III_2 or III_1A with extensive splenic involvement: There is a disagreement whether chemotherapy alone or a combination of chemotherapy and radiation therapy is the preferred treatment modality.

   c. IIIB and IV: The treatment of choice is chemotherapy with or without adjuvant radiation therapy.

4. Various regimens can be used for combination chemotherapy. Most oncologists prefer the combination of doxorubicin plus bleomycin plus vincristine plus dacarbazine (ABVD). Other commonly used regimens are mechlorethamine, oncovin, procarbazine, prednisone (MOPP), MOPP-ABV, MOPP-ABVD, MOPP-BAP (bleomycin, doxorubicin, and procarbazine).

5. In patients with advanced Hodgkin's disease, increased-dose bleomycin, etoposide, doxorubicin, cyclophosphamide, vincristine, procarbazine, and prednisone (BEACOPP) offers better tumor control and overall survival than COPP-ABVD.

Prognosis

1. The overall survival at 10 years is approximately 60%.

2. Cure rates as high as 75% to 80% are now possible with appropriate initial therapy.

3. Poor prognostic features.

   a. Presence of B symptoms.

   b. Advanced age.

   c. Advanced stage at initial presentation.

   d. Mixed cellularity.

   e. Lymphocyte depletion histology.

4. Chemotherapy significantly increases the risk of leukemia.

5. The peak in risk of leukemia is seen approximately 5 years after the initiation of chemotherapy.

6. Mediastinal irradiation increases the risk of subsequent death from heart disease caused by coronary artery sclerosis secondary to irradiation.

7. Both chemotherapy and radiation therapy increase the risk of developing secondary, solid tumors.

SUGGESTED READINGS

Aleman BM, Raemaekers JM, Tirelli U, et al: Involved-field radiotherapy for advanced Hodgkin's lymphoma. *N Eng J Med* 348:2396-2406, 2003.

Ansell SM, Armitage JO: Management of Hodgkin lymphoma. *Mayo Clin Proc* 81:419-426, 2006.

Diehl V, Franklin J, Pfreundschuh M, et al: German Hodgkin's Lymphoma Study Group: Standard and increased-dose BEACOPP chemotherapy compared with COPP-ABVD for advanced Hodgkin's disease. *N Engl J Med* 348:2386-2395, 2003.

NON-HODGKIN'S LYMPHOMA
Fred F. Ferri and Tom J. Wachtel

Definition
Non-Hodgkin's lymphoma (NHL) is a heterogeneous group of malignancies of the lymphoreticular system.

Epidemiology
1. Median age at time of diagnosis: 50 years.
2. Sixth most common neoplasm in the United States.
3. Incidence increases with age.

Clinical Features
1. Lymphadenopathy.
2. Anemia.
3. B symptoms less common than in Hodgkin's.
4. GI symptoms if the site is involved.
5. Hepatomegaly and/or splenomegaly.

Work-up
1. Lymph node biopsy and histologic classification of NHL.
   a. Low grade has a favorable prognosis.
      (1) Small cell lymphocytic.
      (2) Follicular, small cleaved cell.
      (3) Follicular, mixed small cleaved cell and large cell.
   b. Intermediate grade has an unfavorable prognosis.
      (1) Follicular, large cell.
      (2) Diffuse, small cleaved cell.
      (3) Diffuse, large cell.
   c. High grade has an unfavorable prognosis.
      (1) Large cell immunoblastic.
      (2) Lymphoblastic.
      (3) Small noncleaved cell (Burkitt's lymphoma).
2. The 2001 World Health Organization (WHO) Classification is based on a combination of immunologic, genetic, and clinical characteristics.
3. Laboratory tests and staging are the same as for Hodgkin's disease except that lymphangiography and laparotomy are not necessary.

Treatment
1. Low-grade NHL (e.g., follicular cleaved cell, small cell).
   a. Local radiation therapy for symptomatic adenopathy.
   b. Deferment of therapy and observation in asymptomatic patients.
   c. Single-agent chemotherapy with cyclophosphamide or chlorambucil and glucocorticoids.
   d. Combination chemotherapy alone or with radiation therapy.
      (1) Combination chemotherapy is generally indicated only when the lymphoma becomes more invasive, with poor response to less aggressive treatment.
      (2) Commonly used regimens.
         (a) CVP (cyclophosphamide, vincristine, prednisone).
         (b) CHOP (cyclophosphamide, doxorubicin, vincristine, prednisone).
         (c) CHOP-Bleo (bleomycin).

(d) COPP (cyclophosphamide, oncovin, procarbazine, prednisone.
(e) BACOP (bleomycin, epidoxorubicin, cyclophosphamide, vincristine, and prednisone).
(3) Combination regimens.
  (a) Pro-MACE-CytaBOM (prednisone, methotrexate, doxorubicin, cyclophosphamide, etoposide, cytarabine, bleomycin, vincristine).
  (b) MACOP-B (methotrexate, doxorubicin, cyclophosphamide, vincristine, prednisone, bleomycin).
  (c) M-BACOD (methotrexate, bleomycin, doxorubicin, cyclophosphamide, vincristine, dexamethasone).
(4) Addition of recombinant IFN-α at low doses to chemotherapy prolongs remission duration in patients with low-grade NHL.
  e. Monoclonal antibodies.
  (1) Monoclonal antibodies directed against B-cell surface antigens can also be used to treat follicular lymphomas that are resistant to conventional therapy.
  (2) The anti-CD20 monoclonal antibody rituximab is a targeted, minimally toxic treatment effective against low-grade NHL in patients who have not received previous treatment.
  (3) The addition of rituximab to CHOP is generally well tolerated; however, additional studies are necessary to clarify the role of CHOP plus rituximab in patients with indolent NHL.
  (4) Ibritumomab tiuxetan (Zevalin), an immunoconjugate that combines the linker-chelator tiuxetan with the monoclonal antibody ibritumomab, can be used as part of a two-step regimen for treatment of patients with relapsed or refractory low-grade, follicular, or transformed B-cell NHL refractory to rituximab.
  f. New purine analogues (FLAMP, 2CDA) can be used in salvage treatment of refractory lymphomas. They all have activity against follicular lymphomas.
2. Intermediate and high-grade lymphomas (e.g. diffuse histiocytic lymphoma).
  a. Combination chemotherapy regimens (e.g., CHOP, Pro-MACE-CytaBOM, MACOP-B, M-BACOD): An anthracycline-containing regimen (such as CHOP) given in standard doses and schedule is generally the best for treatment of older patients with advanced-stage, aggressive-histology lymphoma who do not have significant comorbid illness.
  b. High-dose sequential therapy is superior to standard-dose MACOP-B for patients with diffuse large-cell lymphoma of the B-cell type. Three cycles of CHOP followed by involved-field radiation therapy may be superior to eight cycles of CHOP alone in patients with localized intermediate- and high-grade NHL.
  c. Monoclonal antibodies.
  (1) The addition of rituximab against CD20 B-cell lymphoma to the CHOP regimen increases the complete response rate and prolongs event-free and overall survival in elderly patients with diffuse large B-cell lymphoma without a clinically significant increase in toxicity.
  (2) Bexxar, a combination of the mononuclear antibody tositumomab and radiolabled ^{131}I tositumomab, can be used for a single treatment

of relapsed follicular NHL in patients who are refractory to rituximab. It results in complete remission in 25% of patients and clinical response in 60% of patients.

d. Granulocyte colony-stimulating factor (G-CSF) may be effective in reducing the risk of infection in patients who have aggressive lymphoma and are undergoing chemotherapy.

e. Treatment with high-dose chemotherapy and autologous bone marrow transplant, compared with conventional chemotherapy, increases event-free and overall survival in patients with chemotherapy-sensitive NHL in relapse.

Prognosis

1. Patients with low-grade lymphoma, despite their long-term survival (6 to 10 years on average), are rarely cured, and the great majority eventually die of the lymphoma. Patients with a high-grade lymphoma can achieve a cure with aggressive chemotherapy.

2. Complete remission occurs in 35% to 50% of patients with intermediate- and high-grade lymphoma. Prognostic factors include the histologic subtype, age of the patient, and bulk of the disease.

SUGGESTED READINGS

Armitage JO, Bierman PJ, Bociek RG, Jose JM: Lymphoma 2006: Classification and treatment. Oncology 20:232-239, 2006.
Landgren O, Porwit MacDonald A, Tani E, et al: A prospective comparison of fine-needle aspiration cytology and histopathology on the diagnosis and classification of lymphomas. Hematol J 5:69-70, 2004.

MULTIPLE MYELOMA

Fred F. Ferri and Tom J. Wachtel

Definition

Multiple myeloma is a malignancy of plasma cells characterized by overproduction of intact monoclonal immunoglobulin or free monoclonal κ or λ chains.

Epidemiology

Annual incidence: 4 cases/100,000 persons.
Ethnic prevalence: Blacks affected twice as frequently as whites.
Multiple myeloma accounts for 10% of all hematologic cancers.
Peak incidence is in the seventh decade at a median age of 69 years.

Clinical Features

1. Bone pain (two thirds of patients).
2. Symptoms of anemia.
3. Renal failure.
4. Hypercalcemia (can cause delirium).
5. Cord or root compression.
6. Infection (especially pneumococcal pneumonia).

Laboratory Findings

1. CBC: Anemia.
2. Elevated ESR.

3. Serum protein electrophoresis.
   a. Monoclonal protein higher than 3 g/dL in 90%.
   b. Hypogammaglobulinemia in 10%.
4. Serum immunoelectrophoresis.
   a. Monoclonal proteins.
   b. IgG (50%).
   c. IgA (20%).
   d. Light chain (17%).
   e. IgD (2%).
5. Urinary electrophoresis shows a globulin peak in 80%.
6. Almost all (99%) patients with multiple myeloma have a monoclonal protein in serum or urine.
7. Serum creatinine, calcium, uric acid levels may be elevated.
8. Alkaline phosphatase level may be normal.
9. Bone x-ray films may show osteoporosis, lytic lesion, or fractures (75% have findings at presentation).
10. Bone scan may be normal.
11. Bone marrow examination reveals at least 10% plasma cells, often more than 20% in sheets.

Differential Diagnosis

1. Bone pain, anemia, renal failure, bone marrow plasmacytosis (>10%), and a greater than 3 g/dL monoclonal serum protein level indicates multiple myeloma.
2. Plasmacytoma.
3. Lymphomas.
4. Waldenström's macroglobulinemia.
5. Heavy-chain diseases.
6. Amyloidosis.
7. Benign monoclonal gammopathies.

Treatment

1. Prevention of renal failure with adequate hydration and avoidance of nephrotoxic agents and dye contrast studies.
2. Patients with a new diagnosis and with good performance status are best treated with autologous stem cell transplantation, resulting in improved survival.
   a. Patients potentially eligible for transplantation should be referred for assessment early after diagnosis and should not be extensively exposed to alkylating agents before collection of stem cells.
   b. Autologous peripheral stem cells should be harvested early in the patient's treatment course (best when performed as part of initial therapy).
   c. A single transplant with high-dose melphalan, with or without total body irradiation, is suggested for patients undergoing transplantation outside a clinical trial.
3. Chemotherapeutic agents effective in multiple myeloma.
   a. Melphalan and prednisone.
      (1) The rates of response to this treatment range from 40% to 60%.
      (2) Adding continuous low-dose interferon (IFN) to standard melphalan-prednisone therapy does not improve response rate or survival.

        (3) Response duration and plateau phase duration are prolonged by maintenance therapy with interferon.

    b. Vincristine, doxorubicin (Adriamycin), and dexamethasone (VAD) can be used in patients not responding or relapsing after treatment with melphalan and prednisone.

    c. High-dose chemotherapy with vincristine, melphalan, cyclophosphamide, and prednisone (VMCP) alternating with vincristine, carmustine, doxorubicin, and prednisone (BVAP) combined with bone marrow transplantation improves the response rate, event-free survival, and overall survival in patients with myeloma (complete response in 25%).

4. Thalidomide, an agent with antiangiogenic properties, is useful to induce responses in patients with multiple myeloma refractory to chemotherapy.

5. Bortezomib (Velcade) is a newer protease inhibitor that is cytotoxic for multiple myeloma. It is indicated for treatment of refractory multiple myeloma.

6. Promptly diagnose and treat infections.

    a. Common bacterial agents are *Streptococcus pneumoniae* and *Haemophilus influenzae*.

    b. Prophylactic therapy against *Pneumocystis jiroveci* with trimethoprim-sulfamethoxazole must be considered in patients receiving chemotherapy and high-dose corticosteroid regimens.

7. Control hypercalcemia and hyperuricemia.

8. Control pain with analgesics.

9. Radiation therapy and surgical stabilization may also be indicated.

10. Treat anemia with epoetin alfa.

11. Skeletal complications.

    a. Monthly infusions of the bisphosphonate pamidronate (Aredia) provide significant protection against skeletal complications and improve the quality of life of patients with advanced multiple myeloma.

    b. Zoledronic acid (Zometa) can be infused over 15 minutes and is more effective than pamidronate for treatment of hypercalcemia of malignancy.

    c. Bisphosphonates (pamidronate, zoledronate, and ibandronate) also appear to have an antitumor effect.

Prognosis

1. Stage I: Median survival is 5 years (Hb >10 g/dL or IgG <5 g/dL or IgA <3g/dL or urinary M spike <4g/24 h; normal calcium; few lytic lesions).

2. Stage II (between stages I and III): Median survival is 4 years.

3. Stage IIIA: Median survival is 3 years (Hb <8.5 g/dL or IgG >7g/dL or IgA >5g/dL or calcium >12 mg/dL or urinary M spike >12 g/24 h; advanced lytic lesion and creatinine <2 mg/dL).

4. Stage IIIB: Median survival is 1 year (same as IIIA except creatinine >2 mg/dL).

5. β_2 Microglobulin at least 2.5 mg/L improves prognosis.

6. Prognosis is better in asymptomatic patients with indolent or smoldering myeloma. Median survival time is approximately 10 years in patients with no lytic bone lesions and a serum myeloma protein concentration less than 3 g/dL.

SUGGESTED READINGS

Attal M, Harousseau JL, Facon T, et al: Groupe Francophone du Myelome: Single versus double autologous stem-cell transplantation for multiple myeloma. *N Engl J Med* 349:2495-2502, 2003.

Imrie K, Esmail R, Meyer RM: Members of the Hematology Disease Site Group of the Cancer Care Ontario Practice Guidelines Initiative: The role of high-dose chemotherapy and stem-cell transplantation in patients with multiple myeloma: A practice guideline of the Cancer Care Ontario Practice Guidelines Initiative. *Ann Intern Med* 136:619-629, 2002.

Rajkumar SV, Gertz MA, Kyle RA, et al: Current therapy for multiple myeloma. *Mayo Clin Proc* 77:813-822, 2002.

Rajkumar SV, Kyle RA: Multiple myeloma: Diagnosis and treatment. *Mayo Clin Proc* 80(10):1371-1382, 2005.

POLYCYTHEMIA VERA

Tom J. Wachtel

Definition

Polycythemia vera is a chronic myeloproliferative disorder characterized by erythrocytosis.

Epidemiology

1. Incidence: 0.5 cases/100,000 persons.
2. Mean age at onset: 60 years.
3. Predominant sex: More common in men.

Clinical Features

1. Asymptomatic.
2. Bruising, bleeding.
3. Headaches.
4. Pruritus.
5. Splenomegaly.

Work-up

1. CBC.
   a. Hct greater than 55%.
   b. Hb greater than 18 g/dL.
   c. Leukocytosis (not seen in secondary polycythemia).
   d. Thrombocytosis (not seen in secondary polycythemia).
2. Bone marrow: Trilinear hyperplasia (not seen in secondary polycythemia).
3. Red cell mass measurement increased.

Differential Diagnosis

1. Relative polycythemia (normal red cell mass, reduced plasma volume).
2. Secondary polycythemia (elevated red cell mass) seen in:
   a. Chronic hypoxemia.
   b. Elevated carboxyhemoglobin level.
   c. Hemoglobinopathy with high oxygen-affinity Hb.
   d. Renal disease (malignant or benign).
   e. Hepatic, ovarian, adrenal, and cerebellar neoplasms.

Treatment

Palliative reduction of Hct.
1. Phlebotomy.

2. Interferon-α-2b.
3. Chemotherapy (hydroxyurea).
4. Chlorambucil is effective at reducing red cell mass but it has leukemogenic potential.

Prognosis
Median survival time is 10 to 15 years.

PROSTATE CANCER
Fred F. Ferri and Tom J. Wachtel

Definition
Prostate cancer is a neoplasm (adenocarcinoma) involving the prostate gland.

Epidemiology
1. Prostate cancer has surpassed lung cancer as the most common cancer in men.
2. More than 100,000 cases are diagnosed yearly and nearly 30,000 men die from prostate cancer each year (second leading cause of death from cancer in U.S. men).
3. Incidence of prostate cancer increases with age. It is uncommon in men younger than 50 years; 80% of new cases are diagnosed in patients 65 years or older.
4. Average age at time of diagnosis is 72 years.
5. Blacks in the United States have the highest incidence of prostate cancer in the world (1 in every 9 male African Americans).
6. Incidence is low in Asians.
7. Approximately 9% of all prostate cancers may be familial.

Clinical Findings
1. Prostate cancer is generally a silent disease until it reaches advanced stages.
2. Bone pain and pathologic fractures may be the initial symptoms of prostate cancer.
3. Local growth can cause symptoms of urinary outflow obstruction.
4. DRE.
   a. DRE might reveal an area of increased firmness.
   b. An asymmetric prostate is also suspicious for cancer.
   c. Ten percent of patients have a negative DRE for cancer. They might have BPH.
5. The prostate may be hard and fixed.
6. The tumor might extend to the seminal vesicles in advanced stages.

Differential Diagnosis
1. BPH.
2. Prostatitis.
3. Prostate stones.

Stage and Grade
1. The degree of malignancy varies with the stage.
   a. Stage A: Confined to the prostate, no nodule palpable.
   b. Stage B: Palpable nodule confined to the gland.

    c. Stage C: Local extension.

    d. Stage D: Regional lymph nodes or distant metastases.

2. In the Gleason grading classification, histologic patterns are independently assigned two scores numbered 1 to 5 (best to least differentiated). These numbers are added to give a total tumor score.

    a. Prognosis is generally good if score is 5 or less.

    b. Score of 6, 7, or 8 carries an intermediate prognosis.

    c. Score of 9 or 10 correlates with anaplastic lesions with poor prognosis.

Work-up

1. Laboratory tests.

    a. PSA level.

        (1) PSA levels may be useful in early diagnosis of prostate cancer (screening) and in monitoring response to therapy, as well as an early sign of recurrence.

        (2) Sensitivity and specificity.

            (a) Normal PSA is found in more than 20% of patients with prostate cancer (lack of sensitivity).

            (b) Only 20% of men with PSA levels between 4 ng/mL and 10 ng/mL have prostate cancer (lack of specificity).

            (c) The most common causes of false-positive PSA are BPH, prostatitis, and ejaculation within 48 hours of testing.

            (d) Rectal exam causes only a minimal rise in PSA (of 0.2 ng/mL over baseline).

            (e) Finasteride and dutasteride reduce PSA values by 50%.

        (3) PSA higher than 10 ng/mL is associated with more advanced prostate cancer. The American Cancer Society recommends offering the PSA test and DRE yearly to men 50 years or older who have a life expectancy of at least 10 years.

        (4) Earlier testing, starting at age 40 is recommended for men at high risk (e.g., African Americans, and men with a family history of prostate cancer).

        (5) There is no evidence yet that screening for prostate cancer and early detection reduce mortality.

    b. PSA velocity.

        (1) Ideally, prostate cancer should be diagnosed when the PSA is between 4 and 10 ng/mL (2.6-10 ng/mL for African American men). Unfortunately, in this range of PSA, many men do not have cancer (false-positive test) and prostate biopsies are invasive, uncomfortable, and themselves subject to false-negative results from sampling.

        (2) Many clinicians therefore use the PSA velocity concept.

            (a) In the absence of cancer, the PSA rises slowly over time in a linear pattern.

            (b) With cancer, the rate of PSA increase can be exponential.

            (c) Instead of repeating the PSA annually when the result is between 4 and 10 mg/mL, it is repeated every 3 months until a pattern of increase can be ascertained.

            (d) Also PSA should not rise by more than 0.85 ng/mL per year and should take 4 years to double in the absence of cancer.

  c. Serum-free PSA.

    (1) The use of serum-free PSA for prostate screening has been proposed by some urologists as a means to decrease unwarranted biopsies without missing a significant number of prostate cancers.

    (2) This approach is based on the higher free PSA in men with prostate cancer.

      (a) For example, in men with total PSA levels of 4 to 10 ng/mL, the cancer probability is 0.25, but if the free PSA is less than 10%, the probability of cancer increases to 0.45 and if the free PSA is higher than 25%, the probability of cancer decreases to 8%.

  d. If the PSA is <2 mg/mL in non–African American men, the frequency of screening can drop from yearly to every 2 years.

  e. Prostatic acid phosphatase can be used to evaluate nonlocalized disease.

2. Imaging studies.

  a. Bone scan.

    (1) Bone scan is useful to evaluate for bone metastasis.

    (2) However, according to the American Urological Association (AUA), the routine use of bone scanning is not required for staging of prostate cancer in asymptomatic men with clinically localized cancer if the PSA level is 20 ng/mL or less.

  b. Transrectal ultrasonography.

    (1) According to the AUA screening recommendations, transrectal ultrasonography adds little to the combination of PSA and DRE.

    (2) It might be useful in selected patients to assess the extent of prostate cancer.

  c. CT scan and MRI.

    (1) CT and MRI imaging are generally not indicated for cancer staging in men with clinically localized cancer and PSA less than 25 ng/mL.

    (2) High-resolution MRI with magnetic nanoparticles has been used to detect small and otherwise undetectable lymph-node metastases in patients with prostate cancer.

3. Biopsy and lymph node dissection.

  a. If the DRE reveals a suspicious prostate for cancer, referral to a urologist for prostate biopsy is appropriate regardless of PSA level.

  b. Transrectal biopsy and fine-needle aspiration of prostate can confirm the diagnosis, but false-negative biopsies are possible as a result of random sampling.

  c. With regard to pelvic lymph node dissection in staging, the AUA states that it might not be required in some patients.

    (1) Patients with PSA levels less than 10 ng/mL.

    (2) Patients with PSA level less than 20 ng/mL and a Gleason score of less than 6.

Treatment

1. Therapeutic approach varies with the following:

  a. Stage of the tumor.

  b. Patient's life expectancy.

  c. Patient's treatment preference.

2. The optimal treatment of clinically localized prostate cancer is unclear.

  a. Radical prostatectomy is generally performed in patients with localized prostate cancer and life expectancy longer than 10 years.

  b. Radiation therapy (external beam irradiation or implantation of radioactive pellets [seeds]) represents an alternative in patients with localized prostate cancer, especially poor surgical candidates, or patients with a high-grade malignancy.

  c. Watchful waiting is reasonable in patients who are too old or too ill to survive longer than 10 years. If the cancer progresses to the point where it becomes symptomatic, palliation can be attempted by several methods.

3. Patients with advanced disease and projected life expectancy less than 10 years are candidates for radiation therapy and hormonal therapy (diethylstilbestrol [DES], luteinizing hormone-releasing hormone [LHRH] analogues, antiandrogens, bilateral orchiectomy).

  a. Androgen-deprivation therapy with a gonadotropin-releasing hormone (GnRH) agonist is the mainstay of treatment for metastatic prostate cancer.

  b. Adjuvant treatment with GnRH agonists (goserelin leuprolide, or triptorelin) plus antiandrogens (flutamide, bicalutamide, or nilutamide), when started simultaneously with external irradiation, improves local control and survival in patients with locally advanced prostate cancer.

  c. Bisphosphonates inhibit osteoclast-mediated bone resorption and prevent bone loss in the hip and lumbar spine in men receiving treatment for prostate cancer with a GnRH.

4. Monitoring.

  a. Patients should be monitored at 3- to 6-month intervals with clinical examination and PSA for the first year, then every 6 months for the second year, then yearly if stable.

  b. For patients who have undergone radical prostatectomy, a rising PSA level suggests residual or recurrent prostate cancer. Chest x-ray examination and bone scan are appropriate in this situation.

Prognosis

1. Prognosis varies with the stage of the disease and the Gleason classification.

2. The ploidy of the tumor also has prognostic value. Prognosis is better with diploid tumor cells, worse with aneuploid tumor cells.

3. For Stage A tumors, the extended 10-year disease-specific survival is similar for patients with prostatectomy (94%), radiation therapy (90%), and conservative management (93%).

4. For Stage B or C localized tumors, survival rate is better with surgery than with radiation therapy or conservative management.

5. Expression of the gene EZH2 has been identified as an important factor in the determination of the aggressiveness of prostate cancer. A recent study revealed that expression of the EZH2 gene may be a better predictor of clinical failure than Gleason score, tumor stage, or surgical

margin status. Testing for EZH2 protein in prostate cancer tissue may be useful to determine prognosis and direct treatment.

SUGGESTED READINGS

Gann PH, Ma J, Catalona WJ, Stampfer MJ: Strategies combining total and percent free prostate specific antigen for detecting prostate cancer: A prospective evaluation. *J Urol* 167:2427-2434, 2002.

Harisinghani MG, Barentsz J, Hahn PF, et al: Noninvasive detection of clinically occult lymph-node metastases in prostate cancer. *N Engl J Med* 348:2491-2499, 2003.

Holmberg L, Bill-Axelson A, Helgesen F, et al: A randomized trial comparing radical prostatectomy with watchful waiting in early prostate cancer, *N Engl J Med* 347:781-789, 2002.

Makinen T, Tammela TL, Stenman UH, et al: Family history and prostate cancer screening with prostate-specific antigen. *J Clin Oncol* 20:2658-2663, 2002.

Nelson WG, De Marzo AM, Isaacs WB: Prostate cancer. *N Engl J Med* 349:366-381, 2003.

Steineck G, Helgesen F, Wolfsson J, et al: Quality of life after radical prostatectomy or watchful waiting. *N Engl J Med* 347:790-796, 2002.

Varambally S, Dhanasekaran SM, Zhou M, et al: The polycomb group protein EZH2 is involved in progression of prostate cancer. *Nature* 419:624-629, 2002.

5.11 Pulmonary Disorders

ASTHMA

Fred F. Ferri and Tom J. Wachtel

Definitions

1. The American Thoracic Society defines asthma as a "disease characterized by an increased responsiveness of the trachea and bronchi to various stimuli and manifested by a widespread narrowing of the airways that changes in severity either spontaneously or as a result of treatment."
2. *Status asthmaticus* can be defined as a severe continuous bronchospasm.

Epidemiology

1. Asthma affects 5% to 12% of the population.
2. It accounts for more than 450,000 hospitalizations and nearly 2 million emergency department visits yearly in the United States.
3. Overall, asthma mortality in the United States is 20 per 1 million persons per year.
4. In older patients, asthma and COPD can overlap.

Clinical Features

1. History.
   a. Typical triad.
      (1) Shortness of breath.
      (2) Cough.
      (3) Wheezing.
   b. These symptoms can occur alone or in any combination.
   c. Exacerbations.
      (1) Episodic.

(2) Sometimes seasonal.

(3) Sometimes associated with specific environmental exposures.

(4) Sometimes associated with exercise.

(5) Sometimes associated with exposure to cold air.

2. Physical findings.

   a. The hallmark physical finding in any patient with active asthma is wheezing (expiratory > inspiratory) and a prolonged expiratory phase during lung auscultation. Between exacerbations (attacks) the exam may be normal.

   b. The physical examination might also reveal:

      (1) Tachycardia and tachypnea.

      (2) Use of accessory respiratory muscles.

      (3) Pulsus paradoxus (inspiratory decline in systolic BP >10 mm Hg).

      (4) Wheezing: Absence of wheezing (silent chest) or decreased wheezing can indicate worsening obstruction.

      (5) Mental status changes are generally secondary to hypoxia and hypercapnia and constitute an indication for urgent intubation.

      (6) Paradoxical abdominal and diaphragmatic movement on inspiration.

         (a) Detected by palpation over the upper part of the abdomen in a semirecumbent patient.

         (b) An important sign of impending respiratory crisis.

         (c) Indicates diaphragmatic fatigue.

      (7) The following abnormalities in vital signs indicate severe asthma:

         (a) Pulsus paradoxus >18 mm Hg.

         (b) Respiratory rate >30 breaths/min.

         (c) Tachycardia with heart rate >120 bpm.

Etiology

1. Intrinsic asthma.

   a. Occurs in patients who have no history of allergies.

   b. May be triggered by upper respiratory infections or psychological stress.

2. Extrinsic asthma (allergic asthma) is brought on by exposure to allergens (e.g., dust mites, cat allergen, industrial chemicals).

3. Exercise-induced asthma manifests with bronchospasm following initiation of exercise and improves with discontinuation of exercise.

4. Drug-induced asthma is often associated with use of NSAIDs, β-blockers, sulfites, or certain foods and beverages.

Differential Diagnosis

1. CHF.

2. COPD.

3. Pulmonary embolism.

4. Foreign body aspiration.

5. Rhinitis with postnasal drip.

6. Pneumonia and upper respiratory infections.

7. Hypersensitivity pneumonitis.

8. Panic disorder with primary hyperventilation.

9. Diffuse interstitial lung disease.

10. GERD.

Work-up

Laboratory tests can be normal if they are obtained during a stable period. The following laboratory abnormalities may be present during an acute bronchospasm:

1. Arterial blood gases (ABGs) can be used in staging the severity of an asthmatic attack.
   a. Mild: Decreased PaO_2 and $PaCO_2$, increased pH.
   b. Moderate: Decreased PaO_2, normal $PaCO_2$, normal pH.
   c. Severe: Marked decreased PaO_2, increased $PaCO_2$, and decreased pH.
2. CBC: Leukocytosis with left shift can indicate a bacterial infection (e.g., bronchitis or pneumonia).
3. Sputum: Eosinophils, Charcot-Leyden crystals, polymorphonuclear neutrophils, and bacteria may be found on Gram stain in patients with pneumonia.
4. Pulmonary function studies with methacholine challenge test.
5. Chest x-ray.
   a. Chest x-ray is usually normal.
   b. It might show evidence of thoracic hyperinflation (e.g., flattening of the diaphragm, increased volume over the retrosternal air space).
   c. It might reveal pneumonia.
6. ECG: Tachycardia, nonspecific ST-T wave changes; might also show cor pulmonale, right bundle-branch block, right axial deviation, counterclockwise rotation.
7. Skin testing for allergens may be appropriate.

Treatment

1. Nonpharmacologic therapy.
   a. Avoidance of triggering factors (e.g., salicylates, sulfites).
   b. Encouragement of regular exercise (e.g., swimming).
   c. Patient education.
      (1) Patients should be taught the warning signs of an attack and proper use of medications (e.g., correct use of inhalers).
      (2) Elderly asthmatics must be observed using the hand-held inhalers.
         (a) A spacer may be helpful and should be ordered routinely.
         (b) Patients who cannot be taught to use metered-dose inhalers should be prescribed nebulizers for routine use at home. Albuterol, ipratropium, and fluticasone are available for nebulizer use.
2. Pharmacologic therapy. The Expert Panel of the National Asthma Education and Prevention Program (NAEPP) recommends the following stepwise approach in the pharmacologic management of asthma in adults:
   a. Step 1 (mild intermittent asthma).
      (1) No daily medications are needed.
      (2) Short-acting inhaled β_2-agonists (e.g., albuterol) should be taken as needed.
   b. Step 2 (mild persistent asthma): Daily treatment is appropriate.
      (1) Low-dose inhaled corticosteroid (e.g., beclomethasone [Beclovent, Vanceril], flunisolide [AeroBid], triamcinolone [Azmacort]), fluticasone (Flovent) or mometasone (Asmanex) can be used. This is usually first-line therapy.

(2) Cromolyn (Intal) or nedocromil (Tilade) may also be used.

(3) The leukotriene receptor antagonist montelukast (Singulair) may be considered for long-term control.

(4) Quick relief of asthma can be achieved with short-acting inhaled β_2-agonists (see earlier). These are often described as "rescue treatment."

c. Step 3 (moderate persistent asthma): Daily medication is recommended.

(1) Low-dose or medium-dose inhaled corticosteroids (see earlier) plus long-acting inhaled β_2-agonist (salmeterol [Serevent]) or long-acting oral β_2-agonists (e.g., albuterol, sustained-release tablets).

(a) Salmeterol is also available as a dry powder inhaler (Discus) that does not require a spacer device; the dosage is one puff bid.

(b) A salmeterol-fluticasone combination for the Discus inhaler (Advair) is available and simplifies therapy for patients with asthma. It generally should be reserved for patients with at least moderately severe asthma not controlled by an inhaled corticosteroid alone.

(c) Use salmeterol with caution given reports of death associated with this drug.

(2) Use short-acting inhaled β-agonists on an as-needed basis for quick relief.

d. Step 4 (severe persistent asthma).

(1) Daily treatment with high-dose inhaled corticosteroids plus long-acting inhaled β-agonists plus long-acting oral β_2-agonist plus long-term systemic corticosteroids (e.g., methylprednisolone, prednisolone, prednisone) can be used.

(2) Short-acting β_2-agonists can be used as needed for quick relief.

e. Treatment of status asthmaticus is as follows:

(1) Oxygen is generally started at 2 to 4 L/min via nasal cannula or large-reservoir mask (Ventimask) at 40% FiO_2; further adjustments are made according to the ABGs.

(2) Bronchodilators.

(a) Various agents and modalities are available.

(b) Inhaled bronchodilators are preferred when they can be administered quickly.

(c) Albuterol 0.5 to 1 mL (2.5 to 5 mg) in 3 mL of saline solution tid or qid via nebulizer is effective.

(3) Corticosteroids.

(a) Early administration is advised, particularly in patients using steroids at home.

(b) Initiation.

i. Patients may be started on hydrocortisone (Solu-Cortef) 2.5 to 4 mg/kg or methylprednisolone (Solu-Medrol) 0.5 to 1 mg/kg intravenous (IV) loading dose, then q6h prn.

ii. Higher doses may be necessary in selected patients (particularly those receiving steroids at home).

iii. Steroids given by inhalation should be (re)initiated after the acute phase. Inhaled steroids are useful for controlling bronchospasm and tapering oral steroids and should be used in all patients with severe asthma.

(c) Tapering.

    i. Rapid but judicious tapering of corticosteroids will eliminate serious steroid toxicity.

    ii. Long-term low-dose methotrexate may be an effective means of reducing the systemic corticosteroid requirement in some patients with severe refractory asthma.

(d) The most common errors regarding steroid therapy in acute bronchospasms are the use of "too little, too late" and too-rapid tapering with return of bronchospasm.

    i. IV hydration: Judicious use is necessary to avoid CHF in elderly patients.

    ii. IV antibiotics are indicated when there is suspicion of bacterial infection (e.g., infiltrate on chest x-ray, fever, leukocytosis).

    iii. Intubation and mechanical ventilation are indicated when IV hydration and antibiotics fail to produce significant improvement.

    iv. General anesthesia: Halothane might reverse bronchospasm in a severe asthmatic who cannot be ventilated adequately by mechanical means.

SUGGESTED READINGS

Diette GB, Krishnan JA, Dominici F, et al: Asthma in older patients: Factors associated with hospitalization. *Arch Intern Med* 162:1123-1132, 2002.

Holgate ST: Therapeutic options for persistent asthma. *JAMA* 285:2637-2639, 2001.

Mintz M: Asthma update: Part I. Diagnosis, monitoring, and prevention of disease progression. *Am Fam Physician* 70:893-898, 2004

National Asthma Education and Prevention Program: *Expert panel report 2: Guidelines for diagnosis and management of asthma.* Bethesda, Md., National Institutes of Health, 1997.

Naureckas ET, Solway J: Clinical practice. Mild asthma. *N Engl J Med* 345:1257-1262, 2001.

Sin DD, Man J, Sharpe H, et al: Pharmacological management to reduce exacerbations in adults with asthma. *JAMA* 292:367-376, 2004.

CHRONIC OBSTRUCTIVE PULMONARY DISEASE

Fred F. Ferri and Tom J. Wachtel

Definitions

1. Chronic obstructive pulmonary disease (COPD) is a disorder characterized by the presence of airflow limitation that is not (fully) reversible. There are two kinds of COPD:

    a. *Emphysema* is characterized by loss of lung elasticity and destruction of lung parenchyma with enlargement of air spaces.

    b. *Chronic bronchitis* is characterized by obstruction of small airways and productive cough for longer than 3 months over more than 2 successive years.

2. Patients with COPD are classically subdivided into two major groups based on their appearance.

    a. *Blue bloaters* are patients with chronic bronchitis.

  (1) The name is derived from the bluish tinge of the skin (secondary to chronic hypoxemia).
  (2) Chronic cough with production of large amounts of sputum is characteristic.
b. *Pink puffers* are patients with emphysema.
  (1) They are often cachectic and have pink skin color (adequate oxygen saturation).
  (2) Shortness of breath may be manifested by pursed-lip breathing and use of accessory muscles of respiration.
3. Both types of COPD can cause hypercapnia and both often coexist.

Epidemiology

1. COPD affects 16 million Americans and is responsible for more than 80,000 deaths per year.
2. COPD is the fourth leading cause of death in the United States and is expected to become the third leading cause of death by 2020.
3. Highest incidence is in men older than 40 years.
4. About 16 million office visits, 500,000 hospitalizations, and more than $18 billion in direct health care costs annually can be attributed to COPD.

Etiology

1. Tobacco exposure.
2. Occupational exposure to pulmonary toxins (e.g., cadmium).
3. Atmospheric pollution.
4. α_1-Antitrypsin deficiency is rare; less than 1% of COPD patients have it.

Clinical Findings

1. Chronic bronchitis (blue bloaters).
   a. Dyspnea.
   b. Peripheral cyanosis.
   c. Productive cough.
   d. Tachypnea.
   e. Tachycardia.
2. Emphysema (pink puffers).
   a. Dyspnea.
   b. Pursed-lip breathing with use of accessory muscles for respiration.
   c. Decreased breath sounds.
3. COPD in general.
   a. Possible wheezing in patients with chronic bronchitis and patients with emphysema.
   b. Many patients with COPD have features of both chronic bronchitis and emphysema in many patients.
4. Acute exacerbation of COPD.
   a. This is mainly a clinical diagnosis.
   b. It generally manifests with worsening dyspnea, increase in sputum purulence, and increase in sputum volume.
5. Complications often involve right-sided heart failure (cor pulmonale) sometimes precipitated by arrhythmias such as atrial fibrillation or multifocal atrial tachycardia.

Differential Diagnosis

1. CHF.
2. Asthma.
3. Respiratory infections.
4. Bronchiectasis.
5. Pulmonary embolism.
6. Obstructive sleep apnea.
7. Pulmonary fibrosis.
8. Other restrictive lung diseases.
9. Anxiety disorders.

Work-up

1. Pulmonary function testing.
   a. The primary physiological abnormality in COPD is an accelerated decline in FEV_1.
      (1) The normal rate of decline in adults older than 30 years is approximately 30 mL/year.
      (2) In COPD patients the FEV_1 declines nearly 60 mL/year.
   b. Pulmonary function testing.
      (1) In patients with emphysema, pulmonary function testing results reveal abnormal diffusing capacity, increased total lung capacity and/or residual volume, and fixed reduction in FEV_1.
      (2) In patients with chronic bronchitis, testing reveals normal diffusing capacity and reduced FEV_1.
   c. Patients with COPD can generally be distinguished from asthmatics by their incomplete response to albuterol (change in FEV_1 <200 mL and 12%) and absence of an abnormal bronchoconstrictor response to methacholine or other stimuli.
   d. However, nearly 40% of patients with COPD respond to bronchodilators.
2. Chest x-ray examination.
   a. Hyperinflation with flattened diaphragm, tenting of the diaphragm at the rib, and increased retrosternal chest space.
   b. Decreased vascular markings and bullae in patients with emphysema.
   c. Thickened bronchial markings and enlarged right heart in patients with chronic bronchitis.
3. ABGs: Hypercapnia and hypoxemia may be present.
4. CBC might reveal leukocytosis with shift to the left during acute exacerbation.
5. ECG and echocardiogram may be appropriate to diagnose associated heart disease (also caused by smoking).

Treatment

1. Nonpharmacologic therapy.
   a. Weight loss in obese patients.
   b. Avoidance of tobacco and elimination of air pollutants.
   c. Supplemental oxygen, usually through a nasal cannula to ensure oxygen saturation greater than 90% measured by pulse oximetry.
   d. Discuss advance directives and end-of-life care issues, especially the use of mechanical ventilation.

2. Pharmacologic therapy.
   a. Inhaled β-agonists.
      (1) Short-acting agents such as albuterol can be used on a schedule (e.g., 2 to 4 puffs every 4 to 6 hours).
      (2) Long-acting agents, such as salmeterol (Serevent), may be given twice daily. Use with caution because of reports of death associated with this medication.
   b. Anticholinergics.
      (1) A short-acting agent such as ipratropium (Atrovent) can be used on a schedule or as needed alone, or in combination with the β-agonist albuterol (Combivent).
      (2) A long-acting agent such as tiotropium (Spiriva) given at one inhalation (18 μg dry powder) qd may be more effective than ipratropium.
   c. An inhaled glucocorticoid drug such as fluticasone is given twice daily alone or in combination with β-agonists or anticholinergic drugs (e.g., Advair combines fluticasone and salmeterol).
   d. Delivery.
      (1) Elderly patients may be unable to coordinate their breathing and hand motion or may otherwise be unable to operate a hand-held metered dose inhaler.
      (2) If such treatment is prescribed, the physician must educate and observe the patient using this therapy. A spacer may be helpful and should be prescribed routinely.
      (3) Elderly patients often do better with a nebulizer than with a hand-held aerosol delivery system.
3. Other therapy.
   a. All patients with COPD should receive pneumococcal vaccine and yearly influenza vaccine.
   b. Pulmonary rehabilitation may improve exercise capacity, reduce dyspnea, reduce hospitalizations, and enhance quality of life.
   c. Lung-volume-reduction surgery in patients with severe upper-lobe emphysema can improve exercise capacity, pulmonary function, and quality of life but not overall survival.

Management of Acute Exacerbation

Patients with acute exacerbations can require hospitalization.
1. Aerosolized β-agonists such as albuterol nebulizer solution 5% 0.3 mL.
2. Anticholinergic agents have equivalent efficacy to inhaled β-adrenergic agonists.
   a. Inhalant solution of ipratropium bromide 0.5 mg can be administered every 4 to 8 hours.
   b. Tiotropium bromide (Spiriva) has a much longer duration of action than ipratropium and produces a more sustained response over time than long-acting β_2-agonists. Usual dose is inhalation of one capsule daily with a breath-activated dry powder inhalation device (Handihaler).
3. Short courses of systemic corticosteroids have been shown to improve spirometric and clinical outcomes.

    a. In the hospital setting give IV methylprednisolone 50 to 100 mg bolus, then q6 to 8h; taper as soon as possible.

    b. In the outpatient setting, oral prednisone 40 mg/day initially, decreasing the dose by 10 mg every other day is generally effective.

4. Judicious oxygen administration.

    a. Hypercapnia and further respiratory compromise can occur after high-flow oxygen therapy.

    b. A large-reservoir mask delivering an inspired oxygen fraction of 24% to 28% is preferred to nasal cannula.

5. Noninvasive positive pressure ventilation delivered by a facial or nasal mask may obviate the need for intratracheal intubation.

6. Inhaled corticosteroids.

    a. The role of inhaled corticosteroids in COPD is controversial.

    b. Some trials have demonstrated mild improvement in patients' symptoms and decreased frequency of exacerbations.

    c. Many pulmonologists believe that these drugs are ineffective in most patients with COPD but should be considered for patients with moderate to severe airflow limitation who have persistent symptoms despite optimal bronchodilator therapy.

7. IV aminophylline administration is controversial. When used, serum levels should be closely monitored to minimize risks of tachyarrhythmias.

8. Antibiotics are indicated in suspected respiratory infection (e.g., increased purulence and volume of phlegm).

    a. *Haemophilus influenzae* and *Streptococcus pneumoniae* are common causes of acute bronchitis.

    b. Oral antibiotics of choice are azithromycin, levofloxacin, amoxicillin-clavulanate, and cefuroxime.

    c. Antibiotics are beneficial in exacerbations of COPD manifesting with increased dyspnea and sputum purulence, especially if the patient is febrile.

9. Mucolytic medications.

    a. Mucolytic medications are generally ineffective.

    b. Their benefits may be greatest in patients with more advanced disease

    c. Guaifenesin can improve cough symptoms and mucus clearance.

10. Cor pulmonale or comorbid heart failure may be exacerbated by hypoxia and must be treated along with pulmonary management (see "Congestive Heart Failure" earlier).

11. Pulmonary toilet.

    a. Careful nasotracheal suction is indicated in patients with excessive secretions and inability to expectorate.

    b. Mechanical percussion of the chest as applied by a physical or respiratory therapist is *ineffective* with acute exacerbations of COPD.

    c. Continuous positive airway pressure (CPAP) can help ventilation and gas exchange during an exacerbation.

    d. Intubation and mechanical ventilation may be necessary if other measures fail to provide improvement.

SUGGESTED READINGS

Aaron S, Vandemheen KL, Hebert P, et al: Outpatient oral prednisone after emergency treatment of chronic obstructive pulmonary disease. *N Engl J Med* 348:2618-2625, 2003.

Anthonisen NR, Connett JE, Murray RP: Smoking and lung function of Lung Health Study participants after 11 years. *Am J Resp Crit Care Med* 166:675-679, 2002.

Celli BR, Cote CG, Marin JM, et al: The body-mass index, airflow obstruction, dyspnea, and exercise capacity index in chronic obstructive pulmonary disease. *N Engl J Med* 350:1005-1012, 2004.

Hogg JC, Chu F, Utokaparch S, et al: The nature of small-airway obstruction in chronic obstructive pulmonary disease. *N Engl J Med* 350:2645-2653, 2004.

Man SF, McAlister FA, Anthonisen NR, Sin DD: Contemporary management of chronic obstructive pulmonary disease: Clinical applications. *JAMA* 290:2313-2316, 2003.

National Emphysema Treatment Trial Research Group: A randomized trial comparing lung-volume-reduction surgery with medical therapy for severe emphysema. *N Engl J Med* 348:2059-2073, 2003.

Sethi S, Evans N, Grant BJ, Murphy TF: New strains of bacteria and exacerbations of chronic obstructive pulmonary disease. *N Engl J Med* 347:465-471, 2002.

Sin DD, McAlister FA, Man SF, Anthonisen NR: Contemporary management of chronic obstructive pulmonary disease: A scientific review. *JAMA* 290:2301-2312, 2003.

Stoller JK: Clinical practice. Acute exacerbations of chronic obstructive pulmonary disease. *N Engl J Med* 346:988-994, 2002.

Sutherland ER, Cherniak RM: Management of chronic obstructive pulmonary disease. *N Engl J Med* 350:2689-2697, 2004.

Vincken W, van Noord JA, Greefhorst AP, et al: Improved health outcomes in patients with COPD during 1 yr's treatment with tiotropium. *Eur Respir J* 19: 209-216, 2002.

5.12 Gastrointestinal Disorders

CHOLELITHIASIS AND CHOLECYSTITIS

Fred F. Ferri and Tom J. Wachtel

Definitions

1. Cholelithiasis is the presence of stones in the gallbladder.
2. Cholecystitis is an acute or chronic inflammation of the gallbladder generally secondary to gallstones (>95% of cases).

Epidemiology

1. About 20 million Americans have gallstone disease.
2. Of these, 2% to 3% (500,000 to 600,000) are treated with cholecystectomy each year.
3. The prevalence of gallstones is 0.6% in the general population and much higher in certain ethnic groups (>75% of Native Americans by age 60 years).
4. The prevalence of gallbladder disease increases with age. Highest incidence is in the fifth and sixth decades.
5. Predisposing factors for gallstones are:
   a. Female sex.
   b. Age >40 years.
   c. Family history of gallstones.
   d. Obesity.
   e. Ileal disease.
   f. History of oral contraceptive use.

g. Diabetes mellitus.

h. Rapid weight loss.

i. Estrogen replacement therapy.

6. Acute cholecystitis occurs most commonly in women during the fifth and sixth decades.

7. Patients with gallstones have a 20% chance of developing biliary colic or its complications at the end of a 20-year period.

Clinical Findings

1. Cholelithiasis.
   a. Physical examination is entirely normal unless the patient is having an attack of biliary colic.
   b. About 80% of gallstones are asymptomatic.

2. Biliary colic.
   a. Typical symptoms of obstruction of the cystic duct include intermittent severe, cramping pain affecting the right upper quadrant (biliary colic).
   b. Pain occurs mostly at night and can radiate to the back or right shoulder. It can last from a few minutes to several hours.

3. Cholecystitis.
   a. Pain and tenderness in the right hypochondrium or epigastrium; pain possibly radiating to the infrascapular region.
   b. Palpation of the right upper quadrant elicits marked tenderness and stoppage of inspired breath (Murphy's sign).
   c. Guarding (right upper quadrant or diffuse).
   d. Jaundice (25% of patients).
   e. Palpable gallbladder (20% of cases).
   f. Nausea and vomiting (>70% of patients).
   g. Fever and chills (>25% of patients).
   h. Medical history may reveal ingestion of a large, fatty meal before the onset of pain.

4. Other complications of cholelithiasis.
   a. Patients with at least one gallstone <5 mm in diameter have a greater than fourfold increased risk of presenting with acute biliary pancreatitis.
   b. A potential serious complication of gallstones is acute cholangitis. Endoscopic retrograde cholangiopancreatography (ERCP) and endoscopic sphincterectomy followed by interval laparoscopic cholecystectomy is effective in acute cholangitis.

5. Given the high prevalence of functional bowel disease and dyspepsia and the high prevalence of gallstones, gastrointestinal (GI) symptoms are often misattributed to cholelithiasis. In this event, elective cholecystectomy does not alleviate the symptoms (sometimes described as postcholecystectomy syndrome).

Etiology

1. Cholelithiasis.
   a. About 75% of gallstones contain cholesterol.
      (1) Cholesterol stones are usually associated with obesity, female sex, and diabetes mellitus.
      (2) Mixed stones are most common (80%).
      (3) Pure cholesterol stones account for only 10% of stones.

   b. Pigment stones.
      (1) About 25% of gallstones are pigment stones (bilirubin, calcium, and variable organic material) associated with hemolysis and cirrhosis.
      (2) These tend to be black pigment stones that are refractory to medical therapy.
2. Cholecystitis.
   a. Gallstones (>95% of cases).
   b. Ischemic damage to the gallbladder; patient is critically ill (acalculous cholecystitis).
   c. Infectious agents, especially in patients with AIDS (cytomegalovirus, cryptosporidium).
   d. Strictures of the bile duct.
   e. Neoplasms, primary or metastatic.

Differential Diagnosis of Right Upper Quadrant Abdominal Pain

1. Hepatic.
   a. Hepatitis.
   b. Hepatic congestion.
   c. Neoplasm.
   d. Trauma.
   e. Liver abscess.
   f. Subphrenic abscess.
2. Biliary.
   a. Neoplasm.
   b. Stricture.
3. Esophageal: GERD.
4. Gastric.
   a. PUD.
   b. Neoplasm.
   c. Gastritis.
5. Pancreatic.
   a. Pancreatitis.
   b. Neoplasm.
   c. Stone in the pancreatic duct or ampulla.
6. Renal.
   a. Calculi.
   b. Infection.
   c. Neoplasm.
   d. Trauma (ruptured kidney).
7. Pulmonary.
   a. Pneumonia.
   b. Pulmonary infarction.
   c. Right-sided pleurisy.
8. Intestinal.
   a. Retrocecal appendicitis.
   b. Intestinal obstruction.
   c. High fecal impaction.
   d. Functional bowel disease.

9. Cardiac.
   a. Myocardial ischemia (particularly involving the inferior wall).
   b. Pericarditis.
10. Cutaneous: herpes zoster.
11. Aortic.
    a. Dissecting aneurysm.
    b. Abdominal aortic aneurysm
12. Musculoskeletal.
    a. Nerve root irritation caused by osteoarthritis of the spine.
    b. Abdominal wall muscle strain.
    c. Incisional hernia.

Work-up

Work-up consists of history and physical examination coupled with laboratory evaluation and imaging studies. No single clinical finding or laboratory test is sufficient to establish or exclude cholelithiasis or cholecystitis without further testing.

1. Laboratory tests.
   a. In cholelithiasis, these are usually normal.
   b. In acute cholecystitis.
      (1) Leukocytosis ($12,000\text{-}20,000/mm^3$) is present in more than 70% of patients.
      (2) Elevated alkaline phosphatase, ALT, AST, bilirubin. Bilirubin elevation >4 mg/dL is unusual and suggests choledocholithiasis.
      (3) Amylase may be elevated (consider pancreatitis if serum amylase elevation exceeds 500 U).
2. Imaging studies.
   a. Plain film of abdomen generally is not useful, because <25% of stones are radiopaque.
   b. Ultrasound of the gallbladder.
      (1) This is the preferred initial test (sensitivity, 95%; specificity, 90%).
      (2) It demonstrates the presence of stones and also dilated gallbladder with thickened wall and surrounding edema in patients with acute cholecystitis.
   c. CT scan of abdomen is useful in cases of suspected abscess, neoplasm, or pancreatitis.
   d. Nuclear imaging (heptobiliary iminodiacetic acid [HIDA] scan) can confirm acute cholecystitis (>90% accuracy) if gallbladder is not visualized within 4 hours of injection and the radioisotope is excreted in the common bile duct.

Treatment

Cholelithiasis

1. Asymptomatic patients do not require therapeutic intervention.
2. Lifestyle changes.
   a. Avoidance of diets high in polyunsaturated fats.
   b. Weight loss in obese patients, but avoid rapid weight loss.
3. Surgical intervention.
   a. Surgery is generally the ideal approach for symptomatic patients.
   b. Laparoscopic cholecystectomy is generally preferred over open cholecystectomy because of the shorter recovery period.

   c. Laparoscopic cholecystectomy after endoscopic sphincterectomy.
- (1) This procedure is recommended for patients with common bile duct stones and residual gallbladder stones.
- (2) Where possible, single-stage laparoscopic treatments with removal of duct stones and cholecystectomy during the same procedure are preferable.

4. Nonsurgical treatment.
   a. Oral bile salts.
- (1) Patients who are not appropriate candidates for surgery because of coexisting illness or patients who refuse surgery can be treated with oral bile salts.
- (2) Candidates for oral bile salts.
  - (a) Patients who have no more than three cholesterol stones (radiolucent, noncalcified stones) with a diameter of ≤15 mm.
  - (b) Candidates for medical therapy must have a functioning gallbladder and must have absence of calcifications on CT scans.
  - (c) Recurrence rate after bile acid treatment is approximately 50% in 5 hours.
  - (d) Periodic ultrasound is necessary to assess the effectiveness of treatment.
  - (e) Drugs and dosing.
    - i. Ursodiol (Actigall) 8 to 10 mg/kg/day in two to three divided doses for 16 to 20 months.
    - ii. Chenodiol (Chenix) 250 mg bid initially, increasing gradually to a dose of 60 mg/kg/day.

   b. Direct solvent dissolution with methyl *tert*-butyl ether (MTBE).
- (1) MTBE can be used in patients with multiple stones with diameter ≥3 cm.
- (2) This method should be used only by physicians experienced with contact dissolution.
- (3) Administration of the solvent.
  - (a) Route is either through percutaneous transhepatic placement of a catheter into the gallbladder or through endoscopic retrograde catheter placement.
  - (b) Continuous infusion and aspiration of the solvent is performed either manually or by automatic pump system.
- (4) MTBE is a powerful cholesterol solvent and can dissolve stones in a few hours (>90% dissolution over a 2-hour infusion).
- (5) Gallstones recur after dissolution therapy with MTBE in >40% of patients within 5 years.

   c. Extracorporeal shock wave lithotripsy (ESWL).
- (1) ESWL can be used in patients who have no more than three stones and whose stone diameter is ≤3 cm.
- (2) Following ESWL, stones recur in approximately 20% of patients after 4 years.

Cholecystitis

1. Nonsurgical treatment.
   a. Intravenous fluids, broad-spectrum antibiotics, and pain management (meperidine) should be used.

b. Gallbladder aspiration in which all fluid visualized by ultrasound is aspirated is a nonsurgical treatment for patients at high operative risk who develop acute cholecystitis. Salvage cholecystectomy is reserved for nonresponders.

2. Surgical treatment.
   a. Laparoscopic cholecystectomy is preferred; open cholecystectomy is acceptable.
   b. Conservative management with IV fluids and antibiotics (ampicillin-sulbactam [Unasyn] 3 g IV q6h or piperacillin-tazobactam [Zosyn] 4.5 g IV q8h) may be justified in some high-risk patients to convert an emergency procedure into an elective one with a lower mortality.
   c. Hospital stay (when necessary) varies from overnight with laparoscopic cholecystectomy to 4 to 7 days with open cholecystectomy.
   d. Patients should be instructed that stones may recur in bile ducts.
   e. Complication rate is approximately 1% (hemorrhage and bile leak) for laparoscopic cholecystectomy and <0.5% (infection) with open cholecystectomy.
   f. ERCP with sphincterectomy and stone extraction can be performed in conjunction with laparoscopic cholecystectomy for patients with choledochal lithiasis. Approximately 7% to 15% of patients with cholelithiasis also have stones in the common bile duct.

SUGGESTED READINGS

Cuschieri A: Management of patients with gallstones and ductal calculi. *Lancet* 360:739-740, 2002.

Trowbridge RL, Rutkowski NK, Shojania KG: Does this patient have acute cholecystitis? *JAMA* 289:80-86, 2003.

CIRRHOSIS

Fred F. Ferri and Tom J. Wachtel

Definition

1. Cirrhosis is defined histologically as the presence of fibrosis and regenerative nodules in the liver.
2. It can be classified as micronodular, macronodular, and mixed; however, each form may be seen in the same patient at different stages of the disease.
3. Cirrhosis manifests clinically with portal hypertension, hepatic encephalopathy, and variceal bleeding.

Epidemiology

1. Cirrhosis is the eleventh leading cause of death in the United States (9 deaths/100,000 persons/year).
2. Alcohol abuse and viral hepatitis are the major etiologies of cirrhosis in the United States; however, nonalcoholic fatty liver disease is emerging as an important cause of cirrhosis.

Clinical Findings

1. Skin.
   a. Jaundice.
   b. Palmar erythema (alcohol abuse).
   c. Spider angiomata.

    d. Ecchymosis (thrombocytopenia or coagulation factor deficiency).
    e. Dilated superficial periumbilical vein (caput medusae).
    f. Increased pigmentation (hemochromatosis).
    g. Xanthomas (primary biliary cirrhosis).
    h. Needle tracks (viral hepatitis).
2. Chest: Possible gynecomastia in men.
3. Abdomen.
    a. Tender hepatomegaly (congestive hepatomegaly).
    b. Small, nodular liver (cirrhosis).
    c. Palpable, nontender gallbladder (neoplastic extrahepatic biliary obstruction).
    d. Palpable spleen (portal hypertension).
    e. Venous hum auscultated over periumbilical veins (portal hypertension).
    f. Ascites (portal hypertension, hypoalbuminemia).
4. Rectal examination.
    a. Hemorrhoids suggest portal hypertension.
    b. Guaiac-positive stools (alcoholic gastritis, bleeding esophageal varices, PUD, bleeding hemorrhoids).
5. Genitalia: Testicular atrophy in men with chronic liver disease or hemochromatosis.
6. Extremities: Pedal edema (hypoalbuminemia).
7. Neurologic.
    a. Flapping tremor.
    b. Asterixis.
    c. Confusion (hepatic encephalopathy).

Etiology

1. Alcohol abuse.
2. Hepatitis.
    a. Chronic hepatitis B or C.
    b. Autoimmune hepatitis.
    c. Steatohepatitis (fatty liver disease) probably accounts for most cases of cryptogenic cirrhosis.
3. Primary biliary cirrhosis.
4. Secondary biliary cirrhosis, usually resulting from obstruction of the common bile duct by:
    a. Stone.
    b. Stricture.
    c. Pancreatitis.
    d. Neoplasm.
    e. Sclerosing cholangitis.
5. Drugs such as acetaminophen, isoniazid, methotrexate, or methyldopa.
6. Hepatic congestion caused by:
    a. CHF.
    b. Constrictive pericarditis.
    c. Tricuspid insufficiency.
    d. Thrombosis of the hepatic vein.
    e. Obstruction of the vena cava.
7. Hemochromatosis.
8. Wilson's disease.
9. α_1-Antitrypsin deficiency.

Work-up

1. History.
   a. Alcohol abuse: alcoholic liver disease.
   b. Hepatitis B or hepatitis C.
   c. Blood transfusions or IV drug abuse.
   d. The metabolic syndrome (obesity, hypertension, hyperlipidemia, diabetes mellitus).
   e. Pruritus, hyperlipoproteinemia, and xanthomas in a woman suggest primary biliary cirrhosis.
   f. Hepatotoxic drug exposure.
   g. CHF.
   h. Diabetes mellitus, hyperpigmentation, and arthritis suggest hemochromatosis.
   i. Inflammatory bowel disease (IBD) suggests primary sclerosing cholangitis.
   j. Neurologic disturbances suggest Wilson's disease.
   k. Family history of "liver disease" suggests hemochromatosis (positive family history in 25% of patients) or α_1-antitrypsin deficiency.
2. Laboratory tests.
   a. Abnormal blood test results.
      (1) Decreased Hb and Hct.
      (2) Elevated mean corpuscular volume.
      (3) Increased BUN and creatinine (the BUN may also be normal or low if the patient has severely diminished liver function).
      (4) Decreased sodium suggests dilutional hyponatremia.
      (5) Decreased potassium suggests secondary aldosteronism.
   b. Decreased glucose in a patient with liver disease indicates severe liver damage.
   c. Elevated transaminases indicate hepatocellular destruction.
      (1) Alcoholic hepatitis and cirrhosis: There may be mild elevation of ALT and AST, usually <500 IU; AST > ALT (ratio >2:3).
      (2) Extrahepatic obstruction: There may be moderate elevations of ALT and AST to levels <500 IU.
      (3) Viral, toxic, or ischemic hepatitis: There are extreme elevations (>500 IU) of ALT and AST.
      (4) Transaminases may be normal despite significant liver disease in patients with jejunoileal bypass operations or hemochromatosis or after methotrexate administration.
   d. Tests of biliary function.
      (1) Alkaline phosphatase can be elevated with extrahepatic or intrahepatic obstruction, primary biliary cirrhosis, and primary sclerosing cholangitis. If bilirubin is normal, intrahepatic obstruction is more likely.
      (2) Serum bilirubin may be elevated in hepatitis, hepatocellular jaundice, and biliary obstruction.
   e. Tests of hepatic synthetic function.
      (1) Serum albumin: Significant liver disease results in hypoalbuminemia.
      (2) Prothrombin time (PT) is elevated in patients with liver disease.

(3) An elevated blood ammonia suggests hepatocellular dysfunction. Serial values, however, are generally not useful in following patients with hepatic encephalopathy because there is poor correlation between blood ammonia level and degree of hepatic encephalopathy or cognitive function.

 f. Etiologic tests.

  (1) Presence of hepatitis B surface antigen implies hepatitis B.

  (2) Hepatitis C viral testing identifies patients with chronic hepatitis C.

  (3) Presence of antimitochondrial antibody suggests primary biliary cirrhosis.

  (4) Antinuclear antibodies may be found in autoimmune hepatitis.

  (5) Elevated serum copper, decreased serum ceruloplasmin, and elevated 24-hour urine copper might indicate Wilson's disease.

  (6) Protein immunoelectrophoresis.

   (a) Decreased α_1 globulins suggest α_1-antitrypsin deficiency.

   (b) Increased IgA suggests alcoholic cirrhosis.

   (c) Increased IgM suggests primary biliary cirrhosis.

   (d) Increased IgG suggests chronic hepatitis or cryptogenic cirrhosis.

  (7) An elevated serum ferritin and increased transferrin saturation suggest hemochromatosis.

3. Imaging and other studies.

 a. Ultrasonography is the procedure of choice for detecting:

  (1) Gallstones.

  (2) Dilating common bile ducts.

  (3) Fatty liver.

 b. CT scan is useful for:

  (1) Detecting mass lesions in liver and pancreas.

  (2) Assessing hepatic fat content.

  (3) Identifying idiopathic hemochromatosis.

  (4) Diagnosing Budd-Chiari syndrome at an early stage.

  (5) Detecting dilation of intrahepatic bile ducts.

  (6) Detecting varices and splenomegaly.

 c. Technetium-99m sulfur colloid scanning is useful for:

  (1) Diagnosing cirrhosis (there is a shift of colloid uptake to the spleen, bone marrow).

  (2) Identifying hepatic adenomas (cold defect is noted).

  (3) Diagnosing Budd-Chiari syndrome (there is increased uptake by the caudate lobe).

 d. ERCP.

  (1) ERCP is the procedure of choice for diagnosing periampullary carcinoma and common duct stones.

  (2) It is also useful in diagnosing primary sclerosing cholangitis.

 e. Percutaneous liver biopsy is useful for:

  (1) Evaluating hepatic filling defects.

  (2) Evaluating persistently abnormal liver function tests.

  (3) Diagnosing hepatocullular disease or hepatomegaly.

  (4) Diagnosing hemachromatosis.

  (5) Diagnosing primary biliary cirrhosis.

(6) Diagnosing Wilson's disease.

(7) Diagnosing glycogen storage diseases.

(8) Diagnosing chronic hepatitis and autoimmune hepatitis.

(9) Diagnosing infiltrative diseases.

(10) Diagnosing nonalcoholic fatty liver, alcoholic liver disease, and drug-induced liver disease.

(11) Diagnosing primary or secondary carcinoma.

Treatment

General Points

1. All patients with cirrhosis should abstain from alcohol and other hepatotoxins.

2. Low-sodium diet and protein restrictions should be considered.

3. Monitor for hypokalemia and provide potassium replacement where indicated.

4. Oral or subcutaneous injection of vitamin K (10 mg/day for 3 days) in patients with elevated prothrombin time.

5. Consider multivitamins and folic acid.

6. Consider liver transplantation for otherwise healthy patients with refractory decompensated cirrhosis, although age >65 is a relative contraindication.

7. Diagnosis and treatment for osteoporosis should be considered.

8. Vitamin A, D, K, and E deficiencies can be clinically important in advanced cases and may respond to oral replacement.

Complications of Cirrhosis

1. Ascites is the most common complication, affecting 50% of cirrhotic patients.

   a. Sequestration of fluid in peritoneal cavity.

      (1) Paracentesis with analysis of ascitic fluid can offer clues to etiology.

         (a) Fluid should be sent for cell count with differential, Gram stain, culture and sensitivity, albumin, and total protein levels.

         (b) Sample of serum for albumin should be obtained on the same day.

      (2) Analysis.

         (a) Infection is suggested by ascitic fluid neutrophil count exceeding 250 cells/mL.

         (b) The finding of organisms on Gram stain is even more compelling.

         (c) The gold standard for diagnosis of spontaneous bacterial peritonitis involves a positive culture of the ascitic fluid. Yield is 85% with bedside inoculation of fluid into blood culture bottles as opposed to 50% if fluid is simply forwarded to the microbiology department.

   b. Portal hypertension.

      (1) Diagnosed or excluded with calculation of the serum albumin-to-ascites albumin gradient (serum albumin level minus ascites albumin level).

         (a) A gradient ≥1.1 is diagnostic of portal hypertension.

      (b) A value <1.1 excludes this diagnosis.

   (2) Portal hypertension occurs with cirrhosis or impaired hepatic venous drainage.

      (a) Budd–Chiari syndrome (hepatic vein thrombosis).

      (b) Severe right-sided heart failure.

      (c) Constrictive pericarditis.

   (3) Ascites in the absence of portal hypertension suggests biliary outflow obstruction or extrahepatic etiology.

      (a) Pancreatitis.

      (b) Extrahepatic neoplasm with peritoneal seeding (e.g., ovarian cancer).

      (c) Tuberculous peritoneal seeding.

      (d) Paracentesis for cytology, acid-fast bacillus smear and culture, amylase, and bilirubin levels should be repeated in these patients.

c. Ascitic fluid total protein level may further clarify etiology or provide prognostic information.

   (1) Ascitic protein >2.5 in patient with portal hypertension is consistent with cardiac cirrhosis.

   (2) Ascitic protein <1.0 imparts high risk of spontaneous bacterial peritonitis because it indicates fluid depleted of all proteins including complement and opsonins.

   (3) Polymicrobial infection with an ascitic protein greater than 1.0 suggests bowel perforation, requiring surgical intervention.

d. Therapy.

   (1) Cefotaxime is the agent of choice for empiric therapy of spontaneous bacterial peritonitis. Quinolones can prevent recurrent episodes.

   (2) Therapy for transudative ascites.

      (a) Sodium restriction to 88 mM/day.

      (b) Initiation of diuresis with a potassium-sparing and potassium-wasting diuretic combination.

         i. Start with spironolactone 100 mg and furosemide 40 mg each morning.

        ii. Dosage may be increased every 2 or 3 days (while keeping this dosage ratio the same to prevent potassium disequilibrium) to a maximum of 400 mg of spironolactone and 160 mg of furosemide daily.

       iii. Ideally, weight should be monitored daily and daily urinary excretion should be estimated by multiplying a spot urine sodium value by the daily urinary volume.

       iv. Optimal dosing is achieved when the patient excretes in excess of 88 mL of sodium per day and is losing 0.5 kg in weight per day.

        v. More aggressive diuresis can lead to the hepatorenal syndrome in patients with ascites who do not have peripheral edema.

   (3) Patients with tense ascites causing dyspnea or dyspepsia should undergo large-volume (i.e., 5 L) paracentesis.

(4) Patients who are refractory to conservative management may be candidates for:
    (a) Surgical or transjugular intrahepatic portosystemic stent shunting.
    (b) Extracorporeal ultrafiltration of ascites fluid.
    (c) Liver transplantation.
2. Esophageal variceal bleeding is the second most common complication of cirrhosis, affecting 30% of patients.
  a. Therapy of acute bleeding.
    (1) Hospitalize.
    (2) Temporizing measures before definitive treatment with endoscopic sclerotherapy in patients with active bleeding and hemodynamic compromise.
      (a) IV vasopressin.
        i. Give 20-U load over 20 minutes followed by 0.4 U/min drip.
        ii. Vasopressin causes splanchnic vasocontriction to reduce portal hypertension.
      (b) IV nitroglycerin.
        i. Give 40 µg/min or dose titrated to a systolic pressure of approximately 100 mg Hg.
        ii. Combats side effects of vasopressin, particularly coronary ischemia.
    (3) Volume replacement with packed red blood cells. IV fluids are contraindicated because they can increase variceal engorgement and exacerbate bleeding.
    (4) For treatment failure, consider balloon tamponade of the bleeding site with a Sengstaken-Blakemore tube.
  b. Definitive therapy for all variceal bleeds, whether active or controlled, is endoscopic intravariceal sclerotherapy. Failure to treat with sclerotherapy leads to an expected 12-month recurrence rate of 70%.
  c. Prophylaxis against initial or recurrent variceal bleeding.
    (1) Oral β-blockers (propranolol, nadolol): Dose titrated to a 20% decrease in heart rate (but not below 55 beats/minute) reduces incidence of initial and recurrent variceal bleeding with a possible mortality benefit.
    (2) Invasive therapy.
      (a) Transjugular intrahepatic porosystemic shunt attempts to reduce portal vein and hepatic vein pressure gradient to <12 mm Hg (level below which esophageal variceal bleeds become uncommon).
      (b) Total portal venous shunting can cause ischemic liver failure, so some portal flow to the liver should be preserved.
3. Hepatic encephalopathy implies altered mental status and neurologic function secondary to hepatic failure.
  a. Precipitants.
    (1) Medications such as central nervous system depressants and benzodiazepines.
    (2) Upper GI bleeding.
    (3) Azotemia.

(4) Infection.

(5) High-protein diet.

(6) Overdiuresis.

(7) Constipation.

(8) Progression of underlying liver disease.

b. Exact biochemical mediators of hepatic encephalopathy are not known.

(1) A cerebrospinal fluid glutamine is useful in diagnosis.

(2) Serum ammonia (NH_3) levels can help monitor therapy somewhat.

c. Treatment.

(1) Dietary protein restriction and substitution of vegetable proteins for animal proteins.

(2) Promotion of GI ammonia excretion with lactulose 30 mL orally several times per day titrated to a production of two loose stools daily.

(3) Reduction of colonic bacteria that produce ammonia with neomycin (1 g orally every 6 hours) for patients unresponsive to lactulose alone.

4. The hepatorenal syndrome is impaired renal function (despite histologically normal kidneys) as a consequence of hepatic disease. The syndrome probably occurs as a result of humoral mediators that promote renal vasoconstriction.

a. Oliguria: A low urine sodium and failure of azotemia to respond to a volume challenge are hallmarks of this condition.

b. Mortality is 90% during hospitalization in which the condition is diagnosed unless the patient is a candidate for liver transplantation, which is the only definitive treatment.

c. Temporizing measures while awaiting liver transplantation include renal dosed IV dopamine in an effort to improve renal perfusion and combat oliguria.

Hemochromatosis

1. Phlebotomy.

a. Weekly phlebotomy.

(1) One or two units of blood, each containing approximately 250 mg of iron.

(2) Continue for several weeks until iron stores are depleted (ferritin level <50 μg/mL and transferring saturation <30%).

b. Subsequent phlebotomies can be performed as needed to maintain a transferrin saturation <50% and a ferritin level <100 μg/L.

2. Desferoxamine (iron-chelating agent).

a. Desferoxamine is generally reserved for patients with severe hemochromatosis with diffuse organ involvement (e.g., liver disease, heart disease) and when phlebotomy is not possible.

b. It is administered in a dose of 0.5 to 1 g IM qd or 20 mg SC over a 12- to 24-hour period with a constant infusion pump.

Primary Biliary Cirrhosis

1. Ursodiol 12 to 15 mg/kg daily, divided or as one bedtime dose.

a. Can extend survival and lengthen the time before liver transplantation in early disease.

  b. Normalizes bilirubin.
  c. Can mask need for transplantation.
  d. Safe and well tolerated.
  e. Relieves pruritus in some patients, although it can initially exacerbate pruritus.
  f. In patients with advanced disease, ursodiol is ineffective and can actually worsen the disease.
2. Colchicine (0.6 mg bid) and methotrexate (15 mg/week).
  a. These drugs yield less impressive results but are still modestly effective.
  b. Patients with primary biliary cirrhosis on methotrexate need to be monitored for development of interstitial pneumonitis, which resolves with discontinuation of the drug.
3. About 20% of patients do not respond to medical therapy and might need liver transplantation.

Nonalcoholic Liver Disease with Fibrosis

1. Diet to lose weight.
2. Exercise.
3. Metformin and thioglitazones appear promising.

Wilson's Disease

1. Penicillamine 0.75 to 1.5 g/day divided bid with pyridoxine 25 mg/day (chelator).
2. Trientine 1 to 2 g/day divided tid (chelator).
3. Zinc 50 mg tid (inhibits copper absorption).

Hepatitis B and C

Treatment of Hepatitis B and C is preferably initiated before cirrhosis develops.
1. Hepatitis B.
  (1) Interferon (IFN)-α.
  (2) Antiviral agents (e.g., lamivudine).
2. Hepatitis C.
  (1) IFN-α monotherapy.
  (2) IFN-α and ribavirin.
  (3) Pegylated interferons.

SUGGESTED READINGS

Bayard M, Holt J, Boroughs E. Nonalcoholic fatty liver disease. *Am Fam Physician* 73:1961-1968, 2006.

Brandhagen DJ, Fairbanks VF, Baldus W: Recognition and management of hereditary hemochromatosis. *Am Fam Physician* 65:853-860, 2002.

Gines P, Cardenas A, Arroyo V, Rodes J: Management of cirrhosis and ascites. *N Engl J Med* 350:1645-1654, 2004.

Kaplan MM, Gershwin ME: Primary biliary cirrhosis. *N Engl J Med* 353:1261-1272, 2005.

Levy C, Lindor KD: Management of osteoporosis, fat-soluble vitamin deficiencies, and hyperlipidemia in primary biliary cirrhosis. *Clin Liver Dis* 7(4):901-910, 2003.

Ong JP, Aggarwal A, Kriger D, et al: Correlation between ammonia levels and the severity of hepatic encephalopathy. *Am J Med* 114(3):188-193, 2003.

Pietrangelo A: Hereditary hemochromatosis—a new look at an old disease. *N Eng J Med* 350:2383-2397, 2004.

Selmi C, Invernizzi P, Keefe EB, et al: Epidemiology and pathogenesis of primary biliary cirrhosis. *J Clin Gastroenterol* 38(3):264-271, 2004.

DYSPHAGIA

Susan Berner, Arvind Modawal, and Tom J. Wachtel

Definition

Dysphagia is difficulty in swallowing. It can be caused by problems in transferring the food bolus from the oropharynx to the upper esophagus or by impairment in transport of the bolus through the body of the esophagus.

Epidemiology

1. Affects 7% to 10% of people older than 50 years.
2. About 30% to 40% of nursing home patients experience some amount of dysphagia.
3. About 25% of hospitalized patients experience problems swallowing.

Clinical Findings

1. History.
   a. A thorough history often gives clues to the site of the lesion and nature of the problem and leads to the diagnosis in 80% to 85% of the cases of dysphagia.
   b. Ask:
      (1) Are symptoms progressive or intermittent?
      (2) What is the duration and course of the dysphagia?
      (3) What type of food causes dysphagia?
      (4) What are the symptoms? Patients often report food "sticking" after swallowing or have to repeat swallows to relieve the dysphagia.
      (5) Is there any substernal pain or heartburn on swallowing?
      (6) What is the medication history?
      (7) Are there any associated symptoms, such as aspiration, weight loss, nasal regurgitation, unilateral wheezing, or chest pain?
2. Physical examination.
   a. Skin exam for signs of collagen vascular disease, such as scleroderma.
   b. Oral cavity and pharynx exam for lesions causing obstruction or painful swallowing (mucositis).
   c. Neck and axillae exam for thyroid swelling, lymph nodes, or tumor.
   d. Pulmonary exam for unilateral wheezing, aspiration pneumonia, foreign body, or mass.
   e. Neurologic exam for signs of a neuromuscular disease, cerebrovascular accident, Parkinson's disease, or tardive dyskinesia.
   f. Abdominal exam for liver and other organomegaly or masses.
   g. Psychiatric exam for evidence of anxiety or depression.

Etiology

1. Oropharyngeal dysphasia may be due to a variety of mechanical and neuromuscular conditions.
2. Esophageal dysphagia may be due to mechanical lesions or motility disorders.

Work-up

1. Laboratory tests are necessary in some cases of metabolic disorders (thyrotoxicosis, Cushing's) to identify infections (candidiasis, herpes).
2. Oropharyngeal dysphagia.
   a. Barium esophagography.
   b. Manometry can be used with barium swallow.
3. Esophageal dysphagia.
   a. Upper endoscopy is the procedure of choice.
   b. Esophageal manometry and pH.

Treatment

1. Oropharyngeal dysphagia.
   a. Treat the underlying neuromuscular or metabolic disorder.
   b. Adjust diet as tolerated.
   c. Show the patient swallowing techniques designed to strengthen muscles used in swallowing.
   d. Eliminate medications known to cause or worsen dysphagia, including NSAIDs, potassium tablets, doxycycline, and bisphosphonates.
   e. Gastrostomy tubes are not proven to reduce the risk of aspiration pneumonia.
2. Esophageal dysphagia.
   a. Motility disorders can be treated with balloon dilators for the lower esophageal sphincter (LES) or injections of botulinum toxin.
   b. Dilation of benign strictures or rings.

SUGGESTED READINGS

American Gastroenterological Association: American Gastroenterological Association medical position statement on management of oropharyngeal dysphagia. *Gastroenterology* 116:452-454, 1999.

Enzinger P, Mayer RJ: Esophageal cancer. *N Engl J Med* 349:2241-2252, 2003.

Lowe RC, Wolfe MM: Esophageal disorders. In Andreoli TE, Carpenter CCJ, Griggs RC, Benjamin IJ (eds.): *Andreoli and Carpenter's Cecil Essentials of Medicine*, 7th ed. Philadelphia, Saunders Elsevier, 2007, pp 384-389.

Spieker MR: Evaluating dysphagia. *Am Fam Physician*, 61:3639-3648, 2000.

FUNCTIONAL GASTROINTESTINAL DISORDERS

Peter S. Margolis, Fred F. Ferri, and Tom J. Wachtel

Nonulcer Dyspepsia

Definitions

1. Dyspeptic pain.
   a. Location.
      (1) Midepigastric.
      (2) Upper abdominal.
      (3) Possible right upper quadrant.
   b. Character is variable.
      (1) Sharp or dull ache.
      (2) Crampy.
      (3) Bloating.
      (4) Burning (most common).

   c. Timing.
     (1) Usually related to meals, either 30 to 60 minutes postprandial or awaking at night.
     (2) Weekly to daily.
2. Nausea.
   a. Very frequent.
   b. Can occur with or without pain.
   c. Postprandial (either immediate or late).
3. Associated symptoms.
   a. Belching.
   b. Bloating.
   c. Flatulence.
   d. Change of appetite.
   e. Changes of weight.

Epidemiology

1. The many symptoms that characterize dyspepsia are very common complaints in the elderly.
2. The prevalence of these symptoms can reach as high as 25% of this population.
3. This prevalence is equal among men and women age 65 years or older.
4. Most elderly persons who experience dyspeptic symptoms report the onset within the previous 5 years.

Etiology

1. The cause is often multifactorial, but functional/motility disorders are the most common.
2. The following are important risk factors or associations:
   a. Smoking.
   b. *Helicobacter pylori* infection.
   c. Alcohol.
   d. Changes in eating arrangements or lifestyle.
   e. Depression.
3. Aspirin and other NSAIDs.
   a. Very important risk factors, with approximately 100 million prescribed annually.
   b. Most likely medication to cause dyspepsia in elderly persons.
4. Medications (excluding NSAIDs).
   a. People 65 years and older represent 10% to 15% of the population yet receive >25% of prescription medication in the United States.
   b. Many medications cause reproducible nausea (side effect).
   c. Other causes include idiosyncratic responses in individual patients.

Work-up

1. History and physical exam.
2. Medication review (prescribed and over-the-counter drugs).
3. Upper endoscopy (EGD).
   a. EGD is more sensitive and specific than upper GI (UGI) studies.
   b. EGD allows biopsy and therapy if needed.
4. Upper GI radiology (UGI).
   a. UGI can complement EGD in selected patients.

b. UGI may be more accessible in rural settings.

Treatment

1. Consensus is to initiate therapy and work-up together.
   a. Discontinue offending agents.
   b. Treat infrequent or mild symptoms with occasional antacid and/or simethicone.
   c. Frequent or more severe symptoms.
      (1) H_2-receptor antagonists (H2RA).
      (2) Proton pump inhibitor (PPI).
   d. Duration of therapy and dosage depends on endoscopic findings.
2. Prophylaxis if NSAIDs are needed.
   a. Remains controversial.
   b. Ranitidine can prevent duodenal ulcer.
   c. Mesoprostil (Cytotech) can prevent both gastric and duodenal ulcers.
3. H. pylori infection.
   a. Cause of PUD.
   b. Eradication recommended for documented ulcer disease.
   c. Possible cause of nonulcer dyspepsia (controversial).

Irritable Bowel Syndrome

Definition

Irritable bowel syndrome (IBS) is a chronic functional disorder manifested by alteration in bowel habits and recurrent abdominal pain and bloating.

Epidemiology

1. IBS occurs in 20% of the population of industrialized countries.
2. It is responsible for >50% of GI referrals.
3. Worldwide adult prevalence is 12%.
4. Female-to-male ratio is 2:1.
5. Nearly 50% of patients have psychiatric abnormalities, with anxiety disorders being most common.
6. Frequent other associated syndromes.
   a. Fibromyalgia.
   b. Chronic fatigue syndrome.
   c. Headaches (migraine or tension).
   d. Temporomandibular joint disorder and bruxism.
   e. Interstitial cystitis.
   f. Dyspareunia and low libido.

Clinical Findings

1. The clinical presentation of IBS consists of abdominal pain and abnormalities of defecation.
   a. Presentation can include loose stools, usually after meals and in the morning, alternating with episodes of constipation.
   b. When diarrhea is present, it almost never wakes up the patient at night.
2. Physical examination is generally normal.
3. Nonspecific abdominal tenderness and distention may be present.
4. Rome II criteria for diagnosis of IBS.
   a. Symptoms at least 12 weeks or more, which need not be consecutive, in the preceding 12 months.

b. Symptoms include abdominal discomfort or pain that has 2 of 3 features:
  (1) Symptoms relieved with defecation.
  (2) Onset associated with a change in frequency of stool.
  (3) Onset associated with a change in form (appearance) of stool.
5. Symptoms that cumulatively support the diagnosis of IBS.
  a. Abnormal stool frequency (>3 bowel movements per day or <3 per week).
  b. Abnormal stool form (lumpy/hard or loose/watery stool).
  c. Abnormal stool passage (straining, urgency, or feeling of incomplete evacuation).
  d. Passage of mucus.
  e. Bloating or feeling of abdominal distention.

Etiology

1. Unknown.
2. Associated pathophysiology includes altered GI motility and increased gut sensitivity.

Differential Diagnosis

1. Inflammatory bowel disease.
2. Diverticulitis.
3. Colon malignancy.
4. PUD.
5. Biliary liver disease.
6. Chronic pancreatitis.

Work-up

1. Diagnostic workup is aimed primarily at excluding the conditions listed in the differential diagnosis.
2. Red flags that signal the possibility of other diseases are important to identify.
  a. Weight loss.
  b. Rectal bleeding.
  c. Onset late in life.
  d. Fever.
  e. Nocturnal pain.
  f. Family history of GI malignancy.
3. In selected cases, some or all of the following may be appropriate:
  a. Blood tests.
    (1) ESR.
    (2) CBC.
    (3) Biochemistry profile.
    (4) Serology for celiac disease.
    (5) TSH.
    (6) Serology for H. pylori.
    (7) Carcinoembryonic antigen.
  b. Stool tests.
    (1) Occult blood.
    (2) Ova and parasites.
    (3) Culture.

   c. Imaging.
     (1) Abdominal ultrasound.
     (2) Abdominal CT.
     (3) Barium enema.
     (4) Upper GI series with small bowel follow-through.
   d. Endoscopy.
     (1) Upper endoscopy.
     (2) Colonoscopy.

Treatment

1. Fiber.
   a. The mainstay of treatment of IBS is a high-fiber diet. Because symptoms are chronic, laxatives should be avoided.
   b. Fiber supplementation may be necessary in some patients.
     (1) Psyllium seed husks (Metamucil) titrated from 1 teaspoon qd to 1 tablespoon bid.
     (2) Calcium polycarbophil (FiberCon) 2 tablets one to four times daily followed by 8 oz of water.
   c. Patients should be instructed that there might be some increased bloating on initiation of fiber supplementation, which should resolve within 2 to 3 weeks.
   d. It is important that patients take these fiber products on a regular basis and not only prn.
2. GI medication.
   a. Antispasmodics and anticholinergics may be useful in refractory cases (e.g., dicyclomine [Bentyl] 10-20 mg up to three times daily).
3. Psychotherapeutic treatment.
   a. Behavioral therapy is recommended, particularly in younger patients, because psychosocial stressors are important triggers of IBS.
   b. Patients who appear anxious can benefit from use of SSRIs.
   c. Tricyclic antidepressants in low doses are also effective in some patients with IBS, but they are constipating.
4. Patients should be reassured that their condition does not lead to cancer.

Prognosis

1. More than 60% of patients respond successfully to treatment over the initial 12 months.
2. However, IBS is a chronic relapsing condition and requires prolonged therapy.

SUGGESTED READINGS

Arents NL, Thijs JC, van Zwet AA, et al: Approach to treatment of dyspepsia in primary care: A randomized trial comparing "test-and-treat" with prompt endoscopy. Arch Intern Med 163:1606-1612, 2003.

Cremonini F, Talley NJ: Irritable bowel syndrome: Epidemiology, natural history, health care seeking and emerging risk factors. Gastroenterol Clin North Am 34: 189-204, 2005.

Fass R, Fullerton S, Naliboff B, et al: Sexual dysfunction in patients with irritable bowel syndrome and non-ulcer dyspepsia. Digestion 59:79-85, 1998.

Fisher RS, Parkman HP: Management of nonulcer dyspepsia. N Engl J Med 339:1376-1381, 1998.

Hadley SK, Gaarder SM: Treatment of irritable bowel syndrome. *Am Fam Physician* 72:2501-2506, 2005.

Jaakkimainen RL, Boyle E, Tudiver F: Is *Helicobacter pylori* associated with non-ulcer dyspepsia and will eradication improve symptoms? A meta-analysis. *BMJ* 319:1040-1044, 1999.

Jackson JL, O'Malley PG, Tomkins G, et al: Treatment of functional gastrointestinal disorders with antidepressant medications: A meta-analysis. *Am J Med* 108:65-72, 2000.

Kay L: Prevalence, incidence and prognosis of gastrointestinal symptoms in a random sample of an elderly population. *Age Ageing* 23:146-149, 1994.

Markowitz M, Harris W, Ricci JF, et al: Comorbid conditions in patients with irritable bowel syndrome: Data from a national IBS awareness registry. *Gastroenterology* 120(Suppl 1):105, 2001.

Mertz HR: Irritable bowel syndrome. *N Engl J Med* 349(22):2136-2146, 2003.

Talley NJ, Boyce P, Jones M: Dyspepsia and health care seeking in a community: How important are psychological factors? *Dig Dis Sci* 43:1016-1022, 1998.

Talley NJ, Silverstein MD, Agreus L, et al: AGA technical review: Evaluation of dyspepsia. *Gastroenterology* 114:582-595, 1998.

Vandvik PO, Aabakken L, Farup PG: Diagnosing irritable bowel syndrome: Poor agreement between general practitioners and the Rome II criteria. *Scand J Gastroenterol* 39:448-453, 2004.

Viera AJ, Hoag S, Shaughnessy J: Management of irritable bowel syndrome. *Am Fam Physician* 66:1867-1874, 2002.

Whitehead WE, Palsson O, Jones KR: Systematic review of the comorbidity of irritable bowel syndrome with other disorders: What are the causes and implications? *Gastroenterology* 122:1140-1156, 2002.

GASTROESOPHAGEAL REFLUX DISEASE

Fred F. Ferri and Tom J. Wachtel

Definition

Gastroesophageal reflux disease (GERD) is an upper GI motility disorder characterized primarily by heartburn and caused by the reflux of gastric contents into the esophagus.

Epidemiology

GERD is one of the most prevalent GI disorders.

1. Nearly 7% of persons in the United States experience heartburn daily, 20% experience it monthly, and 60% experience it intermittently.

2. Nearly 20% of adults use antacids or over-the-counter H_2-blockers at least once a week for relief of heartburn.

Clinical Findings

1. Clinical signs and symptoms.
   a. Heartburn.
   b. Dysphagia.
   c. Sour taste.
   d. Regurgitation of gastric contents into the mouth.
2. Chronic cough and bronchospasm.
3. Nasal congestion, rhinorrhea, and other symptoms of rhinosinusitis.
4. Other symptoms.
   a. Chest pain.
   b. Laryngitis.
   c. Early satiety.
   d. Abdominal fullness and bloating with belching.

5. Symptom response to acid suppressant therapy.
6. Physical examination is generally unremarkable.

Etiology

1. Incompetent LES.
2. Medications that lower LES pressure.
   a. Calcium channel blockers (CCBs).
   b. β-Adrenergic blockers.
   c. Theophylline.
   d. Anticholinergics.
3. Foods that lower LES pressure.
   a. Chocolate.
   b. Yellow onions.
   c. Peppermint.
   d. Tomato sauce.
4. Tobacco abuse, alcohol, coffee.
5. Gastric acid hypersecretion.
6. Hiatal hernia (controversial) is present in more than 70% of patients with GERD; however, most patients with hiatal hernia are asymptomatic.

Work-up

The work-up is aimed at eliminating the conditions noted in the differential diagnosis and documenting the type and extent of tissue damage.

1. Upper GI endoscopy.
   a. Upper GI endoscopy is useful to document the type and extent of tissue damage in GERD and to exclude potentially premalignant conditions such as Barrett's esophagus or esophageal cancer.
   b. The American College of Gastroenterology recommends endoscopy to screen for Barrett's esophagus in patients who have chronic GERD symptoms.
   c. The data demonstrating the cost-effectiveness of endoscopic screening remain controversial.
2. Laboratory tests.
   a. Esophageal pH 24-hour monitoring and the Bernstein test are sensitive diagnostic tests; however, they are not very practical and are generally not done. They are useful in patients with atypical manifestations of GERD, such as chest pain or chronic cough.
   b. Esophageal manometry is indicated in patients with refractory reflux in whom surgical therapy is planned.
3. Imaging studies.
   a. An upper GI series can identify ulcerations and strictures; however, it can miss mucosal abnormalities.
   b. Only one third of patients with GERD have radiographic signs of esophagitis.

Differential Diagnosis

1. PUD.
2. Unstable angina.
3. Esophagitis.
   a. Caused by infections such as herpes or *Candida*.
   b. Induced by medication such as doxycycline or potassium chloride.
4. Esophageal spasm (nutcracker esophagus).

5. Cancer of esophagus.
6. Barrett's esophagus and esophageal cancer.
   a. There is a strong and probably causal relation between symptomatic prolonged and untreated GERD, Barrett's esophagus, and esophageal adenocarcinoma.
   b. GI referral for upper endoscopy is needed when there are concerns about associated PUD, Barrett's esophagus, or esophageal cancer.
   c. A single lifetime esophageal endoscopy is appropriate in any patient with chronic GERD to rule out Barrett's esophagus.
   d. Patients with Barrett's esophagus should probably undergo surveillance endoscopy with mucosal biopsy every 2 years or less because the risk of developing adenocarcinoma of esophagus is at least 30 times greater than that of the general population; however, the effectiveness of such a strategy to reduce esophageal cancer mortality has not been demonstrated.

Treatment

1. Nonpharmacologic therapy.
   a. Lifestyle modifications.
      (1) Avoidance of foods that exacerbate reflux.
         (a) Citrus-based products.
         (b) Tomato-based products.
      (2) Avoidance of drugs that exacerbate reflux.
         (a) Caffeine.
         (b) β-Blockers.
         (c) CCBs.
         (d) α-Adrenergic agonists.
         (e) Theophylline.
   b. Avoidance of tobacco and alcohol.
   c. Elevation of head of bed (4 to 8 inches) using blocks.
   d. Avoidance of lying down directly after late or large evening meals.
   e. Weight reduction, decreased fat intake.
   f. Avoidance of clothing that is tight around the waist.
   g. Lifestyle modification must be followed lifelong, because this is generally an irreversible condition.
2. Pharmacologic treatment.
   a. PPIs are safe, tolerated, and very effective in most patients.
      (1) Esomeprazole 40 mg qd.
      (2) Omeprazole 20 mg qd.
      (3) Lansoprazole 30 mg qd.
      (4) Rabeprazole 20 mg qd.
      (5) Pantoprazole 40 mg qd.
   b. H_2-blockers can be used but are generally much less effective than PPIs.
      (1) Nizatidine 300 mg qhs.
      (2) Famotidine 40 mg qhs.
      (3) Ranitidine 300 mg qhs.
      (4) Cimetidine 800 mg qhs.
   c. Antacids may be useful for relief of mild symptoms; however, they are generally ineffective in severe cases of reflux.

    d. Prokinetic agents (metoclopramide) are indicated only when PPIs are not fully effective. They can be used in combination therapy; however, side effects limit their use.

    e. Recurrence of reflux is common if treatment is discontinued.

3. Surgical management.

    a. Surgery with Nissen fundoplication for refractory cases.

      (1) Potential surgical candidates should have reflux esophagitis documented by EGD and normal esophageal motility as evaluated by manometry.

      (2) Surgery generally consists of reduction of hiatal hernia when present and placement of a gastric wrap around the gastroesophageal junction (fundoplication).

      (3) Laparoscopic fundoplication is now widely used.

      (4) Surgery should not be advised with the expectation that patients with GERD will no longer need to take antisecretory medications or that the procedure will prevent esophageal cancer among those with GERD and Barrett's esophagus.

    b. Newer procedures.

      (1) Endoscopic radiofrequency heating of the gastroesophageal junction (Stretta procedure) is a newer treatment modality for GERD patients unresponsive to traditional therapy, but its mechanism of action remains unclear.

      (2) Endoscopy gastroplasty (EndoCinch procedure) also aims at treating GERD. Initial results appear encouraging.

      (3) Long-term studies are needed before recommending these procedures.

    c. Postsurgical complications.

      (1) Complications occur in nearly 20% of patients.

        (a) Dysphagia.

        (b) Gas.

        (c) Bloating.

        (d) Diarrhea.

        (e) Nausea.

      (2) Long-term follow-up studies reveal that within 3 to 5 years, 52% of patients who had undergone antireflux surgery are taking antireflux medications again.

SUGGESTED READINGS

Heidelbaugh JJ, Nostrant TT, Kim C, Van Harrison R: Management of gastroesophageal reflux disease. *Am Fam Physician* 68:1311-1318, 2003.

Kanrilas PJ: Radiofrequency energy treatment of GERD. *Gastroenterology* 125:970-973, 2003.

Shaheen N, Ransohoff DF: Gastroesophageal reflux, Barrett esophagus, and esophageal cancer: Clinical applications. *JAMA* 287:1982-1986, 2002.

NONALCOHOLIC FATTY LIVER DISEASE

Fred F. Ferri and Tom J. Wachtel

Definition

1. Nonalcoholic fatty liver disease (NAFLD and nonalcoholic steatohepatitis [NASH]) are liver diseases, occurring in patients who do not abuse alcohol.

2. NASH is manifested histologically by mononuclear cells and/or poly-morphonuclear cells, hepatocyte ballooning, and spotty necrosis.

Epidemiology

1. NAFLD affects 10% to 24% of the general population.
2. Prevalence is increased in obese persons (57% to 74%) and in patients with the metabolic syndrome (type 2 diabetes mellitus, obesity, and hyperlipidemia).
3. NASH is the most common noniatrogenic cause of abnormal liver test results in adults in the United States. It accounts for up to 90% of cases of asymptomatic ALT elevations.
4. About 30 million obese adults have steatosis (NAFLD); 8.6 million may have steatohepatitis (NASH). How many patients with NASH progress to cirrhosis is unknown, but it is now believed that most cases of cryptogenic cirrhosis are the long-term outcome of steatohepatitis.
5. Older age is an important risk factor for progression to liver fibrosis and cirrhosis.

Clinical Findings

1. Most patients are asymptomatic.
2. Patients sometimes report a sensation of fullness or discomfort on the right side of the upper abdomen.
3. Nonspecific complaints of fatigue or malaise may be reported.
4. Hepatomegaly is generally the only positive finding on physical examination.

Etiology

Insulin resistance is believed to be causally involved in the development of NAFLD.

Differential Diagnosis

1. Alcohol-induced liver disease.
   a. A daily alcohol intake of 20 g in women and 30 g in men may be enough to cause alcohol-induced liver disease.
   b. Ten grams of alcohol is approximately equivalent to 1 oz of distilled spirits, 12 oz of beer, or 4 oz of wine.
2. Viral hepatitis.
3. Autoimmune hepatitis.
4. Toxin or drug-induced liver disease (including statin therapy).
5. Any other cause of transaminase elevation.
6. All other causes of cirrhosis (see earlier).

Work-up

1. Laboratory tests.
   a. Elevated ALT and AST: AST/ALT ratio is usually less than 1, but it can increase as fibrosis advances.
   b. Negative serology for infectious hepatitis.
      (1) Generally normal γ-glutamyl transpeptidase (GGTP).
      (2) Generally normal serum alkaline phosphatase.
   c. Blood lipids (primarily triglycerides) may be elevated.
   d. Glucose levels may be elevated.
   e. Prolonged PT, hypoalbuminuria, and elevated bilirubin may be present in advanced stages.

2. Imaging studies.
   a. Ultrasound generally reveals diffuse increase in echogenicity as compared with that of the kidneys.
   b. CT scan reveals diffuse low-density hepatic parenchyma.
   c. MRI can conform the fatty nature of any questionable finding on ultrasound or CT but this is usually not necessary.
3. Liver biopsy.
   a. Liver biopsy may show a wide spectrum of liver damage, ranging from simple steatosis to advanced fibrosis and cirrhosis.
   b. It is the only way to differentiate fatty liver, steatohepatitis, and cirrhosis.
   c. Liver biopsy will confirm the diagnosis and provide prognostic information.
   d. Biopsy should be considered in patients with suspected advanced liver fibrosis.
   e. Some clinicians recommend it in all elderly patients (e.g., older than 50 years) with NAFLD.

Treatment

1. Diet and exercise are proven effective.
2. No medications have been proved to directly improve liver damage from NAFLD.
3. Medications to control hyperlipidemia (e.g., fenofibrates for elevated triglycerides) and hyperglycemia (e.g., metformin and thioglitazone) can lead to improvement in abnormal liver test results.

SUGGESTED READINGS

Angulo P: Nonalcoholic fatty liver disease. N Engl J Med 346:1221-1231, 2002.
Bayard M, Boroughs E: Nonalcoholic fatty liver disease. Am Fam Physician 73:1961-1968, 2006.
Clark JM, Diehl AM: Nonalcoholic fatty liver disease: An underrecognized cause of cryptogenic cirrhosis. JAMA 289:3000-3004, 2003.
Neuschwander-Tetri BA, Brunt EM, Wehmeier KR, et al: Improved nonalcoholic steatohepatitis after 48 weeks of treatment with the PPAR-γ ligand rosiglitazone. Hepatology 38:1008-1017, 2003.
Promat K, Lutchman G, Uwaifo G, et al: A pilot study of pioglitazone treatment for nonalcoholic steatohepatitis. Hepatology 39:188-196, 2004.
Shadid S, Jenson MD: Effect of pioglitazone on biochemical indices of non-alcoholic fatty liver disease in upper body obesity. Clin Gastroenterol Hepatol 1:384-387, 2003.

PEPTIC ULCER DISEASE

Fred F. Ferri, with revisions by Tom J. Wachtel

Definition

PUD is an ulceration in the stomach or duodenum resulting from an imbalance between mucosal protective factors and various mucosal damaging mechanisms (see later).

Epidemiology

1. Overall incidence is 250,000 to 500,000.
   a. Incidence of duodenal ulcer is 200,000 to 400,000.
   b. Incidence of gastric ulcer is 50,000 to 100,000.
   c. The ratio of duodenal ulcer to gastric ulcer incidence is 4:1.

2. Anatomic location.
   a. More than 90% of duodenal ulcers occur in the first portion of the duodenum.
   b. Gastric ulcer occurs most commonly in the lesser curvature near the incisura angularis.

Clinical Findings

1. Physical examination is often unremarkable.
2. Symptoms can include:
   a. Epigastric pain often worse in the fasting state and relieved by meals.
   b. GI bleeding (e.g., black stools or occult).
   c. Tachycardia.
   d. Pallor.
   e. Hypotension from acute or chronic blood loss.
   f. Nausea and vomiting if the pyloric channel is obstructed.
   g. Boardlike abdomen and rebound tenderness if the ulcer is perforated.
   h. Hematemesis or melena with a bleeding ulcer.

Etiology

Causes are often multifactorial. The following are common mucosal damaging factors:

1. *Helicobacter pylori* infection.
2. Medications (NSAIDs, glucocorticoids).
3. Incompetent pylorus or LES.
4. Bile acids.
5. Impaired proximal duodenal bicarbonate secretion.
6. Decreased blood flow to gastric mucosa.
7. Acid secreted by parietal cells and pepsin secreted as pepsinogen by chief cells.
8. Cigarette smoking.
9. Alcohol use.

Differential Diagnosis

1. GERD.
2. Cholelithiasis and complications.
3. Pancreatitis.
4. Gastritis.
5. Nonulcer dyspepsia.
6. Neoplasm.
   a. Gastric carcinoma.
   b. Lymphoma.
   c. Pancreatic carcinoma.
7. Cardiac pain.
   a. Angina pectoris.
   b. Myocardial infarction.
   c. Pericarditis.
8. Dissecting aneurysm.
9. Other.
   a. High small bowel obstruction.
   b. Pneumonia.

    c. Subphrenic abscess.

    d. Early appendicitis.

Work-up

1. Imaging.
   a. Esophagogastroduodenoscopy (EGD).
   b. Endoscopy is preferred over upper GI series for the following reasons:
      (1) Highest accuracy (approximately 90% to 95%).
      (2) Useful for identifying superficial or very small ulcerations.
      (3) Essential to diagnose gastric ulcers (1% to 4% of gastric ulcers diagnosed as benign by upper GI series are eventually diagnosed as gastric carcinoma).
      (4) Additional advantages over upper GI series include:
         (a) Biopsy of suspicious looking ulcers.
         (b) Electrocautery of bleeding ulcers.
         (c) Measurement of gastric pH in suspected gastrinoma (e.g., patient with multiple ulcers).
         (d) Diagnosis of esophagitis, gastritis, duodenitis.
         (e) Endoscopic biopsy for *H. pylori*.
   c. Upper GI series should be performed only if EGD is unavailable or refused by the patient. Sensitivity is only 70%, resulting in a substantial possibility of a false-negative test.
2. Laboratory tests.
   a. Anemia may be present in patients with significant GI bleeding.
   b. *H. pylori* testing via endoscopic biopsy.
      (1) Serologic testing for antibodies to *H. pylori* is easy and inexpensive.
      (2) However, the presence of antibodies demonstrates previous but not necessarily current infection. Antibodies to *H. pylori* can remain elevated for months to years after infection has cleared.
   c. Urea breath test.
      (1) The urea breath test documents active infection.
      (2) This test is more expensive and not as readily available as the antibody test.
      (3) Use of proton pump inhibitors within 2 weeks of the urea breath test can interfere with test results.
   d. A stool antigen test (*H. pylori* stool antigen) or specific antibody test may be performed.
   e. Histologic evaluation of endoscopic biopsy samples is currently the gold standard for accurate diagnosis of *H. pylori* infection.
   f. Additional laboratory evaluation is indicated only in specific cases.
      (1) Amylase level in suspected pancreatitis.
      (2) Serum gastrin level in suspected Zollinger-Ellison (Z-E) syndrome.
         (a) Screening for Z-E syndrome should be considered in patients with multiple recurrent ulcers.
         (b) In patients with Z-E, the serum gastrin level is greater than 1000 pg/mL and the basal acid output is usually greater than 15 mEq/h.

Treatment

Lifestyle modification.

    1. Stop cigarette smoking.

       (1) Cigarette smoking increases the risk of PUD.

       (2) Cigarette smoking decreases the healing rate and increases the frequency of recurrence.

  b. Avoid NSAIDs and alcohol.

  c. Special diets have been proved unrelated to ulcer development and healing, but the patient should avoid foods that cause symptoms.

2. Pharmacologic therapy.

  a. In patients testing positive for *H. pylori*, eradication of *H. pylori* can be accomplished with various regimens.

    (1) PPI bid (e.g., omeprazole 20 mg bid or lansoprazole 30 mg bid) plus clarithromycin 500 mg bid and amoxicillin 100 mg bid for 7 to 10 days.

    (2) PPI bid plus amoxicillin 500 mg bid plus metronidazole 500 mg bid for 7 to 10 days.

    (3) PPI bid plus clarithromycin 500 mg bid and metronidazole 500 mg bid for 7 days.

    (4) One-day quadruple therapy regimen consists of:

      (a) Two tablets of 262 mg bismuth subsalicylate qid.

      (b) One 500-mg metronidazole tablet qid.

      (c) One dose of 2 g amoxicillin suspension qid.

      (d) Two capsules of 30 mg lansoprazole.

    (5) A 5-day treatment with three antibiotics (amoxicillin 1 g bid, clarithromycin 250 mg bid, and metronidazole 400 mg bid) plus either lansoprazole 30 mg bid or ranitidine 300 mg bid is an efficacious cost-saving option for patients older than 55 years who have no prior history of PUD.

  b. Patients testing negative for *H. pylori* should be treated with antisecretory agents.

    (1) H_2 receptor antagonists (H_2RAs).

      (a) Cimetidine, ranitidine, famotidine, and nizatidine are all effective.

      (b) They are usually given in split dose or at nighttime.

    (2) PPIs also induce rapid healing. They are given once (or twice) daily.

    (3) Antacids and sucralfate are also effective agents for treating and preventing PUD.

    (4) Maintenance therapy with an H_2RA or a PPI is recommended for the geriatric population.

  c. Patients with gastric ulcers should have repeat endoscopy after 4 to 6 weeks of therapy to document healing and to test exfoliative cytology or to biopsy any suspicious areas for gastric carcinoma.

  d. Misoprostol (Cytotec) therapy (100 μg qid with food, increased to 200 μg qid if well tolerated) is useful for preventing NSAID-induced gastric ulcers in all patients on long-term NSAID therapy.

3. Surgical therapy.

  a. Surgery for refractory ulcers is now only rarely performed.

  b. It consists of highly selective vagotomy for duodenal ulcers or ulcer removal with antrectomy or hemigastrectomy without vagotomy for gastric ulcers.

SUGGESTED READINGS

Graham DY, Agrawal NM, Campbell DR, et al: Ulcer prevention in long-term users of nonsteroidal anti-inflammatory drugs: results of a double-blind, randomized, multicenter, active- and placebo-controlled study of misoprostol vs lansoprazole. *Arch Intern Med* 162:169-175, 2002.

Lai KC, Lam SK, Chu KM, et al: Lansoprazole for the prevention of recurrences of ulcer complications from long-term low-dose aspirin use. *N Eng J Med* 346:2033-2038, 2002.

Lara LF, Cisneros G, Gurney M, et al: One day quadruple therapy compared with 7-day triple therapy for *Helicobacter pylori* infection. *Arch Intern Med* 163:2079-2084, 2003.

Optimal Pharmacotherapy

Marsha D. Fretwell
Deborah Adams Wingate

6.1 Background Statements

1. Parameters used to determine the appropriate medication.
   a. Pharmacodynamic changes related to age.
   b. Potential functional impact of a drug.
   c. Effect medication might have on patient's quality of life.
2. Choosing the correct dose for each medication must incorporate both pharmacokinetic and pharmacodynamic parameters applied to each patient.
   a. Larger volume of distribution for fat-soluble medications.
   b. Reduced renal excretion of medications: The average 85-year-old patient has a creatinine clearance of 35 mL/min.
   c. Multiple medications competing for the same metabolic site in the liver.
   d. Reduced physiologic and functional reserve (in the brain and bladder; cardiovascular and renal function).
3. Educate patient and/or caregiver about expected outcomes and possible side effects. The pharmacist can contribute significantly in this process.
4. Monitor and document the use of medications including PRN and over-the-counter drugs.

SUGGESTED READING

Gurwitz J, Monane M, Monane S, Avorn J: Polypharmacy. In Morris JN, Lipsitz LA, Murphy K, Belleville-Taylor P (eds): *Quality Care in the Nursing Home*. St Louis, Mosby-Yearbook, 1997, pp 13-25.

6.2 Principles of Clinical Management for Optimal Pharmacotherapy

1. Think of medications as external or environmental agents that can have either a positive or negative impact on patient's health and function.
2. Initiate all medication trials within the framework of preserving cognitive function and the patient's quality of life.
3. Use patient functional outcomes as the measure of drug efficacy.
4. Monitor drug levels. This is especially important in:
   a. Patients with impaired renal function.
   b. Patients taking more than two drugs metabolized by the liver.

5. Review all medications regularly.
   a. At every office or nursing home visit.
   b. Every day in the hospital.
6. If the patient is having a new problem, think first what you did to the patient. Do careful reviews of medications for any change.

SUGGESTED READINGS

Owens NJ, Silliman RA, Fretwell MD: A description of the relationship between comprehensive functional assessment and optimal pharmacotherapy in the older patient. *DCIP Ann Pharmacother* 23:847-853, 1989.

Gurwitz J, Monane M, Monane S, Avorn J: Polypharmacy. In Morris JN, Lipsitz LA, Murphy K, Belleville-Taylor P (eds): *Quality Care in the Nursing Home*. St Louis, Mosby-Yearbook, 1997, pp 13-25.

6.3 Assessment for Optimal Pharmacotherapy

1. Collect a comprehensive database.
   a. Interview the patient and family to establish the influence of the family caregiver on the patient's medication use.
   b. Review old charts, document all adverse drug reactions, calculate creatinine clearance (see Appendix I).
   c. List all medications, including over-the-counter drugs.
2. Integrate patient data and organize the problem list.
   a. List all diagnoses.
      (1) Link each medication to a documented diagnosis. Use this process to identify unnecessary medications or to add new diagnoses to the problem list.
      (2) Evaluate for appropriate medication choice (Box 6-1).
         (a) Functional impact of medication.
         (b) Quality of life.
         (c) Pharmacodynamics.
      (3) Evaluate for appropriate medication dosage.
         (a) Pharmacokinetics.
         (b) Pharmacodynamics.

BOX 6-1   **Potentially Inappropriate Medications for the Elderly According to the Revised Beers Criteria**

Alprazolam (Xanax)	Carisoprodol (Soma)
Amiodarone (Cordarone)	Cascara sagrada
Amitriptyline (Elavil)	Chlordiazepoxide (Librium, Mitran)
Amphetamines	
Anorexic agents	Chlordiazepoxide–amitripty-
Barbiturates	line (Limbitrol)
Belladonna alkaloids	Chlorpheniramine
(Donnatal)	(Chlor-Trimeton)
Bisacodyl (Dulcolax)	Chlorpropamide (Diabinese)

BOX 6-1   Potentially Inappropriate Medications for the
Elderly According to the Revised Beers Criteria—cont'd

Chlorzoxazone (Paraflex)
Cimetidine (Tagamet)
Clidinium–chlodizepoxide
  (Librax)
Clonidine (Catapres)
Clorazepate (Tranxene)
Cyclandelate (Cyclospasmol)
Cyclobenzaprine (Flexeril)
Cyproheptadine (Periactin)
Dessicated thyroid
Dexchlorpheniramine
  (Polaramine)
Diazepam (Valium)
Dicyclomine (Bentyl)
Digoxin (Lanoxin)
Diphenhydramine (Benadryl)
Dipyridamole (Persantine)
Disopyramide (Norpace,
  Norpace CR)
Doxazosin (Cardura)
Doxepin (Sinequan)
Ergot mesyloids (Hydergine)
Estrogens
Ethacrynic acid (Edecrin)
Ferrous sulfate (iron)
Fluoxetine (Prozac)
Flurazepam (Dalmane)
Guanadrel (Hylorel)
Guanethidine (Ismelin)
Halazepam (Paxipam)
Hydroxyzine (Vistaril, Atarax)
Hyoscyamine (Levsin,
  Levsinex)
Indomethacin (Indocin,
  Indocin SR)
Isoxsuprine (Vasodilan)
Ketorolac (Toradol)
Lorazepam (Ativan)

Meperidine (Demerol)
Meprobamate (Miltown,
  Equanil)
Mesoridazine (Serentil)
Metaxalone (Skelaxin)
Methocarbamol (Robaxin)
Methyldopa (Aldomet)
Methyldopa–hydrochloro-
  thiazide (Aldoril)
Methyltestoserone (Android,
  Virilon Testrad)
Mineral oil
Naproxen (Naprosyn,
  Avaprox, Aleve)
Neoloid
Nifedipine (Procardia,
  Adalat)
Nitrofurantoin (Macrodantin)
Orphenadrine (Norflex)
Oxaprozin (Daypro)
Oxazepam (Serax)
Oxybutynin (Ditropan)
Pentazocine (Talwin)
Perphenazine–amitriptyline
  (Triavil)
Piroxicam (Feldene)
Promethazine (Phenergan)
Propantheline (Pro-Banthine)
Propoxyphene (Darvon) and
  combination products
Quazepam (Doral)
Reserpine (Serpalan, Serpasil)
Temazepam (Restoril)
Thioridazine (Mellaril)
Ticlopidine (Ticlid)
Triazolam (Halcion)
Trimethobenzamide (Tigan)
Tripelennamine

Data from Fick DM, Cooper JW, Wade WE, et al: Updating the Beers criteria for
potentially inappropriate medication use in older adults: Results of a US consensus
panel of experts. *Arch Inter Med* 163:2716-2724, 2003.

b. Evaluate the functional impact of each medication on each area of concern (see Chapter 4).
   (1) Nutrition (nausea, anorexia, change in bowels).
   (2) Continence.
   (3) Defecation (constipation, diarrhea, bloating).
   (4) Cognition.
       (a) Evaluate whether patient is cognitively able to manage his or her own medications.
       (b) If the patient is impaired, evaluate functional impact of each medication, paying particular attention to any new medications.
   (5) Emotion.
   (6) Mobility.
   (7) Cooperation with care plan: Evaluate for cognitive and emotional impairments.

SUGGESTED READINGS

Fick DM, Cooper JW, Wade WE, et al: Updating the Beers criteria for potentially inappropriate medication use in older adults: Results of a US consensus panel of experts. *Arch Intern Med* 163:2716-2724, 2003.

Simon SR, Chan KA, Soumerai SB et al: Potentially inappropriate medication use by elderly persons in U.S. health maintenance organizations, 2000-2001. *J Am Geriatr Soc* 53:227-232, 2005.

Gurwitz J, Monane M, Monane S, Avorn J: Polypharmacy. In Morris JN, Lipsitz LA, Murphy K, Belleville-Taylor P (eds): *Quality Care in the Nursing Home.* St Louis, Mosby-Yearbook, 1997, pp 13-25.

Tamblyn R, Abrahamowicz M, du Berger R, et al: A 5-year prospective assessment of the risk associated with individual benzodiazepines and doses among new elderly users. *J Am Geriatr Soc* 53:233-241, 2005.

6.4 Adverse Drug Reactions

1. Adverse drug reactions are more common in the elderly because the elderly consume more medications and are more likely to have baseline illness than younger patients, not because of the patient's chronologic age. (see Background Statement 6.1, 2)
2. Drug reactions can be subdivided into four groups.
   a. A primary adverse reaction to a single medication with a narrow toxic-to-therapeutic ratio is responsible for patient's symptoms (e.g., digoxin, theophylline, lidocaine).
   b. A secondary adverse reaction results from interaction between two medications (Table 6-1).
   c. Drug withdrawal syndromes result from sudden cessation of a drug (e.g., angina from β-blocker withdrawal).
   d. Extrapharmacologic effects occur with some drugs (e.g., increased risk of fractured hip with benzodiazepine use).
3. Common types of adverse drug reactions in the elderly.
   a. Primary drug reactions (one drug with one side effect).
      (1) Cimetidine psychosis.
      (2) Narcotic-induced respiratory depression/delirium.
      (3) Lidocaine psychosis.

Table 6-1 Drug Interactions Involving Prescription Drugs

Drugs	Onset	Severity	Effect	Mechanism	Management
Antacids and iron salts	Delayed	Minor	↓ Hematologic response to Fe	↓ Absorption of Fe because of high gastric pH	Give Fe several hours before antacids, liquid preferred
Benzodiazepines and ethanol	Rapid	Minor	↑ Effects of both; ↑ psychomotor dysfunction and sedation	Synergistic effects and ↓ VD; ↓ elimination of benzodiazepines	Avoid ETOH
β-Blockers and prazosin	Rapid	Moderate	↑ Severity and duration; hypotension associated with first dose of prazosin	Blocked cardiovascular reflex because of orthostatic hypotension	First prazosin dose at qhs; monitor orthostatic BP
β-Blockers and indomethacin	Delayed	Moderate	↓ Antihypertensive effect of β-blockers; BP + 5-10 mm Hg	Inhibition of prostaglandin synthesis	Check BP after 7-10 days
Captopril and indomethacin	Rapid	Moderate	↓ Effect of captopril	Inhibition of prostaglandin synthesis	Check BP day 1 of indomethacin Tx; discontinue if BP is too high
Cimetidine and procainamide	Rapid	Moderate	↑ Effect of procainamide, including GI toxicity, weakness, hypotension; ↓ CO, arrhythmias	↓ Renal clearance of procainamide	Decrease procainamide 25%-35% before starting cimetidine; check procainamide and NAPA levels 24 h after cimetidine

Continued

Table 6-1 Drug Interactions Involving Prescription Drugs—cont'd

Drugs	Onset	Severity	Effect	Mechanism	Management
Clonidine and tricyclic antidepressants	Rapid	Moderate	↓ Antihypertensive effect of clonidine; hypertensive crisis possible	Unknown	Avoid concomitant use, or increase clonidine dose; beware of risks of high-dose clonidine
Digoxin and quinidine	Delayed	Major	↑ Toxic effects of digoxin	↓ VD; ↓ renal and nonrenal elimination of digoxin	Check ECG, digoxin level, and effect 27-72 h after starting combination; again 3-5 days; adjust if needed
Digoxin and tetracycline	Delayed	Major	↑ Digoxin toxicity seen in <10% of patients	↑ Bioavailability of digoxin, second-degree change in GI flora	Check digoxin level 5-7 days after starting antibiotic and again in 3-4 mo; adjust dose accordingly
Digoxin and anticholinergics	Delayed	Major	↑ Digoxin toxicity	↑ Bioavailability of slowly dissolving digoxin preparation	Use liquid or rapidly dissolving digoxin preparations
Digoxin and thiazide + loop	Delayed	Major	↑ Digoxin toxicity, especially arrhythmias	Diuretic-induced hypokalemia potentiates arrhythmias	Maintain serum potassium at 4-4.5 mEq/L with potassium supplementation
Lithium and thiazide	Delayed	Major	↑ Levels and toxicity of lithium; polyuria, weakness, lethargy, ECG changes	↓ Renal excretion of lithium	Use loop diuretics or more carefully monitor lithium levels and reduce dose accordingly

Drug combination	Severity	Onset	Effect	Mechanism	Recommendation
Quinidine and rifampin	Moderate	Delayed	↓ Effect of quinidine	↑ Metabolism of quinidine	Monitor quinidine levels 1 wk after starting rifampin; review 3-5 days after discontinuing rifampin
Salicylates and warfarin	Major	Delayed	↑ Anticoagulant effect	Synergistic effect	Avoid combination
Salicylates and antacids	Minor	Delayed	↓ Effect of salicylate	↑ Renal excretion of salicylate	↑ Dose of salicylate; check levels
Sulfonylureas and thiazide diuretics	Minor	Delayed	↓ Hypoglycemic effect	Thiazide-induced glucose intolerance	Monitor glucose, one dose of sulfonylurea
Theophylline and erythromycin	Moderate	Delayed	↓ Effect of erythromycin; ↑ effect of theophylline	Hepatic metabolism of theophylline inhibited	↓ Dose or ↑ dosing interval of theophylline by 60%; monitor levels
Theophylline and β-blockers	Moderate	Delayed	↓ Effect of theophylline	↓ Bronchial resistance caused by β-blockers	Avoid β-blockers in patients with reactive airway diseases
Warfarin and thyroid hormone	Major	Delayed	↑ Hypothrombinemic effect, bleeding	Unknown	Adjust dose according to patient results
Warfarin and quinidine	Major	Delayed	↑ Hypothrombinemic effect	↓ Vitamin K-dependent factor synthesis	↓ Anticoagulant dose; check patient 5-7 days after starting combination

BP, blood pressure; CO, Cardiac output; ETOH, ethanol; GI, gastrointestinal; NAPA, N-acetyl procainamide; Tx, treatment; VD, volume of distribution.
From Day SC, Diserens D, Grisso JA, Lavizzo-Mourey R (eds): Practicing Prevention for the Elderly. Philadelphia, Hanley & Belfus, 1989.

    (4) Theophylline seizures.

    (5) Insulin reaction.

    (6) Chronic salicylism.

  b. Secondary drug interactions (requires at least two drugs to cause an interaction).

    (1) Sulfonylurea and sulfonamide.

    (2) Cimetidine and lidocaine.

    (3) Erythromycin and theophylline.

    (4) Indomethacin and propranolol.

    (5) Tricyclic antidepressant and α-sympatholytic.

    (6) Coumadin and antibiotic therapy.

  c. Drug withdrawal syndromes (addictive and nonaddictive withdrawal).

    (1) β-Blocker withdrawal (angina).

    (2) Calcium channel blocker withdrawal (angina, hypertension).

    (3) Addictive drug withdrawal syndromes (benzodiazepines, narcotics, etc.).

  d. Tertiary extrapharmacologic effects (measurable only by epidemiologic studies).

    (1) Falls caused by tricyclics, benzodiazepines, and antipsychotics.

    (2) Traumatic injuries caused by drug-induced orthostatic hypotension.

4. Physician factors implicated in adverse drug reactions.

  a. The physician prescribes a high-risk drug to a vulnerable host. Examples:

    (1) Acetylsalicylic acid for a patient with peptic ulcer disease.

    (2) Amiodarone for a patient with failure to thrive syndrome.

    (3) Captopril for a patient on a potassium-sparing agent.

    (4) Any anticholinergic medication in a confused patient.

  b. The physician prescribes one drug to treat the side effect of another drug. Examples:

    (1) Tricyclic antidepressant to treat β-blocker depression.

    (2) Major tranquilizer to treat benzodiazepine withdrawal agitation.

    (3) Carbidopa–levodopa to treat extrapyramidal symptoms of an antipsychotic.

  c. Automatic drug prescribing in standing orders.

    (1) Intensive care unit.

    (2) Cardiac care unit.

    (3) Chronic care facilities.

  d. Lack of follow-up on drug effects or poor longitudinal monitoring of drug interactions.

5. Suggestions for preventing drug toxicity are outlined in Box 6-2.

SUGGESTED READINGS

Gurwitz JH, Avorn J: The ambiguous relation between aging and adverse drug reactions. *Ann Intern Med* 114:956-966, 1991.

Gurwitz J, Monane M, Monane S, Avorn J: Polypharmacy. In Morris JN, Lipsitz LA, Murphy K, Belleville-Taylor P (eds): *Quality Care in the Nursing Home.* St Louis, Mosby-Yearbook, 1997, pp 13-25.

Tamblyn R, Abrahamowicz M, du Berger R, et al: A 5-year prospective assessment of the risk associated with individual benzodiazepines and doses among new elderly users. *J Am Geriatr Soc* 53:233-241, 2005.

BOX 6-2   **Suggestions for Preventing Drug Toxicity in the Elderly**

- Strive for an accurate diagnosis before treating
- Take a careful drug history
- Know the pharmacokinetics of the drug or drugs
- Adjust the dose
- Use smaller doses in the elderly
- Work to simplify the regimen
- Regularly review the regimen
- Avoid polypharmacy
- Use medication cards
- Keep a record of the prescription on the problem list
- Use a medication diary (or containers, such as egg cartons) for daily doses
- Have the patient bring in all medicine bottles at every visit
- Check the labels
- Instruct the family
- Destroy old medicines
- Use the services of visiting nurses
- Check serum drug levels when appropriate
- Support community education
- Consider overdose risk in elderly patients with clinically evident psychiatric conditions
- Be sure patients are aware that medicines can cause, as well as cure, illness

From Bosker G, Schwartz GR, Jones JS, Sequeira M (eds): *Geriatric emergency medicine.* St Louis, Mosby, 1990, p 60.

6.5 Drug-Induced Functional Impairments

MALNUTRITION

1. Anorexia: Loss of appetite can be caused by many drugs (e.g., digoxin, theophylline, hydrochlorothiazide, nonsteroidal antiinflammatory drugs [NSAIDs], triamterene).
2. Hypogeusia (loss of taste) may be caused by:
   a. Allopurinol.
   b. Clindamycin.
   c. Antihistamines.
   d. Antibiotics.
3. Malabsorption of vitamins and nutrients can be caused by drug use.
   a. Vitamins A and D: Mineral oil.
   b. Vitamin B_6 and niacin: Isoniazid.
   c. Vitamin C: Salicylates.
   d. Calcium and iron: Tetracycline.

  e. Vitamin D: Anticonvulsants.
  f. Folate: Anticonvulsants, triamterene, trimethoprim.
  h. Vitamin K: Mineral oil, salicylates, anticonvulsants.
  h. Zinc: Diuretics.

CONSTIPATION

1. Drug-induced constipation can set off a cascade of symptoms that result in nausea, anorexia, confusion, urinary tract infection, impaction, and bowel obstruction with paradoxical diarrhea.
2. A variety of medications can cause constipation.
   a. Anticholinergics (narcotics, antidepressants, antihistamines, antipsychotics, antispasmodics).
   b. NSAIDs.
   c. Antacids.
   d. Calcium channel blockers.
   e. Calcium.
   f. Diuretics.
   g. Iron.

URINARY INCONTINENCE

1. The patient is usually predisposed to one of three types of incontinence: overflow, stress, and urge (Table 6-2).
2. Overflow incontinence: Urinary retention can lead to overflow incontinence.
   a. Seen with anticholinergics, smooth muscle relaxants, or α-agonists.
   b. Medications with anticholinergic side effects (rather than pure anticholinergic compounds) (e.g., amitriptyline, imipramine, antihistamines, thioridazine) are often responsible

Table 6-2 **Drug-Induced Urinary Incontinence**	
Type of Incontinence	**Drugs**
Overflow	
Urinary retention	Anticholinergic agents: Benztropine
	Agents with anticholinergic effects: Amitriptyline, imipramine, thioridazine, antihistamines, disopyramide
	Smooth muscle relaxants: Nifedipine
	α-Agonists: Phenylpropanolamine
Stress	
Sphincter relaxation	α-Antagonists: prazosin
Urge	
Central inhibition	Neuroleptics
Polyuria	Diuretics, lithium
Secondary to oversedation	Benzodiazepines, sedatives, or hypnotics

Data from Owens NJ, Silliman RA, Fretwell MD: *DICP* 23:847-854, 1989.

   c. The smooth-muscle relaxant nifedipine can cause overflow incontinence because of its relaxant effect on the detrusor muscle.

   d. α-Agonists such as phenylpropanolamine can cause incontinence by stimulating the proximal urinary sphincter to contract.

3. Stress incontinence: α-Antagonists such as tamsulosin or prazosin can cause incontinence by stimulating proximal urinary sphincter to relax.

4. Urge incontinence.

   a. Urge incontinence is usually associated with drug-induced polyuria caused by diuretics.

   b. A diabetes insipidus-like syndrome can be seen with lithium.

   c. Patients prescribed diuretics or other medications causing hyperglycemia or hypercalcemia (e.g., tamoxifen) can also develop polyuria.

   d. Older patients who have experienced loss of mobility are at greater risk for urge incontinence caused by drug-induced polyuria.

5. Incontinence secondary to oversedation.

   a. Drugs that cause confusional states or delirium in older persons can secondarily cause incontinence.

   b. This association warrants special attention because the delirious incontinent patient is at risk for catheter placement and the use of restraints.

IMPAIRMENTS IN COGNITION

Drug-induced effects on cognitive processes have long been recognized. The subsequent effects of drug-induced cognitive impairment on other functional domains have been described as a cascade effect. The patient who is oversedated with medications loses physical function and may be unable to ambulate, eat, or use the toilet (Table 6-3).

Table 6-3 **Drug-Induced Impairments in Mental State**	
Type of Impairment	**Drugs**
Behavioral Toxicity	
Insomnia, nightmares, sedation, agitation, irritability, restlessness leading to delirium, and/or psychosis, and/or hallucinations	Amantadine, anticholinergics, baclofen, bromocriptine, cimetidine, corticosteroids, digoxin, levodopa, opiate narcotics, ranitidine, sympathomimetics
Depression	β-Blockers, corticosteroids, methyldopa, reserpine
Cognitive Impairment	
Dementia, memory loss	Amantadine, anticonvulsants, benzodiazepines, cimetidine, hydrochlorothiazide, methyldopa, neuroleptics, opiate narcotics, propranolol, reserpine
Metabolic Alterations	
Hyperglycemia or hypoglycemia	β-Blockers, corticosteroids, diuretics, sulfonylureas
Electrolyte disturbances	Diuretics

1. Benzodiazepines have been documented in the literature as a cause of memory impairment, specifically anterograde amnesia, and their use should be avoided in older persons whenever possible.
2. Long-term phenytoin administration can cause reversible memory loss.
3. Anticholinergics.
   a. Atropine and other anticholinergics have been reported to induce delirium.
   b. Patients receiving two or more drugs with anticholinergic effects (e.g., thioridazine with benztropine to prevent extrapyramidal symptoms) are at greater risk for anticholinergic toxicity.
4. H_2 receptor blockers (e.g., cimetidine and ranitidine) can cause confusion or delirium.
5. Digoxin.
   a. Digoxin toxicity can first manifest as confusion or hallucinations.
   b. Nightmares, restlessness or nervousness, hallucinations, and delirium have all been reported as adverse effects of digoxin.
6. Many drugs induce psychoses by their direct effect on dopamine or on the receptors of dopamine and choline (e.g., levodopa, amantadine, baclofen, bromocriptine).
7. Glucocorticoids have been reported to induce psychosis at even low doses.

DEPRESSIVE DISORDERS

1. Many agents used to treat hypertension (e.g., reserpine) may cause depression.
2. Methyldopa and β-blockers (e.g., propranolol) represent well-documented causes of depression.
3. It is especially important to avoid drug-induced depression in older persons because it can manifest as cognitive impairment (pseudodementia) rather than classic depression.

IMPAIRMENTS IN MOBILITY

Medications may impair mobility in older persons as a result of a variety of age-related changes (Table 6-4).

1. Depletion of dopamine in the extrapyramidal center of the brain increases the risk of antipsychotic-induced movement disorders (e.g., tremors, rigidity, akathisia, acute dystonic reactions).
2. Hypotension (and therefore the risk of falling) is more likely to occur in older persons because of diminished baroreceptor sensitivity. The following drugs can contribute to postural hypotension:
   a. Diuretics: From volume depletion and electrolyte abnormalities.
   b. Cardiac medication: From sedation, a decrease in cardiac output, reduced venous return, or decreased peripheral vascular resistance.
   c. Sedative-hypnotics: From sedation or autonomic effects.
   d. Antipsychotics: From α-adrenergic blockade.
3. Some medications can cause mobility problems with short- or long-term use.
   a. Short courses of glucocorticoids can cause proximal muscle wasting. Treated patients can find it difficult to get out of bed or rise from a sitting position.

Table 6-4 Drug-Induced Impairments in Mobility

Type of Impairment	Drugs
Balance	
Neuritis, neuropathies	Metronidazole, phenytoin
Tinnitus, vertigo	Aspirin, aminoglycosides, ethacrynic acid, furosemide
Movement Disorders	
Extrapyramidal symptoms, tardive dyskinesia	Amoxapine, methyldopa, metoclopramide, neuroleptics
Hypotension	Antidepressants, benzodiazepines, β-blockers, calcium channel blockers, diuretics, levodopa, metoclopramide, neuroleptics, vasodilators
Psychomotor retardation	Antidepressants, antihistamines, benzodiazepines, neuroleptics
Supporting Structure	
Arthralgias, myopathies	Corticosteroids, lithium
Osteomalacia, osteoporosis	Corticosteroids, heparin, phenytoin

   b. When taken for a long period of time, glucocorticoids cause osteoporosis by impairing absorption of calcium, enhancing renal excretion of calcium, and decreasing osteoblastic activity in bone.

4. Some medications can affect several areas simultaneously (e.g., atypical antipsychotics can cause psychomotor retardation and postural hypotension and at the same time produce extrapyramidal symptoms such as akathisia, cogwheeling, and muscle rigidity).

5. Risk of falls is increased with any abnormalities in vision, hearing, vestibular function, and proprioception.

   a. Drugs that affect the senses must be avoided if possible.

     (1) Digoxin.

     (2) Aminoglycosides.

     (3) Loop diuretics.

   b. Long-acting benzodiazepines, tricyclic antidepressants, and antipsychotics have been shown to increase risk of falls and hip fractures.

SUGGESTED READINGS

Caterino JM, Emond JA, Camargo CA Jr: Inappropriate medication administration to the acutely ill elderly: A nationwide emergency department study, 1992-2000. J Am Geriatr Soc 52:1847-1855, 2004.

Higashi T, Shekelle PG, Solomon DH, et al: The quality of pharmacologic care for vulnerable older patients. Ann Intern Med 140:714-720, 2004.

Gurwitz J, Monane M, Monane S, Avorn J: Polypharmacy. In Morris JN, Lipsitz LA, Murphy K, Belleville-Taylor P (eds): Quality Care in the Nursing Home. St Louis, Mosby-Yearbook, 1997, pp 13-25.

6.6 Recommendations for Improving Compliance in Older Patients

1. Understand patient's values and beliefs regarding health and medical treatment.
2. Educate patients about their diseases and repercussions of treatment or no treatment.
3. Keep medication regimens as simple as possible.
4. Educate the patient about using over-the-counter medications.
5. Set priorities for which medications are critical to each patient's health.
6. Assure patients that there will be careful monitoring for unexpected and expected adverse reactions. Explain adverse effects in terms of their impact on patient function.
7. Educate patients and family or caregiver about name, dose, and indication for every medication. Reinforce this at every encounter.
8. Ask patients what techniques they have organized to remind themselves to take their medications.
9. Provide printed educational materials to reinforce patient knowledge.
10. Give the patient and family the opportunity to ask questions.
11. Ask patient to repeat medication names and instructions for use to allow reiteration of newly acquired medication knowledge.

SUGGESTED READINGS

Owens NJ, Larrat EP, Fretwell MD: Improving compliance in the older patient. In Cramer JA, Spilker B (eds): *Patient Compliance in Medical Practice and Clinical Trials*. New York, Raven, 1991.

Gurwitz J, Monane M, Monane S, Avorn J: Polypharmacy. In Morris JN, Lipsitz LA, Murphy K, Belleville-Taylor P (eds): *Quality Care in the Nursing Home*. St Louis, Mosby-Yearbook, 1997, pp 13-25.

Long-Term Care

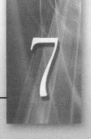

7.1 Home Care and House Calls

John B. Murphy and Tom J. Wachtel

FORMAL HOME CARE

When physicians prescribe home care services for Medicare beneficiaries, they must certify that the patient is homebound; in need of intermittent skilled nursing care or physical, speech, or occupational therapy; and under the physician's ongoing care. By signing a standard authorization form approved for home care services by the Centers for Medicare and Medicaid Services (CMS), the physician verifies that the patient has met the three eligibility criteria and that the physician will review the home care plan periodically but no less than every 2 months and recertify the patient if appropriate. Even though physicians might not have first-hand knowledge that the home care services they prescribe are appropriate and necessary, prescribers of home care need to know that the federal government's position is that "when a physician signs a Medicare certification form, there is an implied representation that all the rules are complied with." In fact, the official form for the home care plan contains a statement that "misrepresentation, falsification or information concealment may be subject to fine, imprisonment or civil penalty."[1]

The eligibility criteria for home care are stringent because the intent of the Medicare program is generally to cover acute care rather than long-term care or preventive care. However, the clinical reality for many patients is that their chronic conditions exacerbate and improve over time, causing them to shift in and out of home care eligibility. These changes in condition complicate the physician's role in determining patients' eligibility for home care services covered by Medicare. The purpose of this section is to discuss the role of the physician in authorizing and monitoring home care services given CMS regulations.

The Homebound Criteria

If the federal Medicare program defined home confinement as absolute, patients who visit doctors in their offices while receiving home care would not be, strictly speaking, confined to their home. Fortunately, CMS does not define home confinement literally. Currently, patients need not be bedridden, but "there should exist a normal inability to leave home and leaving their homes would require a considerable and taxing effort." For practical purposes, Medicare considers patients homebound if they cannot independently leave their residence. However, such patients may leave their home with the aid of assistive devices (crutches, walkers, or wheelchairs), special transportation (e.g., ambulance or van), or another person (e.g., family member). Still, not all patients who use assistive devices are eligible for home care. Medicare also expects that absences from the home be infrequent or relatively short (e.g., a trip to the hairdresser or to church) and that in most instances, absences from the home be for the purpose of medical treatment. Patients may also be considered homebound if leaving the home is medically contraindicated.

The criteria for home confinement are subjective. Therefore, how physicians, home care agencies, patients, and CMS define home confinement may differ. Box 7-1 lists clinical situations that would qualify patients for meeting the Medicare criteria for home confinement.

Skilled Services Requirement

A frail person who is homebound is not considered eligible for home care unless criteria for intermittent skilled care are also met. The criteria for skilled care are even more ambiguous than those for home confinement. Skilled care is care that must be provided by a registered nurse or a physical, occupational, or speech therapist. However, just because a service is provided by one of these health professionals does not necessarily mean the service is a skilled service. To be considered a skilled service, a nurse must be required to provide it because of "its complexity," and

---

BOX 7-1   **Examples of Homebound Cases According to Medicare Criteria**

Mobility restricted by a disease process, such as unsteady gait, draining wounds, or pain.

Poor cardiac reserve, shortness of breath, or activity intolerance as a result of an unstable or exacerbated disease process.

Bedridden or wheelchair-bound patients who require physical assistance to move any distance.

Patients who require caregiver help with assistive devices such as a walker, wheelchair, or other special device to leave home.

A tracheostomy, abdominal drains, colostomy, Foley catheter, or nasogastric tube that restricts ambulation.

Psychotic ideation, confusion, or impaired mental status that restricts functional abilities outside the home.

Fluctuating blood pressure or blood sugar levels that can cause syncope.

Inability to negotiate stairs or uneven surfaces without assistance of a caregiver.

Postoperative patients whose activity has been restricted by the physician.

Patients who are legally blind or cannot drive.

"the patient's condition." The service must also meet "accepted standards of medical and nursing practice." A diagnosis alone is rarely adequate documentation of the need for skilled services. Rather, the relation between a patient's diagnosis, symptoms, and functional status must justify the complexity of services. In addition, the need for skilled services must be intermittent, meaning that the services are required less frequently than 7 days per week, but at least once every 60 days.

Table 7-1 provides examples that do and do not meet the eligibility requirements. The documentation in the medical record should describe the patient's condition and the complexity of required services and should include an assessment of the risk of complications or deterioration should such skilled services become unavailable. These same principles of medical documentation apply for physical, occupational, and speech therapy.

The Physician as Gatekeeper

The home care gatekeeping role may be appropriate for primary care physicians in many cases. However, nurses, therapists, or social workers are sometimes better suited to determine home care eligibility because of the nature of the patient's condition or because, unlike physicians, they visit the patient at home.

Without firsthand knowledge of the patient's homebound status, the physician should not certify the patient in a perfunctory manner as confined to home. The physician should take the time to assess the patient's functional status and need for skilled services before prescribing home care services. In some cases, the physician who prescribes home care has no doubt that the patient meets the Medicare criteria for home confinement. Examples include a patient with a dense hemiparesis, a patient with advanced dementia, or a patient who recently underwent major surgery. These patients are incapable of leaving their home independently or have a medical contraindication to do so; if they need intermittent skilled care, they meet the Medicare criteria for in-home care.

For many patients, however, the physician might not know whether they are eligible to be certified for home care. For example, a diabetic patient with a foot ulcer who is capable of driving her car might benefit greatly from home care for wound management and diabetic teaching by a visiting nurse, but her physician knows or should know that she is able to drive to her doctor's office to receive the wound care and teaching. She is not eligible for home care services. Patients who need physical therapy or daily monitoring of vital signs following hospital discharge might not meet the eligibility criteria for home confinement if they can travel independently to their doctor's office or to a rehabilitation facility. Yet physicians prescribe home care in such situations without much thought because wound care, diabetic teaching, gait training, and blood pressure checks are performed by nurses and physical or occupational therapists. In each of these cases, in order for the patient to receive outpatient nursing care, usually available only through home care agencies, the office-based primary care physician who does not employ a nurse will prescribe home care and certify that patient as home confined, which might be a misrepresentation of the patient's status.

Table 7-1 Clinical Vignettes Related to Medicare Home Care Eligibility Criteria

Vignette	Home Confined	Skilled Care Need	Meets Medicare Eligibility Criteria
Patient with unsteady gait who requires assistance for ambulation and whose blood pressure is 190/110	Yes	Yes	Yes
Patient with a dense hemiparesis who is bedridden or chair bound and who has a pressure ulcer	Yes	Yes	Yes
Patient with severe peripheral neuropathy who is blind and wheelchair-dependent for mobility and whose chronic conditions are well controlled with 12 or more oral medications	Yes	No	No
Patient with advanced Alzheimer's dementia, incontinent of urine, and living in his daughter's home; no other medical problem	Yes	No	No
Patient with a draining venous ulcer who is able to walk and drive her car independently	No	Yes	No
Patient with severe emphysema and cor pulmonale who is ambulatory and stable on home oxygen therapy and medication	No	No	No

Thus physicians are sometimes placed in conflicting roles as advocates for their patients and as gatekeeper for CMS eligibility criteria for home care. This conflict is even more pronounced when patients have chronic conditions such as congestive heart failure (CHF) or chronic obstructive pulmonary disease (COPD) and only meet criteria for skilled services during episodes of exacerbation. Yet, in-home services for those conditions have been shown to reduce exacerbations and hospitalizations.

Physicians should pay sufficient attention to home care certification and plan-of-care forms completed by home care agency staff and mailed to them for signature. Physicians should not rely solely on the recertification plan-of-care forms sent to them because the forms might not contain adequate information about the patient's functional status and condition. Physicians should demand that these forms document not only patients' current needs for skilled care but also the reasons for their homebound status. Copies of these forms should be entered into the medical record and used to justify the in-home skilled services provided. Physicians also should not allow long periods of time to go by (e.g., 6 months for a stable patient) without seeing patients who receive home care services; this might require house calls for some patients. Patients whose chronic diseases are unstable (e.g., those with cardiopulmonary conditions) might require more frequent updates not only to provide good care but also to verify that they remain eligible for needed home care services. Inability to carry out activities of daily living (ADL), cognitive impairment, and urinary incontinence correlate with the need for in-home services. Given that an assessment of functional status is an integral component of geriatric care, the medical record can and should contain up-to-date functional assessments that can be used to justify patients' home confinement and need for skilled services.

HOUSE CALLS AND DOMICILIARY VISITS

A growing number of people in the United States are homebound. Some live at home, and others live in congregate housing arrangements such as elderly housing, independent living, assisted living, boarding houses, and group homes.

House calls in this section refers to the provision of physician services to patients in their home. House calls are provided in lieu of office-based medical care for selected patients. This care may be provided as part of an interdisciplinary care team, as in-home health care following a hospitalization, but it can also exist as ongoing care to patients who are homebound. Furthermore, house calls can be exceptionally helpful in providing the physician with a better understanding of the patient's home situation. The diagnostic house call can provide information about interaction between the patient and the home environment, caregiver burnout, elder mistreatment, use of medications that the primary physician is not aware of, alcohol abuse, and other issues.

For a house call program to be effective and financially viable it is imperative that the program be well planned. Selecting the right patients is also of paramount importance. Current regulations provide reimbursement to physicians, nurse practitioners, and physician assistants, but involvement of other health care services (e.g., laboratory and visiting nurses services) can be helpful.

Strictly speaking, no one is homebound. There is always a way to bring a homebound person to the hospital or to a physician's office. However, except in the case of a medical emergency, transportation by ambulance is not covered by most health insurance plans, and ambulance trips cost several hundred dollars.

The definition of "homebound" that applies to the CMS eligibility criteria for formal home care (see earlier) does not concern house calls by physicians or other health care practitioners. Many physicians who perform house calls use stricter criteria because their offices are better equipped to provide care than patients' homes. Therefore, a patient who is unable to leave his or her home unassisted because of dementia but who has a relative who can provide transportation to the doctor's office might not be a suitable candidate for house calls, although the CMS criterion for "homebound" is met.

For practical purposes, a homebound person can be defined as someone who cannot leave the home, transiently (e.g., after surgery) or permanently, using personal or other resources readily available in the community (e.g., friends, relatives, taxi service, senior citizens' transportation, or public transportation). Such a person might appropriately receive health services at home.

Some programs provide multidisciplinary geriatric assessments within patients' homes. There are no Medicare common procedural terminology (CPT) reimbursement codes to pay providers for such service; therefore, this section describes the provision of care by a single provider.

The House Call

Most first visits at home are scheduled well in advance. Therefore, it is almost always possible for the informal caregiver (most often the patient's daughter) to be present during the visit. Even when a family provides care in shifts, arrangement can be made for a key member of the informal caregiving team to be present. When the patient's condition requires substantial nursing services (e.g., a patient with an active pressure ulcer), every effort should be made for the visiting nurse to be present during the visit; this will enable the whole team to discuss the plan of care.

Taking a history in the patient's home is no different in its content from a history taken in the office, but because it is done on the patient's turf, often over coffee and muffins, the interaction tends to be less formal. Permission should be requested to inspect the living quarters. What does the home look like? Is it clean? Is it orderly? Can the patient get around, go to the kitchen, go to the bathroom? Is the environment safe? Are there loose rugs, nightlights, rails in the bathroom? An office visit, no matter how comprehensive, cannot provide a complete understanding of the patient's daily routine. The cabinet or drawer that contains the medications should be inspected. Outdated and discontinued medications should be discarded. The refrigerator and food cupboards should also be checked, especially when the homebound patient depends on others for his or her food supply. Aside from appearance, what does the home smell like? Incontinence may be immediately detected. Many elderly patients are reluctant to report incontinence in the office. It may be more difficult to hide during a house call ("whiff test").

Observing the interaction between caregivers and patients is also a precious source of information. In the office, patients and families are generally on their best behavior and outbursts are unlikely to occur. In the home setting, people are less inhibited, even in the presence of the physician. Therefore, they are more likely to display their usual pattern of interaction. Moreover, the request for a house call is often placed at a time of crisis. Most often, the crisis is not a new medical problem but rather an exhausted caregiver who needs support or respite.

Although the goal of a house call certainly varies, like any physician–patient interaction, the content of a home visit should include a number of staple items (Box 7-2). Because most candidates for home care are frail or disabled, a functional assessment should always be performed. This includes gathering information on physical function, such as ADL, instrumental activities of daily life (IADL), mobility, and continence; social and role function, such as visits by friends and relatives; and mental function, such as cognition and affect. Unlike the office setting, where these assessments must be done formally by asking specific questions, much of this information can be collected by simple observation during a home visit. A more complete checklist describing the relation between the patient and the home environment is presented in Figure 7-1.

Asking homebound elderly patients to discuss ethical issues such as care intensity should be a routine practice. In the hospital, a common and important question is whether to resuscitate. At home an additional issue is whether to hospitalize. Whatever decision is made, it is entered into the patient's record. Equally important is the question of surrogate decision makers. Competent patients are routinely requested to think about designating someone who will have durable power of attorney for medical decisions. This is also entered into the medical record.

Homebound patients and their informal caregivers should be given a list of community resources.

The physical exam is often less complete at home than in the office or at the hospital. Although technically feasible, a pelvic exam for cancer screening might not be indicated in an elderly patient with Alzheimer's dementia. Although a bimanual exam is possible, expecting to visualize a cervix with an elderly patient lying in a regular bed is unreasonable. Most patients who receive care at home do not expect the same comprehensive services routinely provided to ambulatory patients; nonetheless, it is best to be explicit and explain to patients the medical goals. Blood and urine tests and an occasional electrocardiogram (ECG) can be obtained as readily in the home as in the office (or community-based laboratories). Portable x-rays can be obtained at great expense and poor quality. Typically, a situation that calls for x-rays or other diagnostic procedures requires evaluation in a hospital.

Logistics and Time Management

The logistics of house calls might explain why many physicians, busy with their office and hospital work, find house calls an inefficient use of their time. There is obviously some validity to this argument. However, steps can be taken to reduce travel time. The physician with a substantial number of homebound patients can arrange to make routine visits to a cluster of

BOX 7-2   Problems to Address during a Geriatric Home Visit

Safety

Access to telephone or other means of calling for help
Appliances
Dirt, dust, humidity
Fire alarm
Household risks (e.g., loose rugs, night-lights, bathroom rails)
Security

Psychosocial Situation

Affect (rule out depression)
Financial resources
Mental status
Support (family, friends; rule out loneliness)

Ethical Issues

Decision to (not to) hospitalize
Intensity of care (especially terminal care)
Surrogate decision maker (durable power of attorney) and/or living will

Functional Status

Activities of daily living (ADL)
Instrumental activities of daily living (IADL)
Mobility
Vision and hearing assessment

Continence

Urine and stool

Nutrition

Ability to prepare and eat meals
Alcoholism
Availability of food

Medical Problems

Diagnose and treat acute illness
Primary prevention (vaccination, hygiene)
Prognosis
Skin care, foot care
Tertiary prevention (diagnose, treat, and monitor chronic diseases)

Primary Care

Access to and availability of care
Continuity of care
Coordination of team of health care professionals

patients who live in the same neighborhood. The fact that older members of our society tend to congregate in elderly housing makes clustering easy to accomplish. A photocopy of a map illustrating the location of the patient's home can be placed in the patient's chart.

Except for first encounters, two to four house calls can be scheduled per hour when several visits are arranged in the same apartment building or neighborhood. In addition, routine house calls can be made to replace idle time caused by cancellations in the office. This can actually improve the efficiency of a geriatric practice (e.g., during bad weather).

House calls for urgent problems (e.g., a fever) may be impossible to plan in a physician's schedule. Urgent visits can be made at the end of the day

1. Type of dwelling   ( ) House   ( ) Apartment

2. Previous living situation   ( ) House   ( ) Apartment

3. Who lives at the residence: Name(s), Relation(s) _____

    _____

    ( ) Completely alone   ( ) Alone part of the day   ( ) Rarely/never alone

4. Stairs

    ( ) None (or ramp)   ( ) Stairs to main floor   ( ) Stairs to upstairs

5. Mobility

    ( ) Ambulatory without care   ( ) Ambulatory with care   ( ) Ambulatory with walker

    ( ) Chair bound   ( ) Bed bound

6. ADL

7. IADL

8. Function in the home (*I*, independent; *A*, assistance required; *D*, dependent; *NA*, not applicable)

A. General Obstacle Negotiation	I	A	D	NA
Elevator				
Stairs				

Figure 7-1   Checklist for the traditional home evaluation.

Continued

Ramp					
Uneven terrain					
Thresholds					
Through doorways					
Can patient escape safely (e.g., fire)					

NOTE: Stair covering and railing, smoke alarms, emergency exits, extension cords

B. Entrance	I	A	D	NA	
Driveway					
Walkway					
Landing					
Unlock door					
Open door					
Access mail					

NOTE: Lighting, obstacles

C. Living/Family Room	I	A	D	NA	
Ability to maneuver through room					
Ability to transfer on/off chairs					
Ability to manage TV					
Ability to reach and use phone					

NOTE: Lighting, floors, emergency numbers by phone

Figure 7-1, cont'd.

D. Kitchen	I	A	D	NA	
Ability to maneuver through room					
Ability to use table and chair					
Ability to reach shelves/cabinet					
Ability to use appliances (refrigerator, stove, sink)					
Ability to prepare meals					

NOTE: Lighting, floors, reachability of utensils/dishes/food; the quantity and quality of the food

E. Bathroom	I	A	D	NA	
Ability to maneuver to and through room					
Ability to transfer on/off toilet					
Ability to transfer in/out of tub or shower					
Ability to reach sink, faucet, grooming supplies					

NOTE: Lighting (also between bedroom and bathroom); obstacles; nonskid surface (tub and shower); tub and shower bench; tub, shower, or toilet rails; hot water temperature

F. Bedroom	I	A	D	NA	
Ability to maneuver to and through room					
Ability to transfer in/out of bed					
Ability to reach phone					

Figure 7-1, cont'd.

Continued

Ability to reach light switch					
Ability to use closets and drawers					

NOTE: Lighting, obstacles

_____

_____

_____

G. Medications	I	A	D	NA	
Ability to identify medication					
Ability to follow instructions					
Ability to open containers					

NOTE: What medications are found; outdated, no longer prescribed?

_____

_____

_____

Figure 7-1, cont'd.

on the way home from work. However, it should be made clear to home-bound patients that emergencies cannot always be addressed in the home. The willingness to make house calls should not eliminate use of standard emergency services when necessary.

- Physicians and other health care practitioners who make house calls should specify the conditions under which they will provide this service. For example:
- Patients are eligible for the house calls program if they live within a 15-minute drive and are unable to leave their home.
- Scheduled visits are made every 3 to 4 months. One half-day of a physician schedule per month may be reserved for these visits, and patients are also seen during last-minute unfilled cancellations in the ambulatory practice schedule. Unscheduled visits are made for more urgent problems at the request of the patient, a family member, or a home care nurse.
- Upon enrollment, patients and their caregivers should be given an information sheet stating that although efforts will be made to see patients with acute problems, the practice cannot guarantee the ability to make emergency visits and cannot provide home visits at night or during weekends.

Physicians and other practitioners who provide house calls should have a tool kit (doctor's bag) with the equipment listed in Box 7-3.

BOX 7-3   Contents of Physician's Tool Kit

Basic Supplies

Cell phone
Dictation recorder
Ear syringe and/or cerumen curette
Gloves
Hand disinfectant/wash
Local street map
Lubricating jelly
Otoscope and ophthalmoscope
Patient's chart with directions to the home
Prescription pad
Scale (in patient's home)
Sphygmomanometer
Stethoscope
Stool guaiac cards and developer
Thermometer
Toenail clippers
Tongue depressors

Additional Advisable Supplies

Foley catheter
Lancets and glucometer with alcohol pads, 2×2 gauze, and adhesive
    bandages
Peak flow meter
Portable scale pulse oximeter
Specimen cups
Urine dipsticks
Voice amplifier
Wound debridement kit
Wound dressing materials

Supplies for Special Circumstances

Excisional biopsy kit
Punch biopsy kit
Suture/staple removal kit

The chronic conditions that physicians can expect to manage during
house calls are the same as those seen in the office for an age-matched population with a bias toward conditions that impair mobility such as dementia, post-stroke state, severe arthritis, severe CHF, or COPD. Acute
illnesses include the following:

- Acute musculoskeletal problems (injuries, arthralgia)
- Acute and chronic pain
- Delirium

- End-of-life care
- Exacerbation of CHF or COPD
- Failure to thrive
- Falls
- Gastroenteritis and abdominal pain
- Infections, mostly respiratory and urinary
- Syncope
- Wounds (pressure ulcers, venous ulcers, arterial ulcers, diabetic ulcers)

Payment for House Calls

1. Home visits (includes senior housing and independent living; Table 7-2).
   a. New patient CPT codes: 99341, 99342, 99343, 99344, 99345. The documentation requirements for these codes are similar to office-based new patient evaluation and management (E&M).
   b. Established patient CPT codes: 99347, 99348, 99349, 99350, also similar to office visit codes.
2. Domiciliary visits (include assisted-living and group homes)
   a. New patient CPT codes: 99321, 99322, 99323.
      (1) The documentation requirement for 99321 is a problem-focused history and examination and low-complexity decision making.
      (2) For 99322, the documentation requirement is expanded problem-focused history and examination and moderate-complexity decision making.
      (3) For 99323, the documentation requirement is detailed history and high-complexity decision making.
   b. Established patient CPT codes 99331, 99332 and 99333 come with the same documentation requirements as for follow-up nursing home patients.
3. CMS pays physicians for overseeing the work done by home care agencies. The CPT codes for these services are:
   a. G0180 Certification for home care.

Table 7-2 Payment for House Calls

Code	Visit Type	Approximate Charge ($)*
New Patient		
99341	Low severity	57.87
99342	Moderate severity	84.38
99343	Moderate to high severity	123.21
99344	High severity	161.67
99345	Unstable	200.13
Established Patient		
99347	Minor	44.43
99348	Low to moderate severity	75.42
99349	Moderate to high severity	116.86
99350	High severity	169.89

*2004 Medicare allowable charges before geographic adjustments.
CPT, common procedural terminology.

b. G0179 Recertification for home care.
c. G0181 Care plan overnight for home care (requires at least 30 minutes per month and ability to document the time spent).
d. G0182 Care plan overnight for hospice (same time requirements as for home care).

REFERENCE

1. Wachtel TJ, Gifford DR: Eligibility for home care certification: What clinicians should know. *J Gen Intern Med* 1998;13(10):705-709.

SUGGESTED READINGS

American Academy of Home Care Physicians: Executive Summary, Public Policy Statement, 2005. Edgewood, Md: American Academy of Home Care Physicians, 2005. Available at http://www.aahcp.org/public_policy_2005.pdf (accessed March 1, 2007).
Boling P, Abbey L, Keenan J: Home care. In Ham R, Sloane P, Warshaw G (eds): *Primary Care Geriatrics*, ed 4. St. Louis, Mosby, 2002, pp. 217-228.
Unwin B, Jerant A: The home visit. *Am Fam Physician* 60:1481-1488, 1999.

7.2 Nursing Home Care

Tom J. Wachtel

GENERAL CONSIDERATIONS

Nursing Home Types

Nursing homes have evolved from the almshouses of a century ago into highly regulated institutions providing care to primarily older persons with profound medical, psychiatric, and/or social disabilities. Since the 1980s, the degree of regulation and the level of impairment of nursing home residents have increased dramatically.

In the United States there are roughly 17,000 nursing homes with 1.8 million beds that care for 1.6 million persons receiving custodial care (nursing facility; NF) or skilled care (skilled nursing facility; SNF). Most nursing homes provide both NF and SNF levels of care. Two thirds of the nation's nursing homes are for-profit facilities, and nearly 55% of all homes are part of large regional or national chains. Roughly 25% of nursing homes are voluntary not-for-profit facilities and about 10% are government affiliated. The average nursing home has about 100 beds; fewer than 10% have more than 200 beds.

Nursing Home Staffing

Standard nursing home staff are listed in Box 7-4. Nursing universally accounts for the majority of the staff and minimally trained nurse's aides make up the bulk of the nursing staff. Relatively few licensed nurses are present to conduct assessments, distribute medications, supervise nurse's aides, communicate with physicians, and administer treatments. Only a small percentage of nursing homes, typically the largest nursing homes, have employed physicians. A 1996 Institute of Medicine report recommended

BOX 7-4   Standard Nursing Home Staff

Activities staff
Administrator
Dieticians and other food-service staff
Housekeepers
Maintenance workers
Nurses
Social workers
Therapists*
- Occupational therapists
- Physical therapists
- Speech pathologists

*May be full time or provided by an outside agency.

increased staffing levels as an important step to increase quality of care in nursing homes, but the financial resources to achieve these increases are lacking. The recruitment and retention of nursing staff is a major challenge; turnover rates for licensed nurses are as high as 50% per year and still higher for nursing assistants.

Nursing Home Residents

The lifetime risk of a nursing home stay is currently estimated to be 43%. The prevalent rate of nursing home residence increases with age; 1.5% for Americans age 65 to 74 years and 20% for those 85 years and older. The average length of stay in a nursing home is about 2 years; 25% stay 3 months or less, 50% stay 1 year or longer, and 20% stay as long as 5 years.

As a group, nursing home residents are increasingly disabled. Only 2.8% of nursing home residents are independent in all ADL, and 83% require assistance with three or more ADL. Dementia is one of the most common conditions of nursing home residents, estimated at a prevalence of 50% to 70%. Behavioral problems are common (33%) as are communication problems (seen in more than 50% of residents). Depression is also very likely, estimated at a prevalence of 20%. Most nursing home residents suffer from many chronic illnesses.

One half of nursing home residents are 85 years or older and fewer than 10% are younger than 65 years. The majority of nursing home residents are women (72%). Although 89% are white, black persons are actually at higher risk for a nursing home stay at an earlier age than white persons. Additional factors associated with admission to a nursing home are low income, poor family supports (particularly the lack of a daughter), and cognitive impairment.

Financing of Long-Term Care

Nursing home expenditures currently exceed $100 billion per year and are expected to top $150 billion by 2007. Public expenditures account for about two thirds of all nursing home spending, and Medicaid expenditures are double those of Medicare. Medicare covers only short-term posthospital stays, and Medicaid pays for custodial care for persons who have exhausted their personal finances. The remaining one third of nursing home costs are out-of-pocket expenditures, with a very small amount being covered by long-term care insurance. Nearly one third of persons who enter a nursing home paying privately spend down and end up on Medicaid.

Almost all facilities charge private-pay residents more than Medicaid, often twice as much. Thus, the nursing home with a high self-pay payer mix will be more financially able to provide higher quality services and is more likely to be profitable. The cost of physician payments for nursing home residents is covered by Medicare Part B and, when applicable, Medicaid. The typical nursing home base cost per year is in excess of $60,000, although there is considerable variation.

QUALITY ASSURANCE

Beginning with the nursing home reform act of 1987 (OBRA 87), there have been a number of initiatives to enhance quality of nursing home care. The federal government has established minimum staffing guidelines, training guidelines, basic resident rights, and comprehensive mandatory resident assessments. The standardized resident assessment is known as the Minimum Data Set (MDS) and focuses on clinical issues of quality of care. The MDS will trigger Resident Assessment Protocols (RAPs) for identified problems. Quality indicators (QIs) are a relatively new initiative to enhance quality of care in nursing homes. These quality assurance (QA) measures are described next.

Minimum Data Set

The MDS quantifies current or potential problems in medical, psychological, or functional domains (Figs. 7-2 to 7-17). The MDS is completed for residents admitted for a non-Medicare stay within 14 days of admission, annually, and when a significant change in resident status occurs. In addition, an abbreviated MDS is conducted quarterly. For patients admitted for a stay covered by Medicare Part A, the MDS is completed more frequently. The MDS is completed by the nursing home staff and should be available for the physician to review, but many physicians do not avail themselves of the data. When the MDS is completed, certain item responses identify or trigger one of a number of RAPs.

Resident Assessment Protocols

The RAPs that are triggered by the MDS include issues common to nursing home populations and are listed in Box 7-5. The RAPs highlight areas that need attention and guide the care team through further assessment and intervention (care plan).

Quality Indicators

Quality indicators (QIs) are designed to highlight existing or potential problems as a means to guide each facility's quality assurance program. Quality assurance programs can cover a number of domains that include QIs. Examples are listed in Box 7-6. QIs may be compared among facilities

Text continued on page 528

BOX 7-5   RAPs Triggered by the MDS

Activities
Activities of daily living
Behavioral symptoms
Cognitive loss and dementia
Dehydration and fluid maintenance
Delirium
Dental care
Falls
Feeding tubes
Functional rehabilitation potential
Mood
Nutritional status
Physical restraints
Pressure ulcers
Psychosocial well being
Psychotropic drug use
Urinary incontinence and indwelling catheters
Visual functioning

MDS, minimum data set; RAP, resident assessment protocol.

BOX 7-6   Examples of Nursing Home Quality Indicators

Accidents

Incidence of new fractures
Incidence (prevalence) of falls

Nutrition

Prevalence of dehydration
Prevalence of tube feeding
Prevalence of weight loss

Psychotropic Drug Use

Prevalence of antipsychotic use without appropriate reason
Prevalence of sedative–hypnotic use

Skin Care

Prevalence of pressure ulcers, stage 1-4

		SECTION A. IDENTIFICATION AND BACKGROUND INFORMATION
1.	ASSESSMENT DATE	☐☐ — ☐☐ — ☐☐☐☐ Month Day Year
2.	RESIDENT NAME & I.D.#	(First) (Middle Initial) (Last) ID#_____
3.	SOCIAL SECURITY NO.	☐☐☐ — ☐☐ — ☐☐☐☐
4.	MEDICAID NO. (If applicable)	☐☐☐☐☐☐☐☐☐☐
5.	MEDICAL RECORD NO.	☐☐☐☐☐☐☐☐☐☐
6.	REASON FOR ASSESSMENT	1. Initial admission assess. 4. Annual assessment 2. Hosp/Medicare reassess. 5. Significant change in status 3. Readmission assessment 6. Other (e.g., UR)
7.	CURRENT PAYMENT SOURCE(S) FOR N.H. STAY	(Billing Office to indicate; check all that apply) a. Medicaid ☐a. d. VA ☐d. b. Medicare ☐b. e. Self pay/Private insurance ☐e. c. CHAMPUS ☐c. f. Other ☐f.
8.	RESPONSIBILITY/ LEGAL GUARDIAN	(Check all that apply) a. Legal guardian ☐a. d. Family member responsible ☐d. b. Other legal oversight ☐b. e. Resident responsible ☐e. c. Durable power attrny./ health care proxy ☐c. f. NONE OF ABOVE ☐f.
9.	ADVANCED DIRECTIVES	(For those items with supporting documentation in the medical record, check all that apply) a. Living will ☐a. f. Feeding restrictions ☐f. b. Do not resuscitate ☐b. g. Medication restrictions ☐g. c. Do not hospitalize ☐c. h. Other treatment restrictions ☐h. d. Organ donation ☐d. i. NONE OF ABOVE ☐i. e. Autopsy request ☐e.
10.	DISCHARGE PLANNED WITHIN 3 MOS.	(Does not include discharge due to death) 0. No 1. Yes 2. Unknown/uncertain
11.	PARTICIPATE IN ASSESSMENT	a. Resident b. Family 0. No 0. No 1. Yes 1. Yes ☐a. 2. No family ☐b.
12.	SIGNATURES	Signature & Date of RN Assessment Coordinator _____ Signatures & Dates of Others Who Completed Part of the Assessment _____

Figure 7-2 Minimum Data Set, version 2.0. Identification and background information. (From the Centers for Medicare and Medicaid Services, US Department of Health and Human Services. Available at http://www.cms.hhs.gov/NursingHome QualityInits/downloads/MDS20MDSAllForms.pdf [accessed February 28, 2007].)

		SECTION B. COGNITIVE PATTERNS		
1.	COMATOSE	*(Persistent vegetative state/no discernible consciousness)* 0. No **1. Yes (Skip to SECTION E)**		
2.	MEMORY	*(Recall of what was learned or known)* a. Short-term memory OK—seems/appears to recall after 5 minutes 0. Memory OK 1. Memory problem ▲		a.
		b. Long-term memory OK—seems/appears to recall long past 0. Memory OK 1. Memory problem ▲		b.

3.	MEMORY/ RECALL ABILITY	*(Check all that resident normally able to recall during last 7 days)* Fewer than 3 ✓ = ▲²		
		a. Current season	a.	d. That he/she is in a nursing home	d.
		b. Location of own room	b.	e. *NONE OF ABOVE* are recalled	
		c. Staff names/faces	c.		e.
4.	COGNITIVE SKILLS FOR DAILY DECISION- MAKING	*(Made decisions regarding tasks of daily life)* 0. **Independent**—decisions consistent/reasonable ▲⁴ 1. **Modified independence**—some difficulty in new situations only ▲⁴ ▲² 2. **Moderately impaired**—decisions poor; cues/supervision required ▲⁴ ▲² 3. **Severely impaired**—never/rarely made decisions ▲²		
5.	INDICATORS OF DELIRIUM —PERIODIC DISORDERED THINKING/ AWARENESS	*(Check if condition over last 7 days appears different from usual functioning)*		
		a. Less alert, easily distracted ●¹		a.
		b. Changing awareness of environment ●¹		b.
		c. Episodes of incoherent speech ●¹		c.
		d. Periods of motor restlessness or lethargy ●¹		d.
		e. Cognitive ability varies over course of day ●¹		e.
		f. *NONE OF ABOVE*		f.
6.	CHANGE IN COGNITIVE STATUS	Change in resident's cognitive status, skills, or abilities in last 90 days 0. No change 1. Improved 2. Deteriorated ●¹ ▲¹⁴		

● = Automatic Trigger

1 - Delirium   5 - ADL Functional/Rehabilitation Potential
2 - Cognitive Loss/Dementia   6 - Urinary Incontinence and Indwelling Catheter
3 - Visual Function   7 - Psychosocial Well-Being
4 - Communication   8 - Mood State

▲ = Potential Trigger

9 - Behavior Problems   13 - Feeding Tubes   17 - Psychotropic Drug Use
10 - Activities   14 - Dehydration/Fluid Maintenance 18 - Physical Restraints
11 - Falls   15 - Dental Care
12 - Nutritional Status 16 - Pressure Ulcers

Figure 7-3 Minimum Data Set, version 2.0. Cognitive patterns. (From the Centers for Medicare and Medicaid Services, US Department of Health and Human Services. Available at http://www.cms.hhs.gov/NursingHomeQualityInits/downloads/MDS20MDSAllForms.pdf [accessed February 28, 2007].)

	SECTION C. COMMUNICATION/HEARING PATTERNS		
1.	**HEARING**	*(With hearing appliance, if used)* 0. **Hears adequately**—normal talk, TV, phone 1. **Minimal difficulty** when not in quiet setting 2. **Hears in special situation only**—speaker has to adjust tonal quality and speak distinctly 3. **Highly impaired**/absence of useful hearing	
2.	**COMMUNI-CATION DEVICES/ TECHNIQUES**	*(Check all that apply during last 7 days)* a. Hearing aid, present and used b. Hearing aid, present and not used c. Other receptive comm. technique used (e.g., lip read) d. *NONE OF ABOVE*	a. b. c. d.
3.	**MODES OF EXPRESSION**	*(Check all used by resident to make needs known)* a. Speech ⬜ b. Writing messages to express or clarify needs ⬜ c. Signs/gestures/sounds d. Communication board e. Other f. *NONE OF ABOVE*	c. d. e. f.
4.	**MAKING SELF UN-DERSTOOD**	*(Express information content—however able)* 0. **Understood** 1. **Usually Understood**-difficulty finding words or finishing thoughts 2. **Sometimes Understood**-ability is limited to making concrete requests ▲⁴ 3. **Rarely/Never Understood** ▲⁴	
5.	**ABILITY TO UNDER-STAND OTHERS**	*(Understanding verbal information content-however able)* 0. **Understands** 1. **Usually Understands**-may miss some part/intent of message ▲² 2. **Sometimes Understands**-responds adequately to simple, direct communication ▲² ▲⁴ ▲⁵ 3. **Rarely/Never Understands** ▲² ▲⁴ ▲⁵	
6.	**CHANGE IN COMMUNI-CATION/ HEARING**	Resident's ability to express, understand or hear information has changed over last 90 days 0. No change 1. Improved 2. Deteriorated ●¹	

● = Automatic Trigger

1 - Delirium	5 - ADL Functional/Rehabilitation Potential
2 - Cognitive Loss/Dementia	6 - Urinary Incontinence and Indwelling Catheter
3 - Visual Function	7 - Psychosocial Well-Being
4 - Communication	8 - Mood State

▲ = Potential Trigger

9 - Behavior Problems	13 - Feeding Tubes	17 - Psychotropic Drug Use
10 - Activities	14 - Dehydration/Fluid Maintenance	18 - Physical Restraints
11 - Falls	15 - Dental Care	
12 - Nutritional Status	16 - Pressure Ulcers	

Figure 7-4 Minimum Data Set, version 2.0. Communication/hearing patterns. (From the Centers for Medicare and Medicaid Services, US Department of Health and Human Services. Available at http://www.cms.hhs.gov/NursingHomeQuality Inits/downloads/MDS20MDSAllForms.pdf [accessed February 28, 2007].)

		SECTION D. VISION PATTERNS	
1.	VISION	*(Ability to see in adequate light and with glasses if used)*	
		0. Adequate—sees fine detail, including regular print in newspapers/books	
		1. Impaired—sees large print, but not regular print in newspapers/books ●³	
		2. Highly Impaired—limited vision, not able to see newspaper headlines, appears to follow objects with eyes ●³	
		3. Severely Impaired—no vision or appears to see only light, colors, or shapes ●³	

2.	VISUAL LIMITATIONS/ DIFFICULTIES	a. Side vision problems—decreased peripheral vision; (e.g., leaves food on one side of tray, difficulty traveling, bumps into people and objects, misjudges placement of chair when seating self) ●³	
		b. Experiences any of the following: sees halos or rings around lights, sees flashes of light; sees "curtains" over eyes	a. b.
		c. *NONE OF ABOVE*	c.
3.	VISUAL APPLIANCES	Glasses; contact lenses; lens implant; magnifying glass 0. No 1. Yes	

● = Automatic Trigger

1 - Delirium	5 - ADL Functional/Rehabilitation Potential
2 - Cognitive Loss/Dementia	6 - Urinary Incontinence and Indwelling Catheter
3 - Visual Function	7 - Psychosocial Well-Being
4 - Communication	8 - Mood State

▲ = Potential Trigger

9 - Behavior Problems	13 - Feeding Tubes	17 - Psychotropic Drug Use
10 - Activities	14 - Dehydration/Fluid Maintenance	18 - Physical Restraints
11 - Falls	15 - Dental Care	
12 - Nutritional Status	16 - Pressure Ulcers	

Figure 7-5 Minimum Data Set, version 2.0. Vision patterns. (From the Centers for Medicare and Medicaid Services, US Department of Health and Human Services. Available at http://www.cms.hhs.gov/NursingHomeQualityInits/downloads/MDS20MDSAllForms.pdf [accessed February 28, 2007].)

	SECTION E. PHYSICAL FUNCTIONING AND STRUCTURAL PROBLEMS		

1.	**ADL SELF-PERFORMANCE** *(Code for resident's* **PERFORMANCE OVER ALL SHIFTS** *during last 7 days—Not including setup)*
	
	 0. INDEPENDENT—No help or oversight—OR—Help/oversight provided only 1 or 2 times during last 7 days.
	 1. SUPERVISION—Oversight encouragement or cueing provided 3+ times during last 7 days—OR—Supervision plus physical assistance provided only 1 or 2 times during last 7 days.
	 2. LIMITED ASSISTANCE—Resident highly involved in activity, received physical help in guided maneuvering of limbs, or other nonweight bearing assistance 3+ times—OR—More help provided only 1 or 2 times during last 7 days.
	 3. EXTENSIVE ASSISTANCE—While resident performed part of activity, over last 7-day period, help of following type(s) provided 3 or more times:
	   — Weight-bearing support
	   — Full staff performance during part (but not all) of last 7 days.
	 4. TOTAL DEPENDENCE—Full staff performance of activity during entire 7 days.		

2.	**ADL SUPPORT PROVIDED**—*(Code for MOST SUPPORT PROVIDED OVER ALL SHIFTS during last 7 days; code regardless of resident's self-performance classification)* **0. No setup** or physical help from staff **2. One-person** physical assist **1. Setup help** only **3. Two+ persons** physical assist	**1** SELF-PERFORMANCE	**2** SUPPORT

			1	2
a.	**BED MOBILITY**	How resident moves to and from lying position, turns side to side, and positions body while in bed 3 or 4 for self-perf = ▲⁵		
b.	**TRANSFER**	How resident moves between surfaces—to/from: bed, chair, wheelchair, standing position (EXCLUDE to/from bath/toilet) 3 or 4 for self-perf = ▲⁵		
c.	**LOCO-MOTION**	How resident moves between locations in his/her room and adjacent corridor on same floor. If in wheelchair, self-sufficiency once in chair 3 or 4 for self-perf = ▲⁵		
d.	**DRESSING**	How resident puts on, fastens, and takes off all items of street clothing, including donning/removing prosthesis 3 or 4 for self-perf = ▲⁵		
e.	**EATING**	How resident eats and drinks (regardless of skill) 3 or 4 for self-perf = ▲⁵		
f.	**TOILET USE**	How resident uses the toilet room (or commode, bed-pan, urinal); transfers on/off toilet, cleanses, changes pad, manages ostomy or catheter, adjusts clothes 3 or 4 for self-perf = ▲⁵		
g.	**PERSONAL HYGIENE**	How resident maintains personal hygiene, including combing hair, brushing teeth, shaving, applying makeup, washing/drying face, hands, and perineum (EXCLUDE baths and showers)		
3.	**BATHING**	How resident takes full-body bath, sponge bath, and transfers in/out of tub/shower (EXCLUDE washing of back and hair. Code for most dependent in self-performance and support below.) Bathing Self-Performance codes appear below.) 3 or 4 for (a) = ▲⁵ **0.** Independent—No help provided **1.** Supervision—Oversight help only **2.** Physical help limited to transfer only **3.** Physical help in part of bathing activity **4.** Total dependence	a.	b.

Figure 7-6 Minimum Data Set, version 2.0. Physical functioning and structural problems. (From the Centers for Medicare and Medicaid Services, US Department of Health and Human Services. Available at http://www.cms.hhs.gov/NursingHome QualityInits/downloads/MDS20MDSAllForms.pdf [accessed February 28, 2007].)

Continued

4.	BODY CONTROL PROBLEMS	*(Check all that apply during last 7 days)*			
		a. Balance—partial or total loss of ability to balance self while standing ▲[11]	a.	g. Hand—lack of dexterity (e.g., problem using toothbrush or adjusting hearing aid)	g.
		b. Bedfast all or most of the time ▲[11]	b.	h. Leg—partial or total loss of voluntary movement ▲[11]	h.
		c. Contracture to arms, legs, shoulders, or hands	c.	i. Leg—unsteady gait	i.
		d. Hemiplegia/hemiparesis ▲[11]	d.	j. Trunk—partial or total loss of ability to position, balance, or turn body ▲[11]	j.
		e. Quadriplegia ▲[11]	e.		
		f. Arm—partial or total loss of voluntary movement	f.	k. Amputation	k.
				l. *NONE OF ABOVE*	l.
5.	MOBILITY APPLIANCES/ DEVICES	*(Check all that apply during last 7 days)*			
		a. Cane/walker	a.	d. Other person wheeled	d.
		b. Brace/prosthesis	b.	e. Lifted (manually/ mechanically)	e.
		c. Wheeled self	c.	f. *NONE OF ABOVE*	f.
6.	TASK SEG-MENTATION	Resident requires that some or all of ADL activities be broken into a series of subtasks so that resident can perform them. 0. No 1. Yes			
7.	ADL FUNC-TIONAL REHAB. POTENTIAL	a. Resident believes he/she capable of increased independence in at least some ADLs ▲[5]			a.
		b. Direct care staff believe resident capable of increased independence in at least some ADLs ▲[5]			b.
		c. Resident able to perform tasks/activity but is very slow			c.
		d. Major difference in ADL Self-Performance or ADL Support in mornings and evenings (at least a one category change in Self-Performance or Support in any ADL)			d.
		e. *NONE OF ABOVE*			e.
8.	CHANGE IN ADL FUNCTION	Change in ADL self-performance in last 90 days 0. No change 1. Improved 2. Deteriorated ▲[14]			

● = Automatic Trigger

1 - Delirium	5 - ADL Functional/Rehabilitation Potential
2 - Cognitive Loss/Dementia	6 - Urinary Incontinence and Indwelling Catheter
3 - Visual Function	7 - Psychosocial Well-Being
4 - Communication	8 - Mood State

▲ = Potential Trigger

9 - Behavior Problems	13 - Feeding Tubes	17 - Psychotropic Drug Use
10 - Activities	14 - Dehydration/Fluid Maintenance	18 - Physical Restraints
11 - Falls	15 - Dental Care	
12 - Nutritional Status	16 - Pressure Ulcers	

Figure 7-6,   cont'd.

	SECTION F. CONTINENCE IN LAST 14 DAYS		
1.	**CONTINENCE SELF-CONTROL CATEGORIES** *(Code for resident performance over all shifts.)* 0. **CONTINENT**—Complete control 1. **USUALLY CONTINENT**—BLADDER, incontinent episodes once a week or less; BOWEL, less than weekly 2. **OCCASIONALLY INCONTINENT**—BLADDER, 2+ times a week but not daily; BOWEL, once a week 3. **FREQUENTLY INCONTINENT**—BLADDER, tended to be incontinent daily, but some control present (e.g., on day shift); BOWEL, 2-3 times a week 4. **INCONTINENT**—Had inadequate control. BLADDER, multiple daily episodes; BOWEL, all (or almost all) of the time.		
a.	**BOWEL CON-TINENCE**	Control of bowel movement, with appliance or bowel continence programs if employed	
b.	**BLADDER CONTI-NENCE**	Control of urinary bladder function (if dribbles, volume insufficient to soak through underpants), with appliances (e.g., foley) or continence programs, if employed 2, 3 or 4 = ▲[6]	
2.	**INCONTI-NENCE RELATED TESTING**	*(Skip if resident's bladder continence code equals 0 or 1 AND no catheter is used)* a. Resident has been tested for a urinary tract infection b. Resident has been checked for presence of a fecal impaction, or there is adequate bowel elimination c. *NONE OF ABOVE*	a. b. c.
3.	**APPLIANCES AND PROGRAMS**	a. Any scheduled toileting plan a. b. External (condom) catheter ▲[6] b. c. Indwelling catheter ▲[6] c. d. Intermittent catheter ▲[6] d.	e. Did not use toilet room/commode/urinal e. f. Pads/briefs used ▲[6] f. g. Enemas/irrigation g. h. Ostomy h. i. *NONE OF ABOVE* i.
4.	**CHANGE IN URINARY CONTINENCE**	Change in urinary continence/appliances and programs in last 90 days 0. No change 1. Improved 2. Deteriorated	

● = Automatic Trigger

1 - Delirium
2 - Cognitive Loss/Dementia
3 - Visual Function
4 - Communication

5 - ADL Functional/Rehabilitation Potential
6 - Urinary Incontinence and Indwelling Catheter
7 - Psychosocial Well-Being
8 - Mood State

▲ = Potential Trigger

9 - Behavior Problems
10 - Activities
11 - Falls
12 - Nutritional Status

13 - Feeding Tubes
14 - Dehydration/Fluid Maintenance
15 - Dental Care
16 - Pressure Ulcers

17 - Psychotropic Drug Use
18 - Physical Restraints

Figure 7-7 Minimum Data Set, version 2.0. Continence in the last 14 days. (From the Centers for Medicare and Medicaid Services, US Department of Health and Human Services. Available at http://www.cms.hhs.gov/NursingHomeQuality Inits/downloads/MDS20MDSAllForms.pdf [accessed February 28, 2007].)

7—Long-Term Care

7—Long-Term Care

		SECTION G. PSYCHOSOCIAL WELL-BEING	
1.	SENSE OF INITIATIVE/ INVOLVE- MENT	a. At ease interacting with others	a.
		b. At ease doing planned or structural activities	b.
		c. At ease doing self-initiated activities	c.
		d. Establishes own goals	d.
		e. Pursues involvement in life of facility (i.e., makes/keeps friends; involved in group activities; responds positively to new activities; assists at religious services)	e.
		f. Accepts invitations into most group activities	f.
		g. *NONE OF ABOVE*	g.
2.	UNSETTLED RELATION- SHIPS	a. Covert/open conflict with and/or repeated criticism of staff ●⁷	a.
		b. Unhappy with roommate ●⁷	b.
		c. Unhappy with residents other than roommate ●⁷	c.
		d. Openly expresses conflict/anger with family or friends ●⁷	d.
		e. Absence of personal contact with family/friends	e.
		f. Recent loss of close family member/friend	f.
		g. *NONE OF ABOVE*	g.

3.	PAST ROLES	a. Strong identification with past roles and life status	a.
		b. Expresses sadness/anger/empty feeling over lost roles/status ●⁷	b.
		c. *NONE OF ABOVE*	c.

● = Automatic Trigger

1 - Delirium	5 - ADL Functional/Rehabilitation Potential
2 - Cognitive Loss/Dementia	6 - Urinary Incontinence and Indwelling Catheter
3 - Visual Function	7 - Psychosocial Well-Being
4 - Communication	8 - Mood State

▲ = Potential Trigger

9 - Behavior Problems	13 - Feeding Tubes	
10 - Activities	14 - Dehydration/Fluid Maintenance	17 - Psychotropic Drug Use
11 - Falls	15 - Dental Care	18 - Physical Restraints
12 - Nutritional Status	16 - Pressure Ulcers	

Figure 7-8   Minimum Data Set, version 2.0. Psychosocial well-being. (From the Centers for Medicare and Medicaid Services, US Department of Health and Human Services. Available at http://www.cms.hhs.gov/NursingHomeQualityInits/downloads/MDS20MDSAllForms.pdf [accessed February 28, 2007].)

7—Long-Term Care

SECTION H. MOOD AND BEHAVIOR PATTERNS		
1.	SAD OR ANXIOUS MOOD	*(Check all that apply during last 30 days)*
		a. VERBAL EXPRESSIONS of DISTRESS by resident (sadness, sense that nothing matters, hopelessness, worthlessness, unrealistic fears, vocal expressions of anxiety or grief) ●[8]
		DEMONSTRATED (OBSERVABLE) SIGNS of mental DISTRESS
		b. Tearfulness, emotional groaning, sighing, breathlessness ●[8]
		c. Motor agitation such as pacing, handwringing or picking ●[8]
		d. Failure to eat or take medications, withdrawal from self-care or leisure activities ●[8] ▲[14]
		e. Pervasive concern with health ●[8]
		f. Recurrent thoughts of death—e.g., believes he/she is about to die, have a heart attack ●[8]
		g. Suicidal thoughts/actions ●[8]
		h. *NONE OF ABOVE*
2.	MOOD PERSISTENCE	Sad or anxious mood intrudes on daily life over last 7 days—not easily altered, doesn't "cheer up"
		0. No 1. Yes ●[8]
3.	PROBLEM BEHAVIOR	*(Code for behavior in last 7 days)* 0. Behavior not exhibited in last 7 days 1. Behavior of this type occurred **less than daily** 2. Behavior of this type occurred **daily or more frequently**
		a. WANDERING (moved with no rational purpose; seemingly oblivious to needs or safety) 1 or 2 = ●[9]
		b. VERBALLY ABUSIVE (others were threatened, screamed at, cursed at) 1 or 2 = ●[9]
		c. PHYSICALLY ABUSIVE (others were hit, shoved, scratched, sexually abused) 1 or 2 = ●[9]
		d. SOCIALLY INAPPROPRIATE/DISRUPTIVE BEHAVIOR (made disrupting sounds, noisy, screams, self-abusive acts, sexual behavior or disrobing in public, smeared/threw food/feces, hoarding, rummaged through others' belongings) 1 or 2 = ●[9]
4.	RESIDENT RESISTS CARE	*(Check all types of resistance that occurred in the last 7 days)* a. Resisted taking medications/injection
		b. Resisted ADL assistance
		c. *NONE OF ABOVE*
5.	BEHAVIOR MANAGEMENT PROGRAM	Behavior problem has been addressed by clinically developed behavior management program. (Note: Do not include programs that involve only physical restraints or psychotropic medications in this category.) 0. No behavior problem 1. Yes, addressed 2. No, not addressed
6.	CHANGE IN MOOD	Change in mood in last 90 days 0. No change 1. Improved 2. Deteriorated ▲
7.	CHANGE IN PROBLEM BEHAVIOR	Change in problem behavioral signs in last 90 days 0. No change 1. Improved 2. Deteriorated ●[1]

Figure 7-9 Minimum Data Set, version 2.0. Mood and behavior patterns. (From the Centers for Medicare and Medicaid Services, US Department of Health and Human Services. Available at http://www.cms.hhs.gov/NursingHomeQualityInits/downloads/MDS20MDSAllForms.pdf [accessed February 28, 2007].)

SECTION I. ACTIVITY PURSUIT PATTERNS		
1. TIME AWAKE	*(Check appropriate time periods—last 7 days)* Resident awake all or most of time (i.e., naps no more than one hour per time period) in the:	

		a. Morning	a.	c. Evening	c.
		b. Afternoon	b.	d. *NONE OF ABOVE*	d.

| 2. AVERAGE TIME INVOLVED IN ACTIVITIES | 0. Most—(more than 2/3 of time) ▲10   2. Little—(less than 1/3 of time) ▲10
 1. Some—(1/3 to 2/3 time)   3. None ▲10 | |

3. PREFERRED ACTIVITY SETTINGS	*(Check all settings in which activities are preferred)*	
	a. Own room a.	d. Outside facility d.
	b. Day/activity room b.	e. *NONE OF ABOVE* e.
	c. Inside NH/off unit c.	

4. GENERAL ACTIVITIES PREFER-ENCES (adapted to resident's current abilities)	*(Check all specific preferences whether or not activity is currently available to resident)*	
	a. Cards/other games a.	f. Spiritual/religious activ. f.
	b. Crafts/arts b.	g. Trips/shopping g.
	c. Exercise/sports c.	h. Walking/wheeling outdoors h.
	d. Music d.	i. Watch TV i.
	e. Read/write e.	j. *NONE OF ABOVE* j.

5. PREFERS MORE OR DIFFERENT ACTIVITIES	Resident expresses/indicates preference for other activities/choices.	
	0. No 1. Yes ●10	

● = Automatic Trigger

1 - Delirium
2 - Cognitive Loss/Dementia
3 - Visual Function
4 - Communication

5 - ADL Functional/Rehabilitation Potential
6 - Urinary Incontinence and Indwelling Catheter
7 - Psychosocial Well-Being
8 - Mood State

▲ = Potential Trigger

9 - Behavior Problems
10 - Activities
11 - Falls
12 - Nutritional Status

13 - Feeding Tubes
14 - Dehydration/Fluid Maintenance
15 - Dental Care
16 - Pressure Ulcers

17 - Psychotropic Drug Use
18 - Physical Restraints

Figure 7-10 Minimum Data Set, version 2.0. Activity pursuit patterns. (From the Centers for Medicare and Medicaid Services, US Department of Health and Human Services. Available at http://www.cms.hhs.gov/NursingHomeQualityInits/downloads/MDS20MDSAllForms.pdf [accessed February 28, 2007].)

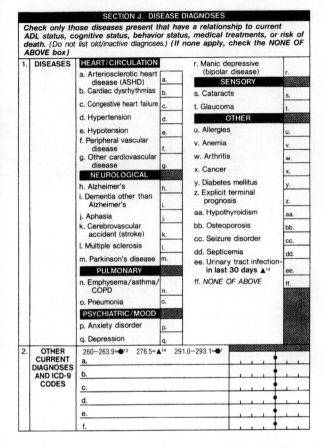

Figure 7-11 Minimum Data Set, version 2.0. Disease diagnoses. (From the Centers for Medicare and Medicaid Services, US Department of Health and Human Services. Available at http://www.cms.hhs.gov/NursingHomeQualityInits/downloads/MDS20MDSAllForms.pdf [accessed February 28, 2007].)

7–Long-Term Care

SECTION K. HEALTH CONDITIONS				
1.	PROBLEM CONDITIONS	*(Check all problems that are present in last 7 days unless other time frame indicated)*		

a. Constipation	a.	j. Pain—resident complains or shows evidence of pain daily or almost daily — j.
b. Diarrhea ▲¹⁴	b.	
c. Dizziness/vertigo ▲¹⁴	c.	
d. Edema	d.	k. Recurrent lung aspirations in last 90 days — k.
e. Fecal impaction	e.	
f. Fever ▲¹⁴	f.	
g. Hallucinations/ delusions	g.	l. Shortness of breath — l.
		m. Syncope (fainting) — m.
h. Internal bleeding ▲¹⁴	h.	n. Vomiting ▲¹⁴ — n.
i. Joint pain	i.	o. *NONE OF ABOVE* — o.

2.	ACCIDENTS	a. Fell—past 30 days ●¹¹	a.	c. Hip fracture in last 180 days	c.
		b. Fell—past 31-180 days ●¹¹	b.	d. *NONE OF ABOVE*	d.

3.	STABILITY OF CONDITIONS	a. Conditions/diseases make resident's cognitive, ADL, or behavior status unstable—fluctuating, precarious, or deteriorating.	a.
		b. Resident experiencing an acute episode or a flare-up of a recurrent/chronic problem.	b.
		c. *NONE OF THE ABOVE*	c.

● = Automatic Trigger

1 - Delirium
2 - Cognitive Loss/Dementia
3 - Visual Function
4 - Communication

5 - ADL Functional/Rehabilitation Potential
6 - Urinary Incontinence and Indwelling Catheter
7 - Psychosocial Well-Being
8 - Mood State

▲ = Potential Trigger

9 - Behavior Problems
10 - Activities
11 - Falls
12 - Nutritional Status

13 - Feeding Tubes
14 - Dehydration/Fluid Maintenance
15 - Dental Care
16 - Pressure Ulcers

17 - Psychotropic Drug Use
18 - Physical Restraints

Figure 7-12 Minimum Data Set, version 2.0. Health conditions. (From the Centers for Medicare and Medicaid Services, US Department of Health and Human Services. Available at http://www.cms.hhs.gov/NursingHomeQualityInits/downloads/MDS20MDSAllForms.pdf [accessed February 28, 2007].)

SECTION L. ORAL/NUTRITIONAL STATUS				
1.	ORAL PROBLEMS	a. Chewing problem [a.] b. Swallowing problem [b.]	c. Mouth pain ●15 [c.] d. *NONE OF ABOVE* [d.]	
2.	HEIGHT AND WEIGHT	*Record height (a) in inches and weight (b) in pounds.* *Weight based on most recent status in* **last 30 days;** measure weight consistently *in accord with standard facility practice—* *e.g., in a.m. after voiding,* before meal, with shoes off, and in nightclothes. HT (in.) [a.] WT (lb.) [b.]		
		c. **Weight loss** (i.e., 5% + in last 30 days; or 10% in last 180 days) 0. No 1. Yes ●12 ▲14		[c.]
3.	NUTRITIONAL PROBLEMS	a. Complains about the taste of many foods ●12 [a.] b. Insufficient fluid; dehydrated ●14 [b.] c. Did **NOT** consume all/almost all liquids provided during last 3 days ▲14 [c.]	d. Regular complaint of hunger ●12 [d.] e. Leaves 25%+ food uneaten at most meals ●12 ▲14 [e.] f. *NONE OF ABOVE* [f.]	
4.	NUTRITIONAL APPROACHES	a. Parenteral/IV ▲14 ●12 [a.] b. Feeding tube ▲14 ●13 [b.] c. Mechanically altered diet ●12 [c.] d. Syringe (oral feeding) ●12 [d.]	e. Therapeutic diet ●12 [e.] f. Dietary supplement between meals [f.] g. Plate guard, stabilized built-up utensil, etc. [g.] h. *NONE OF ABOVE* [h.]	

● = Automatic Trigger

1 - Delirium	5 - ADL Functional/Rehabilitation Potential
2 - Cognitive Loss/Dementia	6 - Urinary Incontinence and Indwelling Catheter
3 - Visual Function	7 - Psychosocial Well-Being
4 - Communication	8 - Mood State

▲ = Potential Trigger

9 - Behavior Problems	13 - Feeding Tubes	17 - Psychotropic Drug Use
10 - Activities	14 - Dehydration/Fluid Maintenance	18 - Physical Restraints
11 - Falls	15 - Dental Care	
12 - Nutritional Status	16 - Pressure Ulcers	

Figure 7-13 Minimum Data Set, version 2.0. Oral/nutritional status. (From the Centers for Medicare and Medicaid Services, US Department of Health and Human Services. Available at http://www.cms.hhs.gov/NursingHomeQualityInits/downloads/MDS20MDSAllForms.pdf [accessed February 28, 2007].)

SECTION M. ORAL/DENTAL STATUS		
1. ORAL STATUS AND DISEASE PREVENTION	a. Debris (soft, easily movable substances) present in mouth prior to going to bed at night ●15	a.
	b. Has dentures and/or removable bridge	b.
	c. Some/all natural teeth lost—does not have or does not use dentures (or partial plates) ●15	c.
	d. Broken, loose, or carious teeth ●15	d.
	e. Inflamed gums (gingiva), oral abscesses, swollen or bleeding gums, ulcers, or rashes ●15	e.
	f. Daily cleaning of teeth/dentures If not checked = ●15	f.
	g. NONE OF ABOVE	g.

● = Automatic Trigger

1 - Delirium	5 - ADL Functional/Rehabilitation Potential
2 - Cognitive Loss/Dementia	6 - Urinary Incontinence and Indwelling Catheter
3 - Visual Function	7 - Psychosocial Well-Being
4 - Communication	8 - Mood State

▲ = Potential Trigger

9 - Behavior Problems	13 - Feeding Tubes	17 - Psychotropic Drug Use
10 - Activities	14 - Dehydration/Fluid Maintenance	18 - Physical Restraints
11 - Falls	15 - Dental Care	
12 - Nutritional Status	16 - Pressure Ulcers	

Figure 7-14   Minimum Data Set, version 2.0. Oral/dental status. (From the Centers for Medicare and Medicaid Services, US Department of Health and Human Services. Available at http://www.cms.hhs.gov/NursingHomeQualityInits/downloads/MDS20MDSAllForms.pdf [accessed February 28, 2007].)

that are similar, as a way to benchmark standards. Each nursing home must conduct a QA program that represents all major disciplines, but the design of such programs is not standardized.

ROLE OF THE ATTENDING PHYSICIAN

Overview

Medical care of nursing home residents offers unique challenges and demands exemplary clinical skills. The physician practicing in a nursing home must embrace interdisciplinary care and be sensitive to ethical issues. Nursing home care includes care that is preventive, curative, and/or palliative. The care requires a biopsychosocial approach, and family communication is a key aspect of care.

The next section discusses the responsibilities of the physician practicing in the nursing home setting. These responsibilities reflect standards of care as well as specific regulations. The regulations encompass several domains, each of which corresponds to a regulatory code known as a tag number. The domains address physician services, resident assessment, resident rights, and quality of care (Table 7-3). Also listed are the CPT codes for physician billing in the nursing home (Table 7-4).

Physician Responsibilities in the Nursing Home

Providing medical care to nursing home patients differs from both the hospital setting and the outpatient setting. Hospitalized patients are acutely ill

	SECTION N. SKIN CONDITION		
1.	STASIS ULCER	(i.e., open lesion caused by poor venous circulation to lower extremities) 0. No 1. Yes	
2.	PRESSURE ULCERS	*(Code for highest stage of pressure ulcer)* 0. No pressure ulcers 1. Stage 1 A persistent area of skin redness (without a break in the skin) that does not disappear when pressure is relieved ●12 ●16 2. Stage 2 A partial thickness loss of skin layers that presents clinically as an abrasion, blister, or shallow crater ●12 ●16 3. Stage 3 A full thickness of skin is lost, exposing the subcutaneous tissues—presents as a deep crater with or without undermining adjacent tissue ●12 ●16 4. Stage 4 A full thickness of skin and subcutaneous tissue is lost, exposing muscle and/or bone ●12 ●16	
3.	HISTORY OF RESOLVED/ CURED PRESSURE ULCERS	Resident has had a pressure ulcer that was resolved/cured in last 90 days 0. No 1. Yes	

4.	SKIN PROBLEMS/ CARE	a. Open lesions other than stasis or pressure ulcers (e.g., cuts)	a.
		b. Skin desensitized to pain/pressure/discomfort	b.
		c. Protective/preventive skin care	c.
	Nothing Checked From C Thru G = ▲16	d. Turning/repositioning program	d.
		e. Pressure-relieving beds, bed/chair pads (e.g., egg crate pads)	e.
		f. Wound care/treatment (e.g., pressure ulcer care, surgical wound)	f.
		g. Other skin care/treatment	g.
		h. *NONE OF ABOVE*	h.

● = Automatic Trigger

1 - Delirium	5 - ADL Functional/Rehabilitation Potential
2 - Cognitive Loss/Dementia	6 - Urinary Incontinence and Indwelling Catheter
3 - Visual Function	7 - Psychosocial Well-Being
4 - Communication	8 - Mood State

▲ = Potential Trigger

9 - Behavior Problems	13 - Feeding Tubes	17 - Psychotropic Drug Use
10 - Activities	14 - Dehydration/Fluid Maintenance	18 - Physical Restraints
11 - Falls	15 - Dental Care	
12 - Nutritional Status	16 - Pressure Ulcers	

Figure 7-15 Minimum Data Set, version 2.0. Skin conditions. (From the Centers for Medicare and Medicaid Services, US Department of Health and Human Services. Available at http://www.cms.hhs.gov/NursingHomeQualityInits/downloads/MDS20MDSAllForms.pdf [accessed February 28, 2007].)

7–Long-Term Care

	SECTION O. MEDICATION USE		
1.	NUMBER OF MEDI-CATIONS	(Record the number of *different medications used in the last 7 days;* enter "0" if none used.)	
2.	NEW MEDI-CATIONS	Resident has received new medications during the **last 90 days** 0. No 1. Yes	
3.	INJECTIONS	*(Record the number of days injections of any type received during the last 7 days.)*	
4.	DAYS RECEIVED THE FOLLOWING MEDICATION	(Record the number of days during last 7 days; *Enter "0" if not used; enter "1" if long-acting meds. used less than weekly)*	
		a. Antipsychotics 1-7 = ▲⁹ ▲¹¹ ▲¹⁷	a.
		b. Antianxiety/hypnotics 1-7 = ▲⁹ ▲¹¹ ▲¹⁷	b.
		c. Antidepressants 1-7 = ▲⁹ ▲¹¹ ▲¹⁷	c.
5.	PREVIOUS MEDICATION RESULTS	*(SKIP this question if resident currently receiving anti-psychotics, antidepressants, or antianxiety/hypnotics— otherwise **code correct response for last 90 days**)* Resident has previously received psychoactive medications for a mood or behavior problem, and these medications were effective (without undue adverse consequences). 0. No, drugs not used 1. Drugs were effective 2. Drugs were not effective 3. Drug effectiveness unknown	

● = Automatic Trigger

1 - Delirium	5 - ADL Functional/Rehabilitation Potential
2 - Cognitive Loss/Dementia	6 - Urinary Incontinence and Indwelling Catheter
3 - Visual Function	7 - Psychosocial Well-Being
4 - Communication	8 - Mood State

▲ = Potential Trigger

9 - Behavior Problems	13 - Feeding Tubes	17 - Psychotropic Drug Use
10 - Activities	14 - Dehydration/Fluid Maintenance	18 - Physical Restraints
11 - Falls	15 - Dental Care	
12 - Nutritional Status	16 - Pressure Ulcers	

Figure 7-16 Minimum Data Set, version 2.0. Medication use. (From the Centers for Medicare and Medicaid Services, US Department of Health and Human Services. Available at http://www.cms.hhs.gov/NursingHomeQualityInits/downloads/MDS20MDSAllForms.pdf [accessed February 28, 2007].)

and are seen every day. Subspecialists in many fields are available for consultation on short notice when help is needed. Ambulatory patients are seen episodically for chronic disease management, health maintenance, or acute conditions, but they are generally independent and mobile and can usually carry out the physician's orders independently or with minimal formal or informal assistance.

Three concepts highlight the nature of nursing home medical care: interdisciplinary, geriatric, and regulated. Nursing home patients are typically sicker than ambulatory patients (admitted following acute care) or more debilitated (admitted for long-term care), but their usual condition does not require daily visits. The schedule of regulatory visits is described in Box 7-7 on page 533. However, this patient population's usual condition requires the services of various professionals such as nurses, rehabilitation

SECTION P. SPECIAL TREATMENTS AND PROCEDURES				
1.	SPECIAL TREAT-MENTS AND PROCE-DURES	**SPECIAL CARE**—*Check treatments received during the last 14 days.*		
		a. Chemotherapy	a.	f. IV meds	f.
		b. Radiation	b.	g. Transfusions	g.
		c. Dialysis	c.	h. O₂	h.
		d. Suctioning	d.	i. Other _____	i.
		e. Trach. care	e.	j. *NONE OF ABOVE*	j.
		THERAPIES—Record the number of days *each of the following therapies was administered (for at least 10 minutes during a day) in the last 7 days:*		
		k. Speech–language pathology and audiology services	k.
		l. Occupational therapy	l.
		m. Physical therapy	m.
		n. Psychological therapy (any licensed professional)	n.
		o. Respiratory Therapy	o.
2.	ABNORMAL LAB VALUES	Has the resident had any **abnormal lab values** during the last 90-day period? **0.** No **1.** Yes **2.** No tests performed		
3.	DEVICES AND RESTRAINTS	*Use the following code for last 7 days:* **0** Not used **1** Used less than daily **2** Used daily		
		a. Bed rails	a.
		b. Trunk restraint 1 or 2 = ▲⁹ ●¹⁸	b.
		c. Limb restraint 1 or 2 = ▲⁹ ●¹⁸	c.
		d. Chair prevents rising 1 or 2 = ▲⁹ ●¹⁸	d.

● = Automatic Trigger

1 - Delirium	5 - ADL Functional/Rehabilitation Potential
2 - Cognitive Loss/Dementia	6 - Urinary Incontinence and Indwelling Catheter
3 - Visual Function	7 - Psychosocial Well-Being
4 - Communication	8 - Mood State

▲ = Potential Trigger

9 - Behavior Problems	13 - Feeding Tubes	17 - Psychotropic Drug Use
10 - Activities	14 - Dehydration/Fluid Maintenance	18 - Physical Restraints
11 - Falls	15 - Dental Care	
12 - Nutritional Status	16 - Pressure Ulcers	

Figure 7-17 Minimum Data Set, version 2.0. Special treatments and procedures. (From the Centers for Medicare and Medicaid Services, US Department of Health and Human Services. Available at http://www.cms.hhs.gov/NursingHomeQualityInits/downloads/MDS20MDSAllForms.pdf [accessed February 28, 2007].)

personnel, dietitians, social workers, personal care attendants, and others with whom the attending physician must interact by phone or in person. This ongoing interaction is necessary both to receive information about the patient's status and to order care. Nursing home physicians must be comfortable with interdisciplinary teamwork in order to perform effectively.

In addition, nursing home physicians must be familiar with geriatric principles to practice competently in this environment. This requires

7—Long-Term Care

Table 7-3 **Regulatory Codes for Physician Responsibilities**	
Domain	**Tag Numbers**
Comprehensively assess each resident Assist in care plan development and coordination of all aspects of care	272, 279
Periodically review the care plan and ensure that the goals and objectives for each care plan are rational and functionally relevant	272, 279, F 250, F 309
Implement treatments and services to enhance or maintain physical and psychological function and to prevent accidents	F 502-F 512, F 310, F 311, F 323, F 324
Physically attend to each resident in a manner consistent with state and federal guidelines (visit every 30 days for the first 90 days following admission, and at least every 60 days thereafter) while ensuring that the appropriate diagnostic tests are performed and followed up in a timely manner	F 387, F 500-F 512
Respond in a timely fashion to a resident's change in function or condition	F 157
Inform residents of their health status and optimize ability for residents to exercise self-determination	F 151, F 152, F 154
Determine each resident's decision-making capacity while establishing advance directives	F151, F152
Ensure that residents are free from unnecessary drugs by periodic review of drug regimens and consultant pharmacist recommendations	F 329-F 331, F 428, F 429

familiarity with geriatric syndromes and with functional concepts (assessments and outcomes).

Finally, nursing homes are highly regulated institutions. Many of the state and federal government regulations are the result of historical (and sometimes current) poor care. Attending physicians might not agree with every regulation (as we do not always agree with every speed limit), but failure to comply results in difficulties for the facility and its managing staff, including the medical director. By agreeing to accept responsibility for the medical care of a nursing home resident, the attending physician agrees implicitly or explicitly (Box 7-7) to comply with the various rules and regulations.

Table 7-4 CPT Codes for Nursing Facility Services

CPT Code	Service
Comprehensive Nursing Facility Assessments, New or Established Patient	
99304	Low complexity (e.g., simple admission or readmission)
99305	Moderate complexity (moderately complex admission or readmission)
99306	High complexity (e.g., complex admission or readmission)
Subsequent Nursing Facility Care, New or Established Patient	
99307	Low (e.g., stable, recertification)
99308	Moderate (e.g., change in treatment, new complaint, not responding)
99309	Complex single problem or multiple chronic conditions, some of which are not controlled
99310	High (e.g., major medical event)
99315	Nursing facility discharge management, less than 30 minutes
99316	Nursing facility discharge management, more than 30 minutes
99318	Comprehensive annual assessment

BOX 7-7   Model Practice Agreement

The attending physician and the nursing facility share a common goal: the highest possible quality of life for the residents. Achieving the highest attainable quality of life for the resident requires the joint efforts of multiple disciplines, which must operate collaboratively.

The attending physician provides medical care (primary function) and interacts with nursing, rehabilitation specialists, dietary, social services, and other professionals (collaborative function) in the context of a highly government regulated environment (regulatory function). This complex structure requires physician knowledge, skills, attitudes and activities that are not typically encountered in other practice settings. This must be understood and accepted.

The attending physicians agree to perform the following:
1. Approve orders on the day of admission (may be done by phone).
2. Visit new patients within 48 hours of admission, unless the patient was examined by a physician within the 5 days prior to admission (e.g., a hospital transfer). In the latter case, with documentation, the attending physician has 7 days to visit the patient.

Continued

BOX 7-7   Model Practice Agreement—cont'd

---

3. The admission visit is comprehensive. It should include a history, a physical examination, a review/assessment of all the diagnoses, a plan of care for each of the diagnoses, a general goal/purpose for the nursing facility stay, and other matters that may need addressing (e.g., advance directives).

4. The attending physician agrees to visit the resident no less than every 30 days for the first 3 months, and then no less than every 60 days (regulatory visits). The attending physician also agrees to visit the resident when a change in condition or an accident requires such a visit (sick visits). Alternate regulatory visits and any sick visits may be performed by a nurse practitioner (NP) or a physician assistant (PA).

5. The progress notes must be legible, indicate the purpose of the visit, document the findings (history and physical [H&P] or subjective and objective [S&O]), contain an assessment (diagnosis) and plan (treatments). The notes must be signed and dated.

6. Over the course of a year, all the resident's medical problems and treatments must be documented in progress notes. This can be done over the course of several visits, or the resident can have an annual comprehensive visit.

7. The attending physician must be available 24 hours a day, 7 days a week, personally or through a coverage arrangement that will be disclosed to the nursing facility.

8. The attending physician agrees to sign all regulatory forms or contact the facility's medical director if she or he believes a form is incorrect or inappropriate.

9. The attending physician will participate in the discharge planning process of residents under his or her care.

10. The attending physician will attend at least one annual meeting with the facility's medical director.

11. The nursing facility agrees to provide high-quality services to its residents.

12. The nursing facility agrees to inform the attending physician and the resident's family of any change in condition in a timely manner.

13. The facility will inform the attending physician of patient-specific problems and systemic issues identified during usual care, quality improvement activities, or state or federal inspections.

14. The nursing facility will make every effort to provide specialty consultants (e.g., psychiatry and podiatry) on site and will arrange for transportation of residents for off-site consultations.

15. The attending physician will inform the medical director of any concerns regarding the care provided to residents by nursing home personnel.

The nuts and bolts of the nursing home attending physician are described in the model practice agreement displayed in Box 7-7. The most notable difference from practice in other settings is the need to work as a member of a care team whose functional captain is the nurse, although the attending physician writes the orders and the nurses and other professionals carry them out. Because physician presence in the facility is intermittent, nursing home nurses have been described as the "eyes and ears" of the physician, but the physician must be aware of the abilities of individual nurses in obtaining accurate clinical information. The most important factor in gauging the quality of this information is prior experience in working with a particular nurse. Interaction with residents' families (and friends) is equally important for transfer of information in both directions. Families need to know what to expect.

Transitions are times of particular patient vulnerability because the patient is new to the care team and because the transfer of information is often incomplete between institutions (e.g., hospital and nursing home). Ideally, direct communication between nurses and between the physicians from both institutions should take place, but in practice many obstacles prevent such interactions. The prevalence of dementia is nearly 50% among long-term care patients who cannot provide reliable medical histories. The quality of the recorded medical information is also variable for many reasons (multiple transitions, low priority, specialty care).

Regulations determine the frequency of routine physician visits, but there are no limitations on the number of sick-patient visits that attending physicians may make so long as such visits are necessary in the judgment of the physician. There also are no regulatory limitations on consultations, but few specialists visit nursing home patients, who therefore must be transported to consultants' offices. This requires nursing home attending physicians to be true generalists and often extend their scope of practice beyond what would be ordinary in their hospital or office practice.

Nursing Home Visits: Documentation and Physician Payment

It is generally expected that patients will be cared for by their attending physician within the nursing home. The availability of consultants or specialists in nursing homes is variable, and nursing home residents often need to be transported to specialists' offices or to hospitals for consultations. In the hospital setting, daily visits by the attending physician are appropriate, expected, and reimbursed by third-party payers. Ambulatory patients are seen episodically by their primary care physician and have some degree of control over the frequency of their office visits. Nursing home patients do not usually need to be seen on a daily basis, but they should be visited by their attending physician according to some schedule.

The CMS has created such a schedule to ensure "reasonable" physician visitation in the long-term care setting. The Medicare Career Manual describes payment of physicians' visits to residents of nursing facilities and nursing facilities in section 15509.1.

1. Nursing home visits must comply with federal regulations (42 CFR 483.40).
2. Resident assessments.

a. Medicare Part B pays for visits necessary to perform all Medicare required assessments.

b. Physicians should use the CPT codes for comprehensive nursing facility assessments (99304-99306) to report these evaluation and management services.

c. Comprehensive assessments must be coupled with the creation of an MDS and resulting RAP. This occurs at the time of admission, readmission, once a year routinely (99318), and whenever a change in condition requires a new MDS (e.g., a stroke).

3. Subsequent visits.

a. Subsequent visits are classified as routine (or regulatory) and sick visits.

b. These visits and all other medically necessary visits for the diagnosis or treatment of illness or injury or to improve the functioning of a body part are covered under Medicare Part B.

c. Physicians should use CPT codes for subsequent nursing facility care (99307-99310) when reporting evaluation and management services that do not involve resident assessments.

d. Medicare pays for visits required to monitor and evaluate residents once every 30 days for the first 90 days after admission and once every 60 days thereafter.

  (1) Medical necessity of a service is key criterion for payment.

  (2) Medical necessity is assumed to exist when regulatory visits are performed.

  (3) The schedule for those visits is determined by the date of admission rather than by the date of the previous visit, and the timing can be difficult to comply with.

    (a) Auditors allow 10 days before or after the scheduled date as "consistent with the requirement."

    (b) A visit "off-schedule" does not reset the clock.

    (c) Sick visits do not reset the clock.

  (4) Sick visits.

    (a) It is not clear whether a sick visit can count as a regulatory visit.

    (b) The physician or practitioner determines the necessity for sick visits. A patient with pneumonia who is managed in a nursing home can be seen appropriately every day while unstable. A patient with onychomycosis treated with an antifungal agent does not need daily visits to monitor progress.

e. Providing unnecessary services is called Medicare abuse (fraud is billing for a service that was not provided).

4. Discharge services.

a. Assessment visits and subsequent regulatory or sick visits require face-to-face contact between the patient and the practitioner/physician.

b. Discharge services (CPT codes 99315 and 99316) do not require face-to-face contact on the day of discharge but require a visit close to the discharge day.

  (1) The billing date should be the date of the face-to-face contact, but the service is typically provided over several days.

(2) The service includes discharge forms, prescriptions, phone calls, a discharge summary, etc.

(3) It is a time-based service: 99315, 30 minutes or less; 99316, longer than 30 minutes. These codes can be used if the reason for discharge is death.

Documentation

1. The volume of documentation should not be the primary influence upon which a specific level of service is billed. Documentation should simply support the level of service reported.
2. Assessment documentation: See Figure 7-18 which can be used for admissions, re-admissions, and annual comprehensive visits.
3. Follow-up regulatory visits: At the minimum, these notes must include:
   a. Date.
   b. Reason for visit (e.g., follow-up for diabetes and CHF).
   c. Relevant interval history (may refer to nurses' notes and telephone calls).
   d. Physical examination.
   e. Interval diagnostic test result acknowledgment.
   f. Assessment, impression, or diagnosis.
   g. Plan of care.
   h. Legible identity (signature) of writer.
4. The 30-day or 60-day regulatory visit should address the medical problems that are under current active management. For example, blood sugar results should be mentioned in diabetic patients, blood pressure should be mentioned in hypertensive patients, mental function and/or behavior should be mentioned in patients treated with psychoactive medication. Because most nursing home residents have multiple comorbid conditions, SOAP (subjective, objective, assessment, plan) notes might not be the most efficient way to document care.
5. Sick visits should be problem-focused and would typically resemble daily progress notes in a hospital record. SOAP notes may be appropriate for such visits.
   a. Chief complaint/reason for visit.
   b. Symptoms.
   c. Examination.
   d. Diagnosis.
   e. Treatment.
6. What E&M CPT code to use?
   a. The national frequency of nursing home visit codes is presented in Table 7-5. Individual physician/practitioner coding profiles should generally reflect these statistics.
   b. All E&M codes have performance and documentation requirements. Each code has standards that pertain to:
      (1) History.
      (2) Examination.
      (3) Medical decision making.
   c. CPT codes 99304, 99305, and 99306 are typically straightforward because of the comprehensive nature of these visits. Documentation requirements for subsequent visit CPT codes 99307, 99308, 99309,

Table 7-5 **Nursing Home Visits, 2000 Codes**		
Old Code	**New Code (2006)**	**%**
99301	99304 and 99318	2.0
99302	99305	2.9
99303	99306	4.8
99311	99307	37.4
99312	99308	41.4
99313	99309	10.3
99315	99315	1.0
99316	99316	0.3

Data from Centers for Medicare and Medicaid Services, U.S. Department of Health and Human Services. Available at http://www.cms.hhs.gov/default.asp? (accessed March 1, 2007).

and 99310 are complex. The same rules apply to regulatory visits and sick visits, which complicates the task of selecting the "correct" CPT code.

7. Assessment/comprehensive visits.
   a. The work and documentation presented on the form included in this chapter will generally satisfy the requirement for these CPT codes (see Fig. 7-18).
      (1) Code 99318 should be used for an overall annual review of the patient's medical problems. This service is not required, but it is desirable and allowed by Medicare. It should occur contemporaneously with a new MDS, but Medicare does not specify how closely the two activities should coincide.
      (2) Code 99306 is used for most new admissions and some readmissions to a long-term care facility (skilled or nonskilled care).
      (3) Code 99305 is used for moderately complex admissions and many (skilled or nonskilled care) readmissions following hospital stays that result in relatively little change in the patient's condition, plan, or care (e.g., noncardiac chest pain or a urinary tract infection [UTI]).
      (4) Code 99304 is used for a simple nursing admission or readmission (e.g., a young patient with an ankle fracture and no chronic conditions being admitted for rehabilitation).
   b. Admission and readmission visits should occur as soon as possible after the admission to the nursing home.
      (1) A phone interaction between the admitting nurse and the admitting physician should occur on the day of admission.
      (2) The physician must review and approve admitting orders as well as certify the patient as requiring nursing home care if the patient requires skilled care.
      (3) The condition of the patient may or may not require a visit within 24 to 48 hours of admission, but waiting longer than 1 week is not advisable.
      (4) Medicare allows up to 30 days to complete the admission.

ATTENDING PHYSICIAN _____ DATE _____

NAME _____ AGE _____

REASON FOR ADMISSION _____

_____

_____

_____

PAST MEDICAL HISTORY _____

_____

_____

Social History/Habits

Marital status _____ Living situation _____

Smoking _____

Alcohol _____ Other _____

Family history _____

Functional Status

Ambulation: Basic ADLs:

__ Unassisted __ With walker

	Independent	Dependent
__ With cane __ Non-ambulatory Transfers	_____	_____
Urine: Feeding	_____	_____
__ Continent __ Incontinent Bathing	_____	_____
Stool: Dressing	_____	_____
__ Continent __ Incontinent Grooming	_____	_____

Review of Symptoms

Informant: Patient __ Staff __ Family __

	NO	YES			ABN	NL
Headache	☐	☐		Hearing	☐	☐
Chest pain	☐	☐		Vision	☐	☐
Abdominal pain	☐	☐		Urination	☐	☐
Pain in limbs	☐	☐		Bowel	☐	☐
Other pain	☐	☐		Sleep	☐	☐
SOB	☐	☐		Appetite	☐	☐
Dizziness	☐	☐		Energy	☐	☐
Fall	☐	☐		Memory	☐	☐

Figure 7-18 Comprehensive history and physical examination. ECG, electrocardiogram; ECHO, echocardiogram; LN, lymph nodes; EOM, extraocular movement; SOB, shortness of breath; TM, tympanic membrane.

Continued

Exam

Vital signs:

BP_____

P _____

Weight _____

Lungs _____

Ears: Hearing _____

TM _____

Heart _____

Abdomen _____

Eyes: Vision (L)_____ (R) _____

EOM_____ Fields _____

Pupils _____

Nose _____

Throat _____

Neck: LN_____

Thyroid _____

Carotids_____

Breasts and axillae _____

Extremities:

Pulses _____

Edema _____

Skin _____

Rectal:

Prostate _____

Mucosa _____

Stool _____

Ortho _____

Neuro:

Motor_____

Reflexes ____

Gait _____

Mental status _____

Affect _____

Laboratory Data   Radiology _____

ECG _____

ECHO _____

Goals of Admission

Rehabilitation/post-acute care ☐   Long-term care ☐

Advance directives _____

Assessment and plan _____

_____

Figure 7-18, cont'd.

(5) A sick visit may precede the admission visit. The CPT code for such sick visit is a subsequent visit code.

(6) Some states and the Joint Commission for the Accreditation of Hospitals (JCAHO) have more stringent time rules for admission visits.

8. Subsequent visit codes.

a. History is divided into:
   (1) History of present illness.
   (2) Past medical history.
   (3) Social history.
   (4) Review of systems.

b. For each of the four history categories, history is divided into:
   (1) Problem focused.
   (2) Expanded problem focused.
   (3) Detailed.
   (4) Comprehensive.

c. Examination is divided into:
   (1) Problem focused.
   (2) Expanded problem focused.
   (3) Detailed.
   (4) Comprehensive.

d. Medical decision making is divided into:
   (1) Number of diagnoses and management options.
   (2) Amount and complexity of data.
   (3) Risk of complication, morbidity, and mortality.

e. Each of the decision-making categories is divided into:
   (1) Straightforward.
   (2) Low.
   (3) Moderate.
   (4) High.

f. The various permutations of all these categories define the CPT level.
   (1) Code 99307 requires (2 of 3) a problem-focused history, a problem-focused exam, and straightforward or low complexity decision making.
   (2) Code 99308 requires (2 of 3) an expanded problem focused history, an expanded problem-focused exam, and moderate-complexity decision making.
   (3) Code 99309 requires (2 of 3) a detailed history, a detailed exam, and moderate- or high-complexity decision making.
   (4) Code 99309 requires (2 of 3) a detailed history, a detailed exam, and highly complex medical decision making.

g. The task of determining the correct CPT code is often more complicated than managing the patient. The fact that Medicare allows a visit to document only a history and examination without decision making (assessment and plan) for these codes makes no clinical sense. Therefore, rather than present the scores of possible permutations, clinical vignettes are more useful for clinicians. CMS has its own set of clinical vignettes.

9. Example of regulatory subsequent visits.
   a. Code 99307: a stable patient with Alzheimer's dementia treated with donepezil.
   b. Code 99308: A patient with dementia, hyperlipidemia, and hypertension who is doing well but whose medication must be adjusted to improve blood pressure control.
   c. Code 99309: A patient with a past stroke, diabetes, hypertension, progressing renal failure, and osteoporosis who visited her nephrologist 2 weeks ago and requires a review of capillary glucose levels, the nephrology consultation, and changes in several chronic condition treatments.
10. Examples of sick visits.
   a. Code 99307: Diagnosis and treatment of pinkeye or eczema.
   b. Code 99308: Evaluation and management of UTI, new pressure ulcer.
   c. Code 99309: Evaluation and treatment of a UTI in a patient with diabetes whose glycemic control also requires attention because of the infection.
   d. Code 99310: Evaluation and management of chest pain, new delirium, a new stroke, pneumonia.
   e. The existence of comorbidities often results in more work and a higher CPT code. For example, as above, a UTI in a diabetic patient has additional clinical implications (e.g., impact of UTI on glycemic control) and would justify the use of CPT code 99309 so long as the documentation accounts for the added complexity of the situation.
   f. Notes.
      (1) A change of physician does not allow for use of a comprehensive CPT code even if the work is comprehensive.
      (2) Advance practice nurses (nurse practitioners) are not allowed to perform the admission work for skilled-care patients. They may admit non–skilled-care patients. They may alternate the subsequent regulatory visits with the attending physician, and there is no limitation on the number of sick visits they may perform. Nurse practitioners will be paid by Medicare for the services they are allowed to perform.
      (3) All consultations must be ordered by the attending physician or practitioner who works with the attending.
      (4) Even professionals with ample experience in coding sometimes disagree about what CPT code to use. The choice between 99308 and 99309 is often difficult because of the interplay of multiple chronic conditions.

MEDICAL DIRECTOR'S ROLE
Introduction

A medical director is a physician who is responsible for overseeing certain aspects of medical care and services for an organization or a health care system. Hospitals have department chairs, chiefs of staff, division directors, or vice presidents for medical affairs. As the needs and the care of nursing home residents became more complex, the expertise of physicians was needed to complement the knowledge and skills of the nursing staff.

Medicare, through the OBRA '87 regulations, requires that all long-term care facilities designate a medical director. Interpretive guidelines describe some of the following duties:

- Help to ensure that the facility provides appropriate medical care.
- Help to establish and implement resident medical care policies.
- Provide oversight of physician services.
- Oversee overall clinical care and make sure it is adequate.
- Help to correct inadequate medical care when such is identified or reported.
- Consult with residents and their attending physicians when needed or requested.

General Statement

From a practical perspective, the role of the medical director can be broken down into two categories: domains of care that fall under physician expertise and domains of care that are the primary responsibility of other health professionals but require some degree of medical director input. Nonmedical domains of services to nursing home residents should not be under medical director oversight.

1. Domains of care that fall under physician expertise.
   a. Physician/practitioner services.
      (1) Timeliness of visits.
      (2) Appropriateness of orders.
      (3) Credentialing of physicians/practitioners.
      (4) Availability of needed consultants.
      (5) Infection control.
      (6) Formulating advance directives.
      (7) Employee health issues.
      (8) Medical record maintenance (e.g., admission notes, progress notes, discharge summaries).
      (9) Treatment protocols.
   b. The medical director should be actively involved in collaboration with the facility's leadership (e.g., the administrator and the director of nursing) in the oversight of these domains.
   c. The medical director shares responsibility with the leadership for satisfactory nursing home performance of those areas.
   d. If problems are discovered during inspections, quality assurance activities, or otherwise, the medical director should provide assistance and recommendations pertaining to corrective action plans.
   e. The medical director might need to intervene directly with staff physicians/practitioners who are not performing according to expectation.
2. Domains of care that are primary responsibility of other health professionals but require some degree of medical director input.
   a. The medical director should be aware of department policies and procedures (e.g., nursing, physical therapy, dietary, social work) and how they are fulfilling their function.
   b. If problems are identified internally (e.g., as a result of a mishap or during the quality assurance process) or by an external party (e.g., by state inspectors), the medical director should be informed and may

be involved in helping the nursing home to formulate plans to correct the problem(s), but should not be held responsible for the actual implementation of the corrective actions, given that the medical director has no authority over any nursing home employees and has no access to nursing home financial resources.

3. Domains of services to nursing home residents that should not be under medical director oversight or responsibility include departments such as laundry services, food services, plumbing, fire, and safety.
   a. Physicians have no training and should not be expected to have any expertise in these areas.
   b. If problems are identified in these areas (e.g., as a "deficiency" during an inspection), the medical director can be informed of these problems (as may be required by the regulatory process), but there should be no expectation from anyone that the medical director has a role in the plan of correction or that she or he can be held responsible for such correction.

Medical Director Job Description

1. Qualifications.
   a. Licensed physician.
   b. Two years of experience in long-term care or specialized training in geriatrics or chronic disease/impaired populations.
   c. Desirable attributes
      (1) Medical director certification by the American Medical Directors Association (AMDA) or equivalent training in management.
      (2) Be the attending physician for a caseload of patients in the facility that one directs (e.g., 10%).
2. Areas of responsibility.
   a. General.
      (1) Overall coordination, execution, and monitoring of physician/practitioner activities.
      (2) Monitoring and evaluating the outcomes of the health care services (e.g., QA).
   b. Physician/practitioner oversight.
      (1) Establish and implement a procedure to review physician/practitioner credentials and grant privileges to be or remain on the list of attending physicians.
      (2) Establish rules that govern the performance of physicians/practitioners.
      (3) Make staff aware of those rules.
      (4) Oversee physician/practitioner performance. Establish a formal procedure for such oversight (QA).
   c. Define the scope of practice for physicians/practitioners (would usually use state or federal regulations).
   d. Ensure physician performance in the following activities:
      (1) Accept responsibility for the care of residents assigned to them.
      (2) Perform timely admissions procedures, including review of medical records.
      (3) Make periodic as well as other pertinent visits.
      (4) Provide adequate ongoing medical coverage (24/7).

(5) Provide appropriate medical care.

(6) Document care and do so legibly.

(7) Formulate and approve advance directives and end-of-life orders.

(8) Other (may be physician, resident, or facility specific).

e. Cover for the attending physician when the latter is unavailable or not performing appropriately.

    (1) The medical director usually becomes the attending physician by default when no other physician on staff is available or willing to accept the patient.

    (2) The medical director might become involved directly in the care of another physician's patient under the following circumstances:

        (a) Request by resident/family.

        (b) Request by nursing home staff (e.g., a nurse).

        (c) Request by another physician.

        (d) When aware of a quality of care concern.

        (e) When aware of a risk-management issue.

    (3) The patient or proxy must consent to involvement by another physician or the medical director as rapidly as possible.

f. Medical policies and procedures.

    (1) The medical director is responsible for the content of policies and procedures that fall under the physician's domain.

    (2) The medical director should sign off on those documents and monitor their implementation even though signing is not required by law.

    (3) The medical director should review policies and procedures that pertain to other types of health care professionals (e.g., nursing) but not be responsible for their implementation.

    (4) Other policies and procedures should not be under medical director oversight.

g. Quality improvement.

    (1) The medical director or his or her designee must attend the quality assurance meetings and be an active participant in the quality improvement process.

    (2) The medical director should review and sign the minutes produced during those meetings.

    (3) The medical director should participate in the facility's overall quality improvement process, including areas that are not in the medical domain, because a physician is often the most knowledgeable member of the QA committee in managing and interpreting statistical data among nursing home personnel.

h. Employee health oversight.

    (1) Nursing homes have varying policies concerning employee health.

    (2) It is not expected that medical directors substitute for employees' primary care physicians.

    (3) What is expected is that the medical director establish or approve policies:

        (a) Covering employee immunization programs.

        (b) Addressing diagnosis and treatment of infectious illnesses that could be transmitted to residents or other employees.

(c) Deal with conditions that could affect the performance of the worker.

(d) Ensure that occupational safety measures are consistent with regulatory requirements.

i. Infection control: The medical director is expected to advise and consult with designated nursing staff regarding communicable diseases, infection control, and isolation procedures, and interact when appropriate with public health officials.

j. Review the reports that describe the findings of formal inspections by the state department of health.

(1) When deficiencies are identified, the medical director must be involved in the plan for correcting problems that are in the medical domain.

(2) The medical director should acknowledge corrective actions concerning problems that exist in other health care domains but not be expected to be accountable for their actual correction.

(3) Medical directors should not be party to corrective measures that have nothing to do with the practice of medicine.

k. Other.

(1) Staff education (physician and other personnel).

(2) Participate in hiring and interviewing key management personnel (e.g., administrator and director of nursing).

(3) Participate in important project development (e.g., a respirator unit).

(4) Occasionally become involved in the decision to admit a patient to the facility, when it is not clear that the potential resident's needs can be met.

(5) Interact as needed with the state's ombudsman.

(6) Interact as needed with residents' families.

3. Medical director oversight plan and authority.

a. The nursing home administrator and medical director will draft a plan that describes how the medical director will carry out her or his responsibilities.

b. This plan should be a written document that is part of the medical director's employment contract.

c. This contract should define the authority of the medical director.

d. The medical director reports to the administrator and usually serves in an advisory capacity.

e. A formal procedure should be created and updated by facility management staff and by the medical director to document performance.

f. Periodic medical director performance evaluations should be carried out.

4. Medical director accountability.

a. Medical directors are held accountable to perform the job described in this chapter.

b. Nursing homes are subjected to considerable oversight by government agencies and other parties (ombudsman, families of residents, etc.).

c. The frail nature of nursing home residents can lead to events such as death, injuries, pressure ulcers, malnutrition, and medication errors, which could generate complaints about nursing homes, their medical directors, and their physicians.

d. The state's department of (public) health and the state's board of licensure and discipline may be asked to adjudicate those complaints.

e. Therefore, medical directors should maintain a written record of their activities; for example, in the form of a quarterly report to the QA committee.

Caveats

The federal and state regulations define a broad outline of nursing home medical director responsibilities; however, those texts are so vague as to preclude a direct translation into a functional and realistic job description. Additionally, the breadth of the regulatory scope of responsibilities of the medical director job within the long-term care setting is unreasonable because it includes areas of involvement where physicians have no expertise. Finally, the authority bestowed upon medical directors is limited by the part-time nature of the position and its advisory status without power to hire or fire any member of the nursing home staff.

Pursuant to the Federal Nursing Home Reform Act of 1987, and specifically 42 CFR 483.75(I), each nursing home covered by the reform act must designate a person to serve as a medical director. The regulations further state that each medical director is responsible for the implementation of resident care policies and the coordination of medical care in the facility. Although these subtopics appear simple and straightforward, the variety of responsibilities included within each subtopic cause concern and call for interpretation. Indeed, taken literally, the job description implied by the regulatory language goes way beyond the role of a hospital chief of staff or department chair. For example, a nursing home medical director's responsibility for the implementation of resident care policies has been interpreted to extend to admissions, transfers, and discharges; infection control; use of restraints; physician privileges and practice; responsibilities of non-physician health care workers in resident care, emergency care and resident assessment and care planning; accidents and incidents; ancillary services such as laboratory, radiology and pharmacy; use of medication; use and release of clinical information; and overall quality of care.

In addition, a director's responsibility as related to the coordination of medical care in the facility has been interpreted to encompass monitoring and ensuring implementation of resident care policies, and providing oversight and supervision of physician services and medical care of residents; overseeing the overall clinical care of residents to ensure that care is adequate and effective; evaluating reports of possible inadequate medical care and taking appropriate action to remedy problems; and assuring the support of essential medical consultants as needed.

Despite the vast amount of responsibility imposed upon each director, the regulations do not provide each medical director with an equivalent amount of authority necessary to ensure compliance with the pertinent regulations. Furthermore, most medical director contracts only require that the director work at the facility for a minimum number of hours (e.g., 2 to 4) each week. In combination with the regulations, such arrangements make the director an easy target for civil liability, investigation by state licensing boards, and even criminal prosecution, but they do not provide an obvious mechanism whereby the director can enforce his or her ideas and strategies. A carefully worded medical director employment contract can offer some protection. Box 7-8 shows a sample medical director contract.

BOX 7-8   Sample Medical Director Contract

WHEREAS, Happy Care Health Center, in order to participate in certain federal and/or state health care programs, is required to engage the services of a medical director and

WHEREAS, Geri Octoplus, MD, hereinafter also referred to as the medical director, is a doctor of medicine licensed to practice his/her profession under the laws of the State of Rhode Island and is willing to provide said services as medical director,

NOW, THEREFORE, said Happy Care Health Center and Dr. Octoplus hereby and herewith mutually agree to the terms and conditions hereinafter set forth:

Happy Care Health Center designates Geri Octoplus, MD, medical director.

The medical director shall devote XX hours per month (more or less) to the performance of his/her nondirect patient care duties under this agreement.

The medical director provides medical expertise and communicates regularly with the administrator, the director of nursing, and other professional staff regarding clinical and administrative issues, specific patient care problems, and professional staff needs.

The medical director will be involved and accountable in the development of medical treatment policies and procedures. The medical director should be aware of other health professionals' policies (e.g., nursing, rehabilitation, dietician, social work). Nonclinical policies and procedures (e.g., cleaning, kitchen, plumbing, fire codes) are not the medical director's responsibility.

The medical director participates in developing and is accountable for policies and procedures regarding the services of the medical and practitioner staff:
1. Credentialing of physicians, advanced practice nurses, and physician assistants.
2. Defining the scope of practice for physicians/practitioners.
3. Establishing rules that govern physician/practitioner performance and monitor compliance:
   - Accepting responsibility for the care of residents assigned to them.
   - Performing timely admission visits, including examinations and writing orders.
   - Being available or providing coverage 24/7.

BOX 7-8   Sample Medical Director Contract—cont'd

- Performing periodic and other pertinent visits.
- Providing appropriate state-of-the-art medical care.
- Documenting care consistent with CMS documentation guidelines.
- Formulating/approving end-of-life orders.

4. In emergency situations, the medical director covers for the attending physician when he or she is unavailable or not performing appropriately.
5. The medical director oversees the implementation of resident medical care policies and medical/practitioner staff performance.
6. The medical director participates in ongoing quality improvement/assurance activities by attending the QI/QA committee meetings and reviewing the minutes.
7. The medical director advises on specific resident care problems identified during the normal process of delivering services to residents.
8. The medical director advises about the identification and management of systemic medical problems that might occur from time to time (e.g., outbreaks and infection-control issues).
9. The medical director assists the facility in identifying needs for new resident care or staff policies/procedures and reviews existing policies from time to time.
10. The medical director advises the administrator and other relevant organization leaders about employee health policies and issues.
11. The medical director must review state and federal survey/inspection reports and help to prepare a response and/or plan of correction when needed (i.e., relevant domains).
12. The medical director helps the facility to coordinate the care provided to residents. This becomes particularly important when a long-term care facility identifies itself as specialized and needs a relevant specialist to provide consultation (e.g., respirator unit, dialysis patients, etc.). The medical director cannot be held responsible for certain services that are unavailable (e.g., dental care).
13. The medical director will work with the facility to promote residents' rights and quality of life and will interact with an ombudsman when needed.
14. The administrator and the director of nursing shall make themselves available to the medical director to discuss relevant matters as needed.
15. Facility personnel will inform the medical director about care issues in a timely manner as such issues arise.
16. The medical director provides a periodic report to the administrator and receives a periodic evaluation from the administrator.

Continued

BOX 7-8   Sample Medical Director Contract—cont'd

17. The center shall pay to the medical director a fee for his/her services in the amount of $XXXX per month. Said amount of money is compensation for his/her services as medical director only and does not include any amounts due him/her for professional fees arising from his/her services to residents or others (e.g., employees) and payable to him/her by residents or third parties. In no case is the professional fee for individual care of a resident a part of the payment for services as medical director.

18. The medical director shall not be considered, and he/she is not, an employee of Happy Care Health Center but is an independent contractor responsible for his/her own acts.

19. The medical director is expected to attend meetings, conferences, seminars, or the like that may be concerned in whole or in part with medical direction in order to remain current with the job. The nursing home will cover up to $XXXX per year in expenses related to the medical director's continuing education activities.

20. This agreement may be amended at any time by mutual agreement, in writing. This agreement shall be for a term of 1 year, but shall automatically renew on the anniversary date of its signing for an additional year each anniversary date thereafter. This agreement may be terminated by the medical director at any time with 60 days' notice or by the nursing home at any time with 180 days' notice (or continued payment for 180 days from the time of termination notice).

21. The medical director shall maintain malpractice insurance at all times in an amount not less than one million dollars ($1,000,000). This insurance will cover the medical director for his/her administrative duties (this is not typically included in standard medical malpractice policies). If the nursing home provides such coverage, the medical director will be identified by name in its policy.

22. Nothing in this contract shall be construed to prohibit either party from entering any other agreement with any other person or entity.

SUGGESTED READINGS

American Medical Directors Association: White paper on the survey process. *J Am Med Dir Assoc* 7:120-123, 2006.

Coleman EA, Berenson RA: Lost in transition: Challenges and opportunities for improving the quality of transitional care. *Ann Intern Med* 140:533-536, 2004.

Dimant J: Roles and responsibilities of attending physicians in skilled nursing facilities. *J Am Med Dir Assoc* 4:231-243, 2003.

Donius M: Comprehensive assessment in an institutional setting. In Ostreweil D, Brummel-Smith, Beck J (eds): *Comprehensive Geriatric Assessment*. New York, McGraw-Hill, 2000, pp 225-251.

Katz P, Karuza J: Nursing home care. In Cobbs E, Duthie E, Murphy JB (eds): *Geriatric Review Syllabus*, ed 5. Malden, Mass, Blackwell, 2003.

Katz P: Nursing home care. In Hazzard W, Blass J, Halter J, et al (eds): *Principles of Geriatric Medicine and Gerontology*, ed 5. New York, McGraw-Hill, 2003, pp 197-209.

Levenson SA: The impact of laws and regulations in improving physician performance and care processes in long-term care. *J Am Med Dir Assoc* 5:268-277, 2004.

Levenson SA: The medical director: Back to basics. *Caring for the aged* 5:46-51, 2004.

Sloane P, Boustani M: Institutional care. In Ham R, Sloane P, Warshaw G (eds): *Primary Care Geriatrics*, ed 4. St. Louis, Mosby, 2002, pp 199-216.

7.3 Hospice

Tom J. Wachtel

OVERVIEW

Hospice is a term that is used for a number of entities and activities. Hospice is offered by Medicare, most Medicaid programs, and many private insurers as a benefit. *Hospice* refers to palliative care provided near the end of life, and it can refer to a physical place where end-of-life (EOL) care is provided. For the purpose of this discussion the focus will be on the Medicare benefit and the services provided under the Medicare hospice benefit.

In 1983, Congress enacted the hospice benefit within the Medicare program. With an aging population, a greater understanding of the place of palliative care in the continuum of care, and growth in the number and quality of hospice organizations, there has been considerable growth in the number of persons enrolled in hospice since the inception of the benefit. That growth has been most dramatic since the 1990s: Annual hospice admissions have risen from 200,000 to almost 1,000,000.

Under Medicare, hospice is a program of care delivered by a Medicare-approved hospice. Reasonable and necessary medical and support services for the management of a terminal illness are furnished under a plan of care established by the beneficiary's attending physician and the hospice team. More than 90% of services are provided in the beneficiaries' homes. Respite and general inpatient services are also provided when socially or medically necessary.

Although most physicians think of hospice and palliation with cancer diagnoses, many other conditions are also appropriate for hospice care. National data show that 50.5% of hospice patients die from cancer. The top five noncancer diagnoses are end-stage heart disease, dementia, lung disease, end-stage kidney disease, and end-stage liver disease. The common thread is that physicians feel their patients are unlikely to survive more than 6 months if their disease runs its natural course. National data also suggest that the referral to hospice is often much later in the course of an illness than may be appropriate.

ELIGIBILITY

Hospice care is available under Medicare in the following circumstances:

- The patient is eligible for Medicare Part A.
- The patient's doctor and the hospice medical director certify that the patient is terminally ill with 6 months or less to live if the disease runs its expected course (Box 7-9).

BOX 7-9   When to Consider Palliative or Hospice End-of-life Care

Palliative/hospice end-of-life care can assist with:
- Pain and symptom control
- Emotional, social, and spiritual suffering
- Home services, medications, nurse case management
- Determining eligibility for supportive services
- Facilitating patient and family conferences to define goals of care, including advance directives

Amyotrophic Lateral Sclerosis

Decubitus ulcers
Impaired breathing at rest
Insufficient nutrition/hydration
Rapid progression in last year
Recurrent aspiration pneumonia
Recurrent fever
Sepsis
Upper urinary tract infection

Multisystem Failure

Albumin <2.5 g/dL
Decubitus ulcers
Frequent emergency department visits
Homebound or confined to bed
Unintentional weight loss

Heart Disease

Cardiac arrest, syncope, or cerebrovascular accident
Congestive heart failure symptoms at rest
Ejection fraction <20%
Frequent emergency department visits for symptoms
New dysrhythmia

Liver Disease

Albumin <2.5 g/dL
Jaundice
Malnutrition and muscle wasting
Prothrombin time >5 sec
Refractory ascites
Spontaneous bacterial peritonitis

Lung Cancer

Advanced disease stage
Albumin <2.5

> **BOX 7-9   When to Consider Palliative or Hospice End-of-life Care—cont'd**

Calcium ≥12.0
Decreasing functional status
Metastasis to brain or bone

Dementia

Albumin <2.5 or decreased oral intake
Fewer than six intelligible words
Frequent emergency department visits
Inability to walk

Diseases with Short Prognosis

Any cancer with generalized metastases to brain, liver, or bone
Any unresectable cancer
Esophageal cancer
Gallbladder cancer
Glioblastoma
Liver cancer
Pancreatic cancer

Pulmonary Disease

Dyspnea at rest
O_2 saturation <88%
P_{CO_2} >50
Signs or symptoms of right heart failure
Unintentional weight loss

Renal Disease

Creatinine clearance <15 mL/min
Not a candidate for dialysis
Serum creatinine >6.0 mg/dL

Stroke

ACUTE
Dysphagia
Secondary coma >3 days

CHRONIC
Poor functional status
Post-stroke dementia
Serum albumin <2.5
Unintentional weight loss

Modified from Bailey FA: *The Palliative Response.* Birmingham, Ala, Menasha Ridge Press, 2005. PDF available at http://www.hospice.va.gov/Amosbaileybook/index.htm (accessed March 1, 2007).

- The patient signs a statement choosing hospice care instead of standard Medicare benefits for the terminal illness.
- The patient receives care from a Medicare-approved hospice program.

Hospice care is a benefit under the hospital insurance program. To be eligible to elect hospice care under Medicare, a patient must be entitled to Part A of Medicare and be certified terminally ill. A patient is considered terminally ill if the medical prognosis is that the patient's life expectancy is 6 months or less if the illness runs its normal course. Section 1814(a)(7) of the Social Security Act specifies that certification of terminal illness for hospice benefits shall be based on the clinical judgment of the hospice physician and the patient's attending physician (if he or she has one) or the medical director regarding the normal course of the patient's illness.

Once a patient enters a hospice program, the first certification is for 90 days. The first recertification is also for 90 days, and all subsequent recertifications are for 60 days. Recertifications require only a single physician signature. A physician may discharge a patient from a hospice program, and patients may revoke or transfer hospice programs at any time. Predicting life expectancy is not exact. The fact that a beneficiary lives longer than expected in itself is not cause to terminate benefits. Once the initial election is processed, the beneficiary remains in hospice status until death or until the patient elects to terminate hospice.

While on hospice, a patient must waive all rights to Medicare payments for the duration of the election of hospice care for the following services:

1. Hospice care provided by a hospice other than the hospice designated by the patient (unless provided under arrangements made by the designated hospice) and any Medicare services that are related to the treatment of the terminal condition for which hospice care was elected or a related condition or services that are equivalent to hospice care, except for services provided by:
   a. The designated hospice (either directly or under arrangement).
   b. Another hospice under arrangements made by the designated hospice.
   c. The patient's attending physician, if that physician is not an employee of the designated hospice or receiving compensation from the hospice for those services.
2. Medicare services for a condition completely unrelated to the terminal condition for which hospice was elected remain available to the patient if he or she is eligible for such care. Nursing home residents are eligible for hospice.

COVERED SERVICES

Once a patient is enrolled in a hospice, the hospice is financially responsible for all diagnostic and therapeutic services related to the terminal disease. This can include palliative treatments, medications, therapies, and any respite or medically related admissions. For conditions totally unrelated to the hospice diagnosis, a patient may be admitted to a hospital, treated at an outpatient facility, or cared for at a physician's office under traditional Medicare.

1. Within hospice, Medicare covers:
   a. Physicians' services.
   b. Nursing care (intermittent with 24-hour on call).

    c. Medical appliances and supplies related to the terminal illness.
    d. Outpatient drugs for symptom management and pain relief.
    e. Short-term acute inpatient care, including respite care.
    f. Home health aide and homemaker services.
    g. Physical therapy, occupational therapy, and speech–language pathology services.
    h. Medical social services.
    i. Counseling, including dietary and spiritual counseling.
    j. Bereavement services.
2. These services are provided as part of symptom control or to enable the patient to maintain ADL and basic functional skills and not as part of a curative care plan.

There are four levels of hospice care: routine home care, continuous home care, respite care, and general inpatient care. Routine home care is provided as medically necessary and involves at least nursing care and social service, with overall direction by a hospice medical director. The frequency and intensity of service depend on medical needs, but they usually increase over time. Continuous home care is 8 or more hours daily, provided to a patient in crisis, with at least 50% of that care performed by licensed nurses. Respite care involves admission to an institution (SNF or other) for up to 5 days when needed to allow the family a temporary break from their caregiving duties. General inpatient care is provided by the hospice under contract with a facility (SNF or other) and is for short-term provision of intensive, aggressive management of acute symptoms that cannot be provided in another setting. In addition, general inpatient care may be provided when a beneficiary's home support system has acutely deteriorated and short-term placement is required while arranging a more permanent placement option.

THE PHYSICIAN'S ROLE IN HOSPICE

The hospice medical director provides administrative and general oversight of the program. The patient's hospice attending physician (who may also be the medical director) is reimbursed for all hands-on care. If the attending is salaried by the hospice, the hospice bills Medicare Part A. If the attending is not employed by the hospice, the Part B carrier is billed using regular E&M codes with the modifier GV (not employed by hospice). The attending physician is listed in the Medicare common working file. Physicians covering for the attending should use locum tenens rules (modifier GV with Q5 or Q6 as appropriate). For non–hospice-related conditions and services, the physician uses regular E&M codes plus the modifier GW (service not related to the hospice patient's terminal condition). The primary medical attending continues to bill Medicare directly for services and may bill under CPT code 99375 for phone management of the hospice patient if it exceeds 30 minutes per month.

Consultations (e.g., with an oncologist) related to the terminal illness must be paid for by the hospice and require prior authorization by the hospice program. Unauthorized testing or treatment for the terminal illness are not covered by Medicare and become the patient's responsibility.

Treatment of disease unrelated to the terminal illness may be independently covered by Medicare, including reimbursement of attending and consulting physician fees. This is more likely to occur for the patient who enrolls in hospice early in the course of the illness.

SUGGESTED READINGS

Fried T, van Doorn C, O'Leary J, et al: Older persons' preferences for site of terminal care. *Ann Intern Med* 131:109-112, 1999.

Lorenz K, Lynn J: Care of the dying patient. In Hazzard W, Blass J, Halter J, et al: *Principles of Geriatric Medicine and Gerontology*, ed 5. New York, McGraw-Hill, 2003, pp 323-334.

Pinderhughes S, Morrison R: Palliative care. In Cobbs E, Duthie E, Murphy JB (eds): *Geriatric Review Syllabus*, ed 5. Malden, Mass, Blackwell, 2003, pp 105-115.

Potash J, Horst P: Palliative care at the end of life. In Ham R, Sloane P, Warshaw G (eds): *Primary Care Geriatrics*, ed 4. St. Louis, Mosby, 2002, pp 229-242.

7.4 Palliative Care

Tom J. Wachtel and Fred F. Ferri

INTRODUCTION

In 1900 most Americans died of unexpected, relatively acute medical illnesses, conditions, and accidents. Currently, most Americans die of complications of chronic illnesses.

1. *Palliative care* as defined by the World Health Organization refers to "the active total care of patients whose disease is not responsive to curative treatments. Control of pain, of other symptoms, and of psychological, social and spiritual problems is paramount. The goal of palliative care is achievement of the best possible quality of life for patients and their families."
2. Palliative care is imperative and most commonly provided at the end of life.
3. For those living with chronic illnesses and disability, palliative care should be an essential component of care even though they might not be imminently dying.
4. Fewer than 20% of Americans are enrolled in hospice prior to death.

PROCESS OF CARE

1. Palliative care is appropriate.
   a. The physician's assessment of the patient's condition can indicate the need for palliative care.
   b. The need for palliative care can come to the physician's attention from other health professionals, patients, family, or friends.
2. Discussion of palliative care and end-of-life decisions with the patient and family.
   a. These discussions often take more than one encounter.
   b. The discussion should include:
      (1) An assessment of what the patient and family understand.
      (2) The patient's and family's beliefs and wishes.
      (3) Information regarding prognosis.
      (4) A sense of confidence in the ability to provide relief from suffering.
3. Care plan.
   a. Establish a plan of care.

   b. Help the family to continue to adhere to the goals of the plan as circumstances change. With adequate support, patients and families can stick to the initial plan and avoid the emotional roller coaster of constantly changing goals.

   c. Establishing a plan of care should include resources to accomplish the goals (e.g., referral to a hospice program, involvement of clergy).

4. Patients (and their families) must be assured that even though their condition is no longer curable, consistent efforts will be made to ensure symptom palliation up to and including the time of death.

5. The goal of symptom palliation is not simply a "good death" but also improvement in the quality of life substantially by helping patients to "live until they die."

COMPONENTS OF PALLIATIVE CARE

Pain Management[1]

Assessment of Pain

1. Like other adults, elderly patients require comprehensive assessment and aggressive management of pain.

2. Older patients are at risk for undertreatment of pain.

   a. Caregivers underestimate their sensitivity to pain.

   b. Caregivers expect that they tolerate pain well.

   c. Patients might be cognitively impaired.

   d. Caregivers have misconceptions about their ability to benefit from opioids.

Issues in Assessing and Treating Pain

1. Issues in assessing and treating cancer pain in older patients include:

   a. Multiple chronic diseases and sources of pain: Complex medication regimens place elderly patients at increased risk for drug–drug and drug–disease interactions.

   b. Visual, hearing, motor, and cognitive impairments.

     (1) Simple descriptive, numeric, and visual analogue pain assessment instruments may be ineffective.

     (2) Cognitively impaired patients might require simpler scales and more frequent pain assessment and response to treatment.

   c. Nonsteroidal antiinflammatory drug (NSAID) side effects.

     (1) Drug reactions such as cognitive impairment, constipation, and headaches in older patients.

     (2) Alternative NSAIDs (e.g., choline magnesium trisalicylate) or coadministration of misoprostol or a proton pump inhibitor should be considered to reduce gastric toxicity.

   d. Opioid effectiveness.

     (1) Older persons tend to be more sensitive to analgesic effects of opioids as well as to side effects (e.g., confusion and constipation).

     (2) Peak opioid effect is higher and duration of pain relief is longer.

   e. Patient-controlled analgesia: Slower drug clearance and increased sensitivity to undesirable drug effects (e.g., cognitive impairment) indicate the need for cautious initial dosing and subsequent titration and monitoring.

f. Alternative routes of administration: The rectal route may be inappropriate for elderly or disabled patients who are physically unable to place the suppository in the rectum.

g. Postoperative pain control: Following surgery, surgeons and other health care team members should maintain frequent direct contact with the elderly patient to reassess the quality of pain management.

h. Change of setting: Reassessment of pain management and appropriate changes should be made whenever the elderly patient moves (e.g., from hospital to home or nursing home).

Pain Assessment

a. Overview.
   (1) Failure to assess pain may lead to undertreatment.
   (2) Assessment should occur at regular intervals.
      (a) After initiation of treatment.
      (b) At each new report of pain.
      (c) At a suitable interval after pharmacologic or nonpharmacologic intervention (e.g., 15-30 min after parenteral drug therapy and 1 hour after oral administration).
   (3) Identifying the etiology of pain is essential to its management.
   (4) Clinicians treating patients with cancer should recognize the common cancer pain syndromes. Prompt diagnosis and treatment of these syndromes can reduce morbidity associated with unrelieved pain (Fig. 7-19).

b. Initial assessment.
   (1) The goal of the initial assessment of pain is to characterize the pain by location, intensity, and etiology.
   (2) Essential to initial assessment are:
      (a) Detailed history.
      (b) Physical examination.
      (c) Psychosocial assessment.
      (d) Diagnostic evaluation.

c. Patient self-report (Fig. 7-20).
   (1) This is the mainstay of pain assessment.
   (2) To enhance pain management across all settings, clinicians should teach families to use pain assessment tools in their homes.
   (3) The clinician should help the patient to describe:
      (a) Pain.
         i. Listen to the patient's descriptive words about the quality of the pain; these provide valuable clues to its etiology.
         ii. Self-report pain intensity scales include simple descriptive, numeric, and visual analogue scales (see Fig. 7-20).
      (b) Location: Ask the patient to indicate the exact location of the pain on his or her body or on a body diagram and whether it radiates.
      (c) Intensity or severity: Encourage the patient to keep a log of pain intensity scores to report during follow-up visits or by telephone.

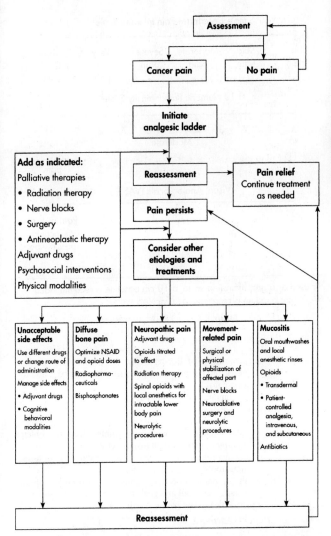

Figure 7-19   The sequence of activities related to pain assessment and management. The flowchart emphasizes the use of multiple modalities concurrently, beginning with the least invasive modalities and advancing treatment to meet the patient's need for pain relief. NSAID, nonsteroidal antiinflammatory drug. (Adapted from Jacox A, Carr DB, Payne R, et al: *Management of cancer pain: Adults quick reference guide No. 9.* AHCPR Pub No. 94-0593. Rockville, Md, Agency for Health Care Policy and Research, US Department of Health and Human Services, Public Health Services, 1994.)

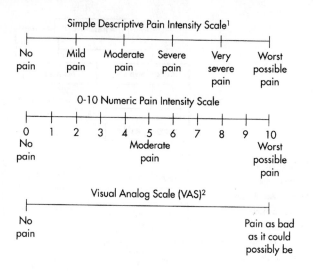

[1]If used as a graphic rating scale, a 10-cm baseline is recommended.
[2]A 10-cm baseline is recommended for VAS scales.

Figure 7-20   Pain intensity scales.

      (d) Aggravating and relieving factors.
         i. Ask when the patient experiences the most pain and the least pain.
         ii. Document responses in patient's chart
      (e) Cognitive response to pain.
         i. Note behavior suggesting pain in patients who are cognitively impaired or who have communication problems relating to education, language, ethnicity, or culture.
         ii. Use appropriate (e.g., simpler or translated) pain-assessment tools.
      (f) Goals for pain control: Document the patient's preferred pain assessment tool and goals for pain control (as scores on a pain scale) in the patient's pain history.

Pharmacologic Treatment

1. NSAIDs.
    (1) NSAIDs are effective for relief of mild pain and have an opioid dose–sparing effect that helps reduce side effects when given with opioids for moderate to severe pain.
    (2) Acetaminophen is included with NSAIDs because it has similar analgesic potency, although it lacks peripheral antiinflammatory activity.

      (3) Tramadol (Ultram) at a dose of 50 to 100 mg q6h may also be used.

2. Opioids.

  a. Opiods can be added for mild to moderate pain.

  b. Table 7-6 describes dose equivalents for opioid analgesics.

  c. The predictable consequences of long-term opioid administration—tolerance and physical dependence—are often confused with the psychological dependence (addiction) that is seen in drug abuse.

    (1) Patient tolerance can lead to ineffective prescribing, administering, or dispensing of opioids for cancer pain, with resultant undertreatment.

    (2) Clinicians may be reluctant to give high doses of opioids to patients with advanced disease because of a fear of serious side effects.

    (3) The clinician's goal of care—to benefit the patient by relieving pain—supports increasing doses, even at the risk of side effects.

    (4) Many patients with cancer pain become opioid tolerant during long-term opioid therapy, and their doses must be increased to provide pain relief. The physician's fear of shortening life by increasing opioid doses is usually unfounded.

    (5) Benefits and risk of using opioids vary among individual patients.

  d. Types of opioids.

    (1) Opioids are classified as full morphine-like agonists, partial agonists, or mixed agonist–antagonists, depending on the specific receptors to which they bind and their activity at these receptors.

    (2) Full agonists.

      (a) Morphine, hydromorphone, codeine, oxycodone, hydrocodone, methadone, levorphanol, and fentanyl are classified as full agonists because their effectiveness with increasing doses is not limited.

      (b) They will not reverse or antagonize effects of other full agonists given simultaneously.

    (3) We do not recommend the use of partial agonists or mixed agonist–antagonists.

  e. Dosing.

    (1) The appropriate dose is the amount of opioid that controls pain with the fewest side effects.

      (a) The need for increased doses of opioid often reflects progression of the disease.

      (b) As patients develop opioid tolerance, they require more frequent dosing.

      (c) Table 7-6 lists equianalgesic initial doses of commonly used opioids for adults.

    (2) Titration: Increase or decrease the next dose by one quarter to one half of the previous dose.

    (3) Route conversion.

      (a) When changing from the oral to the rectal route, begin with the oral dose, then titrate upward frequently and carefully.

      (b) Lower doses are required for parenteral routes and are similar for subcutaneous, intramuscular, and intravenous routes.

Table 7-6 Commonly Used Opioid Analgesics

Drug	Opioid Dose	Usual Oral Dosing Interval	Morphine Equianalgesic Dose
Morphine			
MSIR tablets or capsules	15 mg, 30 mg	q4h	1 to 1
MSIR soluble tablets	10 mg, 15 mg, 30 mg	q4h	1 to 1
Roxanol	10 mg/5mL, 20 mg/5 mL	q4h	1 to 1
MS Contin	15 mg, 30 mg, 60 mg, 100 mg, 200 mg	q12h	1 to 1
Avinza	30 mg, 60 mg, 90 mg, 120 mg	q24h	1 to 1
Parenteral morphine	0.1 to 0.2 mg/kg to as high as necessary SC, IM, or IV	q4h	0.35 to 1
Hydromorphone			
Dilaudid, generic	2 mg, 4 mg, 8 mg	q4h	0.25 to 1
Liquid	5 mg/5 mL	q4h	0.25 to 1
Suppository	3 mg	q4h	0.25 to 1
Oxycodone			
Oxy IR	5 mg	q4h	0.8 to 1
Roxicodone	5 mg	q4h	0.8 to 1
OxyContin	10 mg, 20 mg, 40 mg, 80 mg	q12h	0.8 to 1
Liquid	20 mg/mL	q4h	0.8 to 1

Oxycodone with Acetaminophen			
Percocet, Roxicet	2.5 mg, 5 mg, 7.5 mg, 10 mg	q4h	0.8 to 1
Oxycodone with Aspirin or Ibuprofen			
Percodan	5 mg	q4h	0.8 to 1
Combunox	5 mg/400 mg	q4h	0.8 to 1
Hydrocodone with Acetaminophen			
Lortab	2.5 mg, 5 mg, 7.5 mg, 10 mg	q4h	1 to 1
Lorcet	5 mg, 7.5 mg, 10 mg	q4h	1 to 1
Vicodin	5 mg, 7.5 mg, 10 mg	q4h	1 to 1
Codeine			
Codeine sulfate tablets	15 mg, 30 mg, 60 mg	q4h	7 to 1
Elixir, solution	15 mg/mL	q4h	7 to 1
Codeine with Acetaminophen			
Tylenol No. 2, No. 3, No. 4	15 mg, 30 mg, 60 mg codeine with 300 mg acetaminophen	q4h	7 to 1
Fentanyl (Duragesic)	25, 50, 75, 100 µg/h transdermal patch	q72h	Divide total daily morphine dose (in mg) by 4 to calculate the strength (in µg/h) of fentanyl

IR, instant release; MS, morphine sulfate; MSIR, morphine sulfate instant release.

(4) Schedule.
  (a) Prevent recurring pain rather than having to subdue it.
  (b) Give analgesics on a regular schedule to prevent a loss of effectiveness between doses.
(5) Tolerance: Assume that patients actively abusing heroin or prescription opioids (including methadone) have some pharmacologic tolerance that will require higher starting doses and shorter dosing intervals.
(6) Cessation of opioids: When a patient becomes pain free as a result of cancer treatment or palliation (e.g., nerve destruction), gradually decrease the opioid to prevent withdrawal.
f. Route of administration.
  (1) Oral.
    (a) Oral administration is preferred because it is convenient and usually cost effective.
    (b) When patients cannot take oral medications, other, less invasive (e.g., rectal or transdermal) routes should be offered.
    (c) Parenteral methods should be used only when simpler, less costly methods are inappropriate or ineffective.
    (d) Assessing the patient's response to several different oral opioids is usually advisable before abandoning the oral route in favor of anesthetic, neurosurgical, or other invasive approaches.
  (2) Rectal.
    (a) The rectal route is a safe, inexpensive, and effective route for delivery of opioids (and nonopioids) when patients have nausea or vomiting.
    (b) The rectal route is inappropriate for:
      i. The patient who has diarrhea, anal/rectal lesions, or mucositis.
      ii. The patient who is thrombocytopenic or neutropenic.
      iii. The patient who is physically unable to place the suppository in the rectum.
      iv. The patient who prefers other routes.
  (3) Transdermal (fentanyl).
    (a) Transdermal delivery is not suitable for rapid dose titration.
    (b) Use this route for relatively stable pain when rapid increases or decreases in intensity are not likely.
  (4) Injection or infusion.
    (a) IV and SC routes provide effective opioid delivery.
    (b) Avoid the IM route because of pain associated with injection.
    (c) IV administration provides most rapid onset of analgesia, but duration of analgesia after a bolus dose is shorter than with other routes.
    (d) In patients requiring continuous IV access for other purposes, this route of opioid infusion is cost effective and provides a consistent level of analgesia.

      (e) When IV access is not feasible, SC opioid infusion is practical in the hospital or home.

  (5) Patient-controlled analgesia (PCA).

      (a) PCA helps patient maintain independence and control by matching drug delivery to need for analgesia.

      (b) The opioid may be administered orally or via a dedicated portable pump to deliver the drug IV, SC, or epidurally (intraspinally).

g. Side effects: Clinicians who observe patients during long-term opioid treatment should watch for potential side effects and use adjuvant agents to counteract them.

  (1) Constipation.

      (a) Constipation is an inevitable side effect of opioid therapy.

      (b) Treat it prophylactically with dietary fiber or regularly scheduled doses of a mild laxative.

      (c) Severe constipation may require treatment with a stimulating cathartic (e.g., bisacodyl, standardized senna concentrate, or osmotic agents, orally or via suppository).

  (2) Nausea and vomiting.

      (a) Treat with antiemetics such as phenothiazines or metoclopromide.

      (b) Depending on the antiemetic chosen, monitor the patient for increased sedation.

  (3) Sedation and mental clouding.

      (a) When possible, treat persistent drug-induced sedation by reducing the dose and increasing the frequency of opioid administration.

      (b) Central nervous system (CNS) stimulants such as caffeine, dextroamphetamine, pemoline, and methylphenidate also help decrease opioid sedative effects.

  (4) Respiratory depression.

      (a) Patients receiving long-term opioid therapy generally develop tolerance to the respiratory depressant effects of these agents.

      (b) When indicated for reversal of opioid-induced respiratory depression, administer naloxone, titrated in small increments to improve respiratory function without reversing analgesia.

      (c) Monitor the patient carefully until the episode of respiratory depression resolves.

  (5) Subacute overdose.

      (a) Subacute overdose is far more common than acute respiratory depression.

      (b) Subacute overdose manifests as slowly progressive (hours to days) somnolence and respiratory depression.

      (c) Withhold one or two doses until symptoms have resolved.

      (d) Then reduce the standing dose by 25%.

  (6) Other opioid side effects.

      (a) Dry mouth.

      (b) Urinary retention.
      (c) Pruritus.
      (d) Myoclonus.
      (e) Altered cognitive function.
      (f) Dysphoria, euphoria.
      (g) Sleep disturbances.
      (h) Sexual dysfunction.
      (i) Physiologic dependence, tolerance.
      (j) Inappropriate secretion of antidiuretic hormone

3. Adjuvant drugs are valuable during all phases of pain management to enhance analgesic efficacy, treat concurrent symptoms, and provide independent analgesia for specific types of pain.
  a. Corticosteroids.
    (1) Corticosteroids provide a range of effects.
      (a) Mood elevation.
      (b) Antiinflammatory activity.
      (c) Antiemetic activity.
      (d) Appetite stimulation.
      (e) May be beneficial in managing cachexia and anorexia.
    (2) Corticosteroids reduce cerebral and spinal cord edema.
    (3) Corticosteroids are essential in emergency management of elevated intracranial pressure and epidural spinal cord compression.
  b. Anticonvulsants.
    (1) Anticonvulsants (e.g., gabapentin) are used to manage neuropathic pain, especially lancinating or burning pain.
    (2) Use with caution in cancer patients undergoing marrow-suppressant therapies, such as chemotherapy and radiation therapy.
  c. Antidepressants.
    (1) Antidepressants are useful in pharmacologic management of neuropathic pain.
    (2) Antidepressants have innate analgesic properties and can potentiate the analgesic effects of opioids.
    (3) The most widely reported experience has been with amitriptyline; therefore, it should be viewed as the tricyclic agent of choice.
  d. Local anesthetics.
    (1) Local anesthetics (e.g., transdermal lidocaine) are used to treat neuropathic pain.
    (2) Side effects may be greater than with other drugs used to treat neuropathic pain
4. Placebos should not be used.

Physical and Psychosocial Interventions

1. Overview.
  a. Patients should be encouraged to remain active and participate in self-care when possible.
  b. Noninvasive physical and psychosocial modalities can be used concurrently with drugs and other interventions to manage pain during all phases of treatment.
  c. Effectiveness of these modalities depends on the patient's participation and communication as to which methods best alleviate pain.

2. Types of intervention.
   a. Physical modalities: Generalized weakness, deconditioning, and aches and pains associated with cancer diagnosis and therapy may be treated by:
      (1) Cutaneous stimulation: Noninvasive techniques that can be taught to the patient or family caregiver include:
         (a) Heat.
            i. Avoid burns by wrapping heat source (e.g., hot pack or heating pad) in a towel.
            ii. Use of heat on irradiated tissue is contraindicated.
            iii. Diathermy and ultrasound are not recommended for use on tumor sites.
         (b) Cold.
            i. Apply flexible ice packs that conform to body contours for periods not to exceed 15 minutes.
            ii. Provides longer-lasting relief than heat.
            iii. Should not be used in patients with peripheral vascular disease or on tissue damaged by radiation therapy.
         (c) Massage, pressure, and vibration.
            i. Help the patient through distraction or relaxation but sometimes increase pain before relief occurs.
            ii. Massage should not be substituted for exercise in ambulatory patients.
      (2) Exercise.
         (a) Useful in treating subacute and chronic pain.
         (b) Strengthens weak muscles.
         (c) Mobilizes stiff joints.
         (d) Helps restore coordination and balance.
         (e) Enhances patient comfort.
         (f) Provides cardiovascular conditioning.
      (3) Repositioning.
         (a) Reposition the immobilized patient frequently.
         (b) Helps maintain correct body alignment.
         (c) Prevents or alleviates pain and, possibly, pressure ulcers.
      (4) Immobilization.
         (a) Use restriction of movement to manage acute pain or to stabilize fractures or otherwise compromised limbs or joints.
         (b) Use adjustable elastic or thermoplastic braces to help maintain correct body alignment.
         (c) Keep joints in positions of maximal function rather than maximal range.
         (d) Avoid prolonged immobilization.
   b. Cognitive behavior interventions.
      (1) Cognitive behavior interventions are an important part of a multimodal approach to pain management.
         (a) They help to give the patient a sense of control and to develop coping skills to deal with pain.
         (b) Interventions introduced early in the course of illness are more likely to succeed because they can be learned and practiced by patients while they have sufficient strength and energy.

(c) Patients and their families should be given information about and encouraged to try several strategies and to select one or more of these cognitive behavioral techniques to use regularly.

(2) Relaxation and imagery.

(a) Simple relaxation techniques should be used for episodes of brief pain (e.g., during procedures).

(b) Brief, simple techniques should be used when the patient's ability to concentrate is compromised by severe pain, a high level of anxiety, or fatigue.

(3) Cognitive distraction and reframing: Focusing attention on stimuli other than pain or negative emotions accompanying pain.

(a) Internal distractions (e.g., counting, praying, or making a self-statement such as "I can cope").

(b) External distractions (e.g., music, television, talking, listening to someone read).

(b) Exercises (e.g., rhythmic massage or use of a visual focal point).

(4) Patient education.

(5) Psychotherapy and structured support.

(6) Support groups and pastoral counseling.

Invasive Interventions

With rare exception, less-invasive analgesic approaches should precede invasive palliative approaches. For a minority of patients in whom behavioral, physical, and drug therapy do not alleviate pain, invasive therapies are useful.

1. Radiation therapy.
   a. Local or whole-body radiation enhances effectiveness of analgesic drug and other noninvasive therapy by directly affecting the cause of pain (e.g., reducing primary and metastatic tumor bulk).
   b. The dosage should be chosen to achieve a balance between the amount of radiation required to kill tumor cells and the amount that would adversely affect normal cells or allow repair of damaged tissue.

2. Surgery: Palliative debulking of a tumor can reduce pain directly, relieve symptoms of obstruction or compression, and improve prognosis, even increasing long-term survival.

3. Nerve blocks.
   a. Control of otherwise intractable pain can be achieved by relatively brief application of a local anesthetic or neurolytic agent.
   b. Reasons for nerve blocks.
      (1) Diagnostic: To determine the source of the pain (e.g., somatic vs. sympathetic pathways).
      (2) Therapeutic: To treat painful conditions that respond to nerve blocks (e.g., celiac block for pain of pancreatic cancer).
      (3) Prognostic: To predict outcome of long-lasting interventions (e.g., infusions, neurolysis, rhizotomy).
      (4) Preemptive: To prevent painful sequelae of procedures that can cause phantom limb or regional pain syndrome.
   c. Types of nerve blocks.

(1) A single injection of a nondestructive agent such as lidocaine or bupivacaine, alone or in combination with an antiinflammatory corticosteroid for a longer-lasting effect, can provide local relief from nerve or root compression.

(2) Placement of an infusion catheter at a sympathetic ganglion extends the sympathetic blockade from hours to days or weeks.

(3) Destructive agents such as ethanol or phenol can be used to effect peripheral neurolysis at the sites identified by local anesthesia as appropriate for permanent pain relief.

4. Neurosurgery: Ablation of pain pathways should, like neurolytic blockade, be reserved for situations in which other therapies are ineffective or poorly tolerated.

Nausea And Vomiting

1. Causes of nausea and vomiting can be divided into gastrointestinal (GI) and CNS sources.
   a. GI sources.
      (1) Gastric irritation by iron, alcohol, steroids, NSAIDs, antibiotics, blood.
      (2) Constipation.
      (3) Candidiasis.
      (4) Distal bowel obstruction and gastric outlet obstruction from an enlarging tumor.
   b. CNS causes.
      (1) Narcotics, digoxin, antibiotics.
      (2) Estrogens.
      (3) Uremia.
      (4) Hypercalcemia.
      (5) Chemotherapy.
      (6) Mechanical causes such as increased intracranial pressure and vestibular stimulation.
      (7) Emotional causes.
      (8) Advancing tumor.
2. Treatment begins with eradicating the source of the problem whenever possible and limiting any unnecessary drugs that can complicate the clinical picture.
   a. Patterns of symptoms can help determine the cause; thereafter, treatment focuses on medications.
   b. Although suppositories and injections may be needed initially to get nausea and vomiting under control, oral therapy is best for long-term prophylaxis.
3. Drugs include
   a. Phenothiazines.
      (1) Prochloperazine 10 mg PO or IM or 25 mg PR q4 to 6h.
      (2) Chlorpromazine (Thorazine) 10 to 25 mg PO or 25 to 50 mg IM q4 to 6h.
      (3) Promethazine (Phenergan) 25 to 50 mg PO, IM, or PR q4 to 6h.
      (4) Haloperidol (Haldol) 0.5 to 2 mg PO or SC q6 to 8h.
   b. Others.
      (1) Metoclopramide (Reglan) 10 to 20 mg PO or IM q6 to 8h.

(2) Dexamethasone (Decadron) 4 to 8 mg PO q8 to 12h.
(3) Meclizine (Antivert) 12.5 to 25 mg PO q6 to 8h.
(4) Transdermal scopolamine patch q3d.
(5) Ondansetron (Zofran) 32 mg IV q4h × 3 for chemotherapy-induced vomiting, or 8 mg PO tid for chemotherapy-induced vomiting.

c. Meclizine, scopolamine, and ondansetron are particularly helpful in treating patients with nausea associated with movement.
d. Dexamethasone and other steroids can be particularly useful in treating patients with increased intracranial pressure, hypercalcemia, or malignant pyloric stenosis and for treating severe nausea resistant to other antiemetic therapy.

Constipation

1. Constipation is a source of abdominal distention, pain, anorexia, nausea and vomiting, obstruction, and in some cases confusion.
2. Causes.
   a. Decreased fluid intake and decreased activity.
   b. Narcotics and antidepressants.
   c. Low-residue diets.
   d. Metabolic abnormalities, including hypercalcemia and hypokalemia.
   e. Mechanical obstruction.
   f. Sympathetic and parasympathetic imbalances, resulting in reduced peristalsis.
   g. Weakness, immobility, and confusion.
3. Management.
   a. As with pain, the key to the appropriate management of constipation is prevention, along with constant vigilance. A bowel regimen should be in place at or before the point when opioid narcotics are initiated.
   b. Evacuation should occur at least every 3 days because GI secretions, desquamation, and bacterial matter must be moved despite poor feeding. Constipation can be seen as watery stool oozing around a fixed impaction.
   c. Bowel regimens.
      (1) Bowel regimens should begin with stool softeners (e.g., docusate [Colace] 100 mg qd to bid) and gentle stimulation.
      (2) If bulk agents are used (e.g., psyllium), large amounts of water must be given, or these agents will harden in the GI tract and become a new source of constipation.
      (3) Lactulose 1 tablespoon qd, titrated up until the desired number of stools are produced, and polyethylene glycol (Miralax) 17 gm qd stimulates the large bowel.
      (4) Magnesium salts, such as magnesium sulfate 5 to 10 mL with water, stimulate small-bowel peristalsis.

Diarrhea

1. Etiology.
   a. Radiation malabsorption.
   b. Anxiety.
   c. Tumor infiltration.

   d. Carcinoid tumor.
   e. Bacterial and viral infections.
   f. Laxative imbalance.
   g. Leakage past an impaction.
2. Management.
   a. Frequent gentle cleansing of the perianal area is important to prevent skin breakdown, particularly if there is incontinence.
   b. Antidiarrheal agents include the following:
      (1) Attapulgite (Kaopectate) 30 mL after each loose bowel movement, up to 30 to 60 mL PO q4h.
      (2) Codeine 15 to 60 mg PO q4h.
      (3) Diphenoxylate (Lomotil) 2 tabs q4-6h.
      (4) Loperamide (Imodium) 2 to 4 mg PO q4-6h

Dyspnea

1. Subjective feelings of dyspnea can be particularly distressing for the terminal patient and frightening for the family.
2. Common causes.
   a. Anemia.
   b. CHF.
   c. COPD.
   d. Cardiac arrhythmia.
   e. Myocardial infarction.
   f. Pleural effusion.
   g. Bronchospasm and mucus plugging.
   h. Pulmonary infection.
   i. Enlarging or spreading malignancy in chest.
   j. Lung damage from chemotherapy.
   k. Pulmonary embolus.
   l. Anxiety.
3. Management.
   a. Suctioning and positioning.
   b. Relaxation and breathing exercises.
   c. Medications directed at identifiable causes (e.g., diuretics, antiarrhythmics, bronchodilators, anticoagulants, antibiotics, steroids).
   d. When appropriate, thoracentesis and sclerotherapy.
   e. Oxygen
   f. Medications to suppress air hunger.
      (1) Morphine 5 to 15 mg PO q4h or SR morphine, 15 to 30 mg q12h.
      (2) Hydromorphone 1 to 4 mg q4h.
      (3) Diazepam 5 to 10 mg q6-8h.
      (4) Chlorpromazine 10 to 25 mg PO q4-6h.
   g. Scopolamine 0.4 to 0.6 mg SQ q4h prn to dry pulmonary secretions and relax tracheobronchial smooth muscle.
   h. Synthetic cannabis derivative as a bronchodilator and for sedation.

Dehydration and Anorexia

1. Dehydration and anorexia are often of greater concern to those around the patient than to the patient. Aside from dry mouth, patients rarely complain of subjective feelings of thirst.

2. Etiology.
   a. Nausea and vomiting.
   b. Depression.
   c. Mouth soreness and infection.
   d. Pain.
   e. Dysphagia.
   f. Constipation.
   g. Chemotherapy and radiation.
   h. Increased tumor bulk.
   i. Hyponatremia.
   j. Hypercalcemia.
   k. Uremia.
   l. Hepatic failure.
   m. Many drugs.
3. In most cases, IV fluids and feedings are not appropriate. In some instances there are advantages to decreased oral intake in terms of patient comfort from decreased pulmonary secretions, decreased likelihood of vomiting, decreased urinary output, and possible incontinence. Dehydration and anorexia should be corrected when they are distressing to the patient, not just to the provider.
4. Treatment.
   a. Altering causes whenever possible.
   b. Relining dentures.
   c. Providing frequent small meals.
   d. Providing supplements with or in place of usual meals.
   e. Serving wine before meals.
   f. Prescribing metoclopramide, corticosteroids, or anabolic steroids.
   g. Allowing the patient to eat or drink whenever he or she desires instead of on a fixed schedule.

Anxiety

1. Nonpharmacologic treatment: Cognitive behavior interventions (relaxation, imagery, and psychotherapy).
2. Pharmacologic treatment.
   a. Intermediate-acting benzodiazepines (e.g., lorazepam).
   b. Morphine.

Depression

1. Depression, anticipatory grief, and loss are not uncommon for the terminal patient and his or her significant others. Aggressive symptom management can do much to alleviate depression.
2. For patients in whom the depression persists despite appropriate symptom management, antidepressants should be prescribed.

Confusion or Delirium

1. Misperceptions, disorientation, confusion, and decreasing level of consciousness associated with drug therapy or enlarging tumor are common in the terminal patient.
2. Etiology.
   a. Metabolic derangement (uremia, hypoglycemia, hypercalcemia, hyponatremia, hypomagnesemia, hypoxia, hypercapnia).

    b. Infections.

    c. Sepsis.

    d. Postictal states.

    e. Intracranial malignancy.

    f. Altered environment.

    g. Underlying dementia.

    h. Pain.

    i. Fecal impaction.

    j. Congestive heart failure.

    k. Drug or alcohol withdrawal.

3. Management.

    a. Haloperidol 0.5 to 1 mg qAM and 1 to 2 mg qhs, is the least-sedating medication but carries a significant risk of causing pseudoparkinsonism.

    b. The atypical antipsychotic drugs may be easier to tolerate. They include resperidone, olanzepine, and quietapine.

    c. Prescribing antidepressants and resetting day and night cycles using artificial light often can lessen confusion.

Mouth Care

1. Dry or sore mouth can be a significant source of irritation and pain, resulting in decreased oral intake.

2. Etiology.

    a. Thrush.

    b. Dryness.

    c. Ill-fitting dentures secondary to weight loss.

    d. Local radiation.

    e. Mouth breathing.

    f. Drugs (especially anticholinergics).

    g. Vitamin deficiencies.

3. Management as part of q2h mouth care.

    a. Relining dentures when possible.

    b. Ice chips.

    c. Frequent small sips of fluid.

    d. Hard candies.

    e. Vitamins.

    f. Artificial saliva.

    g. Topical anesthetics such as lidocaine (Xylocaine).

4. Excessive salivation with choking or coughing can be managed with anticholinergic agents such as hyoscyamine.

OTHER ISSUES

1. Caregiver support.

    a. Psychological: Assess for depression and anxiety and treat accordingly.

    b. Spiritual.

        (1) Assess spiritual needs.

        (2) Incorporate spiritual needs into care plan.

        (3) Involve appropriate consultants.

    c. Social.

        (1) Assess for caregiver burnout.

        (2) Identify financial resources.

(3) Consider respite care.

(4) Involve appropriate consultants (e.g., medical social worker).

2. Settings.

a. Home: Most formal hospice care is provided in the patient's home, but this requires able family members or friends to provide most custodial care.

b. Inpatient hospice: Typically for terminal care, acute control of symptoms, or as a bridge in home hospice program.

c. Nursing home: Preferably provided with formal involvement of a hospice program.

d. Hospital: Common, but not optimal, site for terminal care.

3. Financing.

a. Hospice is a benefit of Medicare that covers palliative care when elected by a patient and a physician certifies that the patient has a prognosis of 6 months or less. The certification can be renewed if the patient lives longer than 6 months (see "Hospice" earlier.)

b. Medicare covers physician services related to hospice diagnosis, nursing care, medications, durable medical equipment, social services, short-term respite care, chaplaincy services, physical and occupational therapy, bereavement services, and home health aide services

REFERENCE

1. Adapted from Jacox A, Carr DB, Payne R, et al: *Management of cancer pain: Adults quick reference guide No. 9.* AHCPR Pub No. 94-0593. Rockville, Md, Agency for Health Care Policy and Research, US Department of Health and Human Services, Public Health Services, 1994.).

SUGGESTED READINGS

American Geriatric Society Panel on Chronic Pain in Older Persons: The management of chronic pain in older persons. *J Am Geriatr Soc* 46(5):635-652, 1998.

American Geriatric Society Panel on Persistent Pain in Older Persons: The management of persistent pain in older persons. *J Am Geriatr Soc* 50:5205-5224, 2002.

Hlorenz K, Lynn J: Care of the dying patient. In Hazzard W, Blass J, Halter J, et al (eds): *Principles of Geriatric Medicine and Gerontology,* ed 5. New York, McGraw-Hill, 2003, pp 323-334.

National Comprehensive Cancer Network: Clinical practice guidelines in oncology: Adult cancer pain. Available at http://www.nccn.org/professionals/physician_gls/PDF/pain.pdf (accessed March 1, 2007).

7.5 The Elderly Driver

John B. Murphy

INTRODUCTION

1. Motor vehicle accidents among older drivers have been increasing steadily since 1980, particularly for those 85 and older.

2. Motor vehicle injuries are the leading cause of injury-related death among 65- to 74-year-olds and are second only to falls for those 75 to 84 years of age.

3. The fatality rate per mile driven is higher for older drivers than for any group aside from male drivers younger than 25 years.

4. Older driver involvement in fatal crashes is expected to increase by 155% by 2030, accounting for 54% of the total projected increases in fatal crashes among all drivers.
5. The responsibility for identifying impaired drivers increasingly falls to medical professionals.

ETIOLOGY

1. Vision.
   a. Safe driving requires good visual acuity and adequate visual fields.
   b. Many older drivers have impairments caused by conditions that increase in prevalence with age (e.g., macular degeneration, glaucoma, cataracts, and stroke).
2. Cognition.
   a. Safe driving requires adequate memory, attention, visual processing, and executive functioning.
   b. Many older drivers have impairments caused by conditions that increase in prevalence with age (e.g., stroke and Alzheimer's dementia).
3. Physical function.
   a. Safe driving requires adequate strength and flexibility as well as intact neurologic function (e.g., proprioception and reaction time).
   b. Many older drivers have impairments caused by conditions that increase in prevalence with increasing age (e.g., rheumatologic conditions, peripheral neuropathies, stroke, and deconditioning).

DIAGNOSIS

1. History: Confirm with family member:
   a. Motor vehicle accidents and moving violations.
   b. Copilot phenomenon (physically able, cognitively impaired driver directed by physically impaired, cognitively able passenger).
   c. Past medical conditions.
      (1) Diabetes (vision, peripheral neuropathy).
      (2) Macular degeneration, glaucoma, cataracts.
      (3) Neurologic disability.
         (a) Stroke.
         (b) Transient ischemic attack.
         (c) Dementia.
         (d) Seizures.
         (e) Neuropathy.
   d. Medications.
      (1) Sedative–hypnotics.
      (2) Narcotic analgesics.
      (3) Sedating antidepressants.
      (4) Antihistamines.
      (5) Alcohol.
2. Physical.
   a. Visual testing.
      (1) Acuity.
      (2) Visual field.
   b. Cognitive assessment.
      (1) Mini Mental State Exam (memory and attention deficits).
      (2) Clock drawing (executive function).

    c. Functional assessment.
      (1) Musculoskeletal exam.
      (2) Neurologic exam.

INTERVENTIONS

1. Reversible impairments.
    a. Stop or taper high-risk medications.
    b. Treat musculoskeletal and rheumatologic conditions.
    c. Physical therapy and exercise for deconditioning.
    d. Cataract removal and refraction.
2. Irreversible impairments.
    a. Possibly unsafe driver.
      (1) Refer for driver simulator testing (if available).
      (2) Refer to agency specializing in road-testing older drivers.
      (3) Refer to motor vehicle department for routine road test.
    b. Clearly unsafe driver: Refer to motor vehicle department noting concern.

LEGAL ISSUES

1. Jurisdiction: Dealt with on state level.
2. Liability.
    a. Some states mandate reporting.
    b. Case law suggests there is risk in not reporting patients who have impairments.
    c. Some states have statutes granting immunity to physicians who report in good faith.
    d. Where statutes do not exist, case law suggests physicians are immune if they report in good faith.
    e. At the very least, instruct the patient (or family where appropriate) to stop driving and self-report to the registry of motor vehicles.

SUGGESTED READINGS

American Medical Association: *Physician's Guide to Assessing and Counseling Older Drivers.* 2003. PDF available at http://www.ama-assn.org/ama/pub/category/10791.html (accessed February 26, 2007).

Freund B, Gravenstein S, Ferris R, et al: Clock drawing and driving cars. *J Gen Intern Med* 20:240-244, 2005.

Gilfillan CK, Schwartzberg JG: Addressing the at-risk older driver. *Clin Geriatr* 13:27-34, 2005.

Grabowski D, Campbell AB, Morrisey MA: Elderly licensure laws and motor vehicle fatalities. *JAMA* 291:2840-2846, 2004.

Hogan DB: Which older patients are competent to drive? *Can Fam Physician* 51:362-368, 2005.

Murden RA, Unroe K: Assessing older drivers. A primary care protocol to evaluate driving safety risk. *Geriatrics* 60:20-24, 2005.

7.6 Multicultural Geriatric Care

Michael P. Gerardo

OVERVIEW

1. Population projections estimate that the fraction of the older population who is black, Asian American, Latin American, Alaska Native,

Native American, or other minority will rise dramatically, from 12.3% in 2000 to 34.0% in 2050.
2. The tremendous growth rate of these populations and the decreasing availability of younger generations to provide informal care will result in a greater ethnic and racial mix among those requiring geriatric care and services.
3. The expanded use of health services by older adults with limited English proficiency and culturally distinct backgrounds will have important clinical practice implications, particularly as acute, long-term, and ambulatory care settings deliver more complex medical care.

DEMOGRAPHICS

1. The projected percent increase for the population 65 years and older during the period 1990 to 2030 is shown in Table 7-7.
2. The largest growth is expected to occur in the Latin American and the Asian and Pacific Islander populations.

MULTICULTURAL GERIATRIC ASSESSMENT

This multicultural geriatric assessment provides physicians with a means of understanding each patient's particular preferences and the historical context in which those decisions are made. The use of this comprehensive assessment can improve the patient's adherence to treatment plans, appropriate use of medical services, and satisfaction with care.
1. Ethnicity/race.
   a. Providers should ask the patient which ethnicity or race they associate with.
   b. People often use various terms to describe their personal background. Examples:
      (1) Hispanic or Latin American versus Mexican, Venezuelan, Puerto Rican.
      (2) African American versus black.
2. Acculturation.
   a. A person who is a member of a particular minority group might not share that population's major cultural preferences.
   b. Providers should be aware of certain markers of acculturation.
      (1) Immigration status.
      (2) Years since immigration.

Table 7-7 **Projected Increase in the Population 65 Years and Older, 1990-2030**

Ethnic Group	Increase (%)
Latin American	323
Asian and Pacific Islander	285
American Indian and Alaskan Native	147
African American	131
White, not Latin American	91

(3) Schooling or education.

(4) Composition of ethnic/racial groups in the area of residence.

(5) Fluency in English.

  c. Persons who have adopted the mainstream culture are less likely to practice cultural traditions and beliefs of their ethnic group.

3. Language.

  a. Some patients who speak English as a second language may be more comfortable discussing health care issues in their native language.

  b. The use of interpreter services is an important tool in achieving successful care plans for nonnative English speakers (see later).

4. Decision-making styles.

  a. A common practice in the United States is to place the sole responsibility for health care on the individual patient.

  b. Many older persons, particularly those who are not white, use the family in decision making or have a family member designated as the decision maker.

  c. Physicians should ask all patients about their decision-making style and to what extent the patient would like to know about his or her own health.

  d. This issue might have ethical and legal ramifications that need to be addressed.

5. Historical events.

  a. Experiences like refugee victimization (e.g., torture or genocide), segregation, or the Tuskegee Experiment have discouraged many persons from trusting the health care system.

  b. It is important to identify any historical events that can affect the patient–provider relationship.

6. Rituals and traditions.

  a. Health practices of certain ethnic or racial groups, like folk medicine and ritual purification, should be discussed with patients, because not addressing these issues has been shown to hamper the patient's adherence to care plans.

  b. Ethical and legal boundaries (e.g., Health Insurance Portability and Accountability Act [HIPAA] rules) may need to be addressed and perhaps in some cases involve an ethics committee.

7. Social support.

  a. The social support system of older adults can take any number of forms.

  b. Cultural norms may apply to certain populations, the provider should avoid stereotyping social support systems based on the race/ethnicity of the patient.

  c. Within any one population there are likely to be isolated elders with weak or no family ties.

    (1) Physicians should inquire who lives at home.

    (2) Of those who live at home, determine who helps with care.

  d. The provision of informal services by family has been demonstrated for Mexican American, African American, Filipino American, and Vietnamese American populations.

  e. Fictive kin.

(1) *Fictive kin* are members of the community, most often members of a religious congregation, whom a person can rely on for informal support.

(2) The use of fictive kin is strongest in the African American population.

8. Socioeconomic status.

a. Socioeconomic status is an independent predictor of poor health outcomes.

b. Among the old, the percentage of persons in poverty is higher in any nonwhite community than in any community of white persons of the same age.

c. Physicians should be aware of the patient's financial, educational (quality and quantity of education), and occupational status.

d. Persons who immigrate late in life or undocumented immigrants might not be eligible for Social Security, Medicare and Medicaid, or social services.

9. Disability.

a. Disability, whether reported or observed, is more common for Latin American, African American, and Native American populations than that for white populations.

b. The literature has demonstrated the highest rates of disability to occur in the African American population.

c. Physicians should consider early assessment of disability in these high-risk groups. Examples:

(1) Gait assessment.

(2) Timed Get up and Go test.

(3) Performance-Oriented Mobility Assessment.

d. When appropriate, develop a tailored (e.g. culturally and linguistically sensitive) plan for reducing the risk of future or progressive disability (e.g., chronic disease management, home safety evaluation, physical therapy).

10. Chronic disease.

a. Some chronic diseases disproportionately affect certain populations.

b. Providers should be aware of these differences and be particularly mindful of the influence of mismanaged chronic disease on the prevalence and incidence of disability in older patients.

c. Specific chronic diseases.

(1) Diabetes is 1.5, 1.6, 2.0, and 2.2 times more common in Latin American, African American, Asian American, and Native American populations, respectively, than among whites.

(2) Hypertension is 1.5 times more common in African Americans than among whites.

(3) Depression is more common among Mexican-Americans than among whites. Because diabetic patients who are depressed are more likely to suffer from the macrovascular and microvascular complications of diabetes, physicians should be aware of prevalent comorbid illnesses that preclude effective management of diabetes.

(4) Osteoporosis is more common in the white population than among Latin Americans, African Americans, or Asian Americans.

11. Long-term care and end of life care.
    a. Both of these topics are sensitive in nature for the general population but are particularly sensitive in many nonwhite cultures.
    b. Minority elders might not be familiar with the concepts of life-sustaining measures, long-term care, autopsy, or organ donation.
    c. It is important to develop a relationship with minority elders prior to any discussion of these topics.
    d. The provider should be aware of any unique death rituals, mourning behavior, or preferences for places of death (e.g., the home over an acute-care setting).

MULTICULTURAL CLINICAL SKILLS

1. Interpreter services.
    a. Communication between patients with limited English proficiency and health care providers can be facilitated by the use of interpreter services.
    b. Professional interpreters.
        (1) The provision of professional medical interpreters has had a positive influence on quality of care.
        (2) The use of ad hoc interpreters (hired out as needed), staff not trained in medical interpretation (nurse aides, janitorial staff), and family is inadvisable when professional medical interpreter services are available.
        (3) Use of untrained interpreters has been associated with omission of relevant information, substitution of information, nonadherence to prescriptions, misuse of health services, and poor patient satisfaction.
        (4) A particularly important concern to keep in mind is the obvious loss of patient privacy with the use of family members or friends for interpretation. Under such circumstances, the patient can be expected to withhold important information (e.g., alcohol abuse, sexual history).
2. Cultural brokers may be particularly useful in aligning standards of medical care with various cultural norms, but they are not widely available.
3. Culturally appropriate interviews.
    a. Culturally appropriate interviews can best be accomplished by asking the patient what their particular preference is in relation to the language he or she is most comfortable with and their particular decision-making styles.
    b. Providers should use courtesy title with last name when addressing the patient.
    c. It is tempting to discuss the plan of care with whoever accompanies the older person.
        (1) Providers should acknowledge and greet the older person first.
        (2) When appropriate, providers should avoid obtaining the history solely from a younger family member. This point is important for an interaction with any older person, not just a minority elder, who is accompanied by a family member.
4. Screening tools.
    a. Screening for disease related to memory, mood, or disability is an important component of geriatric care.

   b. Providers should be aware that these assessments have not been standardized or validated for all ethnic or racial groups.
   c. Information regarding the extent to which groups have been evaluated for various screening tools can be found at www.stanford.edu/group/ethnoger.
5. Multicultural staff.
   a. Nursing homes are increasingly staffed with recent immigrants, and the potential for mishaps exists when poor communication occurs between physician and nurses (or nurses' aides).
   b. Physicians should be patient when communicating over the phone with anyone who has a limited fluency in English.
   c. If a physician is unable to communicate verbally with a member of the nursing staff because of a strong accent or inadequate English, it is appropriate to ask politely to speak with another nurse.
   d. When appropriate, medical directors might consider advocating for the training of nursing staff in language proficiency, culturally appropriate nursing care, and the proper use of interpreter services because these educational interventions can improve the quality of care for nursing home residents and can improve the job satisfaction of nursing staff.
6. Other.
   a. The impact of cultural competence on the patient's health status has largely been framed in the sphere of ethnic and racial disparities in health care.
   b. It is important to recognize that the goal of cultural competence is not only to promote the successful interaction of all patients within the health care system but also to decrease cultural and linguistic barriers of access to health services.
   c. Other forms of culture come with their unique set of special needs. Examples:
      (1) Sexual orientation.
      (2) Urban or rural life.
      (3) Historical experiences (war veterans, refugees).
      (4) Physical disability.

SUGGESTED READINGS

Angel J, Angel R: Minority group status and healthy aging: Social structure still matters. *Am J Public Health* 96:1152-1259, 2006.

Angel J, Hogan D: Population aging and diversity in a new era. In Whitfield KE (ed): *Closing the Gap: Improving the Health of Minority Elders in the New Millennium.* Washington, DC, Gerontological Society of America, 2004, pp 1-16.

Brach C, Fraser I: Can cultural competency reduce racial and ethnic health disparities? A review and conceptual model. *Medi Care Res Rev* 57, Suppl 1:181-217, 2000.

Fortier JP, Bishop D: *Setting the Agenda for Research on Cultural Competence in Health Care.* Washington, DC, Office of Minority Health and Agency for Healthcare Research and Quality, 2004. Available at http://www.ahrq.gov/research/cultural.htm

Waldrop J, Stern SM: Disability Status 2000: Census 2000 Brief. Washington, DC, US Department of Commerce, 2003. Available at http://www.census.gov/prod/2003pubs/c2kbr-17.pdf (accessed March 1, 2007).

Xakellis G, Brangman SA, Hinton WL, et al: Curricular framework: Core competencies in multicultural geriatric care. *J Am Geriatr Soc* 52:137-142, 2004.

INTERNET RESOURCES

Administration on Aging (AOA) guidebook for providers of multicultural geriatric care; http://www.aoa.gov/prof/adddiv/cultural/cc-guidebook.pdf

"Diversity, Healing and Care" is a web based resource for providers dealing with religion and culture; www.gasi-ves.org/diversity.htm

Yeo G (ed): Curriculum in Ethnogeriatrics. Core Curriculum and Ethnic Specific Modules. Available at www.stanford.edu/group/ethnoger (accessed March 1, 2007).

Rehabilitation

8

8.1 Introduction to General Rehabilitation Principles

John B. Murphy

OVERVIEW

1. Rehabilitation is critical to geriatric health care.
   a. Disabling conditions are common among older persons.
   b. Disabilities greatly affect quality of life but are often amenable to treatment.
2. Conceptual framework.
   a. Rehabilitation is based upon a conceptual framework wherein a disease results in impairment, which is an alteration in physical function at the organ level.
   b. The impairment then causes a limitation in a person's activities of daily living (ADLs), which is known as a disability.
   c. When a disability prevents a person from fully functioning in society, the person has a handicap.
   d. This framework is shown in Table 8-1, with stroke as an example.
3. Rehabilitation is an approach to care that can be applied anywhere and not just in special units.
4. Rehabilitation is less involved in treating disease and more involved in enhancing function across all domains: physical, psychological, and social.
5. Rehabilitation is based on comprehensive functional assessment and typically is interdisciplinary.

Table 8-1	Conceptual Framework for Rehabilitation		
	Organ Level	**Person Level**	**Societal Level**
Disease→ Stroke→	Impairment→ Left side weakness→	Disability→ Inability to transfer→	Handicap Inability to live alone

PROCESS OF REHABILITATION

1. Overview.
   a. Stabilize the primary problem (e.g., for stroke, treat the hypertension or atrial fibrillation to prevent another stroke).
   b. Prevent secondary complications. Examples:
      (1) Pressure ulcers.
      (2) Deep venous thrombosis (DVT).
      (3) Malnutrition.
      (4) Shoulder subluxation.
   c. Restore lost function. Examples:
      (1) Strength and endurance training.
      (2) Teach stand-pivot transfers from bed to wheelchair.
      (3) Instruct in the use of a walker or wheelchair.
   d. Promote adaptation of the person to the environment. Facilitate physical and psychological acceptance of the changes in function.
   e. Adapt the physical environment.
      (1) Build a ramp for entry into the house.
      (2) Widen doorways to allow a wheelchair to enter.
      (3) Install grab bars in the bathroom.
   f. Adapt the personal environment.
      (1) Assess family strengths.
      (2) Build on strengths.
      (3) Provide supports to bolster weaknesses (e.g., respite care, elderly day care).
2. Rehabilitation professionals.
   a. Physiatrist: Physician trained in physical medicine and rehabilitation (PM&R).
   b. Rehabilitation nurse.
      (1) Provides nursing care.
      (2) Reinforces and adapts techniques taught by other rehabilitation team members.
      (3) Provides psychological support.
      (4) Trains family and other caregivers.
   c. Physical therapist.
      (1) Assesses strength, range of motion, endurance, and mobility.
      (2) Focuses primarily on transfers and ambulation.
   d. Occupational therapist.
      (1) Focuses on assessing and addressing disabilities in ADL.
      (2) Assesses and addresses some instrumental activities of daily living (IADL).
   e. Speech pathologist: Evaluates and treats patients with aphasia, dysphagia, perceptual disorders, speech impairments, and cognitive problems.
   f. Recreational therapist: Identifies and implements satisfying recreational activities to help the patient adjust to the disability.
   g. Audiologist.
      (1) Assesses degree and characteristics of hearing loss.
      (2) Prescribes auditory aids (including hearing aids).
      (3) Conducts aural rehabilitation.

h. Psychologist.
   (1) Assesses psychological function.
   (2) Treats psychological conditions.
i. Neuropsychologist.
   (1) Assesses complex neuropsychological impairments.
   (2) Develops plans for treatment.
   (3) Often assists other rehabilitation team members in adapting their interventions to meet the unique needs of cognitively impaired patients.
j. Social worker.
   (1) Assesses social and psychological strengths and weaknesses of patients and care givers.
   (2) Identifies community resources needed for optimal family function.
k. Orthotist: Fashions complex rehabilitation aids such as a prosthesis or back brace.
3. Rehabilitation settings.
   a. General principles.
      (1) Provided in the least restrictive, most independent, and least costly setting.
      (2) Provided only following a decrement of function, not for maintenance.
      (3) Provided only as long as the patient continues to make progress. Rehabilitation to prevent functional decline (e.g., deconditioning, contractures) is a gray zone and is typically not covered by third party payers.
      (4) Provided only when a patient has sufficient cognitive ability to benefit from therapy.
   b. Acute hospital.
      (1) Immediate phase after illness or an operation.
      (2) Duration: Brief, a few days to a week.
      (3) Focuses on initial assessment and determination of where to provide subsequent care.
      (4) Designed to prevent complications and bridge the patient to the next setting.
      (5) Examples: immediate period following stroke or hip fracture.
   c. Acute level rehabilitation center.
      (1) Patients with complex medical and or rehabilitation needs that require an interdisciplinary team of rehabilitation specialists.
      (2) Duration: Intermediate, generally 1 to 3 weeks.
      (3) Conditions.
         (a) The patient must require two or more therapies.
         (b) The patient must be able to benefit from and participate in therapy for at least 3 hours per day.
      (4) The patient is unable to have needs met in a less intensive (expensive) setting.
      (5) Example: A stroke patient with good endurance, hemiparesis, mild cognitive deficits, and dysphagia.

d. Skilled nursing facility (SNF).
   (1) Patients with all of the following needs.
      (a) Functional losses that would benefit from rehabilitation.
      (b) Can't be cared for at home because of the extent of the functional impairments or the lack of support in the home.
      (c) Can benefit from an interdisciplinary team.
   (2) Duration: Intermediate, weeks to a few months.
   (3) Must need a licensed professional (registered nurse, physical or occupational therapist, or speech pathologist) 5 days per week.
   (4) Example: Patient with hip fracture who lives alone.
   (5) Medicare requires a hospitalization of at least 3 days within the previous 30 days.
e. Home.
   (1) Patients who have functional losses that would benefit from rehabilitation and who have adequate supports in the home or who have mild impairments.
   (2) Duration: Brief to long term, days to months.
   (3) Rehabilitation does not require cumbersome equipment that can't be provided in the home.
   (4) Patient must be homebound (doesn't go out of the house except for medical care).
   (5) Patient might require one or more therapies and might need interdisciplinary team care.
   (6) Example: Patient who has a total hip replacement for osteoarthritis, is otherwise healthy and robust, who has excellent in-home support and a handicapped-accessible home.
f. Outpatient.
   (1) Straightforward rehabilitation needs, with one or more therapies, but commonly only one.
   (2) Duration: Brief to long-term.
   (3) Might require access to sophisticated equipment.
   (4) Commonly follows acute hospital, rehabilitation center, SNF, or home rehabilitation program.
   (5) Example: Gait assessment and prescription of adaptive mobility aid (e.g., cane or walker).
4. Conditions and settings for rehabilitation.
   a. Acute level rehabilitation unit.
      (1) Stroke.
      (2) Amputation.
      (3) Complex fracture (e.g., hip fracture in patient with previous stroke).
   b. SNF.
      (1) Routine hip fracture.
      (2) Total joint replacement.
      (3) Deconditioning.
   c. Home.
      (1) Stroke or major joint repair with excellent in-home supports.
      (2) Deconditioning.

 d. Outpatient.
  (1) Follow-up care after rehabilitation in another setting.
  (2) Small or medium joint surgery.
  (3) Assessment of unstable gait.
  (4) Prescription of adaptive mobility aid (e.g., walker, cane).

PHYSICAL THERAPY

1. Overview.
 a. Physical therapy (PT) is a health profession concerned with the assessment, diagnosis, and treatment of disease and disability through physical means.
 b. PT is performed by a licensed practitioner who works with the physical aspects of a medical illness and specializes in the use of exercise to treat physical conditions.
 c. PT focuses primarily on assessment and treatment of persons with musculoskeletal, neurologic, and cardiopulmonary conditions.
 d. The physical therapist might use a variety of modalities and prescribe devices.
 e. Goals.
  (1) Improve strength, mobility, and function.
  (2) Relieve pain.
  (3) Prevent or minimize disability.
 f. Patient and family education are core components of the practice of PT.
2. Education and licensing.
 a. A physical therapist has at a minimum a bachelor's degree, often a master's degree, and occasionally a doctorate.
 b. A PT assistant generally has an associate's degree.
 c. Physical therapists are licensed at a state level but must pass a national exam administered at the state level.
 d. Physical therapists evaluate and treat primarily under the prescription of a patient's physician.
3. Scope of evaluation capabilities.
 a. Joint range of motion.
 b. Muscle strength and endurance.
 c. Integrity of sensation and proprioception.
 d. Muscle tone.
 e. Functional ability.
 f. Gait assessment.
 g. Performance of ADLs.
4. Techniques.
 a. Therapeutic exercise.
 b. Joint mobilization and range of motion exercises.
 c. Ambulation training.
 d. Cardiovascular endurance training.
 e. Relaxation exercises.
 f. Therapeutic massage.
 g. Biofeedback.
 h. Training in ADL.
 i. Pulmonary physical therapy.

5. Modalities.
   a. Traction.
   b. Ultrasound.
   c. Cryotherapy.
   d. Diathermy.
   e. Electrotherapy.
   f. Hydrotherapy.
6. Physician referral to physical therapists.
   a. Referral can be for assessment, treatment, or both.
   b. Referral needs a specific diagnosis.
   c. Referral should include a statement requesting a specific treatment or that the therapist can evaluate and treat as the therapist determines most appropriate.
   d. Examples.
      (1) Parkinson's disease, ICD-9CM 332.0: Evaluate gait, prescribe and train patient in use of a wheeled walker.
      (2) Adhesive capsulitis, ICD-9CM 726.0: Evaluate and treat as necessary.
   e. Physical therapy is covered under Medicare and most health insurance plans with a physician's prescription, but primarily for recovery, not for maintenance programs.

OCCUPATIONAL THERAPY

1. Overview.
   a. Occupational therapy (OT) is a health profession designed to help people improve their ability to perform tasks in their ADLs and working environments.
   b. Occupational therapists work with patients who have conditions that are mentally, physically, developmentally, or emotionally disabling.
   c. Occupational therapists help persons to improve their basic motor functions and reasoning abilities and to compensate for permanent loss of function.
   d. Their goal is to help clients have independent, productive, and satisfying lives.
   e. Occupational therapists assist patients in performing activities of all types, ranging from using computer to caring for daily needs such as a dressing, cooking, and eating.
   f. Physical exercises may be used to increase strength and dexterity.
   g. Other activities may be chosen to improve visual acuity and the ability to discern patterns.
   h. Therapists instruct those with permanent disabilities, such as spinal cord injuries, cerebral palsy, or muscular dystrophy, in the use of adaptive equipment, including wheelchairs, splints, and aids for eating and dressing.
   i. Family/caregiver education is a core component of the field.
2. Education and licensing.
   a. Until 2007, a registered occupational therapist (OTR) was required to have a bachelor's degree.
   b. Beginning in 2007, to qualify for an OTR, a master's degree has become the minimum requirement.

   c. Occupational therapists must graduate from an accredited educational program and pass a national certification examination.
   d. Licensing is at a state level.
   e. OT Assistants have either an associate's degree or a certificate from a 1-year program.
3. Scope of occupational therapy assessment and treatment techniques.
   a. Perceptual, sensory, and cognitive assessment.
   b. Assessment of ADLs.
   c. Assessment of work readiness.
   d. Assessment of need for assistive technology.
   e. Driving assessments.
   f. Design, fabrication, and training in the use of assistive technology and orthotic or prosthetic devices.
   g. Customized treatment programs to improve a person's ability to perform ADL.
   h. Comprehensive home and job site evaluations with adaptation recommendations.
   i. Cognitive retraining programs.
   j. Guidance to family members and caregivers.
4. Physician referral to occupational therapists.
   a. Referral can be for assessment, treatment, or both.
   b. Referral needs a specific diagnosis.
   c. Referral should include a statement requesting a specific treatment or that the therapist can evaluate and treat as the therapist determines most appropriate.
   d. Examples.
      (1) Stroke, ICD-9CM 436: Evaluate ability to self-feed and provide large-diameter grip eating utensils, a plate guard, and two-handed cup.
      (2) Parkinson's disease, ICD-9CM 332.0: Evaluate and treat as necessary.
   e. Occupational therapy is covered under Medicare and most health insurance plans with a physician's prescription.

SPEECH PATHOLOGY

1. Overview.
   a. Speech pathology is the science concerned with the diagnosis and treatment of functional and organic speech defects and disorders.
   b. Speech and language pathologists evaluate and treat patients with aphasia, dysarthria, cognitive problems, perceptual disorders, and dysphagia.
2. Education and licensing.
   a. Minimum education is a master's degree.
   b. National certification exam administered by the Educational Testing Service (ETS).
   c. Licensing at the state level.
   d. Often works with an audiologist.
3. Common conditions assessed and treated.
   a. Dysphagia, including modified barium swallow examinations.
   b. Aphasias.
   c. Stroke-associated cognitive and communication disorders.

    d. Language-perception disorders.
    e. Hearing impairments and aural rehabilitation.
4. Physician referral to speech pathologists.
    a. Referral can be for assessment, treatment, or both.
    b. A referral needs a specific diagnosis.
    c. The services must be medically necessary.
    d. The plan of care needs to be established by either a speech-language pathologist or the physician.
    e. The patient must be under the care of a physician.
    f. Medicare requires physician review of the plan of care every 30 days but no longer stipulates frequency of physician visits.

SUGGESTED READINGS

American Medical Association: *Health Professions Career and Education Directory.* Chicago, American Medical Association, 2002, pp 289-290.

Hoenig H, Cutson T: Geriatric rehabilitation. In Hazzard W, Blass J, Halter J, et al (eds): *Principles of Geriatric Medicine and Gerontology*, ed 5. New York, McGraw-Hill, 2003, pp 285-302.

Hoenig H, Nusbaum N, Brummel-Smith K: Geriatric rehabilitation: State of the art. *J Am Geriatr Soc* 45:1371-1381, 1997.

Mosqueda L, Brummel-Smith K: Rehabilitation. In Ham R, Sloane P, Warshaw G (eds): *Primary Care Geriatrics*, ed 4. St. Louis, Mosby, 2002, pp 149-163.

8.2 Post-stroke Rehabilitation: Assessment, Referral, and Patient Management

Fred F. Ferri

EPIDEMIOLOGY[1]

1. Each year in the United States, stroke occurs in approximately 550,000 persons.
2. About 3 million Americans are living with varying degrees of disability from stroke.
3. Brain infarctions account for about 75% of all strokes, and intracerebral or subarachnoid hemorrhages account for about 15%. The remainder are due to other or unknown causes.
4. Stroke frequency increases dramatically with advancing age, doubling with every decade after 55 years.
5. Men are more likely to have strokes than women.
6. African Americans are more likely to have strokes than whites.
7. Mortality.
    a. Estimates of stroke mortality range from 17% to 34% in the first 30 days and from 25% to 40% in the first year.
    b. Mortality from stroke has declined because of a combination of factors, including reduced stroke severity, earlier and more accurate diagnosis, and better acute care.
8. Risk factors.
    a. Modifiable or potentially modifiable risk factors for stroke.
        (1) Medical.
            (a) Atrial fibrillation.
            (b) Congestive heart failure.

    (c) Coronary heart disease.
    (d) Diabetes mellitus.
    (e) High serum cholesterol levels.
    (f) Hypertension.
    (g) Left ventricular hypertrophy.
    (h) Transient ischemic attacks.
  (2) Lifestyle.
    (a) Cigarette smoking.
    (b) Cocaine use.
    (c) Heavy alcohol consumption.
    (d) Obesity.
 b. Fixed or nonmodifiable risk factors for stroke.
  (1) Age.
  (2) Gender.
  (3) Family history.
  (4) Previous stroke.
  (5) Race.

CLINICAL EVALUATION

1. Hemiparesis is a presenting finding in about 75% of patients.
2. Acute neurologic impairment often resolves spontaneously, but persisting disabilities lead to partial or total dependence with regard to ADLs in 25% to 50% of stroke patients.
3. Initial treatment.
  a. Acute rehabilitation.
    (1) Most patients who have had a stroke are initially treated in a stroke unit or in the general medical service of an acute care hospital.
    (2) They receive rehabilitation services directed at preventing complications of stroke.
    (3) As medically feasible, mobilization and resumption of self-care activities are encouraged.
  b. Postacute rehabilitation.
    (1) Figure 8-1 outlines the clinical algorithm for stroke rehabilitation.
    (2) When the patient is medically stable, screening for postacute rehabilitation is performed.
      (a) Patients with stroke who recover completely will not need rehabilitation.
      (b) Patients who remain severely incapacitated are not likely to benefit from rehabilitation, although some patients in this group may improve over a further period of recuperation and can be reevaluated at a later date.
      (c) Between these extremes are patients with functional deficits who are candidates for either individual rehabilitation services or an interdisciplinary program.
    (3) The key components of a rehabilitation program include the following factors:
      (a) Medical management.
      (b) Assessment, including use of selected standardized instruments.

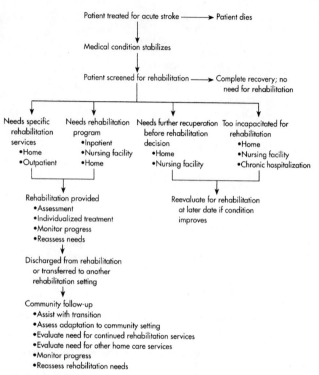

Figure 8-1 Clinical algorithm for stroke rehabilitation. (From Gresham GE, Gresham Duncan PW, Stason WB, et al: *Post-stroke rehabilitation. Clinical practice guideline No. 16.* AHCPR Pub. No. 95-0662. Rockville, Md, U.S. Department of Health and Human Services. Public Health Service, Agency for Health Care Policy and Research, May 1995.)

      (c) Rehabilitation referrals, matching patient needs and program capabilities.
      (d) Provision of rehabilitation according to a well-defined management plan with explicit goals, measurement of progress, and adjustment of the plan or goals as needed.
      (e) Assistance in reintegrating the patient into the community.

MEDICAL MANAGEMENT

1. Setting.
   a. When possible, treat the patient with acute stroke in a setting that provides coordinated, multidisciplinary, stroke-related evaluation and services.
     (1) Acute stroke units.
     (2) Well-staffed neurology or rehabilitation departments.

(3) Other acute hospital settings with coordinated stroke services.

b. Studies have found improved rates of survival and greater likelihood of returning home when acute stroke care is coordinated and multidisciplinary. This improvement may be related to better organization of services, with an emphasis on early mobilization of the patient and early implementation of rehabilitation interventions.

2. Documentation.

a. Fully document the patient's condition and clinical course in the medical record.

b. Thorough documentation of clinical information during the acute hospitalization is essential to making appropriate rehabilitation decisions (Fig. 8-2). The following information should be included in the patient's medical record:

(1) Stroke etiology and areas of the brain involved.

(2) Type(s), severity, and trajectory of neurologic deficits (Box 8-1 describes perceptual deficits in CNS function).

(3) Type(s) and severity of comorbid diseases.

(4) Complications and abnormal health patterns.

(5) Changes in clinical status that might occur over time.

(6) Functional status before the stroke.

3. Timing.

a. Begin rehabilitation-oriented care immediately and increase the patient's activity as soon as medically feasible during the acute phase.

b. Position changes to prevent skin breakdown and careful range-of-motion exercises to prevent contractures should be initiated shortly after admission.

c. Further mobilization should begin when the patient is medically stable, preferably within the first 24 to 48 hours.

d. Transfer techniques should be followed closely and taught to the patient and family.

e. As early as possible, the patient should be encouraged to participate in personal care activities and to communicate and interact with staff and other patients.

f. Attention and gaze need to be directed away from the intact side to prevent unilateral neglect.

g. The benefits of early mobilization include:

(1) Prevention of DVT, skin breakdown, contracture formation, constipation, and pneumonia.

(2) Better orthostatic tolerance.

(3) Earlier return of mental and motor function and ability to perform ADL.

(4) Improved morale of both patient and family.

h. Indications for delaying mobilization or approaching it with caution include:

(1) Coma or severe obtundation.

(2) Progressing neurologic signs or symptoms.

(3) Subarachnoid or intracerebral hemorrhage.

(4) Severe orthostatic hypotension.

Clinical evaluation during acute care
<u>Purposes</u>
Determine etiology, pathology, and severity of stroke
Assess comorbidities
Document clinical course
<u>When</u>
On admission and during acute hospitalization
<u>By whom</u>
Acute care physician
Nursing staff
Rehabilitation consultants

Not referred for rehabilitation

- No or minimal disability
- Too severely disabled to participate in rehabilitation. Provide supportive services; consider rescreening at a future date if condition improves

Screening for rehabilitation
<u>Purposes</u>
Identify patients who may benefit from rehabilitation
Determine appropriate setting for rehabilitation
Identify problems needing treatment
<u>When</u>
As soon as patient is medically stable
<u>By whom</u>
Rehabilitation clinicians

Referred to interdisciplinary rehabilitation program in outpatient facility, home, inpatient unit or facility, or nursing facility

Referred for individual rehabilitation services (rehabilitation nurse, occupational therapist, physical therapist, psychologist, speech-language pathologist)

- Same assessment stages as for interdisciplinary program

Assessment on admission to rehabilitation
<u>Purposes</u>
Validate referral decision
Develop management plan
Provide baseline for monitoring progress
<u>When</u>
Within 3 working days for an intense program;
1 week for a less intense inpatient program;
or three visits for an outpatient or home program
<u>By whom</u>
Rehabilitation clinicians/team

Assessment during rehabilitation
<u>Purposes</u>
Monitor progress
Adjust treatment regimen
Provide basis for discharge decision
<u>When</u>
Weekly for intense program
At least biweekly for less intense programs
<u>By whom</u>
Rehabilitation clinicians/team

Assessment after discharge from rehabilitation
<u>Purposes</u>
Evaluate adaptation to home environment
Determine need for continued rehabilitation services
Assess caregiver burden
<u>When</u>
Within 1 month of discharge
Regular intervals during first year
<u>By whom</u>
Rehabilitation clinicians
Principal physician

Figure 8-2 Stages of assessment for post-stroke rehabilitation. (Redrawn from Gresham GE, Gresham Duncan PW, Stason WB, et al: *Post-stroke rehabilitation. Clinical practice guideline No. 16.* AHCPR Pub. No. 95-0662. Rockville, Md, U.S. Department of Health and Human Services. Public Health Service, Agency for Health Care Policy and Research, May 1995.)

---

    (5) Acute myocardial infarction.

    (6) Acute DVT (until adequate anticoagulation has been achieved).

4. General health.
   a. Manage general health functions throughout all stages of treatment.
   b. Health functions that need to be monitored and managed during acute care and rehabilitation and after return to the community include:
      (1) Dysphagia.
         (a) Physicians should be alert to the possibility of dysphagia.
         (b) If dysphagia is present, consultation should be obtained and an appropriate program initiated.
      (2) Nutrition and hydration: The adequacy of food and fluid intake should be monitored regularly.
      (3) Bladder and bowel function.
         (a) Persistent urinary incontinence should be evaluated to determine its etiology, and appropriate treatment should be provided.
         (b) If possible, the use of indwelling urinary catheters should be avoided.
         (c) Bowel management programs should be implemented in patients with persistent constipation or bowel incontinence.
      (4) Sleep and rest.
         (a) Disturbances in sleep patterns should be evaluated to determine their cause.
         (b) Interventions may include:
            i. Keeping the patient active during the day.
            ii. Teaching relaxation techniques.
            iii. Changing medications.
      (5) Comorbid conditions: Symptoms and signs not clearly attributable to the stroke should be evaluated and treated as indicated.
      (6) Acute illnesses: Patients who develop an acute medical illness during rehabilitation should be evaluated promptly and, if necessary, transferred to an acute care facility.

5. Complications.
   a. Take steps to prevent complications throughout all stages of treatment.
   b. Preventive measures should be initiated during acute care and continued throughout rehabilitation and after the patient's return to the community.
   c. The following potential complications can occur:
      (1) DVT and pulmonary embolism.
         (a) Preventive measures include early mobilization, low-dose heparin, or low-molecular-weight heparin.

BOX 8-1   Perceptual Deficits in Central Nervous System Dysfunction

Left Hemiparesis: Right Hemisphere General Spatial and Global Deficits

VISUAL AND PERCEPTUAL DEFICITS
Figure-ground discrimination
Form constancy
Hand-eye coordination
Position in space
Spatial relationships

BEHAVIORAL AND INTELLECTUAL DEFICITS
Affect lability
Appearance of lethargy
Denial of disability
Difficulty retaining information
Distortion of time concepts
Distraction by verbalization
Disturbances in body image and body scheme
Disturbances in relative size and distance of objects
Feelings of persecution
Fluctuation in performance
Impairment of ability to self-correct
Inability to abstract
Irritability, confusion
Poor judgment, unrealistic behavior
Rigidity of thought
Short attention span
Tendency to see the whole and not individual steps

Right Hemiparesis: Left Hemisphere General Language and Temporal Ordering Deficits

APRAXIA
Ideational
Motor

BEHAVIORAL AND INTELLECTUAL DEFICITS
Compulsive behavior
Difficulty initiating tasks
Directionality deficits
Extreme distractibility
Low frustration levels
Processing delays
Rapid performance of movement or activity
Sequencing deficits
Verbal and manual perseveration

Data from Umphred DA: *Neurological rehabilitation*, ed 2. St Louis, Mosby, 1990.

    (b) Warfarin, intermittent pneumatic compression, and elastic stockings are also effective.

(2) Dysphagia and aspiration.

    (a) Depending on the type of swallowing deficit, treatment may include training to relearn swallowing, compensatory approaches such as changes in food texture, and, if necessary, a gastrostomy tube.

    (b) Dysphagia often resolves spontaneously; however, the condition should be reassessed periodically during rehabilitation, and treatments should be continued or adjusted as necessary.

(3) Skin breakdown: Preventive measures include:

    (a) Daily skin inspection.

    (b) Gentle routine cleansing.

    (c) Minimizing exposure to moisture.

    (d) Avoidance of friction.

    (e) Reduction of pressure.

    (f) Upright sitting posture.

    (g) Proper nutrition and hydration.

    (h) Early mobility.

(4) Prevention of urinary tract infections: If indwelling catheters are used, they should be removed as soon as is feasible.

(5) Seizures.

    (a) Anticonvulsant medications are recommended for preventing recurrent seizures in patients with stroke who have had one or more seizures.

    (b) Anticonvulsants are not recommended for patients who have not had seizures.

(6) Falls.

    (a) Patients who have had a stroke are at increased risk for falls.

    (b) Risk factors include:

        i. Problems with perceptual deficits.

        ii. Visual impairments.

        iii. Impaired communication.

        iv. Confusion.

        v. Drug side effects.

        vi. Environmental hazards.

        vii. Mobility, balance, and coordination.

    (c) The risk is increased by rehabilitation treatments aimed at improving mobility.

    (d) Risk prevention includes:

        i. Supervision of high-risk patients.

        ii. Proper seating and wheelchair modification.

        iii. Regular toileting.

        iv. Supervised transfer and ambulation.

        v. Nurse call systems suited to a patient's abilities.

        vi. Institution-wide fall prevention programs addressing both patient and environmental risk factors.

        vii. Patient and family education for prevention of falls and proper ways to get up after a fall.

(e) Adequate supervision and environmental precautions should continue after the patient returns to the community.

(7) Spasticity and contractures: Methods of prevention and treatment of spasticity and contracture include:

(a) Antispastic pattern positioning.

(b) Range-of-motion exercises.

(c) Stretching.

(d) Splinting.

(e) Nerve blocks.

(8) Shoulder injury.

(a) This is a common cause of pain in stroke patients.

(b) Prevention emphasizes proper positioning and support and avoidance of overly vigorous range-of-motion exercises.

6. Recurrent stroke.

a. Take steps to prevent recurrent stroke throughout all stages of treatment.

b. Persons who have had a stroke are at increased risk for another stroke.

c. The following preventive measures should be taken throughout acute care and rehabilitation and after the patient returns to the community:

(1) Identify and control modifiable risk factors such as hypertension, cigarette smoking, diabetes mellitus, high serum cholesterol, and heavy alcohol consumption.

(2) Oral anticoagulants.

(a) Use oral anticoagulants to prevent embolic strokes in patients with atrial fibrillation or prosthetic cardiac valves.

(b) These medications are not currently recommended for patients with ischemic stroke that is not attributed to embolism from the heart.

d. Use aspirin or Aggrenox or clopidogrel to prevent recurrent stroke secondary to arterial diseases.

e. Carotid endarterectomy.

(1) Use carotid endarterectomy to prevent recurrent strokes following nondisabling strokes or transient ischemic attacks in selected patients with carotid artery stenosis greater than 70%.

(2) Effectiveness of this procedure has been demonstrated to reduce the risk of stroke in patients who have not had previous stroke warning signs but who have greater than 60% stenosis of the carotid artery.

(3) Effectiveness of carotid endarterectomy has not been demonstrated for lesser degrees of stenosis.

f. Use surgery to clip an intracranial aneurysm or resect an arteriovenous malformation.

PATIENT ASSESSMENT

1. Systematically evaluate the patient at key stages throughout acute care and rehabilitation.

a. A patient should be examined on admission to acute care and whenever questions arise concerning the person's condition.

b. In addition, assessments should be performed at the following times:

(1) When screening for rehabilitation.

(2) On admission to a rehabilitation program.

(3) During rehabilitation (to monitor progress).
(4) After discharge from rehabilitation and return to a community residence.
2. Use well-validated standardized measures.
  a. Use of standardized instruments is essential in evaluating stroke patients.
  b. Figure 8-3 describes the FIM (functional independence measure) in more detail.

FIM™ Instrument

LEVELS	7 Complete Independence (timely, safely) 6 Modified Independence (device)	NO HELPER
	Modified Dependence 5 Supervision (subject = 100%) 4 Minimal Assistance (subject = 75%+) 3 Moderate Assistance (subject = 50%+) **Complete Dependence** 2 Maximal Assistance (subject =25%+) 1 Total Assistance (subject = less than 25%)	HELPER

	ADMISSION	DISCHARGE	FOLLOW-UP
Self-Care A. Eating B. Grooming C. Bathing D. Dressing - Upper Body E. Dressing - Lower Body F. Toileting			
Sphincter Control G. Bladder Management H. Bowel Management			
Transfers I. Bed, Chair, Wheelchair J. Toilet K. Tub, Shower			
Locomotion L. Walk/Wheelchair M. Stairs		W Walk C Wheelchair B Both	W Walk C Wheelchair B Both
Motor Subtotal Rating			
Communication N. Comprehension O. Expression		A Auditory V Visual B Both	A Auditory V Visual B Both
Social Cognition P. Social Interaction Q. Problem Solving R. Memory			
Cognitive Subtotal Rating			
TOTAL FIM™ RATING			

NOTE: Leave no blanks. Enter 1 if patient is not testable due to risk.

Figure 8-3 Functional independence measure. Scoring is from 1 (total assistance) to 7 (full independence) for each functional measure. "Dependence" (1 or 2) and "Modified dependence" (3 to 5) both require a helper; no assistance is needed for a score of 6, but the patient uses adaptive equipment. (Copyright © 1997 Uniform Data System for Medical Rehabilitation [UDSMR], a division of UB Foundation Activities, Inc. [UBFA]. Reprinted with the permission of UDSMR. All marks associated with FIM are owned by UBFA.)

THE REHABILITATION REFERRAL

1. Screening.
   a. Screen the patient for formal rehabilitation during the acute hospitalization.
      (1) Screening for rehabilitation should be performed during the acute hospitalization, as soon as the patient's neurologic and medical conditions permit.
      (2) The purposes of this screening are as follows:
         (a) To identify patients who can benefit from a formal rehabilitation program or from individual rehabilitation services.
         (b) To guide selection of the appropriate rehabilitation program.
      (3) The types of information needed are listed in Box 8-2.
         (a) The patient's clinical status.
         (b) Information about the home environment.
         (c) Family circumstances.
         (d) Patient and family preferences regarding rehabilitation.
   b. The use of standardized instruments is recommended to document the extent of impairment and disabilities. These instruments can also be used to detect subtle cognitive problems, which may be missed in the clinical examination.
   c. The person performing the screening examination should be experienced in stroke rehabilitation and should have no direct financial interest in the referral decision.
   d. All screening information should be summarized in the medical record and provided to the rehabilitation setting at the time of referral.
2. Further rehabilitation.
   a. Recommendations.
      (1) Recommend whether the patient should receive further rehabilitation and whether this should consist of individual services or an interdisciplinary program.
      (2) The decision to recommend rehabilitation and whether the choice should be individual services or an interdisciplinary program is based on information obtained during the acute hospitalization and the rehabilitation screening examination.
   b. The most important patient considerations are as follows:
      (1) Medical stability.
      (2) Nature and extent of functional disabilities.
      (3) Ability to learn.
      (4) Physical activity endurance.
   c. Referral criteria for rehabilitation services are as follows:
      (1) Potential candidates for formal rehabilitation.
         (a) the patient has one or more significant disabilities.
         (b) The patient is at least moderately stable medically.
         (c) The patient is able to learn.
         (d) The patient has enough physical endurance to sit supported for 1 hour.
         (e) The patient can participate to at least some extent in active rehabilitation treatments.

BOX 8-2   Screening for Rehabilitation

Current Clinical Status

Comorbid diseases
Functional health patterns
- Ability to swallow
- Activity tolerance
- Bowel and bladder continence
- Nutrition and hydration
- Skin integrity
- Sleep patterns
Neurologic deficits

Special Emphases

Current functional deficits
Emotional status and motivation to participate in rehabilitation
Functional communication
Functional status before stroke
Mental status and ability to learn
Physical activity endurance

Social and Environmental Factors

Adjustment of patient and family to stroke
Characteristics of potential postdischarge environments
Ethnicity and native language
Extent of support by family or others (relationships, number, health, availability)
Measure of disability (ADL)
Mental status screening test
Patient and family preferences for and expectations of rehabilitation
Presence of spouse or significant other
Previous living situation
Standardized instruments
Stroke deficit scale

ADL, Activities of daily living.
Adapted from Gresham GE, Gresham Duncan PW, Stason WB, et al: *Post-stroke reha-bilitation. Clinical practice guideline No. 16.* AHCPR Pub. No. 95-0662. Rockville, Md, U.S. Department of Health and Human Services. Public Health Service, Agency for Health Care Policy and Research, May 1995.

    (2) Patients are candidates for an interdisciplinary rehabilitation program if they meet the criteria for formal rehabilitation and also have significant disabilities in at least two of the following areas of function:
        (a) Mobility.
        (b) Basic ADLs.
        (c) Bowel or bladder control.

(d) Cognition.

(e) Emotional functioning.

(f) Pain management.

(g) Swallowing.

(h) Communication.

(3) Patients with only a single area of disability are candidates for individual rehabilitation services but do not require an interdisciplinary program.

(4) Patients who are too impaired to participate in rehabilitation should receive appropriate supportive services, and their families should receive thorough education regarding care of the patient.

d. Some patients might not be recommended for rehabilitation initially. With time, however, these patients might recover sufficiently to become candidates for rehabilitation. Providers should be alert to such opportunities.

3. Program capabilities.

a. Overview.

(1) Be familiar with local rehabilitation programs and their capabilities.

(2) Rehabilitation programs should maintain and make available information on staffing patterns, services offered, and performance.

(3) Programs vary widely, and physicians and other medical personnel who refer patients for rehabilitation should be knowledgeable about the capabilities of programs in their community.

b. Basic rehabilitation settings are as follows:

(1) Hospital inpatient rehabilitation programs.

(a) Hospital inpatient rehabilitation programs may be located in freestanding rehabilitation hospitals or may be distinct units in acute care hospitals.

(b) These programs are staffed by the full range of rehabilitation professionals, and an interdisciplinary team provides a comprehensive rehabilitation program for each patient.

(c) Hospital inpatient rehabilitation is generally more intense than rehabilitation in other settings and requires greater physical and mental effort from the patient.

(2) Nursing facility rehabilitation programs.

(a) Rehabilitation programs in nursing facilities vary widely in the spectrum of services they provide.

(b) Hospital-based nursing facilities are located in or adjacent to acute care hospitals.

(c) Rehabilitation is designed primarily for patients who have the potential to improve enough during 2 to 3 weeks of treatment to become candidates for inpatient, home, or outpatient rehabilitation.

(d) Programs in community-based nursing facilities vary. Some are as comprehensive as hospital inpatient programs, although usually less intense, and others are very limited.

(3) Outpatient rehabilitation programs.

    (a) Outpatient rehabilitation programs are offered by hospital outpatient departments and freestanding outpatient facilities.

    (b) Outpatient programs can provide either a comprehensive rehabilitation program or individual rehabilitation services.

    (c) An advantage of outpatient programs is that they enable the patient to live at home while still having access to an interdisciplinary program and to rehabilitation equipment.

    (d) Opportunities are also available for the patient to make social contacts and obtain peer support.

    (e) Although typically more intense, day hospital programs are similar to outpatient programs.

    (f) The patient spends several hours, 3 to 5 days each week, in a typical day hospital program.

    (g) Availability of transportation is a prerequisite for both outpatient and day hospital programs.

(4) Home rehabilitation programs.

    (a) Home rehabilitation programs usually provide physical therapy, occupational therapy, and nursing services.

    (b) Some of these programs can also provide speech therapy and social work services.

    (c) Programs are expanding their capabilities, and some now provide comprehensive services, including home visits by physicians and intense rehabilitation.

    (d) Advantages.

        i. New skills are learned in the same environment where they will be applied.

        ii. Many patients function better in a familiar environment.

4. Criteria for choosing a program.

  a. Figure 8-4 shows the step-by-step process of arriving at rehabilitation recommendations on the basis of clinical and social and environmental factors.

  b. For patients who have been identified as candidates for interdisciplinary rehabilitation, the most important patient characteristics in choosing a program are as follows:

    (1) Medical stability.

    (2) Nature and extent of functional disabilities.

    (3) Physical activity endurance.

    (4) Need for assistance.

    (5) Extent of support by family or caregivers.

    (6) Patient and family wishes.

  c. The following are criteria for program choice:

    (1) Patients who meet threshold criteria for an interdisciplinary program and need moderate to total assistance with mobility or basic ADLs are candidates for an intense rehabilitation program, if they can tolerate 3 or more hours of physically demanding rehabilitation activity each day. Otherwise, a less intense program is usually more appropriate.

    (2) Patients who can benefit from intense rehabilitation but have complex medical problems should be treated in inpatient hospital

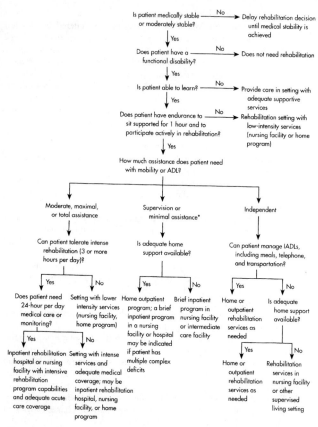

Figure 8-4 Selection of setting for rehabilitation program after hospitalization for acute stroke.* Under special circumstances, inpatient programs may be appropriate for some patients with multiple complex functional deficits. ADL, activities of daily living; IADL, instrumental activities of daily living. (From Gresham GE, Gresham Duncan PW, Stason WB, et al: *Post-stroke rehabilitation. Clinical practice guideline No. 16.* AHCPR Pub. No. 95-0662. Rockville, Md, U.S. Department of Health and Human Services. Public Health Service, Agency for Health Care Policy and Research, May 1995.)

programs that have 24-hour coverage by physicians and nurses skilled in acute medical care and rehabilitation.

(3) Patients who need only supervision or minimal assistance can usually be managed in home or outpatient rehabilitation programs if the home environment and support are adequate. If not, a nursing facility program should be considered.

5. Consensus with patient and family.
   a. To succeed, rehabilitation must have the full support and active participation of the patient and family.
   b. Rehabilitation decisions need to be agreed on by the patient, family, treating physician, and accepting rehabilitation program to the maximum extent possible.
   c. To this end, health care providers should carry out the following recommendations:
      (1) Explain clearly the reasons for the recommendations concerning rehabilitation.
      (2) Listen carefully to any concerns of the patient or family that might dictate a different choice.
      (3) Point out the possibility of transfer to a different program in the future (if the patient's condition changes).

SUGGESTED READING

Duncan PW, Zorowitz R, Bates B, et al: Management of adult stroke rehabilitation care: A clinical practice guideline. *Stroke* 36(9):3100-e143, 2005. Available at http://stroke.ahajournals.org/cgi/content/full/36/9/e100 (accessed March 1, 2007).

8.3 Geriatric Rehabilitation Following Hip Fracture

Fred F. Ferri

1. Good postoperative care begins preoperatively. A functional assessment involving physical, cognitive, and psychosocial aspects (in addition to a system-oriented medical assessment) should be performed preoperatively on all geriatric patients.
2. Elderly persons are particularly susceptible to the adverse effects of medications.
   a. Preoperative medications should be closely reviewed and unnecessary drugs should be discontinued.
   b. Serum levels of selected drugs (e.g., digoxin, theophylline) should be measured preoperatively and frequently monitored postoperatively.
   c. Codeine should be avoided for pain control (increased constipation and confusion). Acetaminophen 650 mg q4h around the clock is preferred.
   d. Use of nonsteroidal antiinflammatory drugs (NSAIDs) can result in gastrointestinal bleeding, delirium, and renal failure.
   e. Use of sedatives can cause delirium, urinary retention, and pulmonary or cardiac abnormalities.
   f. Immediate resumption of antihypertensives postoperatively can result in hypotension.
   g. Sudden discontinuation of antianginal medications (e.g., β-blockers) can result in unstable angina and myocardial infarction.
   h. Sulfonylureas must be temporarily discontinued. Glucose should be monitored every 6 hours and hyperglycemia should be treated with regular insulin in the immediate preoperative and postoperative period.

i. Patients receiving long-term steroids are at risk for developing relative hypoadrenalism if steroid doses are not augmented.

j. Antiseizure medications should be continued and the levels frequently monitored to avoid postoperative seizures or toxicity.

k. Antiparkinsonian drugs should be reinstituted as soon as possible postoperatively to prevent significant bradykinesia.

l. Vigorous bronchodilator therapy and monitoring of arterial blood gases should be initiated preoperatively and postoperatively in all patients with asthma or chronic obstructive pulmonary disease.

3. The following medical complications should be rapidly identified and treated:

   a. Anemia.

   (1) Hematocrit should be monitored daily in the immediate postoperative period.

   (2) Transfusion is indicated only if there is significant blood loss and the patient is symptomatic.

   (3) Patients with compromised cardiovascular status should receive a small dose of furosemide between units of blood to prevent fluid overload.

   (4) If oral iron replacement is started, a laxative should be added to minimize its constipating effect.

   b. Urinary tract infections.

   (1) Prolonged catheterization should be avoided.

   (2) Intermittent postoperative catheterization is preferred if urinary retention develops.

   (3) In the elderly, urinary tract infections might have nonspecific symptoms such as delirium.

   (4) Suspicion of incontinence should be investigated and situational factors (e.g., difficulty in gaining access to the toilet, slow staff response time to the patient's request to urinate) should be eliminated before labeling the patient incontinent.

   c. Constipation.

   (1) Constipation is usually multifactorial (inactivity, poor fluid intake, opiates).

   (2) Scrupulous bowel care must be instituted preoperatively with enemas, bulking agents, lactulose, glycerin suppositories, and other agents.

   (3) Fecal impaction can result in urinary retention and spurious diarrhea (caused by intermittent bowel blockage with leakage of feces).

   (4) Digital examination should be done in any cases of suspected constipation.

   (5) Manual disimpaction may be required in severe cases of obstipation.

   d. Pressure ulcers (see Chapter 4, section 8).

   (1) Skin care must be carefully addressed.

   (2) Unnecessary pressure on heels and sacrum should be avoided.

   (3) Frequent repositioning and avoidance of incontinence are necessary to prevent decubitus ulcers.

   (4) Early postoperative mobilization is critical.

e. Venous thromboembolism: Adequate prophylaxis of DVT in patients undergoing hip surgery involves external pneumatic compression of lower extremities (intermittent pneumatic compression boots) plus low-dose warfarin started 1 to 2 days before surgery.

f. Fluid and electrolyte imbalance.

(1) Hypovolemia, congestive heart failure, and electrolyte abnormalities are very common in the postoperative period and can significantly alter cognitive function.

(2) Daily monitoring of electrolytes and renal function is recommended in the early postoperative period.

4. Physical therapy varies with the postoperative period.

a. Initially, only isometric exercises of the involved hip should be allowed.

b. This is followed by gradual mobilization, ambulatory exercises 1 to 10 days postoperatively, and stair climbing after 10 to 12 days.

c. A sample of post–hip fracture gait training is described in Table 8-2.

5. Functional outcome varies with the presence of comorbid illness, social support, and type of surgery performed.

a. Functional outcome is generally better with prosthetic hip replacement than nail-and-plate or pin-and-plate fixation.

Table 8-2 Sample Post–Hip Fracture Gait Training

Fracture Type	Fixation Type	Gait-Training Program
Stable intertrochanteric or subtrochanteric	Nail plate or medullary nail	Progressive weight bearing within first postoperative week initially PWB in standing Then WBAT during ambulation
Femoral neck	Multiple pins	From day 1: OOB in wheelchair Day 5-7: Begin standing, ambulation with walker, WBAT Continue walker until healed Cane later
	Screw plate, pin and plate combination, or compression screw	From day 1: OOB in wheelchair From day 3-4: Begin bedside standing, then ambulation with walker, WBAT From week 6-12: FWB with walker

FWB, full weight bearing allowed on affected limb during ambulation; OOB, out of bed; PWB, some (partial) weight bearing on affected limb allowed during standing or ambulation; WBAT, weight bearing allowed to tolerance of patient (usually limited by pain), may be partial or full.

Modified from Sisk DT: Fractures of the hip and pelvis. In Crenshaw AH (ed): *Campbell's Operative Orthopedics*. St Louis, Mosby, 1992.

b. Poor recovery is associated with older age, rehospitalization, longer hospital stays, presence of depressive symptoms, and cognitive deficits (acute or chronic).

c. Greater contact with a social network following discharge enhances the probability of a good recovery.

d. Most recovery occurs within the first 6 months.

Socioeconomic and Legal Issues

Marsha D. Fretwell
Deborah Adams Wingate

9.1 Competence for Self-Care and Informed Consent

1. The issue of competency arises most often in two specific situations in the care of frail older patients.
   a. It may be raised by family members or neighbors if there is a concern about a person's capacity for self-care and making appropriate social and financial decisions.
   b. It may be raised by the physician or another health care provider during an acute illness when informed consent for a treatment or procedure must be obtained.
2. In both cases, there is the assumption that at an earlier time, the older individual was able to care for himself or herself and/or make rational decisions about medical treatment.

COMPONENTS OF INFORMED CONSENT

1. The patient must have the capacity to make the decision.
2. The medical provider must disclose information on the treatment or procedure, including expected risks and benefits and the likelihood the risks and benefits will occur.
3. The patient must comprehend the information.
4. The patient must voluntarily grant consent.

EVALUATION OF COMPETENCE FOR SELF-CARE AND INFORMED CONSENT

Step 1

What cognitive, emotional, or perceptive impairments underlie this change in capacity for self-care and/or medical decision making?

1. Evaluation of competence in older persons should begin with an in-depth exploration of perceptive, cognitive, and emotional functions fundamental to the ability to make appropriate decisions.
2. Consultation with a psychiatrist, neurologist, or psychologist is helpful if difficulties or inconsistencies are found in the evaluation of cognitive function.
3. Cognitive functions that underlie competency (Fig. 9-1).
   a. Attention.
      (1) Ask the patient to perform tasks such as counting down from 10 to 1 or listing the days of the week backward.

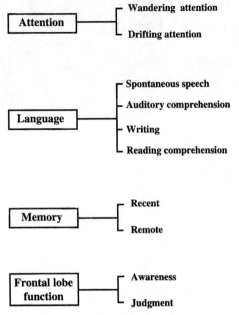

Figure 9-1   Cognitive functions underlying competency. (From Freedman M, Stuss DT, Gordon M: *Ann Intern Med* 115:203-207, 1991.)

(2) If the patient is unable to complete these tasks, evaluate for metabolic disorders, adverse drug reactions, or any other causes of acute confusional states or delirium (see Chapter 4).

(3) The patient who cannot sustain adequate attention to take in or retain instructions and questions will not be able to complete further elements of cognitive testing and, for the moment, must be considered incompetent.

(4) Because most causes of isolated attention deficits are reversible, the incompetency should not be labeled permanent. After appropriate medical interventions, the patient's attention span should be frequently reevaluated.

b. Language.

(1) Disorders in language function (aphasia) are seen in patients with:

(a) Alzheimer's disease.

(b) Cerebrovascular accidents.

(c) Severe head injury.

(2) Patients who are deaf, blind, or intubated have significant difficulty in communication.

(3) When barriers to effective communication exist, physicians and families must make a concerted effort to overcome them before declaring a patient incompetent.

c. Memory.
   (1) Loss of short-term memory is the most common impairment of cognition seen in older patients.
   (2) Depression must be ruled out as a cause of memory disorder.
   (3) If the attention span is intact, a deficit in short-term memory will not necessarily impair the ability to read and understand a consent form for medical or surgical treatment.
   (4) A consistent response to the consent process on two separate occasions implies competency; an inconsistent response implies incompetency.
d. Frontal lobe dysfunction.
   (1) Frontal lobe dysfunctions are seen in:
       (a) Alzheimer's disease.
       (b) Cerebrovascular accidents.
       (c) Chronic alcoholism.
       (d) Parkinson's disease.
       (e) Frontal lobe dementia.
   (2) The patient might have knowledge of appropriate facts but be unable to evaluate the impact of the facts or to respond appropriately.
   (3) Frontal lobe assessment should include information and observations from both the patient and significant others.

Step 2

1. Maximize the patient's residual capacity to make decisions by addressing the treatable causes underlying the change in capacity.
2. Except in an emergency, no statement about incompetency should be made until this process is completed.

Step 3

Examine for competency in each area of decision making.
1. Areas of decision making.
   a. Place of residence.
   b. Choice of guardian or caretaker.
   c. Financial affairs.
   d. Informed consent in medical treatments.
2. Overlap in areas of decision making.
   a. A person who is incompetent to manage financial affairs may be capable of making informed decisions about medical treatments.
   b. A person incapable of making a decision about medical treatment may be competent to choose the place of residence and caretakers.
3. When a person is declared incompetent, it should always be in the least restrictive manner and linked to a specific situation of decision making.

Step 4

Legally, a person can only be declared "incompetent" by a court of law.

SUGGESTED READINGS

Adelman RD, Breckman R: Mistreatment. In Abrams WB, Berkow R (eds): *The Merck Manual of Geriatrics*. Rahway, NJ, Merck Sharp & Dohme, 1990.

Freedman M, Stuss DT, Gordon M: Assessment of competency: The role of neurobehavioral deficits. *Ann Intern Med* 115:203-208, 1991.

9.2 Patient Self-Determination Act, Health Care Proxy, Living Will, and Physician Orders for Scope of Treatment

PATIENT SELF-DETERMINATION ACT

In December 1991 the Patient Self-Determination Act was implemented in all institutions reimbursed by Medicare, Medicaid, or both. This law was designed to increase patient involvement in decisions regarding life-sustaining treatment. Its purpose is to help implement a right that has been universally recognized: the right to refuse any and all medical interventions, even life-sustaining interventions. The act requires health care providers in hospitals, skilled nursing facilities, home care agencies, hospice programs, and health maintenance organizations (HMOs) to:

1. Develop written policies concerning advance directives.
2. Ask all new patients whether they have prepared an advance directive and include this information in the patient's chart.
3. Give patients written materials regarding the facility's policies on advance directives and the patient's right to prepare such documents.
4. Educate staff and the community about advance directives.

HEALTH CARE DIRECTIVES

Before the Patient Self-Determination Act, the use of advance health care directives by patients was limited. Advance health care directives are legally binding documents that allow currently competent patients to document what medical treatments they would want if they become incompetent in the future. Two types of advance directives are currently in use: the living will and the health care proxy or durable power of attorney.

1. The living will.
   a. The living will is defined by statutes in about three quarters of the states.
   b. Statutes vary from state to state but usually allow a terminally ill person to have life-sustaining treatments withheld or withdrawn should the patient be unable to direct the physician to do so.
   c. Some states have statutes providing immunity to health care providers who execute the living will.
2. The health care proxy or durable power of attorney.
   a. The health care proxy or durable power of attorney for health care is a written document (see Appendix III) that allows the patient to designate a person to act on the patient's behalf if, in the future, the patient is unable to speak or act.
   b. It is based in the ethical principle of substituted judgment, which assumes that other persons (the proxy) can make decisions that approximate the patient's values.
   c. It is referred to as *durable* because it is not invalidated (as is the traditional power of attorney) when the individual becomes incompetent.
   d. Currently, not all states specifically authorize the durable power of attorney for health care.
   e. With the impetus of the Self-Determination Act, it is likely that supporting statutes will soon follow.

3. Physician orders for scope of treatment (POST).*
   a. The POST form is primarily intended for patients in health care facilities: Nursing homes, extended care facilities, and acute care hospitals.
   b. POST is designed to help health care providers establish the end-of-life treatment wishes of patients.
   c. POST translates a patient's wish into physician orders that are portable from one care setting to another.
   d. POST includes cardiopulmonary resuscitation.
      (1) Code or no code status.
      (2) Level of intervention (comfort care, intermediate, or full treatment).
      (3) Use or withholding of antibiotics and feeding tubes.

STEPS IN SECURING ADVANCE DIRECTIVES

1. Clarify what type of advance directive meets the legal requirements of the state.
2. Initiate the conversation with patients before the onset of acute illnesses and/or cognitive impairments.
3. Include the children and the spouse of the older patient in the discussion.
4. Secure a copy of advance directive for the patient's chart.
5. Instruct the patient to carry a copy of the directive.

SUGGESTED READINGS

Annas GJ: The health care proxy and the living will. *N Engl J Med* 324:1210-1213, 1991.

Greco PJ, Schulman KA, Lavizzo-Mourey R, Hansen-Flaschen J: The Patient Self-Determination Act and the future of advance directives. *Ann Intern Med* 115:639-643, 1991.

Hickman SE, Tolle SW, Brummel-Smith K, Carley MM: Use of the Physicians Orders for Life-Sustaining Treatment program in Oregon nursing facilities: Beyond resuscitation status. *J Am Geriatr Soc* 52:1424-1429, 2004.

9.3 Elder Abuse

1. Epidemiology.
   a. Each year, approximately 500,000 persons older than 60 years experience abuse or neglect.
   b. Of these, 21% are reported and substantiated by adult protective services.
2. Types of abuse or neglect (Box 9-1).
   a. Neglect (48.7%).
   b. Emotional/psychological (35.5%).
   c. Financial/material exploitation (30.2%).
   d. Physical (25.6%).
   e. Abandonment (3.6%).
3. Risk factors for abuse: Although any older person may become a victim of abuse, certain characteristics or attributes appear to be associated with an increased risk (see Box 9-1).
4. Characteristics of abusers.
   a. Approximately 50% of abuse is committed by an adult child of the victim who is living in the same home and is usually financially dependent on the victim.
   b. About 20% of abuse is committed by one spouse against another.

---

*A sample copy of the POST form is available at http://www.hsc.wvu.edu/chel/wvi/POST%20Information/POST%20Form%202006%20Sample.pdf

BOX 9-1 **Characteristics of Abuse Victims**

The frail elderly
Female
White
Severe cognitive and/or physical impairment
Dependent on caretaker for most daily care needs
Exhibits problematic behavior: incontinence, shouting, paranoia
Socially isolated
Stress of caretaker

From Bosker G, Schwartz GR, Jones JS, et al (eds): *Geriatric Emergency Medicine.* St Louis, Mosby, 1990, p 534.

  c. About 9% of abuse is committed by other relatives; 8.6% were grandchildren.
  d. Abuse occurs at all economic levels, in all age groups, and to men as well as women.
5. Assessment and treatment.
  a. Abuse is most often the result of interacting medical, psychological, and social problems in both victim and abuser.
  b. Abuse requires a comprehensive and functional orientation to diagnosis and treatment.
    (1) Have a low threshold for suspecting abuse, particularly when there is unexplained physical trauma or unexplained loss of physical, cognitive, and emotional function.
    (2) Create an opportunity to interview the patient in the presence of the caretaker.
    (3) Complete a comprehensive geriatric assessment (see Chapter 2). Consider physical and psychological neglect or abuse as a potential etiologic factor underlying problems or changes in each area of concern.
    (4) Diagnosis.
      (a) Falls, fractures.
      (b) Absence of eyeglasses, hearing aids, dentures, prosthesis.
      (c) Signs of physical restraints.
      (d) Genital infections.
      (e) Decubitus ulcers, skin lesions, or infections.
    (5) Medications: Evidence of noncompliance or misuse of medications (overdosing or underdosing).
    (6) Nutrition.
      (a) Evidence of malnutrition or dehydration.
      (b) Unexplained weight loss or gain.
      (c) Increased alcohol intake.
      (d) Loss of appetite.
    (7) Continence: Unexplained urinary incontinence.
    (8) Defecation: Unexplained fecal incontinence or impaction.
    (9) Cognition.
      (a) Unexplained confusion.
      (b) New onset of disruptive behavior.

(10) Emotion.
    (a) Unexplained insomnia or hypersomnia.
    (b) Anxiety.
    (c) Agitation.
    (d) Paranoia.
    (e) Depression.
(11) Mobility: Unexplained change in social patterns and ambulatory activities out of the home.
(12) Cooperation with care plan: Unexplained or new onset of lack of cooperation with care plan.

c. Establish competency of the victim, inform a protective service agency, and decide whether emergency intervention is needed. Need for emergency intervention is indicated by:
    (1) Urgent need for medical or psychiatric care.
    (2) Life-threatening or permanently damaging abuse.
    (3) Impairment of the abuser to the degree that he or she is unable to care for the victim.

d. Reduce stresses in the care-taking situation.
    (1) Treat all reversible medical disorders.
    (2) Minimize or simplify medications.
    (3) Reverse such functional impairments as urinary and fecal incontinence, immobility, confusion, and anxiety, depression, and paranoia.
    (4) Secure outside agencies to provide respite for housekeeping, personal care, or transportation needs.
    (5) Assist abusing caretaker in seeking appropriate medical or psychological support.

e. If the problem is likely to be ongoing and the victim is not competent, contact a protective services agency for consideration of guardianship and a change in the living situation.

f. A recent study of geriatric assessment for victims of elder mistreatment reveals the following types of interventions:
    (1) Home care services: 46.4%.
    (2) Institutional placement: 35.4%.
    (3) Guardianship: 35.4%.
    (4) Urgent medication initiated: 25.8%.
    (5) Acute medical hospitalization: 19.6%.

SUGGESTED READING

Adelman RD, Breckman R: Mistreatment. In Abrams WB, Berkow R (eds): *The Merck Manual of Geriatrics*. Rahway, NJ, Merck Sharp & Dohme, 1990.

9.4 Financing of Health Care

MEDICARE

1. Medicare is the U.S. government's health insurance.
2. It is available to all Americans aged 65 years and older who are eligible for Social Security and to younger people who receive Social Security disability benefits.
3. It is funded by a federal tax on income that is paid partly by the employee and partly by the employer.

4. Medicare benefits (Tables 9-1 to 9-3).
    a. Part A: Hospital and skilled nursing care benefits.
    b. Part B: Physician and additional services.
    c. Part C: Managed care demonstration project.
    d. Part D: Medication benefits.

MEDIGAP

1. Medigap, or Medicare supplement insurance, covers some of the health care costs not paid by Medicare.
2. Medigap policies are purchased out of pocket and offer a variety of benefits.
3. In 1992, the National Association of Insurance Commissioners created 10 standardized packages of coverage, designated by the letters A through J (Table 9-4).

MEDICARE PRESCRIPTION DRUG AND MODERNIZATION ACT

1. Basic drug benefit.
    a. Medicare beneficiaries sign up for a drug plan or join a private health plan (Medicare managed care/HMO plan) that offers drug coverage.
    b. There is a gap in coverage after $2250 in total drug costs.
    c. Medicare (the drug insurance plan) pays nothing more until the beneficiary has paid $3600 out of pocket.
2. Low-income assistance.
    a. Medicare beneficiaries with annual incomes less than 135% of the federal poverty level ($12,123 for an individual or $16,362 for a couple) and assets less than $6000 (individual) or $9000 (couple) are eligible for additional assistance.
    b. No premium payment.
    c. No deductible.
    d. No gap in coverage.
3. Increase in Part B deductible and premium.
    a. Part B deductible will increase annually by the same percentages as the Part B premium increases.
    a. For beneficiaries earning more than $80,000.00 a year, the percentage of the subsidy paid by Medicare (usually 70% of the premium cost) will be reduced.
4. Medicare Advantage and Comparative Cost Adjustment (CCA) program.
    a. Medicare Advantage program will replace Medicare+ Choice currently offered under Medicare Part C.
    b. The Comparative Cost Adjustment program will examine the efficiency of private managed care plans (Medicare Advantage) versus traditional (fee-for-service) Medicare.
5. Cost Containment.
    a. Any time general revenue funding (i.e., taxes) of Medicare exceeds 45%, the President and Congress are required to respond.
    b. This might result in a higher out-of-pocket expenditure for beneficiaries.
6. Expansion of Medicare benefits.
    a. Initial physical examination.
    b. Cardiovascular screening blood test.

Table 9-1 **Medicare Part A**		
Type of Care	**Covered Services**	**Patient Pays**
Hospital stay	Semi-private room, meals General nursing and other hospital services and supplies Not television, telephone, private duty nurse, or private room	For each benefit period: Total of $912 for 1-60 days $228 per day for days 61-90 $456 per day for days 91-150 All costs for each day beyond 150 days
Skilled nursing facility	Semiprivate room, meals Skilled nursing and rehabilitative services and other services and supplies	For each benefit period: Nothing for the first 20 days Up to $114 per day for days 21-100 All costs beyond the 100th day in the benefit period
Home health care	Intermittent skilled nursing care, physical therapy, occupational therapy, home health aide services Speech and language pathology services Durable medical equipment (such as wheelchairs, hospital beds, oxygen, and walkers) and supplies and other services.	Nothing for home health care services 20% of approved amount for durable medical equipment
Hospice care	Pain and symptom relief and supportive services for the care of a terminal illness Home care is provided Necessary inpatient care and a variety of services otherwise not covered by Medicare	Limited costs for outpatient drugs and inpatient respite care
Blood	From a hospital or skilled nursing facility during a covered stay	For the first 3 pints

Table 9-2 Medicare Part B

Type of Care	Covered Services	Patient Pays
Medical expenses	Doctors' services, inpatient and outpatient medical and surgical services and supplies Physical, occupational, and speech therapy Diagnostic tests Durable medical equipment	$110 deductible (once per year) 20% of approved amount after the deductible, except in the outpatient setting 50% for most outpatient mental health 20% for all outpatient physical, occupational, and speech and language services.
Clinical laboratory	Blood tests, urinalysis, and more	Nothing for services
Home health care	Intermittent skilled care, home health aide services Durable medical equipment (such as wheelchairs, hospital beds, oxygen, and walkers) and supplies and other services.	Nothing for services 20% of approved amount for durable medical equipment
Outpatient hospital services	Services for the diagnosis or treatment of an illness or injury	A coinsurance or fixed copayment amount, which can vary according to service
Blood	As an outpatient, or as part of a Part B covered service	For the first 3 pints plus 20% of approved amount for additional pints (after the deductible)

    c. Diabetes screening test.
    d. Screening and diagnostic mammography.
    e. Intravenous γ-globulin.
  7. Employer subsidy.
    a. The employer subsidy is an $88 billion dollar subsidy to encourage them not to drop existing retiree drug plans.
    b. It is anticipated that many employers will drop the drug plans for retirees.
  8. Health savings accounts.

Table 9-3 Medicare Part D Prescription Drug Benefit

Yearly Cost of Drugs ($)	Amount Paid by Recipient ($)	Amount Paid By Medicare ($)
250	250	0
500	313	186
1000	438	563
1500	563	938
2000	688	1313
2500	1000	1500
3000	1500	1500
4000	2500	1500
5000	3500	1500
7500	3720	3780
10,000	3845	6155
15,000	4095	10,905

    a. Health savings accounts (HSA) provide tax incentives for wealthier people to make tax-free contributions to an HSA if they have high-deductible medical insurance.

    b. Lost tax revenues are estimated at $6.4 billion between 2004 and 2013.

9. Subsidies for insurance companies and HMOs: Subsidies will be provided for insurance companies and HMOs to establish the Medicare Advantage programs.

10. Concessions to Drug Companies: No cost-containment provisions.

Table 9-4 Medigap Comparison

Medigap Benefit	A	B	C	D	E	F	G	H	I	J
Medicare A and B coinsurance	✓	✓	✓	✓	✓	✓	✓	✓	✓	✓
365 days extra hospital stay	✓	✓	✓	✓	✓	✓	✓	✓	✓	✓
3 pints blood	✓	✓	✓	✓	✓	✓	✓	✓	✓	✓
Part A deductible		✓	✓	✓	✓	✓	✓	✓	✓	✓
Foreign travel emergency			✓	✓	✓	✓	✓	✓	✓	✓
Skilled nursing coinsurance			✓	✓	✓	✓	✓	✓	✓	✓
Medicare Part B deductible			✓			✓				✓
Medicare Part B excess						✓	✓		✓	✓
At-home recovery			✓				✓		✓	✓
Preventive care					✓					✓
Prescription drug benefit								✓	✓	✓

MEDICAID

1. Medicaid is a program that helps pay medical bills for very low income patients of any age.
2. Eligibility requirements vary from state to state but can be established by contacting the Social Security Office or Office of Social Services.
3. Services required by the federal government.
   a. Inpatient and outpatient hospital care.
   b. Services of physicians.
   c. Laboratory services.
   d. Skilled nursing facilities for adults.
4. Services covered by states.
   a. As of 1992, states pay Medicare premiums, deductibles, and copayments for beneficiaries whose incomes are at or below 100% of the federal poverty level.
   b. States have the option to cover prescribed drugs, care in an intermediate care facility, physical therapy, and dental care.
5. Drug coverage: Under The Medicare Prescription Drug and Modernization Act, Medicaid beneficiaries now receive drug coverage under Medicare Part D.
6. Medicaid is the major public payer for long-term care.
   a. Medicaid contributes close to 41% of the dollars spent for nursing home care.
   b. As more people live to old age, Medicaid has become the de facto long-term care insurance for both the poor and the elderly.
   c. Some patients divest their assets to qualify for Medicaid when they enter a nursing home.
   d. Some patients enter nursing homes as private patients but spend their savings down and thus qualify for Medicaid reimbursement for such services.

VETERANS ADMINISTRATION

1. In the Veterans Administration (VA) system, health care services are provided without charge on a space-available basis, with priority going to veterans with service-connected disabilities.
2. Free from the restrictions of the Medicare fee-for-service structure of reimbursement, the VA has launched several innovative geriatric programs.
   a. Geriatric assessment units.
   b. Interdisciplinary research and education centers.
   c. Hospital-based home health care programs.
3. All of these programs focus on continuity of services for older patients.

SUGGESTED READING

The Medicare Prescription Drug and Modernization Act: The Good, the Bad, the Ugly Overview. Available at www.medicare.gov.

Alcohol Use Disorders in Older Adults

10

Marsha D. Fretwell
Deborah Adams Wingate

10.1 Definition

1. Alcoholism is a chronic disease, with genetic, psychosocial, and environmental factors influencing its development and manifestations.
2. Characteristics.
   a. Impaired control over drinking.
   b. Preoccupation with the drug alcohol.
   c. Use of alcohol despite adverse consequences.
   d. Distortions in thinking, most notably denial.
3. In the elderly, the onset or continuation of drinking can become problematic because of physiologic and psychosocial changes that occur with aging, including increased sensitivity to the effects of alcohol.

10.2 Epidemiology

1. About 50% of persons older than 65 years drink daily.
2. Estimated prevalence of alcohol abuse in community-dwelling elderly persons is 3% to 4%.
3. Prevalence in hospitalized elderly persons is considerably higher, estimated at 20%.
4. The rate of alcohol abuse is four times higher for elderly men than for elderly women. Some studies show that alcohol abuse in elderly women (compared to elderly men) is less likely to be detected by physicians.
5. An estimated 5% to 10% of cases of dementia are related to alcohol abuse.
6. About 15% of older adults may be experiencing health risks due to alcohol.
7. An estimated one third of persons in Alcoholics Anonymous are older than 50 years.

10.3 Diagnostic Approach

SCREENING RECOMMENDATIONS

All patients 65 years and older should be screened annually, especially patients with the following risk factors:
1. Emotional and social problems.
   a. Bereavement.
   b. Losses.
   c. Retirement.
   d. Social isolation.
   e. Boredom.

2. Medical problems.
   a. Pain.
   b. Vision and hearing loss.
   c. Disability.
   d. Insomnia.
   e. Memory loss.
   f. Depression and anxiety.
3. History: Past personal or family history of an alcohol use disorder.

RATIONALE
1. Age-related physiologic changes that affect risks associated with alcohol.
   a. Higher blood alcohol levels for the amount consumed.
      (1) Decreased gastric alcohol dehydrogenates.
      (2) Lower volume of distribution (less muscle mass).
   b. Increased central nervous system sensitivity to alcohol.
2. Medications that can interact with alcohol.
   a. About 90% of older adults use medication.
   b. Up to 100% of medications can interact adversely with alcohol.
   c. Examples of medication interactions with alcohol.
      (1) Increased blood alcohol levels.
         (a) Acetylsalicylic acid (ASA; aspirin).
         (b) H_2 blockers.
      (2) Increased sedation and impaired motor function.
         (a) Antihistamines.
         (b) Barbiturates.
         (c) Benzodiazepines.
         (d) Narcotics.
         (e) Tricyclic antidepressants.
      (3) Increased bleeding time.
         (a) Aspirin.
         (b) Nonsteroidal antiinflammatory drugs (NSAIDs).
      (4) Increased gastric inflammation and bleeding.
         (a) Aspirin.
         (b) NSAIDs.
      (5) Disulfiram response, with nausea and vomiting.
         (a) Metronidazole.
         (b) Sulfonamides.
      (6) Hypotension.
         (a) Hydralazine.
         (b) Methyldopa.
         (c) Nitroglycerin.
         (d) Reserpine.
      (7) Hepatic toxicity: Acetaminophen.
      (8) Exacerbation of the underlying disease: Drugs for:
         (a) Diabetes.
         (b) Gout.
         (c) Heart failure.
         (d) Hypertension.
         (e) Ulcers.

    (9) Altered drug metabolism.
       (a) Benzodiazepines.
       (b) Isoniazid.
       (c) Narcotics.
       (d) Propranolol.
       (e) Warfarin.
3. Chronic conditions that may be triggered or worsened by alcohol use in 30% of older adults.
   a. Cirrhosis, gastrointestinal bleeding, ulcers, and gastroesophageal reflux disease.
   b. Gout.
   c. Hypertension.
   d. Diabetes mellitus.
   e. Depression, anxiety, or other mental conditions.

SCREENING

1. CAGE questions:
   a. Have you ever felt you should Cut down on your drinking?
   b. Have people ever Annoyed you by criticizing your drinking?
   c. Have you ever felt Guilty about your drinking?
   d. Have you ever had a drink (Eye opener) in the morning to get rid of a hangover?
2. Classification of drinking behavior.
   a. Low risk.
      (1) No more than 1 drink per day and a maximum of 2 drinks on any drinking occasion.
      (2) CAGE score of 0.
      (3) No evidence of physical, social, or psychological dysfunction related to alcohol.
      (4) No medical conditions that alcohol could trigger or worsen.
   b. High risk.
      (1) On average, more than 1 drink or day or more than 7 drinks per week on heavier drinking occasions.
      (2) Any amount of drinking and CAGE score other than 0.
      (3) Evidence of physical, social, or psychological dysfunction related to alcohol.
      (4) Use of alcohol and medication in combinations that can interact adversely.
      (5) Use of alcohol and having conditions that can be triggered or worsened by alcohol.

GENERAL MEDICAL HISTORY

Clues from the general medical history can signal the presence of alcoholism.
1. Memory loss.
2. Symptoms of depression or anxiety.
3. Neglect of hygiene or appearance.
4. Poor appetite, nutritional deficits.
5. Sleep disruption.
6. Hypertension and resistance to therapy.
7. Blood sugar control problems.

8. Seizures.
9. Impaired balance and gait, frequent falls and bruises.
10. Recurrent gastritis and esophagitis.
11. Difficulty managing warfarin dosing.
12. Incontinence.
13. Change in behavior or social isolation.
14. Prescription drug abuse.
15. Evidence of drug and alcohol interactions.

PHYSICAL EXAMINATION

The physical exam should include a search for signs of alcohol abuse such as systolic hypertension, evidence of trauma, evidence of chronic liver disease, gastrointestinal bleeding, peripheral neuropathy, or cardiomyopathy.

1. General.
   a. Routine evaluation for pulse and blood pressure.
   b. Examination of skin for bruises.
   c. Actual observation of gait, mobility, and balance as the patient enters the room and gets in and out of a chair.
   d. Actual observation of the patient performing the basic or instrumental activities of daily living.
2. Head, ears, eyes, nose, and throat.
   a. Evaluation for evidence of recent trauma or fall.
   b. Carotid bruits.
   c. Intraoral dryness.
3. Upper body.
   a. Full range of motion of the arms.
   b. Routine cardiopulmonary, carotid, and peripheral vascular evaluation.
   c. Routine abdominal examination for hepatomegaly and ascites.
   d. Rectal examination for gastrointestinal bleeding.
4. Neurologic.
   a. The Mini Mental State Exam.
      (1) Orientation, registration, short-term memory, attention, and language.
      (2) Clock drawing.
      (3) Fast animal naming (average normal is naming 33 in one minute).
   b. Any focal changes in muscle strength and reflexes.
   c. Balance.
   d. Vibratory sensation and light touch sensation.

LABORATORY TESTS

1. Blood alcohol level.
2. Tests for hepatocellular injury. The most sensitive tests are γ-glutamyl transpeptidase (GGTP) and aspartate aminotranferase (AST).
3. Anemia (often multifactorial and macrocytic) and thrombocytopenia.
4. Electrolytes.
5. Blood sugar levels.
6. Albumin.
7. Prothrombin time, international normalized ratio.

10.4 Treatment

1. Treat coexisting condition such as depression, anxiety, dementia, metabolic, or nutritional problems.
2. Overcome patient denial.
   a. Report findings to the patient.
      (1) State the data, conclusions, and opinion clearly but nonjudgmentally.
      (2) Explain how alcohol is affecting the patient's health, interpersonal relationships, and family.
   b. Identify the patient's needs.
      (1) Sleep disorder.
      (2) Mood disorder.
      (3) Energy depletion.
   c. Provide empathic discussion.
   d. Initiate direct advice.
   e. Enlist support of family members.
3. Drug therapy.
   a. Naltrexone 25 mg × 2 days, then 50 mg daily.
   b. Monitor liver enzymes.
   c. Contraindicated in renal failure.
4. Plan for long-term treatment.
   a. Residential.
   b. Outpatient.
   c. Self-help for the patient (e.g., Alcoholics Anonymous).
   d. Self-help for the patient's family (e.g., Al-Anon).

10.5 Resources

1. Alcoholics Anonymous.
   a. Listed in local telephone directories.
   b. http://www.alcoholics-anonymous.org/.
2. National Association of State Alcohol and Drug Abuse Directors.
   a. 202–783–6868.
   b. http://www.nasadad.org/.
3. National Association of Addiction Treatment Providers.
   a. 202–371–6731.
   b. http://www.naatp.org/index.php.

SUGGESTED READINGS

American Geriatrics Society: AGS position paper: Alcohol use disorders in older adults. AGS Clinical Practice Guidelines. *Annals of Long-Term Care* 14(1):23-26, 2006.

Kaempf G, O'Donnell C, Oslin DW: The BRENDA model: A psychosocial addiction model to identify and treat alcohol disorders in elders. *Geriatr Nurs* 20(6):302-304, 1999.

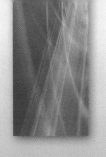

Appendices

Marsha D. Fretwell
Deborah Adams Wingate
Aman Nanda
Tom J. Wachtel

Frequently Used Clinical Formulas

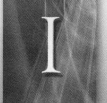

1. **Calculation of creatinine clearance (CCr):**

$$CCr \text{ (male)} = \frac{(140 - \text{age}) \times \text{weight (kg)}}{\text{Serum creatinine} \times 72}$$

$$CCr \text{ (female)} = 0.85 \times CCr \text{ (male)}$$

2. **Alveolar-arterial oxygen gradient (Aa gradient):**

$$\text{Aa gradient} = \left[\left(713 \times (\text{FiO}_2) - \left(\frac{\text{PaCO}_2}{0.8} \right) \right) \right] - \text{PaO}_2$$

Normal Aa gradient = 5-15 mm
FiO_2 = Fraction of inspired oxygen (normal = 0.21-1.0)
PaCO_2 = Arterial carbon dioxide tension (normal = 35-45 mm Hg)
PaO_2 = Arterial partial pressure oxygen (normal = 70-100 mm Hg)
Differential diagnosis of Aa gradient:

Abnormality	15% O_2	100% O_2
Diffusion defect	Increased gradient	Correction of gradient
Ventilation/perfusion mismatch	Increased gradient	Partial or complete correction of gradient
Right-to-left shunt (intracardiac or pulmonary)	Increased gradient	Increased gradient (no correction)

3. **Anion gap (AG):**

$$AG = Na^+ - (Cl^- + HCO_3^-)$$

4. **Fractional excretion of sodium (FE_{Na}):**

$$FE_{Na} = \frac{U_{Na} / P_{Na}}{U_{Cr} / P_{Cr}} \times 100$$

5. **Serum osmolality (Osm):**

$$Osm = 2(Na^+ + K^+) + \frac{\text{Glucose}}{18} + \frac{\text{BUN}}{2.8}$$

6. **Corrected sodium in hyperglycemic patients:**

$$\text{Corrected } Na^+ = \text{Measured } Na^+ + 1.6 \times \frac{\text{Glucose} - 140}{100}$$

7. **Water deficit in hypernatremic patients:**

$$\text{Water deficit (in liters)} = 0.6 \times \text{Body weight (kg)} \times \left(\frac{\text{Measured serum Na}^+}{\text{Normal serum Na}^+} - 1 \right)$$

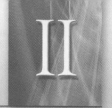

Functional Assessment Instruments

Instrument	Source
Alcohol Abuse	
Michigan Alcoholism Screening Test (MAST)	Selzer ML: The Michigan Alcoholism Screening Test: The quest for a new diagnostic instrument. *Am J Psychiatry* 127:1653-1658, 1971.
Cognition	
Blessed Dementia Scale and Information-Memory Concentration (IMC) Test	Blessed G, Tomlinson BF, Roth M: The association between quantitative measures of dementia and of senile change in the cerebral grey matter of elderly subjects. *Br J Psychiatry* 114:797-811, 1968.
Clock Drawing Test (CLOX), an executive clock-drawing task	Royall DR, Cordes JA, Polk M: CLOX: An executive clock drawing task. *J Neurol Neurosurg Psychiatry* 64:588-594, 1998. (http://jnnp.bmj.com/cgi/reprint/64/5/588.pdf)
Hachinski Ischemic Score (HIS) for multi-infarct dementia	Hachinski VC, Iliff LD, Silhka E, et al: Cerebral blood flow in dementia. *Arch Neurol* 32:632-637, 1975.
Severe Mini Mental State Examination	Harrell LE, Marson D, Chatterjee A, Parrish JA: The severe mini-mental state examination: A new neuropsychologic instrument for the bedside assessment of severely impaired patients with Alzheimer disease. *Alzheimer Dis Assoc Disord* 14(3):168-175, 2000.
Confusion Assessment Method for the Intensive Care Unit (CAM-ICU)	Ely EW, Margolin R, Francis J, et al: Evaluation of delirium in critically ill patients: Validation of the Confusion Assessment Method for the Intensive Care Unit (CAM-ICU). *Crit Care Med* 29(7):1370-1379, 2001.
Depression and Anxiety	
Center for Epidemiologic Studies Depression Scale (CES-D)	Radloff LS: The CES-D Scale: A self-report depression scale for research in the general population. *Appl Psychol Measure* 2:385-401, 1977.
Cornell Scale for Depression in Dementia (CSDD)	Alexopoulos GS, Abrams RC, Young RC, Shamoian CA: Cornell Scale for Depression in Dementia. *Biol Psychiatry* 23(3):271-284, 1988.
Hamilton Anxiety Rating Scale (HARS)	Hamilton M: The assessment of anxiety states by rating. *Brit J Med Psychol* 32:50-55, 1959.

Continued

Appendix II

Instrument	Source
Falls	
Abnormal Involuntary Movement Scale (AIMS), screening for tardive dyskinesia	Guy W: *ECDEU Assessment Manual for Psychopharmacology*, rev. ed. Washington, DC, US Department of Health, Education, and Welfare, 1976. Modified by Munetz MR, Benjamin S: How to examine patients using the Abnormal Involuntary Movement Scale. *Hospital Com Psychiatry* 39(11):1172-1177, 1988.
Berg Balance Scale	Berg KO, Wood-Dauphinee SL, Williams JI, Maki B: Measuring balance in the elderly: Validation of an instrument. *Can J Pub Health* 83(suppl 2):S7-S11, 1992.
Timed Up and Go Test	Podsiadlo D, Richardson S: The timed "Up & Go": A test of basic functional mobility for frail elderly persons. *J Am Geriatric Soc* 39:142-148, 1991.
Tinetti Balance and Gait Evaluation, performance-oriented assessment of mobility	Tinetti ME: Performance-oriented assessment of mobility problems in elderly patients. *J Am Geriatric Soc* 34:119-126, 1986.
Nutrition	
Body Mass Index	National Heart, Lung, and Blood Institute: *Clinical Guidelines on the Identification, Evaluation, and Treatment of Overweight and Obesity in Adults: The Evidence Report.* Washington, DC, National Heart, Lung, and Blood Institute, 1998. PDF available at http://www.nhlbi.nih.gov/guidelines/obesity/ob-gdlns.pdf (accessed March 1, 2007).
Mini Nutritional Assessment (MNA)	Nestlé Nutrition Institute: MNA Mini Nutritional Assessment. Vevey, Switzerland, Societé des Produits Nestlé S.A, 1994, revision 1998. Available at http://www.mna-elderly.com/index.htm (accessed March 1, 2007).
Physical Function	
Instrumental Activities of Daily Living Scale (IADL)	Lawton MP, Brody EM: Assessment of older people: Self-maintaining and instrumental activities of daily living. *Gerontologist* 9:179-186, 1969.

Preoperative Cardiac Risk Assessment

Stepwise approach to preoperative cardiac assessment	Eagle KA, Berger PB, Calkins H, et al: ACC/AHA guideline update for perioperative cardiovascular evaluation for noncardiac surgery—executive summary. A report of the American College of Cardiology/American Heart Association Task Force on Practice Guidelines (Committee to Update the 1996 Guidelines on Perioperative Cardiovascular Evaluation for Noncardiac Surgery). *Circulation* 105:1257-1267, 2002.
Indications for coronary angiography in perioperative evaluation before (or after) noncardiac surgery	American College of Cardiology/American Heart Association Task Force on Practice Guidelines (Committee on Coronary Angiography): ACC/AHA guidelines for coronary angiography: Executive summary and recommendations. *Circulation* 99:2345-2357, 1999.
Clinical predictors of increased perioperative cardiovascular risk (myocardial infarction, congestive heart failure, death)	Eagle KA, Berger PB, Calkins H, et al: ACC/AHA guideline update for perioperative cardiovascular evaluation for noncardiac surgery—executive summary. A report of the American College of Cardiology/American Heart Association Task Force on Practice Guidelines (Committee to Update the 1996 Guidelines on Perioperative Cardiovascular Evaluation for Noncardiac Surgery). *Circulation* 105:1257-1267, 2002.
Cardiac risk stratification for noncardiac surgical procedures	Eagle KA, Berger PB, Calkins H, et al: ACC/AHA guideline update for perioperative cardiovascular evaluation for noncardiac surgery—executive summary. A report of the American College of Cardiology/American Heart Association Task Force on Practice Guidelines (Committee to Update the 1996 Guidelines on Perioperative Cardiovascular Evaluation for Noncardiac Surgery). *Circulation* 105:1257-1267, 2002.
Estimated energy requirements for various activities	Wachtel TJ: *Geriatric Clinical Advisor: Instant Diagnosis and Treatment.* Philadelphia, Mosby, 2007.

Continued

Appendix II

Appendix II

Instrument	Source
Pressure Ulcers	
Braden Scale for Predicting Pressure Sore Risk	Braden B, Bergstrom N: Braden Scale for Predicting Pressure Sore Risk. 1988. PDF available at http://www.bradenscale.com/braden.PDF (accessed March 1, 2007).
Risk	
National Pressure Ulcer Advisory Panel (NPUAP) staging system for pressure ulcerations	National Pressure Ulcer Advisory Panel: Pressure ulcer stages, definitions, and descriptions, 2007. PDF available at http://www.npuap.org/documents/NPUAP2007_PU_Def_and_Descriptions.pdf (accessed March 1, 2007).
Norton Pressure Ulcer Prediction Scale	Norton D, McLaren R, Exton-Smith AN: *An investigation of geriatric nursing problems in hospital.* London, Churchill Livingstone, 1962.
Pressure Ulcer Scale for Healing (PUSH): PUSH Tool 3.0	National Pressure Ulcer Advisory Panel: Pressure Ulcer Scale for Healing (PUSH): PUSH Tool 3.0. PDF available at http://www.npuap.org/PDF/push3.pdf (accessed March 1, 2007).
Quality of Life	
Medical Outcomes Study Short Form 36 (MOS SF-36)	Co-copyright and trademark holders for the Medical Outcomes Study Short Form 36 (MOS SF-36) and Medical Outcomes Study Short Form 12 (MOS SF-12) are the Medical Outcomes Trust (MOT), the Health Assessment Lab, and QualityMetric Incorporated. Information regarding licensing, use, and ordering may be found online at http://www.qualitymetric.com. The forms may be viewed at http://www.qualitymetric.com/products/sfsurvey.aspx. The MOS SF-36, MOS SF-12, and other quality-of-life forms may also be viewed at http://www.rand.org/health/surveys.html.
Missoula-VITAS Quality of Life Index (MVQOLI)	VITAS Healthcare Corporation, Miami, Florida, and Ira R. Byock, MD, Missoula, Montana, 2001. The form may be viewed online at http://www.dyingwell.com/MVQOLI.htm. For permission for use, contact: Dr. Stephen McKenna, Galen Research, Enterprise House, Manchester Science Park, Lloyd Street North, Manchester M15 6SE, UK, or e-mail kfirth@galen-research.com. This tool may be viewed online at http://
Nottingham Health Profile (NHP)	www.galen-research.com/documents/68is021%20NHP4.pdf.

Sexual Function

Androgen Deficiency in Aging Males (ADAM) questionnaire — Morley JE, Perry HM: Androgen deficiency in aging men. *Med Clin North Am* 83(5):1279-1289, vii, 1999.

Swallowing Evaluation

Burke Dysphagia Screening Test — DePippo KL, Holas MA, Reding MJ: The Burke dysphagia screening test: Validation of its use in patients with stroke. *Arch Phys Med Rehabil* 75(2):1284-1286, 1994. Described online at http://www.medal.org in Chapter 8 Section.

Urinary Incontinence

American Urological Association (AUA) symptom index — Widely available online for downloading and can be found at http://www.prostate-cancer.org/tools/forms/aua_symptom_form.html.

Incontinence Impact Questionnaire (IIQ-7) — Shumaker SA, Wyman JF, Uebersax JS, et al: Health-related quality-of-life measures for women with urinary incontinence, *Qual Life Res* 3(5):291-306, 1994.

Urogenital Distress Inventory (UDI-6) — Shumaker SA, Wyman JF, Uebersax JS, et al: Health-related quality-of-life measures for women with urinary incontinence, *Qual Life Res* 3(5):291-306, 1994.

POWER OF ATTORNEY FOR HEALTH CARE INSTRUCTIONS

CAUTION:

THE ATTACHED POWER OF ATTORNEY FOR HEALTH CARE IS PROVIDED FOR YOUR CONVENIENCE. IT MAY OR MAY NOT FIT THE REQUIREMENTS OF YOUR PARTICULAR STATE. A GROWING NUMBER OF STATES HAVE SPECIAL FORMS OR SPECIAL PROCEDURES FOR CREATING HEALTH CARE POWERS OF ATTORNEY. IF POSSIBLE, SEEK LEGAL ADVICE BEFORE SIGNING ANY POWER OF ATTORNEY. IF NOT CLEARLY RECOGNIZED BY LAW IN YOUR STATE, THE DOCUMENT MAY STILL PROVIDE THE BEST EVIDENCE OF YOUR WISHES IF YOU SHOULD BECOME UNABLE TO SPEAK FOR YOURSELF.

Page 1 Instructions

Section 1—Designation of Health Care Agent: Print your full name here as the "principal" or creator of the power of attorney.

Print the full name, address and telephone number of the person (over age 18) you appoint as your health care "attorney-in-fact" or "agent." Appoint *only* a person whom you trust to understand and carry out your values and wishes. Do not name any of your health care providers as your agent, since some states prohibit them acting as your agent.

Section 2—Effective Date and Durability: The sample document is effective if and when you become unable to make health care decisions. That point in time is determined by your agent and your doctor. You can, if you wish, specify other effective dates or other criteria for incapacity (such as requiring two physicians to evaluate your capacity). You can also specify that the power will end at some later date or event before death. In any case, you have the *right to revoke* the agent's authority at any time by notifying your agent or health care provider orally or in writing. If you revoke, it is best to notify both your agent and physician in writing and to destroy the power of attorney document itself.

Section 3—Agent's Powers: This grant of power is intended to be as broad as possible so that your agent will have authority to make any decision you could make to obtain or terminate any type of health care.

(continued on next instruction page)

POWER OF ATTORNEY FOR HEALTH CARE

1. Designation of Health Care Agent.

I, _____hereby appoint:
(principal)

_____
(Attorney-in-fact's name)

_____
(Address)

Home:_____ Work:_____

as my attorney-in-fact (or "Agent") to make health and personal care decisions for me as authorized in this document.

2. Effective Date and Durability.

By this document I intend to create a durable power of attorney effective upon, and only during, any period of incapacity in which, in the opinion of my agent and attending physician, I am unable to make or communicate a choice regarding a particular health care decision.

3. Agent's Powers.

I grant to my Agent full authority to make decisions for me regarding my health care. In exercising this authority, my Agent shall follow my desires as stated in this document or otherwise known to my Agent. In making any decision, my Agent shall attempt to discuss the proposed decision with me to determine my desires if I am able to communicate in any way. If my Agent cannot determine the choice I would want made, then my Agent shall make a choice for me based upon what my Agent believes to be in my best interests. My Agent's authority to interpret my desires is intended to be as broad as possible, except for any limitations I may state below. Accordingly, unless specifically limited by Section 4, below, my Agent is authorized as follows:

A. To consent to, refuse, or withdraw consent to any and all types of medical care, treatment, surgical procedures, diagnostic procedures, medication, and the use of mechanical or other procedures that affect any bodily function, including (but not limited to) artificial respiration, nutritional support and hydration, and cardiopulmonary resuscitation;

Page 1 of 5.

Page 2 Instructions

Section 3—Agent's Powers, continues on this page

Even under this broad grant of authority, your agent still must follow your desires and directions, communicated by you in any manner now or in the future. You can specifically limit or direct your agent's power, if you wish, in Section 4.

Section 4—Statement of Desires, Special Provisions, and Limitations:

Paragraph A. Here you may include any limitations you think are appropriate, such as instructions to refuse any specific types of treatment that are against your religious beliefs or unacceptable to you for any other reasons, such as blood transfusion, electroconvulsive therapy, sterilization, abortion, amputation, psychosurgery, admission to a mental institution, etc. State law may not allow your agent to consent to some of these procedures, regardless of your health care power of attorney. Be very careful about stating limitations, because the specific circumstances surrounding a future health care decision are impossible to predict. If you do not want any limitations, simply write in "No limitations."

B. To have access to medical records and information to the same extent that I am entitled to, including the right to disclose the contents to others;

C. To authorize my admission to or discharge (even against medical advice) from any hospital, nursing home, residential care, assisted living, or similar facility or service;

D. To contract on my behalf for any health care related service or facility on my behalf, without my Agent incurring personal financial liability for such contracts;

E. To hire and fire medical, social service, and other support personnel responsible for my care;

F. To authorize, or refuse to authorize, any medication or procedure intended to relieve pain, even though such use may lead to physical damage or addiction or hasten the moment of (but not intentionally cause) my death;

G. To make anatomical gifts of part or all of my body for medical purposes, authorize an autopsy, and direct the disposition of my remains, to the extent permitted by law;

H. To take any other action necessary to do what I authorize here, including (but not limited to) granting any waiver or release from liability required by any hospital, physician, or other health care provider; signing any documents relating to refusals of treatment or the leaving of a facility against medical advice, and pursuing any legal action in my name, at the expense of my estate to force compliance with my wishes as determined by my Agent, or to seek actual or punitive damages for the failure to comply.

1. **Statement of Desires, Special Provisions, and Limitations.**

A. The powers granted above do not include the following powers or are subject to the following rules of limitations:

_____
_____
_____
_____
_____
_____

Appendix III

Page 3 Instructions

Section 4—Statement of Desires, Special Provisions, and Limitations continues on this page.

Paragraph B: Because the subject of "life-sustaining treatment" is particularly important to many people, this paragraph provides a place for you to give general or specific directions on the subject, if you want to do so. The different paragraphs are options— choose only *one,* or write your desires or instructions in your own words (in the last option). If you already have a "Living Will," you can simply refer to it by choosing the first option. Or, the instructions you provide here can do what a Living Will would do.

Paragraph C: Because people differ widely on whether nutrition and hydration is something that ought to be refused or stopped under certain circumstances, it is important to make your wishes clear on this topic. Nutrition and hydration means food and fluids provided by a nasogastric tube or tube into the stomach, intestines, or veins. This paragraph allows you to include or not include these procedures among those that may be withheld or withdrawn under the circumstances described in the preceding paragraph. Either choice still permits nonintrusive efforts such as spoon feeding or moistening of lips and mouth.

B. With respect to any *Life-Sustaining Treatment,* I direct the following:

(Initial Only One of the Following Paragraphs)

☐ REFERENCE TO LIVING WILL. I specifically direct my Agent to follow any health care declaration or "living will" executed by me.

☐ GRANT OF DISCRETION TO AGENT. I do not want my life to be prolonged nor do I want life-sustaining treatment to be provided or continued if my Agent believes the burdens of the treatment outweigh the expected benefits. I want my Agent to consider the relief of suffering, the expense involved, and the quality as well as the possible extension of my life in making decisions concerning life-sustaining treatment.

☐ DIRECTIVE TO WITHHOLD OR WITHDRAW TREATMENT. I do not want my life to be prolonged and I do not want life-sustaining treatment:
  a. if I have a condition that is incurable or irreversible and, without the administration of life-sustaining treatment, expected to result in death within a relatively short time; or
  b. if I am in a coma or persistent vegetative state that is reasonably concluded to be irreversible.

☐ DIRECTIVE FOR MAXIMUM TREATMENT. I want my life to be prolonged to the greatest extent possible without regard to my condition, the chances I have for recovery, or the cost of the procedures.

☐ DIRECTIVE IN MY OWN WORDS: _____

_____

_____

_____

C. With respect to *Nutrition and Hydration* provided by means of a nasogastric tube or tube into the stomach, intestines, or veins, I wish to make clear that . . .

(Initial Only One)

☐ I intend to include these procedures among the "life-sustaining procedures" that may be withheld or withdrawn under the conditions given above.

☐ I do not intend to include these procedures among the "life-sustaining procedures" that may be withheld or withdrawn.

Page 3 of 5.

Page 4 Instructions

Section 5—Successors: If you wish to name alternate agents in case your first agent becomes unavailable, print the appropriate information in this paragraph. You can name as many successors in the order you wish.

Section 6—Protection of Third Parties Who Rely on My Agent: In most states, health care providers cannot be compelled to follow the directions of your agent, although in some states, they may be obligated to transfer your care to another provider who is willing to comply. This paragraph is intended to encourage compliance with the power of attorney by waiving potential civil liability for good faith reliance on the agent's statements and decisions.

Section 7—Nomination of Guardian: The use of a health care power of attorney is intended to *prevent* the need for a court-appointed guardian for health care decision-making. However, if for any reason, court involvement becomes necessary, this paragraph expressly names your Agent to serve as guardian. A court does not have to follow your nomination, but it will normally comply with your wishes unless there is good reason not to.

Section 8—Administration Provisions: These items address miscellaneous matters that could affect the implementation of your power of attorney.

5. **Successors**

   If any Agent named by me shall die, become legally disabled, resign, refuse to act, be unavailable, or (if any Agent is my spouse) be legally separated or divorced from me, I name the following (each to act alone and successively, in the order named) as successors to my Agent:

   A. First Alternate Agent _____
      Address: _____
      Telephone: _____

   B. Second Alternate Agent _____
      Address: _____
      Telephone: _____

6. **Protection of Third Parties Who Rely on My Agent.**
   No person who relies in good faith upon any representations by my Agent or Successor Agent shall be liable to me, my estate, my heirs or assigns, for recognizing the Agent's authority.

7. **Nomination of Guardian.**
   If a guardian of my person should for any reason be appointed, I nominate my Agent (or his or her successor) named above.

8. **Administrative Provisions.**

   A. I revoke any prior power of attorney for health care.

   B. This power of attorney is intended to be valid in any jurisdiction in which it is presented.

   C. My Agent shall not be entitled to compensation for services performed under this power of attorney, but he or she shall be entitled to reimbursement for all reasonable expenses incurred as a result of carrying out any provision of this power of attorney.

   D. The powers delegated under this power of attorney are separable, so that the invalidity of one or more powers shall not affect any others.

Page 5 Instructions

Signing the Document: Required procedures for signing this kind of
document vary from signature only to very detailed witnessing
requirements, or, in some states, simply notarization. The suggested procedure here is intended to meet most of the various
state requirements for signing by noninstitutionalized persons.
The procedure here is likely to be more detailed than is required
under your own state's law, but it will help ensure that your
Health Care Power is recognized in other states, too. First, sign
and date the document in front of *two witnesses.* Your witnesses
should know your identity personally and be able to declare that
you appear to be of sound mind and under no duress or undue
influence. Further, your witnesses should not be:

- Your treating physician, health care provider, or health facility
  operator, or an employee of any of these.
- Anyone related to you by blood, marriage, or adoption.
- Anyone entitled to any part of your estate under an existing will
  or by operation of law. Even a creditor of yours should not be
  used under these guidelines.

If you are in a nursing home or other institution, be sure to consult
state law, because a few states require that an ombudsman or patient
advocate be one of your witnesses.

Second, have your signature *notarized.* Some states permit notarization as an alternative to witnessing. Others may simply apply the
rules for signing ordinary durable powers of attorney. Ordinary durable
powers of attorney are usually notarized. This form includes a relatively typical notary statement, but here again, it is wise to check state
law in case a special form of notary acknowledgement is required.

BY SIGNING HERE I INDICATE THAT I UNDERSTAND THE CONTENTS OF THIS DOCUMENT AND THE EFFECT OF THIS GRANT OF POWERS TO MY AGENT.

I sign my name to this Health Care Power of Attorney on this _____ day of _____, 20_____

My current home address is: _____

_____

      Signature: _____

      Name: _____

Witness Statement

I declare that the person who signed or acknowledged this document is personally known to me, that he/she signed or acknowledged this durable power of attorney in my presence, and that he/she appears to be of sound mind and under no duress, fraud, or undue influence. I am not the person appointed as agent by this document, nor am I the patient's health care provider or an employee of the patient's health care provider. I further declare that I am not related to the Principal by blood, marriage, or adoption, and, to the best of my knowledge, I am not a creditor of the Principal or entitled to any part of his/her estate under a will now existing or by operation of law.

Witness #1:

Signature: _____ Date: _____

Print Name: _____ Telephone: _____

Residence Address: _____

_____

Witness #2:

Signature: _____ Date: _____

Print Name: _____ Telephone: _____

Residence Address: _____

_____

Notarization

STATE OF _____)

) ss.

COUNTY OF _____)

On this ____ day of _____, 20___, the said _____, known to me (or satisfactorily proven) to be the person named in the foregoing instrument, personally appeared before me, a Notary Public, within and for the State and County aforesaid, and acknowledged that he or she freely and voluntarily executed the same for the purposes stated therein.

My Commission Expires: _____

_____   *NOTARY PUBLIC*

Geriatric Depression Scale (GDS)

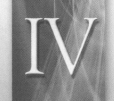

Choose yes or no.

1. Are you basically satisfied with your life?   N = 1
2. Have you dropped any of your activities or interests?   Y = 1
3. Do you feel that your life is empty?   Y = 1
4. Do you often get bored?   Y = 1
5. Are you hopeful about the future?   N = 1
6. Are you bothered by thoughts you can't get out of your head?   Y = 1
7. Are you in good spirits most of the time?   N = 1
8. Are you afraid that something bad is going to happen to you?   Y = 1
9. Do you feel happy most of the time?   N = 1
10. Do you often feel helpless?   Y = 1
11. Do you often get restless and fidgety?   Y = 1
12. Do you prefer to stay at home, rather than going out and doing new things?   Y = 1
13. Do you often worry about the future?   Y = 1
14. Do you feel you have more problems with memory than most?   Y = 1
15. Do you think it is wonderful to be alive now?   N = 1
16. Do you often feel downhearted and blue?   Y = 1
17. Do you feel pretty worthless the way you are now?   Y = 1
18. Do you worry a lot about the past?   Y = 1
19. Do you find life very exciting?   N = 1
20. Is it hard for you to get started on new projects?   Y = 1
21. Do you feel full of energy?   N = 1
22. Do you feel that your situation is hopeless?   Y = 1
23. Do you think that most people are better off than you are?   Y = 1
24. Do you often get upset over little things?   Y = 1

25. Do you often feel like crying?   Y = 1

26. Do you have trouble concentrating?   Y = 1

27. Do you enjoy getting up in the morning?   N = 1

28. Do you prefer to avoid social gatherings?   Y = 1

29. Is it easy for you to make decisions?   N = 1

30. Is your mind as clear as it used to be?   N = 1

A score of 11 has been shown to be useful in the diagnosis of depression.

Modified from Yesavage JA, Brink TL, Rose TL, et al: Development and validation of a geriatric depression screening scale: A preliminary report. *J Psychiatr Res* 17:37-49, 1983.

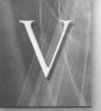

Recommendations

Cancer Screening Modality	US Preventive Services Task Force	American Cancer Society	Canadian Task Force
Breast Cancer			
Self-examination	No evidence	No evidence	No evidence
Clinical examination	Every 1-2 y to 75	Yearly	Yearly
Mammogram	Every 1-2 y to 75	Yearly	Yearly
Cervical Cancer			
Pap smear	NR if consistently normal up to age 65	Yearly; less frequently if consistently normal 3 times or more	Every 5 y; more or less depending on clinical judgment
Colon Cancer			
Fecal occult blood	No evidence*	Yearly	No evidence*
Sigmoidoscopy	No evidence*	Every 3-5 y according to physician	No evidence*
Prostate Cancer			
Digital rectal examination	No evidence	Yearly	No evidence
Prostate-specific antigen	NR	No evidence	NE

Continued

Appendix V

Recommendations

Cancer Screening Modality	US Preventive Services Task Force	American Cancer Society	Canadian Task Force
Ovarian Cancer			
Pelvic examination	NR	Yearly after age 40	NE
Oral Cancer			
Clinical examination	NR except if high risk	Yearly	No evidence
Skin Cancer			
Self-examination	No evidence	NE	NE
Clinical examination	If high risk	Yearly	If high risk
Testicular Cancer			
Clinical examination	NE	Yearly	No evidence
Thyroid Cancer			
Clinical examination	Regularly if exposed to upper body radiation	Yearly	NE

*There is insufficient evidence for or against the use of a test in asymptomatic persons aged 65 years and older who have no risk factors. Further data are needed (*for low-risk groups only).

NE, not evaluated; NR, not recommended.

From Yoshikawa TT, Cobbs EL, Brummel-Smith K (eds): *Ambulatory Geriatric Care.* St Louis, Mosby, 1993.

Katz Index of Activities of Daily Living

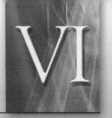

1. **Bathing (sponge bath, tub bath, or shower)**

    a. Receives no assistance (gets in and out of tub by self if tub is usual means of bathing)

    b. Receives assistance in bathing only one part of body such as the back or a leg

    c. Receives assistance in bathing more than one part of body or is not bathed

2. **Continence**

    a. Controls urination and bowel movement completely by self

    b. Has occasional accidents

    c. Needs supervision to keep urine or bowel control, uses catheter, or is incontinent

3. **Dressing (gets clothes from closets and drawers, including underclothes, outer garments; uses fasteners, including braces, if worn)**

    a. Gets clothes and gets completely dressed without assistance

    b. Gets clothes and gets dressed without assistance except in tying shoes

    c. Receives assistance in getting clothes or getting dressed or stays partly or completely undressed

4. **Eating**

    a. Feeds self without assistance

    b. Feeds self except for assistance in cutting meat or buttering bread

    c. Receives assistance in feeding or is fed partly or completely by using tubes or intravenous fluids

5. **Toileting (going to the "toilet room" for bowel and bladder elimination; cleaning self after elimination and arranging clothes)**

    a. Goes to the "toilet room," cleans self, and arranges clothes without assistance (may use object for support, such as cane, walker, or wheelchair and may manage night bedpan or commode and emptying same in morning)

    b. Receives assistance in going to the "toilet room," cleaning self, or arranging clothes after elimination or receives assistance in using night bedpan or commode

    c. Does not go to the "toilet room" for the elimination process

6. **Transferring**
   a. Moves in and out of bed or chair without assistance (may use object for support such as cane or walker)
   b. Moves in and out of bed or chair with assistance
   c Does not get out of bed

Response a., 3 points; b., 2 points; c., 1 point; maximum score, 18 points.

From Yoshikawa TT, Cobbs EL, Brummel-Smith K (eds): *Ambulatory Geriatric Care*, St. Louis, Mosby, 1993.

Mini-Cog Scoring Algorithm

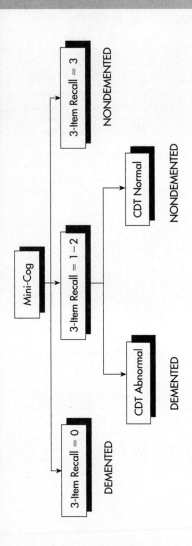

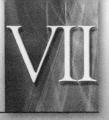

CDT, Clock drawing test.
From Borson S, Scanlon J, Brush M, et al.: The mini-cog: a cognitive "vital signs" measure for dementia screening in multi-lingual elderly. Int J Geriatr Psychiatry 15:1021-1027, 2000.

Index

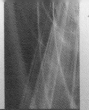

Note: Page numbers followed by the letter b refer to boxes, those followed by the letter f refer to figures, and those followed by the letter t refer to tables.

Index

Index

Index

Index

1

Key Telephone Numbers

This is a listing of the phone numbers of departments and individuals in the hospital who might be needed for immediate consultation.

Department

Admitting _____

Anesthesia _____

CCU _____

ECG _____

EEG _____

ER _____

ICU _____

Information _____

IV Team _____

Laboratory _____

    Chemistry _____

    Hematology _____

    Microbiology _____

    Other _____

Medical Records _____

Nuclear Medicine _____

Paging _____

Pathology _____

Pharmacy _____

Physical Therapy _____

Pulmonary Function _____

Radiology _____

Recovery Room _____

Respiratory Therapy _____

Security _____

Social Service _____

Sonography _____

Other _____

Nursing Stations

_____
_____
_____
_____
_____
_____
_____
_____

House Staff

_____
_____
_____
_____
_____
_____
_____

Attending Staff

_____
_____
_____
_____
_____
_____
_____
_____
_____
_____
_____